NEW HORIZONS
IN ALLERGY
IMMUNOTHERAPY

ADVANCES IN EXPERIMENTAL MEDICINE AND BIOLOGY

NEW HORIZONS IN ALLERGY IMMUNOTHERAPY

Edited by

Alec Sehon
University of Manitoba
Winnipeg, Manitoba, Canada

Kent T. HayGlass
University of Manitoba
Winnipeg, Manitoba, Canada

and

Dietrich Kraft
Institute of General and Experimental Pathology
Vienna, Austria

PLENUM PRESS • NEW YORK AND LONDON

Library of Congress Cataloging-in-Publication Data

New horizons in allergy immunotherapy / edited by Alec Sehon, Kent T.
  HayGlass, and Dietrich Kraft.
      p.   cm. -- (Advances in experimental medicine and biology ; v.
  409)
    "Proceedings of the 2nd International Conference on the Molecular
  Biology of Allergens and the Atopic Immune Response, held February
  18-22, 1995, in Quebec City, Canada"--T.p. verso.
    Includes bibliographical references and index.
    ISBN 0-306-45498-X
    1. Allergy--Immunotherapy--Congresses.   I. Sehon, Alec H.
  II. HayGlass, Kent T.   III. Kraft, Dietrich.   IV. International
  Conference on the Molecular Biology of Allergens and the Atopic
  Immune Response (2nd : 1995 : Québec City, Québec) V. Series.
    [DNLM: 1. Hypersensitivity, Immediate--congresses.
  2. Immunotherapy--congresses. 3. Allergens--genetics--congresses.
  4. Recombinant Proteins--immunology--congresses.   W1 AD559 v.409
  1996 / WD 300 N5317 1996]
  RC588.I45N48   1996
  616.97'06--dc21
  DNLM/DLC
  for Library of Congress   96-50090
                                                                  CIP

Proceedings of the Second International Conference on the Molecular Biology of Allergens and the Atopic
Immune Response, held February 18 – 22, 1995, in Quebec City, Canada

ISBN 0-306-45498-X

© 1996 Plenum Press, New York
A Division of Plenum Publishing Corporation
233 Spring Street, New York, N. Y. 10013

10 9 8 7 6 5 4 3 2 1

Printed in the United States of America

FOREWORD

One of the main attractions of research into hypersensitivity disorders is that it brings together scientists from a very broad range of disciplines. As the most common human immunologic disorder, it excites the interest and concern of clinicians, geneticists, basic and clinical immunologists, molecular biologists, biochemists, and physiologists. General agreement has been forged on the the pathophysiology of the disease and the mechanisms responsible for its maintenance, but many areas remain as black boxes for which we have only hypotheses.

In 1992 Vienna hosted an international symposium to consider the explosion of information being generated by the identification, cloning, and expression of common environmental allergens.[*] The present second international conference on the MOLECULAR BIOLOGY OF ALLERGENS AND THE ATOPIC IMMUNE RESPONSE, again jointly organized and co-chaired by Professors Alec Sehon (Winnipeg) and Dietrich Kraft (Vienna), provided an exciting opportunity for many leaders in this field to share data, argue hypotheses and seek future opportunities to enlarge our understanding of these very complex diseases. This symposium was co-sponsored by the International Union of Immunological Societies (I.U.I.S.) and the International Association of Allergology and Clinical Immunology. It was held in the hospitable and comfortably elegant surroundings of Quebec City.

Over five days, data and opinions on many topical, often controversial, issues were presented which addressed (i) genetic factors predisposing, or perhaps protecting, any given individual from development of atopic disease; (ii) detailed molecular characterization of many of the major allergens known to be associated with atopic disease; (iii) examination of the characteristics of environmental antigens that lead to their (functional) definition as allergens in some individuals; (iv) mechanisms of allergic sensitization and the role played by different cell populations and cytokines in this process; and (v) novel approaches for therapy of atopic disease ranging from antigen-specific tolerization or prophylaxis to methods resulting in inhibition of IgE synthesis or function across the board, and a host of other topics critically reviewed in this volume.

Tremendous progress has been made in identifying, cloning, and expressing the major allergens responsible for atopic diseases. The implications that our increasing access to such well-defined materials has for diagnosis, experimental studies, and therapy of ongoing hypersensitivity disease were thoroughly explored. The field has clearly progressed from the cloning of a handful of the major allergens by pioneers in this area, beginning

---

[*] *Molecular Biology and Immunology of Allergens.* Eds. Dietrich Kraft and Alec Sehon, CRC Press, Inc., Boca Raton, Florida, 1993

only in 1988 with publication of the cDNA sequence of Der p1, to the current situation, where the widespread availability of a multitude of allergens allows us to pose questions about the physiological and practical relevance of different allergen isoforms. Clearly, with the current availability of these molecular tools, our ability to probe the induction, maintenance, expression, and suppression of allergic disease enters a new era.

The co-chairmen and the participants of this symposium express their gratitude for the generous support of the listed sponsors who made it possible to organize this conference. Special thanks for the splendid organization and hospitality are expressed to Professor Jacques Hébert (Québec) and his colleague Dr. Yvan Boutin who were responsible for the splendid planning of the scientific program and the Symposium Secretariat.

Kent T. HayGlass, Ph.D.
Winnipeg, Canada

ACKNOWLEDGMENTS

The financial assistance in support of this Symposium from the following agencies and companies is gratefully acknowledged.

Allergen Standardization Committee	(I.U.I.S.)
ALK Laboratories	(Denmark)
ASAHI Breweries Ltd.	(Japan)
CIBA-GEIGY LTD.	(Switzerland)
Connaught Laboratories Ltd.	(Canada)
Medical Research Council of Canada	
Fujisawa Pharmaceutical Co., Ltd.	(Japan)
Glaxo Canada	(Canada)
Glaxo Nippon Ltd.	(Japan)
Hoechst-Roussel Canada Inc.	(Canada)
Hokuriku Seiyaku Co., Ltd.	(Japan)
Immuno Aktiengesell Schaft	(Austria)
ImmuLogic Pharmaceutical Corporation	(U.S.A.)
Kabi Pharmacia	(Sweden)
Kirin Brewery Co., Ltd.	(Japan)
Kyorin Pharmaceutical Co., Ltd.	(Japan)
Merck Frosst Canada	(Canada)
Miles Inc., Pharmaceutical Division	(U.S.A.)
Nippon Boehringer Ingelheim Co., Ltd.	(Japan)
Marion Merrel Dow, Inc.	(U.S.A.)
Nordic Merrel Dow	(Canada)
Sandoz Canada Inc.	(Canada)
Sanofi Diagnostics Pasteur, Inc.	(U.S.A.)
Schering	(Canada)
Torii Pharmaceutical Co., Ltd.	(Japan)
Wakamoto Pharmaceutical Co., Ltd.	(Japan)

CONTENTS

FOOD ALLERGY IN ATOPIC DOGS

O. L. Frick

University of California
San Francisco, California

OVERVIEW

The aim was to develop an animal model for food allergy. Twenty inbred allergic dogs were immunized as newborns and infancy with 1 µg food allergen-soy, cow's milk, wheat, beef, rice in alum 2mg, after 3 monthly injections of 0.5ml distemper-hepatitis live virus vaccine. At 4 months, most animals made IgE antibodies to these foods. At 6 months on, food challenges with 200–500g amounts caused significantly increased fecal index scores, and in some-facial edema, rash, and vomiting. Via gastroendoscopy, 0.1ml food extracts were injected into gastric mucosa after giving intravenous 0.5% Evans blue dye (0.25ml/kg). Within minutes, blue wheals and erythema occurred at injection sites on mucosa, none at saline control sites. Punch biopsies were taken within 10–15min. and again at 24 or 48hr. Aliquots of biopsy specimens were used for histology. Immediate reaction specimens showed edema and neutrophils. The 24 and 48hr. samples showed eosinophil and mononuclear cells infiltrations. With soy allergens-gly m-1 and Kunitz trypsin inhibitor glycinins-thioredoxin incubation for 1hr. at 25C which reduced intrachain disulfide bonds, caused marked reduction in allergenicity evidenced by reduction in skin reaction threshold with serial dilutions of allergens. The food allergic dog is a useful model for food allergy research.

A large animal model for chronic food allergy reactions is desirable to study the mechanisms of sensitization and reactions utilizing serial biopsies over days or weeks and developing possible treatment regimens. Dogs have an incidence of spontaneous food and inhalant allergies of about 10% comparable to that in human beings.

We have established such a canine food allergy model using anti-canine IgE RAST and immunodot assays to measure IgE antibodies to foods; food challenges following by fecal index scores for severity of reactions; mucosal "skin-testing" via gastric endoscopy with serial biopsies; and finally reducing allergenicity of foods using thioredoxin treatment.

From our inbred atopic dog colony at UC Davis, we selected three litters of 20 pups which were immunized by a similar protocol to that we had used previously for inducing allergies to pollens. (1) On newborn day 1, pups were injected subcutaneously with 2 µg each of soy, wheat, cow's milk, and beef extracts in 2mg alum. At 3, 7, and 11 weeks of age, they received injections of 0.5ml live attenuated distemper-hepatitis vaccine followed

New Horizons in Allergy Immunotherapy
edited by Sehon et al. Plenum Press, New York, 1996

1

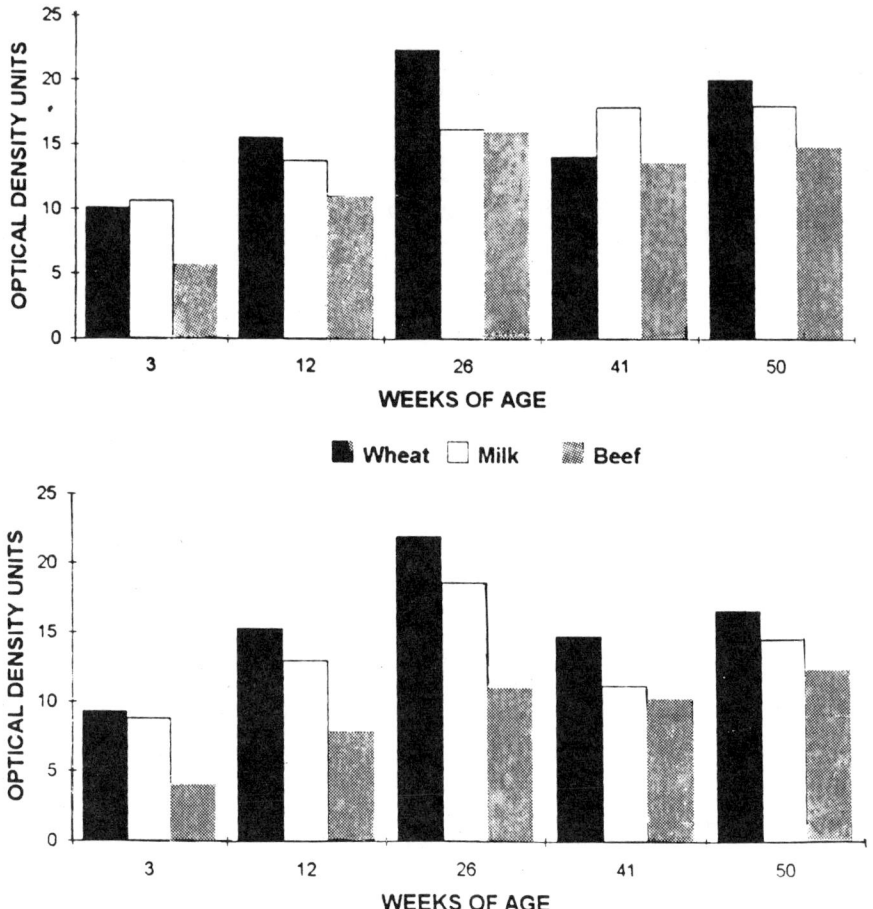

Figure 1. Histogram of the IgE anti-wheat, cow's milk, and beef antibody titers of the dog litters CGB (upper, n = 7) and GCB (lower n = 7) at different ages obtained by the immunodot method.

by repeat injections of the same food allergens. By 3 - 4 months of age, most animals made IgE antibodies measured by RAST or Immunodot assays to the four foods. (2) Fig. 1 is a histogram showing development of specific IgE antibodies to foods in two litters of atopic dogs.

At 6 months, they were fed 200 - 500g of the food to which they had been sensitized. For 3 days prior and 5 days post-challenge, stools were carefully monitored for quality on a 1 - 5+ scale times number/d to give a fecal index score. The mean daily pre-challenge score was subtracted from the 3 day post-challenge score to a change in score rating. Fig. 2 shows significant correlations occurred between change in fecal index scores versus RAST titers to both soy and cow's milk (r = 0.63, p <.01 for soy and r = 0.38, p <.01 for cow's milk, respectively). On several occasions, the feeding challenge, especially in Dog 5CB4, caused almost immediate rubbing and swelling of the muzzle, sneezing, retching, vomiting, explosive diarrhea, and collapse that required epinephrine injections. Two other dogs had milder forms of such reactions, so no further oral challenges were done on these animals.

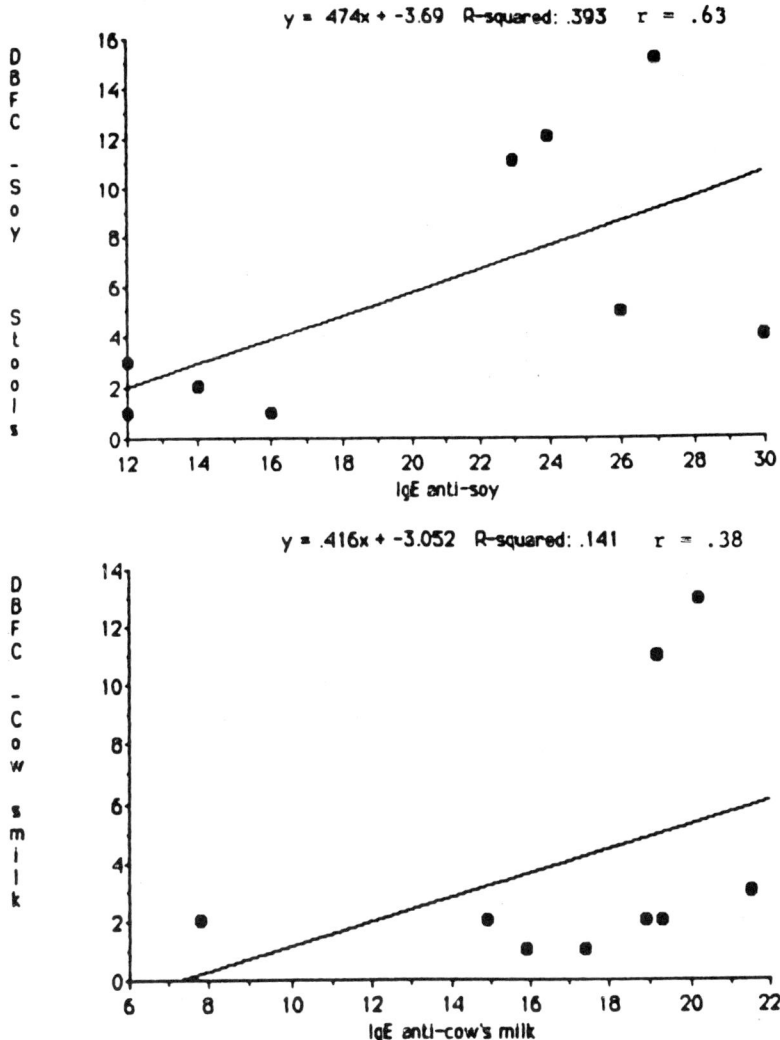

Figure 2. Regression analysis of anti-soy (top) and anti-cow's milk (bottom) IgE antibodies with change in number of stools over 3 days post-food allergen challenge.

Because late-phase allergic reactions have been described in skin (3), bronchi (4), nose (5), and eyes (6) in sensitized animals and human beings, we wondered if the late-phase allergic reactions occurred in the gastrointestinal tract after food challenges in sensitized dogs. With Dr. Grant Gilford, previously (7), we had demonstrated a localized wheal reaction when concentrated food allergen was dropped onto the gastric mucosa during endoscopy. With Dr. Rick Ermel (8), and dogs under light 1% Isoflurane anesthesia, we injected via endoscope through a catheter with a 23 gauge variject sclerotherapy needle attached, 0.1ml of 10-fold dilutions of food allergens (wheat, cow's milk, and soy) into the mucosa of greater curvature of the stomach. Just prior to this, the dog was injected i.v. with 0.25ml/kg of 0.5% Evans blue dye to better visualize the reactions.

Within 1 to 3 minutes localized edema and erythema occurred at the antigen injection sites always larger than minimal edema at saline injection sites. After 3 minutes, blue-

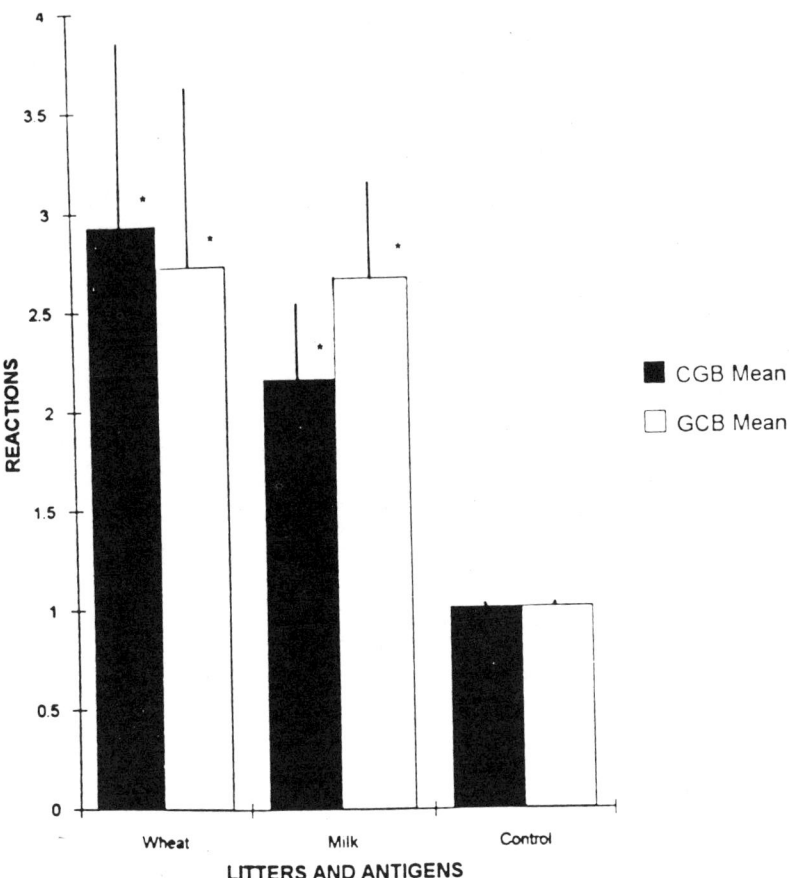

Figure 3. Histograph of the mean and standard deviations of gastric mucosal reactions to food allergenic extracts injected endoscopically into the gastric mucosa of sensitized dogs. Comparison between two dog liters (CGB, n = 7 and GCB, n = 7). * p < 0.05.

ing of the reaction sites occurred. We followed the reactions by videoendoscopy for 10–20 minutes. At 10–15 minutes post-injection, with a 2.2mm radial jaw biopsy, forceps four punch biopsies were taken around the left side of the reaction site. Aliquots of the biopsy tissue were snap frozen in N2, others were placed in formalin or glutaraldehyde for histology. Three-6 injections with different foods or dilutions and controls were made at one experimental time. The gastric mucosal responses were graded on a 1 to 4+ scale according to the amount of edema, erythema, and blue patching that occurred post-injections. Fig. 3 is a histogram of such reactions with wheat and cow's milk in 14 atopic dogs showing significantly greater reactions with foods than in control injection sites.

At 24 or 48hr. post-food challenge, upon repeat endoscopy the old reaction sites were located by persistent blue spot and biopsy wounds, (several sites that had been injected with allergen were not biopsied initially). Upon locating these blue reaction sites, these sites were rebiopsied on the opposite (right) side of the reaction site. We tried in vain to stain sections for eosinophils EG1 and EG2 and anti-ECP stains; apparently these anti-human eosinophil monoclonals are species specific.

Histologic examination showed in the immediate reactions mucosal edema and some neutrophils. The 24 and 48hr. post-challenge sections showed eosinophil and lymphocyte infiltration. One sensitized animal developed a sarcoma of the tongue and had to be euthanized. However, 48hr. prior to this he received an oral challenge feeding of 200g soy followed by diarrhea. Histological sections of the entire gastrointestinal tract and other organs were made. In the GI tract, stomach, jejunum, and ileum showed great infiltration of the deeper submucosal layers with eosinophils and lymphocytes. We concluded that injection of food allergen into gastric mucosa resulted in an immediate edema reaction followed in 24 - 48 hours by a late-phase reaction with accumulation of eosinophils and lymphocytes.

Dr. Bob Buchanan, Professor of Plant Biology, UCB, has developed a thioredoxin treatment of plant proteins that reduces their allergenicity. Originally, he used thioredoxin to increase the cross-linking in cereals-wheat, oat- to increase plasticity in bread and for making rising bread from non-glutinous flours such as rice, corn, and sorghum. Thioredoxin is a small ubiquitous dithiol protein that reduced intrachain disulfide (S-S) bonds to sulfhydryl (S-H) state (9). Thioredoxin achieves this reduction when activated (reduced) either enzymatically by NADPH-thioredoxin reductase (NTR) or chemically dithiothreitol (DTT), a synthetic reductant

$$\text{NADPH} + \text{H}^+ + \text{thioredoxin h}_{ox} \xrightarrow{\text{NTR}} \text{NADP} + \text{thioredoxin h}_{red}$$

After reduction samples were derivatized with monobromobimate (nBBr), a reagent that reacts specifically with SH groups to form a covalent complex. This derivative becomes highly fluorescent, as seen in treated reduced soy and wheat extracts subjected to SDS-PAGE. A number of fluorescent protein bands are allergens, such as gly m-l and Kunitz trypsin inhibitor bands in soy and glycinin and gliadin in wheat. A quantitative analysis of the extent of reduction of such proteins in wheat indicated that NTS and DTT systems were effectively reduced, but similar treatment with a glutathione system was not effective.

When food allergens (soy, wheat, cow's milk, and beef extracts) were treated with thioredoxin, allergenicity was markedly diminished or eliminated, as evidenced by diminished skin tests and feeding challenge scores. To each 1mg soy, wheat or cow's milk extracts was added 4.8 µg thioredoxin, 4.2 µg NTR and 1mM NADPH which was reacted for 1hr. at 25C or 37C. Other aliquots of 1mg antigen were reacted with 4.8 µg thioredoxin and 1.5mM dithiothereitol (DTT) for similar times. Half log dilutions of untreated and treated food allergen (soy, wheat, cow's milk, and beef) were injected intradermally into ventral abdominal skin of sensitized dogs after they received 0.25ml/kg of 0.5% Evans blue dye i.v. Generally, there was 10^3 to 10^5 reaction in end-point titration reaction with the treated vs untreated allergen.

In soy, gly m-1 (mw 30kd) and Kunitz trypsin inhibitor (mw 20.5kd) were the primary allergens - skin reactions to these were reduced by 10^3 or more by thioredoxin treatment. Similarly, in wheat glycinin and gliadin were the principle allergens; skin reactions to these were similarly reduced by thioredoxin treatment.

For oral challenges, 200g of food allergen was treated with 9.6g thioredoxin + 8.4g NTR and 1M NADPH for 1hr. at 25C. In 6 soy, milk, and wheat sensitive littermate dogs, 3 pairs with matched skin reactivity to the food were given either untreated soy or thioredoxin-treated soy and observed for immediate or delayed reactions to the food for 3 days as evidenced by changes in fecal index. Similar challenges were repeated 4 weeks later on

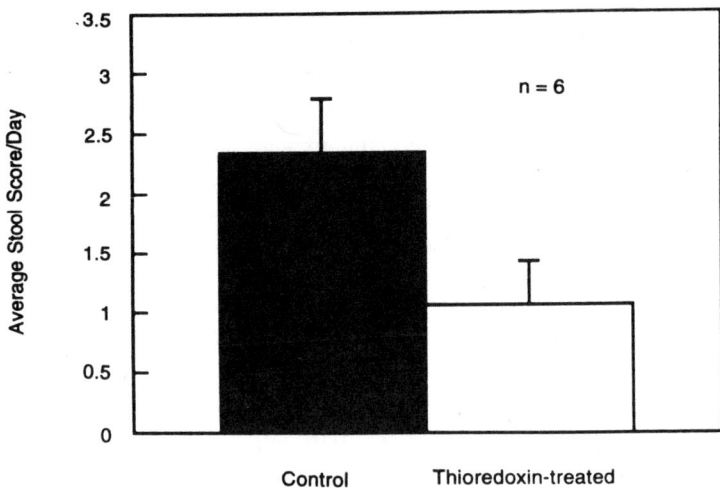

Figure 4. Mitigation of allergic response to feeding by treating soy formula with thioredoxin.

the same animals with wheat or cow's milk. Fig. 4 shows comparisons of fecal scores in dogs challenged with thioredoxin-treated or untreated food allergens showing lesser reactions with the treated food allergens. Once we can obtain sufficient quantities of purified allergens fractions, we plan similar challenges with these in the food sensitive dogs.

SUMMARY

The food sensitive dog provides a good animal model for food allergy, whose allergic reaction can be followed serially with repeated challenges both in skin and by oral challenges and by endoscopic direct visualization and serial biopsies. This model is proving useful in showing reduced allergenicity in food allergens-soy, wheat, cow's milk by thioredoxin treatment. Recently Dr. Buchanan has cloned the gene for the NADP-thioredoxin reductase (NTR) which he transferred into barley seeds with a bacterial vector. He is attempting to do the same with wheat and soy seeds to produce genetically hypoallergenic foods. The canine model for food allergy provides an excellent model in which to test such bio-engineered potentially hypoallergenic foods.

REFERENCES

1. Frick, O.L., Brooks, D.L., 1983, Immunoglobulin E antibodies to pollens augmented in dogs by viral vaccines. Am J Vet Res, 44:440–445.
2. Frick, O.L., Derer, M., Bigler, B., deWeck, A.L., 1993, Immunodot assay for IgE antibodies in atopic dogs. J Allergy Clin Immunol, 91:316.
3. Dolovich, J., Hargreave, F.E., Chalmers, R., Shier, K.J., Gauldie, J., Bienenstock, J., 1973. Late cutaneous allergic responses in isolated IgE-dependent reactiions. J Allergy Clin Immunol, 52:38–46.
4. Robertson, D.G., Kerigan, A.T., Hargreaves, F.E., Chalmers, R., Dolovich, J., 1973. Late asthmatic responses induced by ragweed allergen, J Allergy Clin Immunol, 54:244–254.
5. Pelikan, Z., 1978. Late and delayed responses of the nasal mucosa to allergen challenge. Ann Allergy, 41:37–47.

6. Bonini, S., Bonini, S., 1993. IgE and non-IgE mechanisms in ocular allergy. Ann Allergy, 71:296–299.

7. Guilford, W.G., Strombeck, D.R., Rogers, Q. Frick, O.L. Lawoka, C., 1994. Development of gastroscopic food sensitivity testing in dogs. J Vet Int Med, 8:414- 422.

8. Ermel, R.W., Frick O.L. Reinhart, G.A., 1994. Does the gastrointestinal tract have a late- phase inflammatory response to a food allergen? J Allergy Clin Immunol., 93:208.

9. Buchanan, B.B., Schurman, P., Decottignies, P., Lozano, R.M., 1994. Thioredoxin: A multifunctional regulating protein with a bright future in technology and medicine. Arch Biochem Biophys 314:257–260.

2

MECHANISMS OF ALLERGIC BRONCHOCONSTRICTION IN THE RAT[*]

James G. Martin

Meakins-Christie Laboratories
McGill University
3626 St-Urbain Street
Montreal, Quebec, Canada H2X 2P2

1. INTRODUCTION

A number of animal models of allergic bronchoconstriction have been developed in order to better understand the mechanisms of airway narrowing induced by inhalation of allergen and the underlying immunobiology of the reaction to allergen. The Brown Norway (BN) rat has been extensively characterized and appears to be among the best models thus far described, showing high levels of specific immunoglobulin E (IgE) on active sensitization (9,15), early and late allergic responses in high prevalence (4), airway eosinophilia and cholinergic hyperresponsiveness after inhalations of allergen (5,10). Further to the striking similarity of the responses of the BN rat to human allergic subjects, there are several practical advantages of the BN rat, namely, its highly inbred nature which reduces inter-animal variability, commercial availability and its size which is such that it is large enough for reliable measurements of pulmonary function, but small enough to offer the advantages associated with the study of small animals. Although we have a reasonable understanding of some of the characteristics of the BN that make it responsive to allergen, the ultimate genetic basis for its atopic nature has yet to be evaluated.

2. IMMUNOGLOBULIN E

Active sensitization of the BN rat leads to a high IgE response in contrast to other rat strains (7,9,15). Various regimens have been used to sensitize the rat but following a single dose of ovalbumin with adjuvant (aluminum hydroxide and Bordetella pertussis) IgE reaches high levels by two weeks after sensitization. The peak level is reached by 2 to 3 weeks after sensitization and thereafter declines to reach baseline levels at twenty

[*] Supported by the Medical Research Council of Canada and the Respiratory Health Network of Centres of Excellence of Canada.

New Horizons in Allergy Immunotherapy
edited by Sehon et al. Plenum Press, New York, 1996

9

weeks. IgG levels rise more slowly than IgE and reach a peak by 3 weeks and also gradually decline somewhat more slowly than IgE (15). Pertussis serves to boost total IgE synthesis, whereas alum adsorbs antigen and subsequently releases it slowly in such a way as to lead to enhancement of specific IgE levels.

3. MAST CELLS

There is no comprehensive study of either mast cell phenotype or the density of distribution of airway mast cells among various rat strains. There are a few reports of the numbers of mast cells in a few strains of rat and the results suggest that the BN rat may have more mast cells than some other strains (13,21). Insofar as the number of mast cells may be determined by cytokine expression by the T lymphocytes of the T helper 2 (TH_2) type, it is plausible that the number of mast cells may be linked to the factors that also account for high IgE levels on sensitization. However the Wag rat which is a low IgE producing strain has an equivalent number of mast cells in its airways (20), suggesting that the two characteristics do not necessarily go together. Furthermore whether the predominant mast cell phenotype, connective tissue type or mucosal type, is different in the BN from other rats does not seem to have been investigated but is potentially of importance given the fact that the profile of mediators produced by each phenotype differs. Of particular pertinence is the fact that mucosal mast cells produce more leukotriene C4 than connective tissue mast cells (6) because cysteinyl-leukotrienes are critical mediators of the allergic airway responses.

4. ALLERGEN INDUCED AIRWAY RESPONSES

The development of immediate hypersensitivity reactions (early responses) following allergen challenge has been well documented in a variety of strains of rat. The prevalence of such responses is approximately 70% in the BN rat (4) and from personal experience this is higher than in many other strains. The prevalence of late responses is also approximately 70% in the BN rat (4) whereas late responses are infrequently identified in other rat strains (14).

Typical early and late responses are illustrated in Figure 1. The early response is usually characterized by a brisk increase in pulmonary resistance within minutes of challenge and resolution within 1 hour. The late response is a rather variable perturbation in pulmonary resistance which occurs most frequently about 5 hours after challenge, but perturbations frequently occur around 3 hours after challenge, suggesting the possibility that more than one event may account for the response. Much of the early response and late response can be attributed to smooth muscle contraction (2,3), although microvascular leak occurs (8) and may also contribute to airway narrowing.

Following allergen challenge there is an influx of leukocytes to the airways which takes place within a few hours of challenge. This is a predominantly neutrophilic influx, although movement of eosinophils and lymphocytes can be detected also within the same time frame (11). The importance of the inflammatory cells to the late response is as yet uncertain, but a relationship between BAL total cellularity and the late response is present and is suggestive evidence of a link between the two. It seems likely that airway leukocytes contribute to the biochemical mediators responsible for airway narrowing, of which leukotriene D_4 appears to be the predominant one (12). Serotonin also contributes to the early response, but whether it also contributes to the late response has not been examined. The completeness of the blockade of the late response by LTD_4 antagonists suggests that it

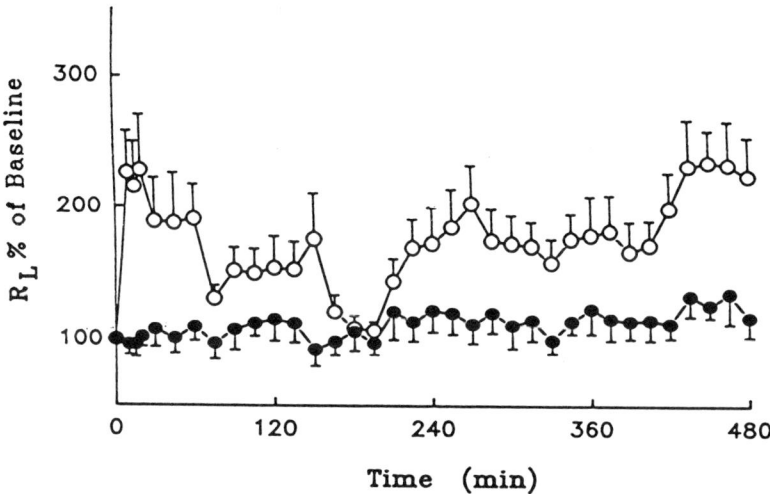

Figure 1. The time course of pulmonary resistance (R_L) from challenge with aerosolized ovalbumin (OA) to 8 hours after challenge. The open circles show OA-challenged sensitized rats (n=14) and closed circles are saline-challenged animals (n=13). Vertical bars indicate one standard error of the mean. Note the persistent elevation of R_L in the 4 to 8 hour period following challenge. Reproduced with permission from Am J Respir Crit Care Med 1995;151:470–474.

may well be the only significant mediator involved. Interestingly, late responses can occur in isolated airways in culture (1), suggesting that de novo influx of leukocytes is not necessary for the response and raises the possibility that resident airway cells such as macrophages may be responsible for the late response.

5. SERUM IMMUNOGLOBULINS AND ALLERGIC AIRWAY RESPONSES

Although active sensitization of the BN rat leads to an increase in IgE and also the appearance of early and late responses following inhalational challenge, there is no relationship between the magnitude of either of these airway responses and the level of serum IgE (15). It is possible that the level of circulating specific IgE to ovalbumin is supramaximal and therefore variations in its level would not necessarily be expected to be related to the magnitude of the airway responses. Interestingly, there is an inverse correlation between the level of ovalbumin-specific IgG and the magnitude of the early response suggesting that it may have a blocking effect (15), but no such relationship is found with the late response. Early and late responses are themselves weakly correlated.

6. THE ROLE OF THE T LYMPHOCYTE IN LATE ALLERGIC RESPONSES

6.1. Peripheral Mononuclear Cell Responses to Allergen

The lack of significant relationships between IgE and allergic airway responses prompted us to examine the relationship between T lymphocyte function and allergic air-

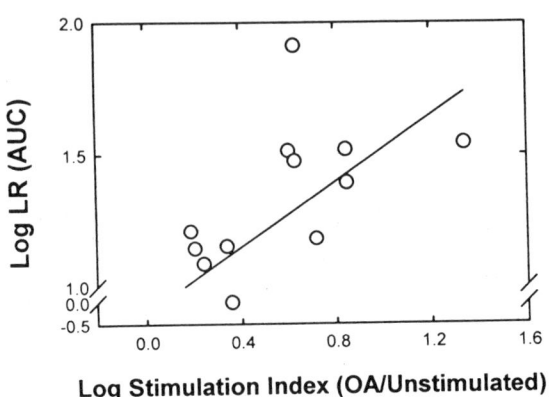

Figure 2. The late response (LR) measured as the area under the curve of R_L against time from 4 to 8 hours after challenge is correlated with the stimulation index (^{3}H-thymidine incorporation after OA/^{3}H-thymidine incorporation by unstimulated mononuclear cells). Both LR and the stimulation index were log transformed. The Spearman rank correlation was significant at p<0.05.

way responses. We were interested in particular in the possibility that the late response might relate more closely to the magnitude of the pool of ovalbumin-responsive T cells than circulating immunoglobulins. The rationale for this idea was based on the assumption at the time that the T cell was responsible for much of the associated airway inflammation. We first examined the relationship between the proliferative response of mononuclear cells isolated from the peripheral blood of sensitized animals to ovalbumin and the relationship between this magnitude of this response and the late airway response (16). The peripheral blood mononuclear cell response (largely T lymphocytes) measured as thymidine incorporation was quite variable from animal to animal, and was unrelated to the level of circulating immunoglobulins. However, the mononuclear cell proliferative response was significantly correlated with the magnitude of the late response (Figure 2), suggesting that the level of sensitization as reflected by the T cell response is a more pertinent determinant of late responses than measures of the humoral response.

6.2 Adoptive Transfer of the Late Response by Purified T Cells

In the view of the above suggestive evidence that the T lymphocyte might relate more closely to the late response than the human immune response, we more directly examined the hypothesis by isolating T cell populations from the lymph nodes (intrathoracic and cervical) of sensitized rats, subsequently transferring these cells to unsensitized recipients and challenging these latter with ovalbumin (17,18). Recipients of T cells from sensitized animals demonstrated late responses of comparable magnitude to those registered from actively sensitized animals. Experiments using immunomagnetic selection confirmed that CD4[+] T cells transferred the late response, but not CD8[+] T cells (Figure 3).

The cells retrieved by bronchoalveolar lavage of CD4[+] recipients that underwent airway challenge with ovalbumin demonstrated increased expression of IL-5 messenger RNA (mRNA) by *in situ* hybridization (19). This increase in mRNA was associated with bronchoalveolar lavage eosinophilia. The latter was evident only after immunohistochemical identification of major basic protein using a specific monoclonal antibody and was not

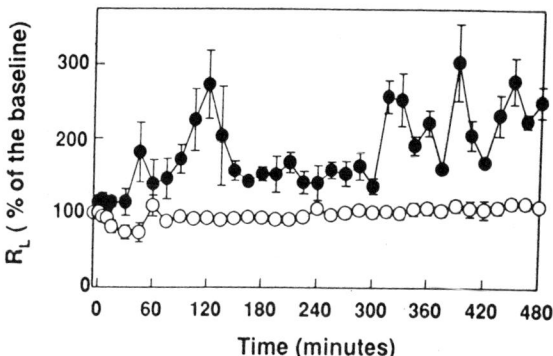

Figure 3. Time course of changes in lung resistance (R_L) after OA challenge in the recipients of either CD4+ or CD8+ T cells from sensitized rats. Naive BN rats received either purified 2 million CD4+ T cells (CD4+(2) group) or CD8+ cells (CD8+(2) group), which were obtained from OA-sensitized donors 14 days after the sensitization. Two days later the recipients were inhalationally challenged with OA (5% solution) for 5 minutes. Rats were analyzed for changes in R_L before, at 5, 10, and 15 minutes after the OA challenge, and at 15 minute intervals for a total period of 8 hours. The baseline value of R_L in the CD4+(2) group (closed circles, n=6) was 0.186±0.017 $cmH_2O/ml/s$, and 0.203±0.08 $cmH_2O/ml/s$ in the CD8+ group (open circles, n=6). A significant effect between groups was demonstrated by ANOVA (p<0.001). Reproduced by permission from *J Clin Invest* (in press).

evident with conventional staining (18). This suggests the possibility that activated eosinophils were present in the BAL and that the loss of granule proteins was responsible for the failure to identify the cells. The recipients of CD8[+] T cells showed no significant expression of IL-5 mRNA, but did show interferon gamma expression that exceeded that seen in CD4[+] T cell recipients. This observation suggests that CD8[+] T cells are not bystanders in the airway response, but are potential modulators of the response.

6.3. Independence of the Adoptively Transferred Late airway Response on IgE

Although the absence of early responses in recipients of CD4[+] T cells undergoing ovalbumin challenge was strong *a priori* evidence against significant levels of ovalbumin-specific IgE, in order to exclude the possibility that IgE participated in the triggering of late response, the sera of the recipients of sensitized CD4[+] cells were tested for IgE by ELISA. There was no evidence of ovalbumin-specific IgE by this test. Likewise, neither passive cutaneous anaphylaxis nor intradermal skin tests revealed any evidence of significant IgE in the serum of these animals (18). Presumably T cell activation results from antigen presentation by airway antigen presenting cells.

7. CONCLUSIONS

Allergic-induced airway reactions can be readily induced in actively sensitized BN rats. The high prevalence of these reactions makes them a suitable animal for study of the mechanisms of allergic airway narrowing. It has also been possible to demonstrate an important potential role for CD4[+] T cells in the late allergic response, which may account for the lack of a more obvious relationship between responses that have been generally considered to be IgE-dependent and circulating IgE levels. Preliminary evidence suggests that the BN rat responds to sensitization with a TH$_2$ profile of cytokines, making the association with atopic human disease even stronger and supporting the relevance of this model to allergen asthma.

ACKNOWLEDGMENTS

The contribution of my collaborators, Drs. D. Eidelman, S. Sapienza, P. Renzi, S. Waserman, A. Watanabe, H. Mishima and Q. Hamid in the above-cited studies is gratefully acknowledged.

REFERENCES

1. Dandurand, R. J., C. G. Wang, S. Laberge, J. G. Martin, and D. H. Eidelman. In vitro allergic bronchoconstriction in the brown Norway rat. *Am J Respir Crit Care Med* 149: 1499–1505, 1994.

2. Du, T., S. Sapienza, D. H. Eidelman, N. S. Wang, and J. G. Martin. Morphometry of the airways during late responses to antigen challenge in the rat. *Am Rev Respir Dis* 143: 132–137, 1991.

3. Du, T., L. J. Xu, M. Lei, N. S. Wang, D. H. Eidelman, H. Ghezzo, and J. G. Martin. Morphometric changes during the early airway response to allergen challenge in the rat. *Am Rev Respir Dis* 146: 1037–1041, 1992.

4. Eidelman, D. H., S. Bellofiore, and J. G. Martin. Late airway responses to antigen challenge in sensitized inbred rats. *Am Rev Respir Dis* 137: 1033–1037, 1988.

5. Elwood, W., P. J. Barnes, and K. Fan Chung. Airway hyperresponsiveness is associated with inflammatory cell infiltration in Brown-Norway rats. *Intl Arch Allergy & Immunol* 99: 91–97, 1992.

6. Lichtenstein, L. M. and B. S. Bochner. The role of basophils in asthma. [Review]. *Annals of the New York Academy of Sciences* 629: 48–61, 1991.

7. Murphey, S. M., S. Brown, N. Miklos, and P. Fireman. Reagin synthesis in inbred strains of rats. *Immunology* 27: 245–253, 1974.

8. Olivenstein, R., T. Du, L. J. Xu, and J. G. Martin. Microvascular leakage in the airway wall and lumen during allergen-induced responses in rats. *Am J Respir Crit Care Med* 1995.(submitted)

9. Pauwels, R., H. Bazin, B. Platteau, and M. van der Straeten. The influence of antigen dose on IgE production in different rat strains. *Immunology* 36: 151–157, 1979.

10. Renzi, P. M., R. Olivenstein, and J. G. Martin. Effect of dexamethasone on airway inflammation and responsiveness after antigen challenge of the rat. *Am Rev Respir Dis* 148(4): 932–939, 1993.

11. Renzi, P. M., R. Olivenstein, and J. G. Martin. Inflammatory cell populations in the airways and parenchyma after antigen challenge of the rat. *Am Rev Respir Dis* 147: 967–974, 1993.

12. Sapienza, S., D. H. Eidelman, P. M. Renzi, and J. G. Martin. Role of leukotriene D4 in the early and late pulmonary responses of rats to allergen challenge. *Am Rev Respir Dis* 142: 353–358, 1990.

13. Sorden, S. D. and W. L. Castleman. Brown Norway rats are high responders to bronchiolitis, pneumonia, and bronchiolar mastocytosis induced by parainfluenza virus. *Experimental Lung Research* 17: 1025–1045, 1991.

14. Sorkness, R., K. Johns, W. L. Castleman, and R. F. Lemanske,Jr. Late pulmonary allergic responses in actively but not passively IgE-sensitized rats. *J Appl Physiol* 69: 1012–1021, 1990.

15. Waserman, S., R. Olivenstein, P. Renzi, L. J. Xu, and J. G. Martin. The relationship between late asthmatic responses and antigen-specific immunoglobulin. *Journal of Allergy & Clinical Immunology* 90: 661–669, 1992.

16. Waserman, S., L. J. Xu, R. Olivenstein, P. M. Renzi, and J. G. Martin. Association between late allergic bronchoconstriction in the rat and allergen-stimulated lymphocyte proliferation in vitro. *Am J Respir Crit Care Med* 151: 470–474, 1995.

17. Watanabe, A., H. Mishima, P. M. Renzi, Q. Hamid, and J. G. Martin. Adoptive transfer of allergic airway responses with sensitized lymphocytes in BN rats. *Am J Respir Crit Care Med* 1995. (In Press)

18. Watanabe, A., H. Mishima, P. M. Renzi, L. J. Xu, Q. Hamid, and J. G. Martin. Transfer of allergic airway responses with antigen-primed CD4+ but not CD8+ T cells in Brown Norway rats. *J. Clin. Invest.* 1995. (In Press)

19. Watanabe, A., H. Mishima, E. Schotman, P. M. Renzi, J. G. Martin, and Q. Hamid. Adoptively transferred late allergic airway responses are associated with Th2 type cytokines in the rat. *Am J Respir Crit Care Med* 1995. (Abstract)

20. Wilkes, L. K., C. McMenamin, and P. G. Holt. Postnatal maturation of mast cell subpopulations in the rat respiratory tract. *Immunology* 75: 535–541, 1992.

21. Xu, L. J., S. Sapienza, T. Du, S. Waserman, and J. G. Martin. Comparison of upper and lower airway responses of two sensitized rat strains to inhaled antigen. *J Appl Physiol* 73: 1608–1613, 1992.

3

THE ROLE OF NEBULIZED IFN–γ IN THE MODULATION OF ALLERGIC RESPONSES

Gideon Lack and Erwin W. Gelfand[*]

Divisions of Basic Sciences
Department of Pediatrics
National Jewish Center for Immunology and Respiratory Medicine
Denver, Colorado 80206

Cytokines are required for B-cell proliferation and differentiation and additionally, direct Ig isotype switching. Interleukin-4 causes both murine and human B cells to undergo isotype switching to IgE synthesis; IL-4 also induces IgG1 and IgG4 production by murine and human B cells, respectively. More recently IL-13 has been shown to induce Ig isotype switching to IgE and IgG4 humans. Interferon-γ (IFN–γ) is an important regulator of IgE production; it antagonizes IL-4 directed Ig isotype switching to IgE in both murine and human B cells (1–4). Additionally, IFN–γ inhibits IL-13 driven IgE synthesis by human B cells (5). *In vitro,* IFN–γ selectively inhibits the proliferation of T_H2 cells and favors the differentiation of precursor T_H0 cells into cells with a T_H1 phenotype (6).

Human allergic diseases are characterized by high circulating IgE levels, allergen-specific IgE and allergic inflammation (eosinophils and mast cells) in target organs. There are numerous studies demonstrating an excess of IL-4 production and a deficiency of IFN–γ in human allergic disease. CD4$^+$ T cell clones from allergic patients show skewing towards a T_H2 profile in that they produce high amounts of IL-4 and low amounts of IFN–γ. We recently showed in human atopic PBMC that there is deficient IFN–γ production and localized this defect to the CD4 population (7).

The rationale for the treatment of atopic disease with IFN–γ has therefore, two objectives: First, the inhibition of IgE production; second, the correction of the cytokine imbalance. Several clinical trials have been carried out attempting to modify allergic disease with IFN–γ. However, the results of most of these studies were generally equivocal. One trial showed no improvement in seasonal allergic rhinitis and no changes in serum IgE following IFN–γ treatment. In atopic dermatitis, IFN–γ resulted in some improvement in inflammation and symptom scores in a sub-group of patients, but did not affect total IgE production. A study of IFN–γ treatment in asthmatic individuals showed only slight im-

---

[*] **Address Correspondence to:** Dr. Erwin W. Gelfand, National Jewish Center for Immunology and Respiratory Medicine, 1400 Jackson St., Denver, CO 80206.

New Horizons in Allergy Immunotherapy
edited by Sehon et al. Plenum Press, New York, 1996

provement over placebo without affecting IgE synthesis. There was, however, a decrease in circulating eosinophils.

A major limitation in the design of these studies was that they were unable to address certain issues. First, there is evidence in humans that the local delivery of IFN–γ is more bioavailable to the lungs than is systemic treatment (8). Parenteral treatment was the only route employed in most of the clinical trials. Second, the critical element of timing of IFN–γ treatment was not studied. There are data indicating that the late addition of IFN–γ treatment to PBMC cultured with IL-4 is ineffective in preventing IgE synthesis. Third, clinical studies cannot compare the effect of IFN–γ treatment on primary allergic sensitization with secondary and subsequent allergic responses. Finally, these studies did not differentiate between polyclonal and allergen-specific IgE production. Allergic disease is characterized both by raised total serum IgE and allergen-specific IgE as well as by allergen-specific cutaneous reactivity.

In order to address these important issues, we employed a murine model that should permit the analysis of these components (9–11). IgE high responder BALB/c mice were sensitized through the airways and the lungs by ultrasonic nebulization of OVA. Mice exposed to daily OVA over 10 days, developed high anti-OVA IgE responses in the serum and immediate cutaneous reactivity to OVA. Exposure of tracheal smooth muscle to electrical field stimulation showed that OVA-exposed mice developed altered airway function. Increased airway responsiveness (AR) was observed in sensitized compared to non-sensitized controls and this correlated with increased acetylcholine release and impaired M2 receptor function (12). To assess the ability of IFN–γ to modify these responses, mice were treated with IFN–γ using different routes of administration, dosages, and timing schedules (13).

PARENTERAL IFN-γ DECREASES TOTAL BUT NOT ALLERGEN-SPECIFIC IGE PRODUCTION

Mice were treated with 25,000 units of IFN–γ via the intraperitoneal (i.p.) route, daily during the period of OVA sensitization and for three days prior to that. The use of higher dosages was abandoned because of toxicity and no apparent benefits over the lower doses. Mice sensitized to OVA developed an increase in serum total IgE levels (13) (Table 1). IFN–γ treatment given i.p. resulted in a 50% decrease in total serum IgE, to levels equivalent to those seen in PBS-treated controls. In contrast, i.p. IFN–γ failed to decrease anti-OVA IgE responses that follow OVA sensitization via the airways. These mice had anti-OVA IgE levels, cutaneous reactivity to OVA and increased AR comparable to animals that received OVA alone (Table 1). Even intravenous IFN–γ failed to inhibit anti-OVA IgE responses.

NEBULIZED IFN-γ BUT NOT I.P. IFN-γ IS BIOAVAILABLE TO THE LOCAL LYMPHOID TISSUE OF THE AIRWAYS

When given by the i.p. route, IFN–γ was bioavailable to inhibit systemic polyclonal IgE production but may not have been available to the local lymphoid tissue of the airways, where allergen-specific IgE production was occurring. We hypothesized that the local delivery of nebulized IFN–γ unlike i.p. IFN–γ would be active in the airways and thus

Table 1. Comparison of the effects of intraperitoneal (i.p.) and nebulized (neb) IFN-γ

Treatment	OVA	OVA/IFN-γ i.p.	OVA/IFN-γ neb
Total IgE	↑	↓	↑
Anti-OVA-IgE	↑↑	↑↑	↓↓
Anti-OVA-IgG2a	↓	↓	↑↑
Cutaneous reactivity OVA	↑↑	↑↑	↓↓
Airway responsiveness	↑↑	↑↑	↓↓

IFN-γ was administered intraperitonially or by nebulization to BALB/c animals for 3 days prior to and during the 10-day period of OVA sensitization via the airways. On day 12, serum for IgE levels was obtained and testing for immediate cutaneous reactivity and airway function was monitored.

modulate the local production of anti-OVA IgE. Nebulized IFN–γ (250,000 units dissolved in 7 ml of PBS) was found to retain its bioactivity (13). Aerosolized particles were collected by condensation and the condensate was found to effectively inhibit IgE production by IL-4-stimulated MNC in 14-day cultures. Determination of particle size by laser nephelometry revealed that more than 60% of the nebulized IFN–γ particles were in the respirable range (0.5 to 2 μm).

Having established the bioactivity of nebulized IFN–γ and the appropriateness of particle size, we compared the bioavailability of nebulized and i.p. IFN–γ to the peribronchial lymphoid tissue (PBLN) draining the trachea and upper airways. We found that nebulized IFN–γ increased class II MHC (Ia) expression in PBLN-derived MNC and to a lesser extent in the spleen as determined by surface staining and flow cytometry (13). In contrast, i.p. IFN–γ caused a large induction of Ia expression in the spleen but not in the PBLN (13). Additionally, we found that nebulized but not i.p. IFN–γ was able to inhibit *in vitro* IgE production by PBLN-derived MNC (13). These data demonstrate that nebulized IFN–γ was effective in the local milieu of the airways where sensitization to OVA was occurring, likely accounting for the inability of systemic IFN–γ to modulate local allergic sensitization. As further confirmation, we found that nebulized IFN–γ but not i.p. IFN–γ was able to inhibit subsequent *in vitro* IgE production by PBLN-derived MNC.

NEBULIZED INF-γ PREVENTS ALLERGIC SENSITIZATION TO OVA

Nebulized IFN–γ administered for thirteen days, for three days prior to sensitization and daily during the ten day period of OVA exposure, decreased anti-OVA IgE by more than 60% compared to OVA-treated controls (13) (Table 1). Additionally, IFN–γ treated mice developed a significant anti-OVA IgG2a response not observed in OVA treated animals and non-sensitized controls. There was a significant inverse correlation between anti-OVA IgE and anti-OVA IgG2a, confirming the reciprocal regulation of these isotypes by IFN–γ (13). The dosage of 250,000 units IFN–γ per nebulization was found to be optimal and it was estimated that each mouse only received a maximum of 5000 units per nebulization. Treatment regimens that consisted of thirteen days and included pre-treatment produced the greatest decline in anti-OVA IgE.

Using this treatment regimen, we found that IFN–γ also prevented the development of cutaneous reactivity to OVA (Table 1). This has been shown to result from allergen-triggered mast cell degranulation and the responses correlated with allergen-specific IgE in the serum (10).

Additionally, thirteen days of nebulized IFN–γ prevented the development of increased AR (13) (Table 1). Shorter IFN–γ treatments that started on the first day of OVA sensitization or were delayed further were less effective than the thirteen day course of IFN–γ treatment in inhibiting anti-OVA IgE. Initiation of IFN–γ treatment after day 6 of OVA sensitization failed to inhibit anti-OVA IgE.

IFN-γ INHIBITS THE PRODUCTION OF SECONDARY IgE RESPONSES

Whether or not IFN–γ can prevent IgE responses to secondary allergen challenge and subsequent allergen exposure has important implications for the treatment of human allergic disease. The answer depends in part on the cellular interactions and signaling requirements for secondary IgE production by B cells. If secondary IgE production is derived from a pool of IgE committed memory B cells, then clearly it is too late for IFN–γ to prevent Ig isotype switching to IgE. If alternatively, the secondary response is derived from IgM⁺ memory B cells that undergo *de novo* isotype switching to IgE, there is a window of opportunity for IFN–γ to inhibit IgE production. In the mouse, there is evidence that B cells require IL-4 and a signal from CD4⁺ T cells to generate both primary and secondary IgE responses *in vivo* (14). This suggests that isotype switching to IgE is also necessary for the generation of a secondary IgE response.

To examine the control of secondary IgE responses *in vivo*, mice that had been initially sensitized to OVA received a secondary OVA challenge. Following 10 days of OVA sensitization, we found that serum anti-OVA IgE levels declined to less than 30% of the peak response (days 12–18) by day 30. At that point, animals lost their cutaneous reactivity to OVA and had normal AR. Secondary OVA challenge on days 30 and 31 induced a secondary anti-OVA IgE response measured on day 37 which was accompanied by cutaneous reactivity to OVA and increased AR. Nebulized IFN–γ administered for thirteen days during primary OVA sensitization, as well as inhibiting the primary allergic response, prevented the development of a secondary IgE response, cutaneous reactivity to OVA and increased AR following secondary OVA challenge (Table 2). If nebulized IFN–γ was administered for only five days, days 26–30, but after normal allergen sensitization had been achieved, it prevented the development of secondary IgE and immediate hypersensitivity responses following secondary OVA challenge. Therefore, treatment with nebulized IFN–γ can prevent the development of secondary allergic responses, even if treatment is initiated after normal primary allergic responses were established.

NEBULIZED IFN-γ TREATMENT ALTERS T-CELL FUNCTION AND SHIFTS CYTOKINE PRODUCTION FROM A T$_H$2 TO A T$_H$1-LIKE PATTERN

Lymphocytes from the PBLN of mice sensitized to OVA develop *in vitro* proliferative responses to OVA. Treatment of mice with nebulized IFN–γ significantly inhibited the proliferative responses and shifted the dose-response curve to the right. A likely explanation for this anti-proliferative effect is that IFN–γ was able to selectively inhibit the proliferative response of T$_H$2-like OVA reactive T cells. IFN–γ treatment did not affect the proliferative response to non-specific mitogen stimulation.

Table 2. Effects of IFN-γ on primary and secondary responses to OVA

	Anti-OVA IgE		ST		AR
Groups	1°	2°	1°	2°	2°
OVA 10 days	↑	↑↑	↑	↑	↑
IFN-d3→10	↓	↓↓	↓	↓↓	↓
IFN-d26→30	↑	↓↓	↑	↓	↓

Mice were exposed to OVA via the airways from days 1-10 (1° sensitization) or on days 30,31 (2° challenge). IFN-γ treated animals received nebulized IFN-γ on days -3 to +10 or from day 26 to day 30. Primary responses were assessed on day 12 and secondary responses on day 37.

In order to examine the effect of IFN–γ on the profile of cytokine production by T cells, we examined *in situ* production of IL-4 and IFN–γ in T cells obtained from PBLN and spleen. We found that T cells from naive animals had very low frequencies of IL-4 and IFN–γ production following mitogen stimulation. OVA sensitization caused a marked increase in the frequency of IL-4 and IFN–γ producing T cells, both in the spleen and PBLN (Table 3). IL-4 was produced almost exclusively by CD4$^+$ T cells whereas IFN–γ was produced by both CD4$^+$ and CD8$^+$ T cell subsets. Nebulized IFN–γ significantly decreased the frequency of IL-4 producing T cells both in the PBLN and spleen (Table 3). Thus, *in vivo* treatment with IFN–γ was able to decrease the capacity of T cells to produce T$_H$2-type cytokines as measured at the single cell and shifted the T cell response toward a T$_H$1 pattern of cytokine production.

THE INHIBITION OF ALLERGEN RESPONSES BY IFN–γ REQUIRES THE PRESENCE OF ALLERGEN DURING IFN–γ TREATMENT

There are data showing that IFN–γ inhibits IgE production through its action on B cells and conflicting data showing that it acts on T cells as well. In order for IFN–γ to influence lymphocyte function it must bind to the IFN–γ receptor on the cell surface. Constitutive IFN–γ receptor (IFN–γR) expression is very low on B cells and is only expressed on 5% of resting T cells. IFN–γ can only alter lymphocyte function once lymphocytes have been pre-activated and expression of IFN–γR is upregulated. There are several different lines of evidence in our model that point to a requirement for the presence of allergen for IFN–γ responses to occur. First, we found that there was no reduction in IL-4 production by lymphocytes from animals that were treated with IFN–γ alone. Inhibition of

Table 3. Frequency of cytokine producing cells/10^3 CD4$^+$ T Cells

Sensitization	Cell Population	IFN	IL-4
PBS	CD4$^+$	34.1 ± 6.0	32.3 ± 4.1
IFN–γ	CD4$^+$	6.4 ± 2.1	28.4 ± 4.1
OVA	CD4$^+$	56 ± 11.3	149.4 ± 25.5
OVA/IFN–γ	CD4$^+$	71 ± 15.2	24.6 ± 3.2

Mice were sensitized to OVA via the airways on 10 consecutive days. IFN-γ treatment was by nebulization from day -3 to day 10. Spleens were harvested on day 12 and *in situ* staining for IFN-γ and IL-4 carried out as described in (15). Results are from 3 separate experiments. Similar results were obtained with PBLN.

IL-4 production by CD4⁺ T cells only occurred in mice that had the combination of IFN–γ and OVA exposure. Secondly, we found that CD4⁺ T cells from OVA-sensitized/IFN–γ-treated mice were able to inhibit polyclonal and anti-OVA IgE production *in vitro* whereas CD4⁺ T cells from mice that had been exposed to IFN–γ alone did not inhibit IgE production. There is supportive evidence in humans that immunotherapy with an allergen induces IFN–γ production and allergen-specific IgE but results in inhibition of *in vitro* lymphocyte proliferation to the injected allergen but not to an irrelevant allergen. These specific changes may similarly be explained in terms of the anti-proliferative effects of IFN–γ on T_H2 type cells and its ability to prevent isotype switching. The fact that these changes are allergen-specific suggests that IFN–γ produced during immunotherapy only influences allergen-specific T cells and B cells that have been specifically activated by allergen.

In summary, we have shown in a murine model of allergic sensitization via the airways that nebulized IFN–γ can inhibit both primary and secondary IgE responses and immediate hypersensitivity reactions. There are three critically important factors that appear to be necessary for successful immunomodulation with IFN–γ. IFN–γ must be delivered early during the course of a primary or secondary response. It must be delivered to the site of allergic sensitization i.e., the lungs, in order to inhibit allergen-specific IgE production induced by aerosolization of allergen. Thirdly, it must be delivered in the presence of the allergen in order to influence antigen-specific lymphocyte cell function. In light of these observations, the relative lack of success with IFN–γ in clinical trials is not surprising. Recognition of the requirements for optimal times of administration as well as route of exposure may reveal the therapeutic potential of this important regulatory cytokine.

ACKNOWLEDGMENTS

This work was supported by Grants PO1-HL36577, AI-26490 and AI 29704 from the National Institutes of Health. We gratefully acknowledge the contributions of our many colleagues to this work. We thank Debbie Remley for preparation of the manuscript.

REFERENCES

1. Snapper, C. M., and W. E. Paul. 1987. Interferon-γ and B cell stimulatory factor-1 reciprocally regulate Ig isotype production. *Science* 236:944–947.
2. Coffman, R. L., and J. Carty. 1986. A T cell activity that enhances polyclonal IgE production and its inhibition by interferon-γ. *J. Immunol.* 136:949–954.
3. Pene, J., F. Rousset, F. Briére, I. Chrétien, J. Y. Bonnefoy, H. Spits, T. Yokota, N. Arai, K. I. Arai, J. Banchereau, and J. E. De Vries. 1988. IgE production by normal human lymphocytes is induced by interleukin 4 and suppressed by interferons α, γ and prostaglandin E₂. *Proc. Natl. Acad. Sci. USA* 85:6880–6884.
4. Chrétien, I., J. Péne, F. Briére, R. De Waal-Malefijt, F. Rousset, and J. E. DeVries. 1990. Regulation of human IgE synthesis. I. Human IgE synthesis *in vitro* is determined by the reciprocal antagonistic effects of interleukin 4 and interferon-γ. *Eur. J. Immunol.* 20:243–251.
5. deVries, J. E. and Zurawski, G. 1995. Immunoregulatory properties of IL-13: Its potential role in atopic disease. *Int. Arch. Allergy Immunol.* 106:175–179.
6. Bradley, L. M., K. Yoshimoto, and S. L. Swain. 1995. The cytokines IL-4, IFN-g, and IL-12 regulate the development of subsets of memory effector/helper T cells *in vitro*. *J. Immunol.* 155:1713–1724.
7. Jung, T., G. Lack, U. Schauer, W. Uberück, H. Renz, E. W. Gelfand, C. H. L. Rieger. 1995. Decreased frequency of interferon-γ and interleukin-2-producing cells in patients with atopic diseases measured at the single cell level. *J All Clin Immunol*, in press, 1995.

8. Jaffe, H. A., R. Buhl, A. Mastrangeli, K. J. Holroyd, C. Saltini, D. Czerski, H. S. Jaffe, S. Kramer, S. Sherwin, and R. G. Crystal. 1991. Organ specific cytokine therapy. Local activation of mononuclear phagocytes by delivery of an aerosol of recombinant interferon-γ to the human lung. *J. Clin. Invest.* 88:297–302.

9. Renz, H., H. R. Smith, J. E. Henson, B. S. Ray, C. G. Irvin, and E. W. Gelfand. 1992. Aerosolized antigen exposure without adjuvant causes increased IgE production and increased airway responsiveness in the mouse. *J. Allergy Clin. Immunol.* 89:1127–1138.

10. Saloga, J., H. Renz, G. Lack, K. L. Bradley, J. L. Greenstein, G. Larsen, and E. W. Gelfand. 1993. Development and transfer of immediate cutaneous hypersensitivity in mice exposed to aerosolized antigen. *J. Clin. Invest.* 91:133–140.

11. Larsen, G. L., H. Renz, J. E. Loader, K. L. Bradley, and E. W. Gelfand. 1992. Airway response to electrical field stimulation in sensitized inbred mice. *J. Clin. Invest.* 89:747–752.

12. Larsen, G. L., T. M. Fame, H. Renz, J. E. Loader, J. Graves, M. Hill and E. W. Gelfand. 1994. Increased acetylcholine release in tracheas from allergen-exposed IgE-immune mice. *Am. J. Physiol.* 266:L263-L270.

13. Lack, G., Renz, H., Saloga, J., Bradley, K. L., Loader, J., Leung, D. Y. M., Larsen, G., and Gelfand, E. W. 1994. Nebulized but not parenteral IFN-γ decreases IgE production and normalizes airways function in a murine model of allergen sensitization. *J. Immunol.* 152:2546–2554.

14. Finkelman, F. D., I. M. Katona, J. F. Urban, Jr., J. Holmes, J. O'hara, A. S. Tung, J. G. Sample and W. E. Paul. 1988. IL-4 is required to generate and sustain *in vivo* IgE responses. *J. Immunol.* 252:2335–2341.

15. Renz, H., G. Lack, J. Saloga, R. Schwinzer, K. Bradley, J. Loader, A. Kupfer, G. L. Larsen and E. W. Gelfand. Inhibition of IgE production and normalization of airways responsiveness by sensitized CD8 T cells in a mouse model of allergen-induced sensitization. *J Immunol,* 152:351–360, 1993.

MURINE ANIMAL MODELS TO STUDY THE CENTRAL ROLE OF T CELLS IN IMMEDIATE-TYPE HYERSENSITIVITY RESPONSES

Udo Herz,[1] Uschi Lumpp,[1] Angelika Daser,[1] Erwin W. Gelfand,[2] and Harald Renz[*1]

[1]Institute of Clinical Chemistry and Biochemistry
Virchow Klinikum of the Humboldt University
Augustenburger Platz 1, 13353 Berlin, FRG
[2]National Jewish Center for Immunology and Respiratory Medicine
Department of Pediatrics
1400 Jackson Street, Denver, Colorado 80206

1. SUMMARY

The development of allergic sensitization and inflammation is dependent on activation and stimulation of T cells that exhibit pro-allergic functions. A mouse model system was developed to study the role of T cells in allergic sensitization in more detail. Local sensitization of mice stimulates an allergen specific IgE/IgG1 response that is associated with the development of immediate type skin test responses and increased airway responsiveness (AR). Strains of mice are identified that are high or low responder animals for allergens including ovalbumin and house dust mite. Each allergen stimulates a different pattern of T-cell receptor Vβ expressing T cells in local draining lymph nodes. To induce a state of increased AR, at least two separate events are required. The first event is the presence of allergen specific IgE/IgG1. The second event is characterized as a local allergen challenge at the site of the response. These T cells play a critical role in the regulation of the allergic immune response including IgE production and increased AR. Based on these results intervention strategies can be developed which specifically target the development and function of these allergen specific T-cell populations and modify their pro-allergic activities.

* To whom correspondence should be addressed.

New Horizons in Allergy Immunotherapy
edited by Sehon et al. Plenum Press, New York, 1996

25

2. DEVELOPMENT OF ALLERGIC INFLAMMATION IS T-CELL DEPENDENT

It is widely accepted that T lymphocytes play a central role in the development of allergic sensitization and inflammation. Detailed analysis of inflammatory lesions of airway mucosa in patients suffering from bronchial asthma and of the skin of patients with atopic dermatitis revealed the presence of a mononuclear cell infiltrate that mainly consists of T lymphocytes and some monocytes/macrophages. In allergic lesions, T-cells are activated and express the CD45RO isoforme suggesting effector cell functions, whereas quiescent T cells expressing the CD45RA isoforme, are not detected. In addition to T cells, allergic inflammation is also characterized by an influx of effector cells, such as eosinophils and mast cells, to the site of inflammation (1–3).

Analysis of cytokine production by T cells in allergic diseases revealed an imbalanced release of cytokines characterized by an increased production of interleukin (IL)-4 and IL-5 compared to interferon (IFN)-γ. The cytokines IL-4 and IL-5 play an important role as pro-allergic interleukins. IL-4 controls the production of IgE together with IL-13 (in the human immune system), and activates mast cells and basophils. IL-5 promotes eosinophil activation and more recent data suggest that IL-5 also prevents apoptosis in eosinophils. The latter finding may explain the development of eosinophilia in allergic diseases. On the other hand, IFN-γ is known as a potent inhibitor of IL-4 induced IgE production. Overproduction of IL-4 and IL-5 together with a reduced secretion of IFN-γ was observed in T cells from the peripheral blood of allergic patients as well as in T cells derived from atopic lesions. In addition, allergen-specific T cell clones from lesional skin also exhibit a similar pattern of cytokine production (4–9). Recent data (10) indicate that the pattern of cytokine production by T cells in skin lesions from patients with atopic dermatitis is dependent on the stage of inflammtion. During acute exacerbation of the disease, an exclusive increase of IL-4 mRNA was observed. Only in chronic lesions the increased production of IL-4 was accompanied by an increase of IL-5 production together with a small rise in IFN-γ. These results suggest that IL-4 plays an important and dominant role during the initial stages of allergic inflammtion and presumably during the intial phase of allergic sensitization. In contrast, when inflammation has reached a more chronic stage, a mixed pattern of cytokine production could be observed (10).

These findings raise the question about the signals and cellular events that control T-cell activation in allergic diseases. T-cells are activated in an allergen/antigen dependent fashion implying an interaction of antigen presenting cells (APC) with T-cells. APC phagocyte or internalize antigen or allergen and present linear peptides (T-cell epitopes) on MHC- class II molecules to T-cells. T-cells recognize these epitopes in a MHC dependent and restricted fashion via the T cell receptor (TCR). This trimolecular complex that consisting of MHC-class II molecule, peptide and TCR, provides the initial signal for T-cell activation. This level of T-cell- APC interactions ensures that only T-cells with a specificity for the presented T-cell epitope can become activated (11).

For a complete activation of T cells additional signals are required. For example, to induce IgE production at least two additional events are essential. As a consequence of the allergen-specific signal, the T cell starts to express the CD40 ligand (CD40L) which binds to the CD40 receptor that are constitutively expressed on B cells (12). Recently we reported that B cells from atopic dermatitis patients express the CD40 receptor with increased intensity as compared to non atopic B cells (13). However, interaction of CD40L with CD40R seems to represent an universal signal that is required for any immunoglobulin isotype switch from IgM towards other Ig isotypes and subclasses including (14) IgE. Secondly, CD28 molecules on T cells interact with B7 molecules, their counterpart expressed on B cells. As a consequence of complete T-cell activation, the interleukin production machinery is turned on. In allergy, the allergen specific T cell is characterized by the production of IL-4 that provides signals required to promote IgE isotype switching in B cells. Why a certain T cell starts to selectively produce IL-4 (or any other cytokine) remains still unclear.

3. MURINE ANIMAL MODEL SYSTEM TO STUDY ALLERGIC SENSITIZATION EVENTS IN VIVO

Since the access to immune cells from the local site of allergic inflammation is limited and ethical reasons prevent many functional cell-cell interaction studies under in-vivo conditions, development of animal model systems is required to study the cellular and molecular events that result in allergic sensitization. Several years ago we set out to develop a murine model of allergic inflammation. It was the aim that such a model system should mimic the development of allergic sensitization observed in human as closely as possible. Since the most important route of sensitization in human is via the airways and the lung, mice were sensitized by nebulization of allergens. Aerosolization of allergens generates particles that are in the respiratory range. Initially this model was established for ovalbumin (OVA) that represents a well characterized model antigen used in many in vitro and in vivo systems (15). Many immune functions dependent on OVA and OVA derived peptides have been studied in the past. Recently, this model of allergic sensitization was expanded to other clinically more relevant allergens, including ragweed pollen (16), house dust mite and cat allergen.

Several protocols of allergic sensitization were compared. Short term sensitization by daily exposure of the allergen for 20 min each day over a period of 10 days already induced the induction of an allergen specific IgE/IgG1 response that is detectable in the serum of the animals. In addition, a rise of specific IgE/IgG1 antibodies is also achieved by long term sensitization once a week over several consecutive weeks. Long term exposure has the advantage that not only events of primary sensitization can be studied but also effects of secondary and tertiary responses are analyzed.

The induction of an allergen specific immune respnse is dependent on the mice strain used in these studies. For example, BALB/c mice are high responder animals for OVA and ragweed sensitization. In contrast, SJL/J mice do not develope an IL-4 dependent allergic response to OVA (17). Furthermore, C57Bl/6 mice develop an allergen specific immune response to house dust mite allergen, whereas BALB/C mice are low/no responder for this allergen. It is possible that differences in the MHC between these strains are responsible for the differential effects in terms of induction of an allergen specific immune response to a given allergen, but further experiments are required to exactly determine the reason for strain differences in the induction of an allergic response (Table 1).

A functional consequence of the induction of an allergen specific Ig response is the development of immediate-type skin test responses to the allergen. A skin test technique was established, where the intracutaneous injection of small quantities of the allergen stimulates the development of wheal responses in IgE/IgG1 positive mice. The kinetic of these responses parallels the pattern of skin prick test responses in allergic patients. Maximal wheal formation was observed within 15 - 20 min, and within the following 15 min

Table 1. Development of immediate type hypersensitivity responses to allergens
in different strains of mice

Strain	H-2	OVA	Ragweed	House dust mite
BALB/C	$H\text{-}2^d$	high	high	low
C57Bl/6	$H\text{-}2^b$	high	n.d.	high
CBA	$H\text{-}2^k$	n.d.	n.d.	high
SJL/J	$H\text{-}2^s$	low	low	n.d.

Mice of different strains were sensitized to allergens by ultrasonic nebulization as described (15). The
following concentrations of allergens were used: 0.1 % (w/v) OVA, 500 µg/ml ragweed, 7 µg/ml house
dust mite extract. Immediate hypersensitivity responses were assessed by measurement of allergen-specific serum IgE/IgG1 antibody titers (15), determination of airway responsiveness by electrical stimulation (17) and analysis of skin test responses (18). Animals were considered as "high responder" mice, if
all three read out systems gave positive results. Low responder mice were mice that did not mount a
specific IgE response and had a normal airway response to electrical stimulation.

they completely disappeared. Immediate type skin responses to the allergen were compared to the effects of the application of positive and negative control solutions. Compound 48/80, an unspecific mast cell degranulator, always yields positive responses within
the same time frame, whereas application of PBS, the allergen diluent, is ineffective. Additional histological examination of site of wheal responses indicated that the formation of
the immediate type skin responses were due to mast cell degranulation. Furthermore, only
IgE/IgG1 positive mice developed these responses, whereas mice that did not mount an allergen-specific immune response or produced Ig of other Ig isotypes and subclasses, had a
negative response (18).

Since mice were sensitized via the airways and the lung, it was of interest to study
possible changes in airways responsiveness (AR). In mice, AR can be measured in several
ways. In OVA sensitized BALB/c mice we compared in-vivo measurement of airway resistance and conductance with the results of the analysis of in-vitro AR using electrical
stimulation of tracheas from sensitized and non-sensitized control animals. Using both
techniques, it was found that sensitization via the local route induced a state of airway hyperresponsiveness (15, 17). These results prompted the question whether the induction of
increased AR is IgE dependent or not. To analyze the role of allergen-specific Ig production in more detail, C57Bl/6 mice were sensitized either via the local route by repeated
aerosolization of house dust mite allergen extract or by intraperitoneal allergen injections
emulsified in $Al(OH)_3$ (systemic sensitization). Systemic sensitization with adjuvant
mounted an allergen specific immune response that was associated with the development
of positive skin test responses. Measurement of AR in these mice by electrical stimulation
revealed a completely normal dose response curve to increased electrical frequencies (Hz)
suggesting a normal state of AR as comapred to non-sensitized animals. Following systemic sensitization these mice were then challenged with house dust mite extract by two
consecutive aerosolizations prior to analysis. Under these conditions, a shift of AR was
detected indicating a half maximal constriction of tracheal segments at an electrical frequency significantly lower compared to mice sensitized without local allergen challenge.
From these experiments it is concluded that in an allergen specific model system induction
of increased AR is dependent on two events. The first event is provided by the presence of
an allergen-specific antibody response. It is of minor importance whether the IgE/IgG1 response is induced via local or systemic sensitization. The second event is provided by the

Table 2. Development of increased airway responsiveness requires allergen-specific IgE/IgG1 production and local allergen challenge

Route of sensitization	Airway challenge	IgE/IgG1 plus positive IST	Airway responsiveness
Airway	+	+	increased
i.p.	−	+	normal
i.p.	+	+	increased
−	+	−	normal

C57Bl/6 mice were sensitized with house dust mite extract (kindly provided by Dr. H. Lowenstein, ALK Laboratories, Hörsholm, DK) by repeated intraperitoneal injection of 5 μg/mouse/day emulsified in Al(OH)₃, or by ultrasonic nebulization of 7 μg per nebulization. Sensitization was performed once a week for 4 weeks, and the local challenge with allergen was applied by two nebulizations of allergen prior to analysis. All read out systems were carried out as described (17). IST: Immediate type skin test responses.

local allegen exposure at the site of the allergic response. To induce increased AR, local allergen exposure via the airwys is required (Table 2).

4. ALLERGEN SENSITIZATION STIMULATES T CELLS EXPRESSING A RESTRICTED TCR Vβ REPERTOIRE

As a consequence of local sensitization increases in the size of local draining lymph nodes were detected (15). Further analysis revealed that changes in the size of local lymph nodes were due to a preferential influx or expansion of CD4 T cells. To examine whether the increased frequency of CD4 T cells was a result of a randome expansion of these T cells or whether a selected expansion of T cells occured during allergic sensitization, we analyzed the TCR repertoire before and after allergen sensitization in local lymph nodes. The usage of variable elements on the TCR β chain can be relatively easily studied since monoclonal antibodies against Vβ families and some individual members of families are available that cover about two thirds of the TCR Vβ repertoire expressed on mature T cells.

In local draining lymph nodes of BALB/c mice sensitized to OVA an increased frequency in Vβ8.1 and Vβ8.2 positive T cells was detected. This analysis was compared to the distribution of TCR VβT cells in the spleen of sensitized and non-sensitized animals. The results revealed that in the spleen, an immunological organ distant from the site of sensitization, a different group of T cells was found expanded upon stimulation. Here OVA sensitization favoured the expansion of Vβ 2, Vβ8 and Vβ 14 positive T cells (19). To examine whether these T cell subgroups were indeed OVA specific, Vβ2, Vβ8 and Vβ14 positive T cells were purified from OVA sensitized animals and subjected to in-vitro proliferation experiments with OVA. Stimulation gave a comparable dose dependent proliferative response curve in each subgroup. It was then asked whether these T-cells would be able to provide help for Ig production. For this purpose purified Vβ2 and Vβ8 T cells from OVA sensitized animals were cocultured with purified B cells from OVA primed mice and the production of Ig isotypes and subclasses was measured following in-vitro stimulation with OVA. Only Vβ8.1/8.2 positive T cells were able to provide help for IgE production in this culture system, whereas Vβ2 T cells did not stimulate the production of IgE. Furthermore, when Vβ8 and Vβ2 T cells were simultaneously cocultured with B cells, the stimulatory effect on IgE production by Vβ8 T cells was abolished in the pres-

Table 3. Allergen dependent stimulation of TCR-Vβ T-cells in different immunological compartments

Vβ	OVA		Ragweed	
	Local LN	Spleen	Local LN	Spleen
2				
3				
4				
5				
6				
7				
8.1	↑	↑	↑	↑
8.2	↑	↑	↑	↑
8.3				↑
9				↑
10				
11				
13			↑	
14		↑		↑
17				

BALB/c mice were sensitized to OVA and ragweed as described (15, 16) and the TCR repertoire was analyzed in local draining lymph nodes and spleen by flow cytometry. Data summarize previously published results (16, 19).

ence of Vβ2 T cells. These results indicate that TCR-Vβ T cells play a differential role in the regulation of IgE production under in vitro conditions.

To evaluate the role of these T cells on in vivo IgE production and development of immediate type hypersensitivity responses, transfer experiments were performed (20). Vβ 8.1/8.2 and Vβ2 T cells were purified from OVA sensitized and control animals and transfered into syngeneic naive recipients that were then challenged with OVA via the airways. Analysis of IgE production, skin test responsiveness and AR revealed that transfer of Vβ8 T cells together with a local allergen challenge stimulated an allergic response in the recipients to a similar degree as observed in donor animals. In addition, the inhibitory role of Vβ2 T cells on in vitro IgE production could be confirmed vy in vivo transfer experiments. Simultaneous transfer of Vβ8 together with Vβ2 T cells from OVA sensitized mice inhibited and prevented the development of all tested immediate hypersensitivity responses.

Only Vβ8 T cells from allergen primed mice were able to exhibit their pro-allergic activity. In contrast, when Vβ8 T cells were purified from non-sensitized naive mice and transfered into naive recipients, stimulation of IgE production or changes in AR were not observed despite local allergen challenge. It is concluded from these experiments that priming of T cells induces a state of T cell activation that promotes pro-allergic T-cell functions. This view is compatible with the concept of naive and effector T cell functions. Naive (unprimed) T cells produce only IL-2 and do not provide help for Ig production. Antigen exposure triggers the development of effector T cells which will then develope into T cell subsets that produce a differential pattern of cytokines, including IL-4. It is the effector T cell population that provides help for Ig production.

Different allergens stimulate a differential pattern of TCR Vβ expressing T cells. This conclusion is based on results from sensitization experiments of BALB/c mice with different allergens. The results summerized above were obtained in the OVA animal model. Mice of the same strain were also sensitized to a different allergen, an extract of ragweed pollen. Using different protocols of sensitization it was shown that local sensitization to ragweed stimulates an allergen specific IgE/IgG1 response that was paralleled by positive allergen specific skin test responses and accompanied by the development of increased AR. The analysis of the TCR Vβ repertoire in local lymphe nodes and spleen revealed striking differences as compared to OVA sensitized mice. In ragweed sensitized mice, an increased frequency in Vβ8.1, Vβ8.2 and Vβ13 positive T cells was found compared to an increase in Vβ8.1, Vβ8.2, Vβ8.3, Vβ9 and Vβ14 T cells in the spleen. These differences in the two systems are most likely due to the presentation of different T cell epitopes that are recognized by different TCR phenotypes. That different T cells are stimualted in the lymph nodes and the spleen may be a result of the presentation capacity of different sources of antigen presenting cells. It is possible that APC in the spleen present antigens in a different way than antigen presenting cells in the airway mucosa or in local draining lymph nodes.

5. CONCLUSION

The development of allergic sensitization is dependent on the state of T cell activation. T cells are stimulated in an allergen-dependent fashion in the local immune environment. Local sensitization through the airways and the lung stimulates T cells expressing a TCR-Vβ repertoire that is unique for each allergen. The stimulation of TCR Vβ T cells is MHC dependent and restricted, and may depend on the source of antigen presenting cell. T cells activated in this fashion deliver signals to B cells which stimulate an allergen specific IgE/IgG1 response. IgE/IgG1 antibodies plus local allergen exposure trigger the development of immediate hypersensitivity responses. These responses can be detected as a wheal formation on the skin following intradermal allergen challenge, or as a shift in airway responsiveness in the lung. These data indicate that T cells play the central role in the development of the allergic response. Based on these results therapeutic intervention strategies can be developed which are aimed to modify or prevent the stimulation of T cells with pro-allergic activities.

REFERENCES

1. Lever, R., Turbitt, M., Sanderson, A., MacKie, R. Immunophenotyping of the cutaneous infiltrating and of the mononuclear cells in the peripheral blood in patients with atopic dermatitis. Invest. Dermatol. 89: 4–7 (1987)
2. Zachary, C.B., Poulter, L.W., MacDonald, D.M. Cell-mediated immune responses in atopic dermatitis: the relevance of antigen-presenting cells. Br. J. Dermatol. 113 (suppl. 28): 10–16 (1985)
3. Bos, J.D., Hagenaars, C., Das, P.K., Krieg, S.R., Voorn, W.J., Kapsenberg, M.L.
4. Vollenweider, S., Saurat, J.-H., Röcken, M. and Hauser, C. Evidence suggesting involvement of interleukin-4 (IL-4) production in spontaneous in vitro IgE synthesis in patients with atopic dermatitis. Allergy Clin. Immunol. 87: 1088–1095 (1991)
5. Parronchi, P., De Carli, M., Menetti, R., Simonelli, C., Piccini, M.-P., Macchia, D., Maggi, E., Del Prete, G., Ricci, M., Romagnani, S. Aberrant interleukin (IL)-4 and IL-5 production in vitro by CD4+ helper T cells from atopic subjects. Eur. J. Immunol., 22: 1615–1620 (1992)
6. Parronchi, P., Macchia, D., Piccini, M.-P., Biswas, P., Simonelli, C., Maggi, E., Ricci, M., Ansari, A.A. and Romagnani, S. Allergen- and bacterial antigen-specific T-cel clones established from atopic donors show a different profile of cytokine production. Proc. Natl. Acad. Sci. 88: 4538–4542 (1991)
7. Jujo, K., Renz, H., Abe, J., Gelfand, E.W., Leung, D.Y.M. Decreased IFN-g and increased IL-4 in atopic dermatitis. J. Allergy Clin. Immunol. 90: 323–331 (1992)

8. Romagnani, S., Maggi, E., Del Prete, P., Parronchi, P., Macchia, D., Tiri, A., Ricci, M. Role of Interleukin-4 and Gamma Interferon in the Regulation of Human IgE Synthesis: Possible alterations in atopic patients. Int. Arch. Allergy Appl. Immunol. 88: 111–113 (1989)

9. Durham, S.R., Ying, S., Varney, V.A., Jacobson, M.R., Sudderick, R.M., Mackay, I.S., Kay, B., and Hamid, Q.A. Cytokine messenger RNA expression for IL-3, IL-4, IL-5, and granulocyte/macrophage-colony-stimulating factor in the nasal mucosa after local allergen provocation: Relationship to tissue eosinophilia. J. Immunol. 148: 2390–2394 (1992)

10. Hamid, Q., Bogumiewica, M., Leung, D.Y.M. Differential in situ cytokine gene expression in acute versus chronic atopic dermatitis. J. Clin. Invest. 94: 870–876 (1994)

11. Mosse, P.A., Rosenberg, W.M.C. and Bell, J.I. The human T-cell receptor in health and disease. Annu. Rev. Immunol. 10: 71–96 (1992)

12. Jabara, H.H., Fu, S.M., Geha, R.S., and Vercelli, D. CD40 and IgE: Synergism between anti-CD40 monoclonal antibody and interleukin 4 in the induction of IgE synthesis by highly purified human B cells. J. Exp. Med. 172: 1861–1864 (1990)

13. Renz, H., Brodie, Ch, Bradley, K., Leung, D.Y.M., and Gelfand, E.W. Enhancement of IgE production by anti-CD40 antibody in atopic dermatitis. J. Allergy Clin. Immunol. 93: 658–668 (1994)

14. Fuleihon, R., Ramesh, N., Loh, R., Jabara, H., Rosen, F., Chatila, T. Fu, S.M., Stamenkovic, I., and Geha, R.S. Defective expression of the CD40 ligand in X chromosome-linked immunoglobulin deficiency with normal or elevated IgM. Proc. Natl. Acad. Sci. USA 90: 2170–2173 (1993)

15. Renz, H., Smith, H.R., Henson, J.E., Ray, B.S., Irvin, C.G., Gelfand, E.W. Aerolized antigen exposure without adjuvant causes increased IgE production and airway hyperresponsiveness in the mouse. J. All. Clin. Immunol., 89: 1127–1138 (1992)

16. Renz, H., Saloga, J., Bradley, K.L., Loader, J., Greenstein, J.L., Larsen, G.L., Gelfand, E.W. Specific Vβ T-cell subsets mediate the immediate hypersensitivity response to ragweed allergen. J. Immunol., 151: 1907–1917 (1994)

17. Larsen, G.L., Renz, H., Loader, J.E., Bradley, K., Gelfand, E.W. Airway response to electrical field stimulation in sensitized inbred mice: passive transfer of increased responsiveness with peribronchial lymph nodes. J. Clin. Invest. 89: 747–752 (1992)

18. Saloga, J., Renz, H., Lack, G., Bradley, K., Larsen, G., Gelfand, E.W. Development and transfer of immediate cutaneous hyersensitivity in mice exposed to aerosolized antigen. J. Clin. Invest. 91: 133–140 (1993)

19. Renz, H., Bradley, K., Marrack, P., Gelfand, E.W. T cells expressing variable elements of T-cell receptor β8 und β2 chain regulate murine IgE production. Proc. Natl. Acad. Sci. USA, 89: 6438–6442 (1992)

20. Renz, H., Bradley, K., Saloga, J., Loader, J., Larsen, G.L., Gelfand, E.W. T-cells expressing specific V elements regulate IgE production and airways responsiveness in vivo. J. Exp. Med. 177: 1175–1180 (1993)

GLUTATHIONE S-TRANSFERASE INDUCES MURINE DERMATITIS THAT RESEMBLES HUMAN ALLERGIC DERMATITIS

Ching-Hsiang Hsu,[1] Kaw-Yan Chua,[1*] Shau-Ku Huang,[4] I-Ping Chiang,[3] and Kue-Hsiung Hsieh[1,2]

[1]Graduate Institutes of Microbiology and Immunology
[2]Departments of Pediatric and
[3]Department of Pathology
College of Medicine, National Taiwan University
Taipei, Taiwan, Republic of China
[4]Johns Hopkins Asthma and Allergy Center
Johns Hopkins University School of Medicine
Baltimore, Maryland

INTRODUCTION

Atopic dermatitis (AD) is a common pruritic disorder that most often begins in early infancy and frequently occurs in patients with a personal or family history of atopic disease. The incidence of atopic dermatitis, like asthma, has been increasing.[1] Larsen *et al.* found that the cumulative incidence rate of atopic dermatitis in children up to 7 years of age increased from 3% in the cohort born between 1960 and 1964 to 10% in the cohort between 1970 and 1974.[2]

Histological features of AD are non-specific but generally show epidermal spongiosis and mononuclear cell infiltration in the dermis, suggesting a type IV hypersensitivity reaction. However, different studies point to the importance of IgE-mediated reactions and the occurrence of the late cutaneous reaction which is characterized by allergic inflammation with prominent eosinophilia and T cells with a Th2 cytokine profile.[3–5] However, the precise sequence of events leading to the inflammatory responses is still unclear. The molecular and functional basis of allergen-induced inflammation seen in AD remain undefined. One of the main difficulties is probably the lack of suitable animal model for definitive study *in vivo*. The objective of this study is, therefore, to establish a murine

* Correspondence and reprint requests: Kaw-Yan Chua Ph.D., Graduate Institute of Immunology, College of Medicine, National Taiwan University Hospital, No.1, Jen Ai Road, 1st Section, Taipei, Taiwan, Republic of China, 10018. FAX: 886–2–3217921; TEL: 886–2 3217510.

New Horizons in Allergy Immunotherapy
edited by Sehon et al. Plenum Press, New York, 1996

33

model to further dissect the pathological mechanisms of inflammatory reactions leading to the development of atopic dermatitis and provide an experimental model for exploring the potential efficacy of various therapeutic interventions. In this communication, we report the establishment of the first animal model that fulfills criteria for atopic dermatitis seen in humans.

Mr 26000 antigen of *Schistosoma japonicum* adult worms (Sj26) is a functional glutathione S-transferase.[6] The glutathion S-transferase is capable of detoxifying a variety of targets through the conjugation of reduced glutathione to electrophilic centers in such molecules. Sj26 binds to hematin and inhibits the formation of large hematin crystals which could block the evacuation of the parasite gut. A cDNA encoding Sj26 has been cloned and expressed in *Escherichia coli*.[7] This rSj26 was weakly immunogenic in early vaccination studies in mice, especially in BALB/c strain. However, when rSj26 conjugated to the hapten azobenzenearsonate was used as immunogen, BALB/c mice produced substantial amount of anti-Sj26 antibodies, compared to CFA adjuvant.[8] Furthermore, when we were in the process of studying the *in vivo* responses of mice to dust mite allergen, *Der p* V as an GST fusion protein, we unexpectedly found that rSj26 could induce allergy-like immune responses in BALB/c strain, and therefore has prompted us to perform further studies in order to understand the immunological responses of rSj26 to BALB/c mice.

MATERIALS AND METHODS

Animals. Female BALB/c, C57BL/6 and (C57BL/6 × BALB/c)F1 mice, aged between 6 and 8 weeks, were obtained from the animal-breeding center of College of Medicine, National Taiwan University. Mice were age- and sex- matched for each experiment.

Purification of Recombinant Sj26. Recombinant Sj26 (rSj26) was purified from *E. coli* containing a plasmid (pSj26) that directs synthesis of rSj26.[7] The methods to purify rSj26 from *E. coli* were according to the descriptions in [9].

Sensitization. Animals were sensitized by intraperitoneal injection of 30 μg of rSj26 with 4 mg of aluminum hydroxide. Age-matched control mice received PBS only or 30 μg of OVA with aluminum hydroxide. Mice were boosted 21 days after the first immunization. Venous blood was obtained weekly from the tail vein under anesthesia by injecting 0.2 mg of PromAce® (Ayerst Laboratories) intraperitoneally. Blood was clotted at room temperature for 1 h, and serum was collected after centrifugation.

Determination of rSj26 Specific Serum IgE and IgG Titer. The amounts of rSj26-specific IgE, IgG1 and IgG2a were determined by ELISA according to the standard methods.

Histological Evaluation. Skin was carefully excised from animal under anesthesia. Each biopsy specimen was fixed with formaldehyde (4%) and paraffin embedded. 5 μm sections were cut for staining with hematoxylin-eosin staining. Immunostainings were performed according to the instructions of Histomouse-SP™ Kits (Zymed).

Intradermal Skin Testing. Skin tests were performed as described.[10] Briefly, the skin of the belly was carefully shaved with an electric clipper. For each skin test 20 μl (20 μg/ml of rSj26) of test solution were injected intradermally with a 30-gauge needle while the skin was stretched taut in animals anesthetized with PromAce®. At least a 1.5-cm distance was kept between the sites of injection to avoid confluence of solutions. PBS was used as a negative control and the mast cell degranulation compound 48/80 (Sigma) at a concentration of 1 ug/ml served as a positive control. Wheal reactions were assessed after 30 min. A reaction was scored as positive if the size of the wheal was more than 0.3 cm in diameter in any direction measured with a transparent ruler. Evaluation of wheal formation was always carried out in a blinded fashion in which the evaluator was unaware of the sensitization status of each individual animals.

Epicutaneous Patch Test. Epicutaneous patch tests were performed as described.[11] Briefly, the skin of animal's back was carefully shaved with an electric clipper. 100 µg of rSj26 protein in 100 µl of PBS was applied to gauze which was then fixed tightly to the skin by tapping for 24 h. After 24 h, gauze was removed and skin was excised for histological study as described above.

RESULTS AND DISCUSSION

Immunization of animals was carried out by injecting peritoneally with 30 µg of rSj26 in conjunction with aluminum hydroxide. Serum collected from animals before rSj26 exposure contained no rSj26-specific IgE or IgG antibodies. Sj26-specific IgE antibody could be detected 2 wk after immunization. The antibody titer raised gradually and was boostable at 3 wk after immunization. In control animals receiving OVA solution alone for the same period of time, there were no detectable Sj26-specific IgE or IgG antibodies. Sj26-specific T cells responses were also detected prior to IgE production. Skin lesions were grossly noted between 2 wk and 3 wk after immunization. Hair became sparse and skin got erythmatous. Then the skin lesions became progressively worse after the booster injection of rSj26.

In addition to BALB/c mice, similar immunization protocol using rSj26 was also performed with C57BL/6 and (BALB/c × C57BL/6)F1 hybrid. Serological data revealed that in contrast to BALB/c mice, C57BL/6 mice produced a low level of IgE, whereas the F1 hybrid showed an intermediate IgE responses between that of BALB/c and C57BL/6. Furthermore, skin lesions were not found in both poor IgE responder (C57BL/6) and F1 hybrids. Interestingly, these data appear to be in good accordance with the etiological observations of human AD, which has been shown to be dependent on a genetic predisposition [2]. More extensive genetic studies are required to confirmed the involvement of such genetic elements in theimmunopathogenesis of this murine dermatitis model. Moreover, mice receiving booster injections of rSj26 at wk 3 showed a corresponding boost in IgE production. These increased IgE production was accompanied by an increase in the severity of skin lesions. Taken together, it is obvious that in this animal model, the skin lesions formation paralleled the IgE production. For years various lines of evidence have been advanced supporting the role of allergen -specific IgE antibodies in the pathogenesis of human AD.[12–13]

To investigate the pathology of skin lesions, we excised skin from animals 21d after rSj26 immunization. Hematoxyline-eosin staining of skin biopsy specimens revealed mild spongiosis secondary to intercellular edema and intracellular edema of the keratinocytes was present in the epidermis layer. As compared to normal skin of control animals, increased number of inflammatory infiltrating cells including monocytes, lymphocytes and eosinophils were noted in the dermis. Immunohistochemical studies showed that infiltrating lymphocytes were predominantly CD4$^+$ cells, and CD8$^+$ T lymphocytes were rarely found (data not shown). The histological changes were not distinctive and generally mild like those of AD in human. Further immnohistochemical studies showed deposits of IgE on cells within the dermal infiltrate. The number of IgE bound cells ranged from 20% to 25% of the number of infiltrating cells. It has been demonstrated that, skin from patients with AD contain a significant number of IgE-bearing dendritic cells which are specific for AD.[14] Furthermore, in vitro studies showed that these IgE-bearing cellswere capable of allergen presentation in an IgE-dependent manner.[15] Since both type I and type IV hypersensitivity reactions have been implicated in the pathogenesis of atopic dermatitis.[16] It is suggested that the finding of IgE-bearing antigen presenting cells specific for AD in the skin biopsies may provide a link between the two types of hypersensitivity reactions.

To further characterized this animal model, we performed skin test and epicutaneous skin test in sensitized mice to provide evidences of rSj26-specific acute and late phase responses. Most sensitized mice (4 out of 6) showed erythmatous wheals 20 min after rSj26 intracutaneous injection. The histological studies of skin biopsies from epicutaneuos patch test demonstrated prominent eosinophils infiltration in the dermis. The number of eosinophils increased from 3% to 15%, representing a 5-fold increase as compared to controls after 24 h challenge with rSj26. On the other hand, mononuclear cells infiltrate into the antigen challenge site was less impressive (increase from 15% to 20%). It is , therefore, apparent that eosinophils were specifically attracted to the site , and involved in the pathogenesis of the late phase responses. Similar differential cellular changes with a significant increase in eosinophils have been observed in studies of cutaneous late phase response to allergen in human.[17–18] In addition, we found that peripheral venous blood sampled 21 days after immunization revealed 3–4% of eosinophils, as compared to control animals immunized with OVAwhich showed less than 1% eosinophil in peripheral blood. It has been documented that there was a positive correlation between blood eosinophil levels and disease activity in AD patients.[19] Taken together, our data clearly suggested that eosinophils were actively participated in the pathogenesis of dermatitis induced by rSj26.

In summary, our results demonstrated that rSj26 could induce allergic responses in BALB/c strain mice including production of high level of rSj26-specific IgE, epidermal spongiosis and mononuclear cell infiltration in the dermis, eosinophilia, and rSj26-specific immediate and late phase responses. Further experiments including the characterization of T cell cytokine profiles by *in situ* hybridization and skin lesion tissue RT-PCR as well as cells and serum transfer experiments are now underway to unravel the mechanisms involved in the pathogenesis of rSj26 in BALB/c mice. We believed that this animal model can serve as a good experimental model for elucidating the immunopathogenesis of allergen-induced atopic dermatitis and the development of possible therapeutic interventions for this disorder.

ACKNOWLEDGMENT

We thank Dr. P.G. Holt (Perth, Australia) for helpful discussions and suggestions.

This work was supported by grants from National Science Council (NSC 82–0412-B-002–183) and Institutional grant of Academia Sinica (IBMS-CRC84-T11) of Republic of China.

REFERENCES

1. Taylor, B., M. Wadsworth, F. Wadsworth., and C. Peckham. 1984. Changes in the reported prevalence of childhood eczema since the 1939–45 war. Lancet II:1255.
2. Larsen, F.S., N.V. Holm, and K. Henningsen. 1986. Atopic dermatitis: a genetic epidemiological study in a population-based twin sample. J. Am. Acad. Dermatol. 15:487.
3. Sampson, H.A. 1989. Role of immediate hypersensitivity in the pathogenesis of atopic dermatitis. Allergy 44[Suppl 9]: 52.
4. Frew, A.J., and A.B. Kay. 1988. The pattern of human late phase skin reactions to extracts of aeroallergens. J. Allergy Clin. Immunol. 73:116.
5. Sager, N., A. Feldman, and G.Schilling 1992. House dust mite-specific T cells in the skin of subjects with atopic dermatitis: frequency and lymphokine profile in the allergen patch test. J. Allergy Clin. Immunol. 89: 801.
6. Smith, D.B., K.M. Davern, P.G. Board, W.U. Tiu, E.G. Garcia, and G.F. Mitchell. Mr 26000 antigen of Schistosoma japonicum recognized by resistant WEHI 129/J mice is a parasite glutathione S-transferase. Proc. Natl. Acad. Sci. USA 1986, 8703.
7. Smith, D.B., M. R. Rubira, R. M. Rubira, R. M. Simpson, K. M. Davern, P. G. Borard, W. U. Tiu and G.F. Mitchell. 1988. Expression of an enzyme-active parasite molecule in Escherichia coli: Schistosoma japonicum glutathione S-transferase. MOl. Biochem. Parasitol. 14, 173.
8. Davern, K.M., W.U. Tiu, G. Morahan, M.D. Wright, E.G. Garcia, and G.F. Mitchell.1987. Responses in mice to Sj26, a glutathione S-transferase of Schistosoma japonicum worms. Immuno. Cell. Biol. 65, 473.
9. Chua, K.Y., R.J. Dilworth,and W.R. Thomas. 1990. Expression of Dermatophagoides pternyssinus Allergen, Der p II, in Escherichia coli and the binding studies with human IgE. Int. Arch. Allergy. Appl. Immunol. 91, 124.
10. Saloga, J., H. Renz, G. Lack, K. Bradley, G. larsen, and E. W. Gelfand. 1993. Development and transfer of immediate cutaneous hypersensitivity in mice exposed to aerosolized antigen. J. Clin. Invest. 912:133.
11. Desager, G., H.P. Van Bever, and W.J. Stevens. 1987. Contact sensitivity to aeroallergens in children with atopic dermatitis demonstrated by patch test. J. Allergy Clin. Immunol. 52:38.
12. Pasternack, B. 1965. The prediction of asthma in infantile eczema. J. Pediatr. 66, 164.
13. Stone, S.P., S.A. Muller, G.J. Gleich, and R. Minn. 1973. IgE levels in atopic dermatitis. Arch. Dermatol. 108, 806.
14. Jonathan, N.W.N, Barker., V.A. Alegre, and D.M. MacDonald. 1988. Surface-bound immunoglobulin E on antigen-presenting cells in cutaneous tissue of atopic dermatitis. J. Invest. Dermatol. 90:117.
15. Mudde, G.C., F.C. Van Reijsen, G.J. Boland, G.C. De Gast, L.B. Bruijnzeel, and C.A.F.M. Bryijnzeel-Koomen. 1990. Allergen presentation by epidermal langerhans' cells from patients with atopic dermatitis is mediated by IgE. Immunology 69:335.
16. Sampson, H.A. 1990. Pathogenesis of eczema. Clin. Exp. Allergy. 20:459.
17. Charlesworth, E.N., A.F. Hood, N.A. Soter, A. Kagey-Sobotka, P.S. Norman, and L.M. Lichtenstein. 1989. Cutaneous late-phase response to allergen. J. Clin. Invest. 83:1519.
18. Ott, N.L., G.L. Gleich, P.T. Fujisawa, S. Sur, and K.M. Leiferman. 1994. Assessment of eosinophil participation in atopic dermatitis: comparison with the IgE-mediated late-phase reaction. J. Allergy Clin. Immunol. 94:120.
19. Kägi, M.K., H. Joller-Jemelka, and B. Wüthrich. 1992. Correlation of eosinophils, eosinophil cationic protein and soluble interleukin-2 receptor with the clinical activity of atopic dermatitis. Dermatology 185:88.

6

EFFECTS OF rIL-12 ADMINISTRATION ON AN ANTIGEN SPECIFIC IMMUNE RESPONSE

Julia D. Rempel-Chin, Ming Dong Wang, and Kent T. HayGlass

Department of Immunology
University of Manitoba
Winnipeg, Canada

I. INTRODUCTION

Many *in vivo* immune responses can be broadly categorized as either T_h1 or T_h2-like. Murine T_h1-like responses are characterized by increased IFNγ, IL-2 and IgG_{2a} production; whereas, T_h2-like responses are dominated by IL-4, IL-10, IgG_1 and often IgE. IL-12 has been reported to promote T_h1-like responses *in vitro* among naive T cells (1) and to stimulate both T_h1 (2) and T_h2 (3) clones to produce IFNγ, although the latter was determined to be transient. In addition, IL-12 was proposed as a powerful adjuvant, useful in driving protective T_h1-like responses during primary *Leishmania major* infection (4).

Immunization of C57Bl/6 mice with ovalbumin (OVA) in $Al(OH)_3$ adjuvant induces strong antigen specific IL-4, IL-10 and IgE responses in a widely used model of human immediate hypersensitivity. Since the cytokine microenvironment at the time of T cell activation is considered paramount in determining the resulting cytokine constitution (5, 6), we examined the ability of *in vitro* and *in vivo* administration of exogenous rIL-12 to commit the OVA-specific response in a T_h1-like direction.

II. METHODS AND MATERIALS

rIL-12 was administered at 200 ng i.p. for 5 days simultaneously with primary OVA $Al(OH)_3$ immunization of C57BL/6 mice. Secondary and tertiary immunizations were given at 28 day intervals. Mice were bled 10 days after primary immunization for antigen specific IgE analysis by PCA. IgG's were determined by ELISA from d. 14 sera. Upon subsequent immunizations mice were bled 7 days later. Mice were also bled during the course of IL-12 administration for sera IFNγ.

Five days after immunization, whole spleen cells were cultured with and without OVA, +/- IL-12 (100 pg/ml) and IL-2 (10 U/ml). Supernatants were harvested at 24, 48 and 96 h, then analyzed for IL-4, IFNγ and IL-10 respectively. IL-4 was determined by CT.4S bioassay, while IL-10 and IFNγ were assayed by ELISA.

New Horizons in Allergy Immunotherapy
edited by Sehon et al. Plenum Press, New York, 1996

The frequency of CD4+ T cells producing these cytokines was examined in limiting dilution analysis. Highly enriched CD4 spleen cells were cultured at 312.5 to 40,000 cells/well in the presence of IL-2 (20 U/ml), irradiated antigen presenting cells (APC) and OVA (1 mg/ml). Control cultures were done with IL-2 in the absence of OVA. Cultures were restimulated with OVA and APC two weeks after they were established. Supernatants were harvested 48 h later. Cytokine analyses were performed as stated.

III. RESULTS

As previously demonstrated (1) the addition of exogenous IL-12 to antigen stimulated cultures substantially increased IFNγ, while IL-10 was largely unchanged. Though a decrease in IL-4 production was observed, it proved not to be significant (p>0.05, Student's t test).

In contrast to control OVA (alum) immunized mice, which exhibited undetectable (<0.5 U/ml) levels of serum IFNγ, OVA (alum)/IL-12 treated mice produced transient serum IFNγ levels of approximately 27 U/ml.

Notwithstanding the increases in serum IFNγ, or IFNγ production *in vitro*, rIL-12 administration *in vivo decreased* peak IFNγ, IL-10 and IL-4 intensities as measured by bulk culture. Moreover, limiting dilution analysis failed to demonstrate an increase in the frequency of CD4 mediated IFNγ production. This raises the possibility that much of the impact of exogenous IL-12 in this system is due to NK cell derived, rather than CD4/OVA specific T cell mediated, IFNγ.

Administration of rIL-12 at the time of primary immunization resulted in 100 fold inhibition of OVA-specific IgE production. Specific IgG_1 titres were marginally decreased (5 fold) while IgG_{2a} titres were substantially increased (24 fold). Toxicity was observed following administration of substantially higher IL-12 concentrations, while use of lower concentrations (100 ng, 20 ng) elicited qualitatively similar but less intense changes in the OVA specific response.

To determine whether the exogenous IL-12 induced changes in antibody production were transient or stable, mice received secondary and tertiary OVA (alum) booster immunizations in the absence of further IL-12 administration. With each subsequent exposure to antigen the differences in antibody production between control and rIL-12 treated mice decreased. Thus, by the tertiary immunization IgE and IgG_1 levels were equivalent in both groups and the IgG_{2a} response of the treatment group was decreased to a 5 fold increase.

IV. CONCLUSION

Although the administration of IL-12 to naive mice at the same time as initial antigen exposure can strongly promote T_h1-like responses, these effects appear to be transient in that upon subsequent immunizations there was minimal impact on antibody responses. Therefore, the potential efficacy of IL-12 as a therapeutic agent used to redirect long term responses and to act as an adjuvant in the management of immediate hypersensitivity should be viewed with caution.

REFERENCES

1. Brunda, M. J. 1994. Interleukin-12. *J. Leukoc. Biol. 55:280.*

2. Germann, T., M. K. Gately, D. S. Schoenhaut, M. Lohoff, F. Mattner, S. Fischer, S-C. Jin, E. Schmitt, and E. Rude. 1993. Interleukin-12/T cell stimulating factor, a cytokine with multiple effects on T helper type 1 (T_h1) but not on T_h2 cells. *Eur. J. Immunol. 23:1826.*

3. Yssel, H., S. Fasler, J. E. de Vries, and R. de Waal Malefyt. 1994. IL-12 transiently induces IFN-γ transcription and protein synthesis in human CD4+ allergen-specific T_h2 T cell clones. *Int. Immunol. 6:1091.*

4. Alfonso, L. C., T. M. Scharton, L. Q. Vieira, M. Wysocka, G. Trinchieri, and P. Scott. 1994. The adjuvant effect of interleukin-12 in a vaccine against *Leishmania major. Science 263:235.*

5. DeKruyff, R. H., Y. Fang, S. F. Wolf, and D. T. Umetsu. 1995. IL-12 inhibits IL-4 synthesis in keyhole limpet hemocyanin-primed CD4+ T cells through an effect on antigen-presenting cells. *J. Immunol. 154:2578.*

6. Seder R. A. and W. E. Paul. 1994. Acquisition of lymphokine-producing phenotype by CD4+ T cells. *Annu. Rev. Immunol. 12:635.*

7

MAPPING THE GENES FOR IgE PRODUCTION AND ALLERGY

David G. Marsh

Johns Hopkins Asthma and Allergy Center
5501 Hopkins Bayview Circle
Baltimore, Maryland 21224

1. INTRODUCTION

1.1. Atopic Allergy Is a Complex Disease

Human beings are complex organisms living in a complex environment. Not surprisingly, common human diseases like atopic allergy, and especially asthma, are complex. First, allergy is *multifactorial*, that is to say, the expression of the disease is influenced by interactions between multiple major and minor genes as well as by non-genetic factors such as the degree of allergen exposure. Second, like many other complex human diseases, allergy is likely to be *genetically heterogeneous* (many distinct genes, or groups of genes, lead to similar clinical phenotypes). Two levels of genetic heterogeneity should be considered: (i) the different categories of allergic disease (asthma, allergic rhinitis, eczema, etc.) may be associated with different groups of genes, and (ii) for each characteristic disease sub-phenotype (such as asthma) several distinct groups of major genes may be involved in the expression of the particular condition. Thus, the picture of allergic disease that is emerging is one comprised of overlapping *constellations* of genes that interact in an indefinitely large number of ways with a wide variety of environmental factors. Such interactions often lead to the expression of allergic rhinitis and, less commonly, to asthma.

However, the genetics of this disease may well be even more complicated; the allergic phenotype is probably also influenced by different mutations in individual major genes. There are certainly numerous examples in the literature relating to Mendelian diseases that illustrate the point that different mutations in a single gene can lead to quite different phenotypes. For example, different mutations in the receptor tyrosine kinase gene, *RET*, can lead to the expression of at least four different diseases as diverse as familial medullary thyroid carcinoma and Hirchsprung's disease (absence of parasympathetic innervation of the lower intestine); see ref 1. A situation that is perhaps more analogous to the allergic diseases is found in ocular diseases, where different mutations in the peripherin/RDS gene can lead to the expression of four types of ocular diseases (2).

New Horizons in Allergy Immunotherapy
edited by Sehon et al. Plenum Press, New York, 1996

43

1.2. Explanations for the Complexity

Why are the common diseases like allergy so complex? The interactive pathways involving component genes and their products probably look something like the diagram shown in Figure 1 which illustrates a theoretical case of a system containing 20 genes with 40 interactions, taken from Stuart Kauffman's book, *The Origins of Order* (3). An example of this type of interactive network is the inflammatory system which is typical of complex networks seen in higher organisms. Under normal physiology, this system plays an important role in protecting the host from infection, but it disfunctions in asthmatic subjects and 'turns against' the host. The first point to emphasize is the marked *redundancy* of the inflammatory network, which has arisen by gene duplication, recombination and mutation (*cf*, the *IL4* cytokine cluster on chromosome 5 which constitutes an important part of this network; see below). Secondly, such systems are remarkably resistant to perturbation: a mutation in a gene involved in one of the multiple redundant pathways would not usually perturb the system unduly, because other pathways could help compensate for loss in functionality (3, 4). However, the circumstances under which a 'new' mutation produces a near-neutral or disease-predisposing outcome depends on the *context* in which the mutated gene finds itself, including the presence of genetic polymorphisms in other genes within the interactive network. The final outcome is conditioned by the influence of non-genetic factors.

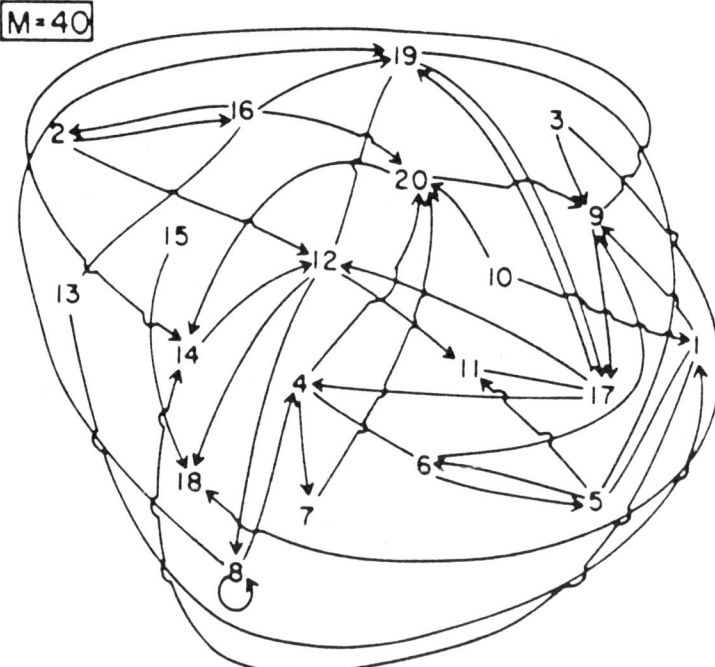

Figure 1. A theoretical interactive model containing 20 genes (indicated by numbers) and 40 interactive pathways (arrows) connected at random to the genes. As the ratio of arrows to genes increases, more and more interlocking cycles form, to produce the complex webbed structure indicated in the figure. Taken from Kauffman SA, "The Origins of Order," New York, Oxford University Press, p 423, 1993, with permission.

Environmental and other non-genetic influences are considered to be key components of the complex mosaic that determines the expression of allergic disease: evidence for this proposition is provided particularly by twin studies. Monozygotic (MZ) twins are more concordant for atopic allergy (of any type) than are dizygotic twins; nevertheless, the concordance for allergic disease in MZ twin pairs, where at least one member is allergic, averages only about 50–60% (5). The corresponding concordance for asthma is still lower; if one member of MZ twin pair has asthma, the chance of the other having asthma is only 26% (based on 451 MZ twin pairs living in California; TM Mack, personal communication, 1994). Furthermore, the risk that a sibling of an asthmatic subject also has asthma is only about twice the risk that a totally unrelated individual has asthma, *i.e.*, the relative risk for sibs, λ_s is approximately 2; furthermore, λ_s for the more common condition, atopic allergy is probably even lower. Such low λ_s values are in a range that is not considered favorable for finding genes involved in complex diseases (6). To emphasize the problem, it is noteworthy that for the monogenic disease, cystic fibrosis $\lambda_s \approx 500$: for the complex diseases, insulin-dependent diabetes and schizophrenia, $\lambda_s \approx 15$ and 8.6, respectively (6). The aforementioned considerations suggest that it will not be easy to define asthma and atopy genes by genomic scanning and positional cloning in the absence of biological information regarding the genes that map in a region showing evidence of linkage.

1.3. Approaches Toward Defining the Genes

The genetic analysis of complex diseases has been largely based on the philosophy of reductionism, namely, that each disease can be analyzed as a linear combination of a series of single-gene components involved in the disease expression. This approach has proved to be useful where familial, early-onset components of the disease can be broken out as predominantly single, autosomal dominant traits, as in the cases of Alzheimer's disease (7–9) and breast cancer (10, 11), but has proved to be more problematic for the more common, later-onset forms of these diseases, where genetic influences are probably more subtle. A more sophisticated analytic approach has been to develop optimized models based on the presumption of two major genes which interact (12, 13). Such reductionist models are, however, based on a number of simplifying assumptions, and the conclusions may be less relevant if one steps outside the context of the narrowly defined hypotheses that are implicit in the gene-by-gene approach. Here, one can draw an analogy with the numerous 'surprises' that have turned up in gene 'knock-out' experiments in mice: the disruption of genes like NFκB that were thought to be essential for host survival produced not dead fetuses but healthy mice, once again illustrating the robust nature of the redundant interactive networks of complex organisms.

Although theories and experimental approaches relating to the behavior of complex biological systems are under development (3, 4, 14), their adaptation to studies of the genetics of complex diseases are only just beginning. In the meantime, we are left with analyzing the genetics of diseases like allergy with reductionistic approaches – looking at model systems down narrowly focused 'analytical tunnels,' and trying to draw conclusions that have general validity concerning the etiology of the disease. With these caveats in mind, we will now consider two sets of data that relate to the analysis of genes associated with the expression of the allergic diseases. The first example concerns *HLA*-linked immune response (*Ir*) genes, which are located within the *HLA-D* region in chromosome 6p21.3 (15); the second relates to evidence for a gene(s) located in chromosome 5q31–q33 (16, 17). Members of the former type of gene (*HLA-D*) are structurally homologous, and most genes are highly polymorphic, which is reflected in the diversity of immune recognition. Each *HLA-D* gene encodes an individual polypeptide, and pairs of these peptides associate to form heterodimeric class II molecules, eg, HLA-DRαβ. Individual class II molecules are able to bind to particular peptide epitopes (T-cell epitopes) of an antigen (Ag) molecule and 'present' the epitopes to compatible T-cell receptors (TcRs), thereby regulating specific immune responsiveness, including IgE (15). Evidence for the influence of *HLA-D* genes in the expression of specific atopic allergies presently seems overwhelming, so much so that it is appropriate to name this group of genes *AA1* (for atopy-and-asthma-1). The latter group of genes (mapping within chromosome 5q31–q33) appears to be associated with a more general control of IgE production and the expression of asthma. Here, there are multiple candidate genes in the same chromosomal region, several of which are structurally and functionally related (the *IL4* cytokine cluster in 5q31.1). We will argue that both types of gene are relevant in controlling allergic disease, including asthma.

2. GENETIC ANALYSIS OF SPECIFIC IMMUNE RESPONSIVENESS

2.1. Rationale

Our first analytical focus concerns the role of *HLA-D* genes in specific IgE antibody (Ab) responsiveness and allergic disease. Most biologically complex allergens (pollens, mites, etc) contain large numbers of components toward which different genetically susceptible individuals produce different patterns of specific IgE Abs in their sera (18). We hypothesize that the wide variety of different immune response 'fingerprints' that one can observe within outbred human populations reflects different host genetic and environmental factors, including the presence or absence of particular *HLA-D* genes. We propose, further, that the analysis of *HLA-D* genes is relevant in understanding the genetic basis of complex allergic diseases, such as ragweed pollen hay fever. In such case, the recognition of a specific T-cell epitope(s) on one or more ragweed allergens facilitates specific IgE Ab response(s), which leads to expression of ragweed allergy following further exposure to the same allergen complex. By a similar reasoning, the recognition by particular *HLA-D*-encoded class II molecules of specific T-cell epitopes on individual molecular components of 'indoor' allergens, such as *Dermatophagoides pteronyssinus* (19, 20), leads to specific IgE responses to these allergens. The expression of allergen-induced acute allergic inflammation, followed by chronic inflammation and asthma, appears, however, to be *dependent on* prolonged exposure to the offending allergen and/or the individual being genetically susceptible to asthma (perhaps requiring other, asthma-specific genes).

2.2. Experimental Results and Conclusions

In order to examine the role of specific *HLA-D* genes in specific IgE responsiveness, we first chose to use, as models, short ragweed Amb a 5 (M_r = 5000) and its Amb 5 homologues from other ragweed species. We postulated that, in the case of the low molecular weight allergen, Amb a 5, immune recognition would potentially involve a single major T-cell epitope that might interact with a single class II molecule (18). In unrelated Caucasian ragweed-atopic subjects, we analyzed the associations between specific Ab responsiveness (primarily IgE) and specific HLA-DR and DQ types. Our early observations (21–22), and similar findings of other laboratories (23, 24), showed striking associations between HLA-DR2 and Dw2 (DR2.2) and immune responsiveness to Amb a 5 (Table 1).

Table 1. Associations of HLA with specific antibody responsiveness toward highly purified Amb 5 ragweed pollen allergens atopic US Caucasoid subjects living in the Baltimore area

Allergen	M_r	Major HLA Association	Westinghouse Subjects*		Clinic Patients		Overall p values‡
			+ve **	−ve **	+ve	−ve	
Amb a 5	5,000	DR2/Dw2	9/9 (100%)	20/83 (24%)	27/29 (93%)	10/56 (18%)	−9
Amb t 5	4,400	DR2/Dw2	3/4 (75%)	0/13 (0%)	3/3 (100%)	1/7 (14%)	−3

* Atopic subjects from an epidemiologic study of Westinghouse Electric Corporation employees in the Baltimore area.
** Positive (+ve) or negative (−ve)with respect to the patient having detectable serum IgE Ab prior to immunotherapy, except in the case of Amb t 5 where the data refer to serum IgG Ab in patients who had received immunotherapy with extracts containing giant ragweed in the past.
‡ p values by Fisher's Exact Test for analysis of the combined groups of Westinghouse and clinic subjects.

Analysis of immune responsiveness to Amb t 5 and Amb p 5 (from giant and western ragweeds, respectively) also revealed significant associations with DR2.2 (23, 25–27), with the Amb p 5 association being of similar significance to that for Amb a 5, and the Amb t 5 being less striking (Table 1). These consistent DR2.2 associations with responsiveness to three Amb 5 species suggest that a single, related major T-cell epitopes are present on the three different Amb 5 molecules.

For further analysis of the class II specificities involved in Amb a 5 recognition, we amplified the polymorphic second exons of the *HLA-D* genes in responder and non-responder subjects using the polymerase chain reaction (PCR). We employed sequence-specific oligonucleotides (SSOs) and dot-blot analysis, as well as sequencing, to examine the regions of the *HLA-D* genes which encode the Ag-binding regions of the class II molecules (28, 29). This approach allowed us to define more precisely the HLA class II specificity likely to be involved in 'presenting' the major T-cell epitopes of the Amb 5 molecules to specific T-cell receptors (TcRs). Our analyses showed that, in Caucasians, the most likely candidate was a DR2.2-associated class II molecule that is encoded either by DRA and DRB1, or by DRA and DRB5 [known as DR(α,β1*1501) or DR(α,β5*0101), respectively].

In order to investigate further which class II molecule is actually involved in the presentation of the major Amb a 5 T-cell epitope, we isolated a series of Amb a 5-specific human T-cell clones from Amb a 5-atopic subjects having the DR2.2 phenotype (30). These T cells express Th2-associated cytokines and are able to induce Amb a 5-specific IgE synthesis *in vitro* (31). In experiments using Amb a 5 and DR2.2$^+$ Ag-presenting cells (APCs), all of these clones showed clear evidence of Amb a 5-induced proliferation (Fig. 2). When monoclonal Abs (MAbs) directed against HLA-DQ or DP, were included in the stimulation assays, we found no evidence of inhibition of T-cell proliferation relative to the Ag control (Figs 2a and 2b). However, with the addition of a MAb to HLA-DR, there was clear evidence of inhibition. These experiments confirmed that an HLA-DR molecule is actually involved in the presentation Amb a 5 to the T cells. In order to resolve whether the DR $\alpha\beta$1 or $\alpha\beta$5 class II molecule was involved, we used MAb Hu30 which is specific for DR($\alpha\beta$1*15) group [(DRα,β1*1501) and DR(α,β1*1502)]. This MAb strongly inhibited T-cell proliferation (Figs 2a, b and c), clearly showing that the DR$\alpha\beta$1 molecule is involved in Amb a 5 presentation to these T-cell clones. These and further experiments defined the HLA-DRβ residues 67, 70 and 71 as being important for in immune recognition of the Amb 5 T-cell epitope.

These results provide a clear demonstration of the role of *HLA-D*-encoded molecules in a well-defined immune response. We and others have made similar findings in regard to specific immune responses to other purified allergens from several pollens, mites,

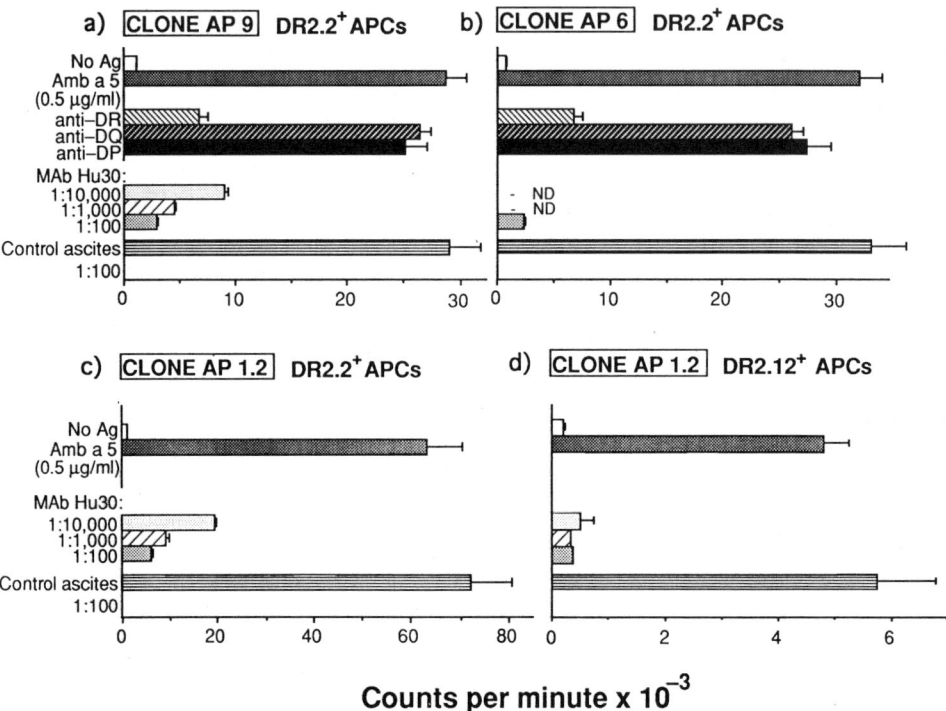

Figure 2. Inhibition of Amb a 5-induced proliferation of human T-cell clones clones AP9, AP6 and AP1.2 by anti-HLA-DR, DQ and DP MAbs. MAb Hu30, which is specific for the DR(α,β1*1501) and DR(α,β1*1502) class II molecules, was also used in all experiments. T-cell proliferation was measured by the uptake of ^{3}H-thymidine. Autologous APCs from the HLA-DR2.2$^+$ donor were used in experiments a, b and c: APCs from an HLA-DR2.12 donor were used for experiment d. Taken from reference 30 with permission of the copyright owners.

etc (15, 19, 32), which establishes a general role for *HLA-D* genes in controlling specific IgE responses that are relevant in the expression of various specific allergic diseases. Localized inflammatory allergic responses are induced by individual allergens interacting with their specific IgE Abs on mast cells and basophils; but exactly how the these responses lead, in susceptible individuals, to the up-regulation of immune responsiveness to multiple component allergens within an allergenic matrix, and more generalized and chronic inflammation in asthmatic subjects is presently unclear.

3. GENETIC ANALYSIS OF TOTAL SERUM IGE, BRONCHIAL HYPERRESPONSIVENESS (BHR) AND ASTHMA AND CHROMOSOME 5Q

3.1. Rationale

Human chromosome 5q31–33 contains multiple genes that are candidates for allergy and asthma (16, 17; Fig 3). These include a family of related cytokine genes, *IL3, IL4, IL5, IL13* and *CSF2* (*GMCSF*) clustered in human chromosome 5q31.1 (16, 33), which

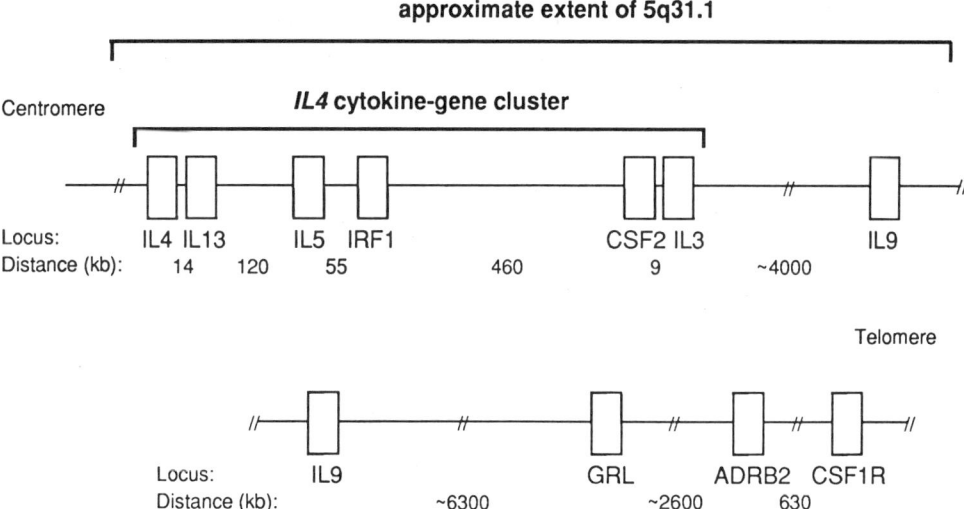

Figure 3. Some candidate genes for allergy and asthma that map to chromosome 5q31–q33. Pysical map based on information kindly supplied by Dr. Edward Rubin, Lawrence Berkeley Laboratory, CA.

play important interactive roles in the allergic inflammatory response (34, 35). Notably, IL-4 is known to be important in immunoglobulin class-switching to IgE and in the differentiation of naïve T cells into Th2/Th0 cells that are involved in IgE-mediated inflammation (36–38). The glucocorticoid receptor and β2-adrenergic receptor genes, *ADRB2* and *GRL* respectively, are located approximately 11 and 13.5 million bases telomeric of *IL4* (personal communication, E Rubin, 1995). Certain polymorphisms within these genes have been implicated in asthma (39–41). Thus, it seems appropriate to analyze for linkage of asthma or of asthma/allergy-associated phenotypes, such as total serum IgE and bronchial hyperresponsiveness (BHR) to this region. The advantage of this approach is that one can test for linkage to a large ensemble of genes important in allergic inflammation and asthma. The disadvantage is that, if one finds evidence of genetic linkage, or an association of a particular phenotype within a population of affected individuals, it is difficult to sort out which of several individual genes, or combinations of genes, may be involved.

In a large epidemiologic study, Burrows et al (42) showed that the log of the risk for asthma is directly *linearly* related to the log[total serum IgE], after adjustment for age, sex, smoking habits and, importantly, the subject's specific skin-test responsiveness to common inhalant allergens. They also found that, even in skin-test negative subjects, the presence of asthma is correlated with total IgE, and no asthma was reported by 7% of the study population having the lowest IgEs (≤ 2 IU/ml, or ≤ 5 ng/ml). Other groups, including our own, have reported similar findings (43–45). These data suggest that 'non-Ag-cognate' IgE production (polyclonal upregulation of IgE that is not directly Ag-driven) is somehow associated with the elevated IgE levels seen in asthmatic subjects.

3.2. Analysis of the Total Serum IgE Phenotype for Linkage to Chromosome 5q31–33

Marsh et al (16) studied the genetic regulation of serum IgE in the Pennsylvania Old Order Amish, a religious isolate group that has several desirable attributes for genetic studies, including a high degree of intermarriage, large family size and relatively uniform environment. They found evidence for linkage with total IgE, but not specific IgE, within the 5q31.1 region, but not for three markers lying just outside this region. These and further studies studies suggested that *IL4* and/or nearby gene(s) in 5q31.1 regulates IgE production in a non-cognate fashion. Basophils, in particular, may be implicated in this non-cognate IgE production, although other FcεRI-positive cells may also be involved (46). It seems likely that a generalized up-regulation of IL-4 could induce B cells (that are precommitted to make IgG Ab to a broad array of Ags) to switch to IgE. Under normal physiology, such 'polyclonal' IgE would not be specific for common environmental allergens.

Linkage of total IgE concentrations to *IL4* and to 5q31–q33 is supported by recent studies of Meyers and collaborators (17, 47) as well as unpublished reports from the laboratories of Borish, Holgate and Cookson. The studies of Meyers show the strongest evidence for linkage for marker D5S436, which maps within about 100 kb of *GRL*, and about 11Mb telomeric of *IL4* (personal communication, E Rubin, 1995). Interestingly, the Meyers' studies were in 'asthma' families collected by Postma and collaborators in Holland, and the enrichment for asthma may help explain the differences in the results in comparison with those of Marsh, Holgate and Cookson which, for largely non-asthmatic subjects, all point to the region in or around *IL4*. A study by Borish, Rosenwasser and collaborators (unpublished), that shows an association between a polymorphism at position −590 in *IL4* (upstream of the promoter) and total serum IgE level, seems to point directly to *IL4*.

In another study (41), there is evidence for a reduction in the affinity of glucocorticoids for the glucocorticoid receptor (GRL) in the order: normals > steroid-sensitive asthmatics > steroid-resistant asthmatics, which suggests that polymorphic variation in *GRL* may be important in the expression of asthma. Ohe et al (40) have evidence that a restriction fragment length polymorphism (RFLP) in the β_2-adrenergic receptor *ADRB2* gene is associated with asthma, and Turki et al (39) have found evidence that a specific polymorphism in the *ADRB2* gene, Gly16, is associated with the expression of 'nocturnal asthma' within the asthmatic population. This polymorphism is just as common in non-asthmatics as in asthmatics, however, suggesting that it may provide a modulating influence in regard to the type of disease that is expressed in subjects who are already predisposed toward asthma.

Taken together, these observations pose the possibility that multiple functional polymorphisms exist within several genes of the 5q31–q33 region, each of which play important roles in IgE production and in the expression of asthma and variants of asthma. Extensive analysis of genetic polymorphisms in numerous genes, in relation to biological function, will likely be needed in many different types of affected individuals and their families in order to resolve the location of critical functional mutations.

4. CONCLUSIONS AND FUTURE DIRECTIONS

In the present review we have presented evidence that two regions of the human genome, chromosomes 6p21.3 and 5q31–33, contain genes implicated in the expression of allergy and asthma. Clearly, there is much work to be done in defining the functional polymorphisms of genes in these regions. Further chromosomal regions containing genes associated with the expression allergic disease are also being investigated. Already candidate regions in chromosomal regions 11q13 and 14q11.2 (*TCRA/D*) have been identified by Cookson and collaborators (48, 49), which are the topics of another chapter in this book. Several more candidate regions will no doubt be identified in the near future as genetic analytical studies of allergy and asthma gather pace in many centers around the world, and as the mapping and sequencing of the human genome develops. As more and more candidate genes are defined and functional relationships established with allergy, the main task will be to evaluate the relative importance of each gene in disease expression, and to try to put together the complex series of genes and environmental factors into a coherent whole. Presently, this possibility looks to be rather remote if a purely reductionist approach is used. A breakthrough is needed in understanding complex biological systems and, more specifically, in developing mathematical approaches to evaluate complex diseases, based on knowledge about genetic polymorphisms and environmental factors involved in disease expression. In the meantime, headway will be made by defining as least some of the major genes, and their polymorphisms, that are involved the expression of asthma and other allergic diseases, and using existing models of gene interaction to try to define the relative functional importance of each gene.

5. ACKNOWLEDGMENTS

I would like to thank many collaborators, especially Shau-Ku Huang, John Neely, Daniel Breazeale, Terri Beaty, Linda Freidhoff and Carsten Schou. This work was supported by NIH Grants Nos AI 20059 and HL/AI49612.

6. REFERENCES

1. van Heyningen V. One gene – four syndromes. Nature 367:319–320, 1994.
2. Davies K. Peripherin and the vision thing. Nature 362:92, 1993.
3. Kauffman SA. The Origins of Order. New York, Oxford University Press, 1993.
4. Depew DJ, Weber BH. Darwinism Evolving. Cambridge, MA, MIT Press, 429–457 and 477–495, 1995.
5. Blumenthal MN, Bonini S. Immunogenetics of specific immune responses to allergens in twins and families. In: Marsh DG, Blumenthal MN (eds), Genetic and Environmental Factors in Clinical Allergy. Minneapolis, University of Minnesota Press, 132–142, 1990.
6. Lander ES, Schork NJ. Genetic dissection of complex traits. Science 265:2037–2048, 1994.
7. Goate A, Chartier-Harlin MC, Mullan M, et al. Segregation of a missense mutation in the amyloid precursor protein gene with familial Alzheimer's disease. Nature 349:704–706, 1991.
8. Sherrington R, Rogaev EI, Liang Y, et al. Cloning of a gene bearing missense mutations in early-onset familial Alzheimer's disease. Nature 375:754–760, 1995.
9. Levy-Lahad E, Wasco W, Poorkaj P, et al. Candidate gene for the chromosome 1 familial Alzheimer's disease locus. Science 269:973–977, 1995.
10. Miki Y, Swensen J, Shattuck-Eidens D, et al. A strong candidate for the breast and ovarian cancer susceptibility gene BRCA1. Science 266:66–71, 1994.
11. Wooster R, Neuhausen SL, Mangion J, et al. Localization of a breast cancer susceptibility gene, BRCA2, to chromosome 13q12–13. Science 265:2088–2090, 1994.
12. Hasstedt SJ, Meyers DA, Marsh, DG. Inheritance of IgE. Amer J Med Genet 14:61–66, 1983.
13. Schork NJ, Boehnke M, Terwilliger JD, et al. Two-trait-locus linkage analysis: a powerful strategy for mapping complex genetic traits. Am J Hum Genet 53:1127–1136, 1993.
14. Langton CG. Life at the edge of chaos. In: Langton CG, Taylor C, Farmer JD, Rasmussen S, Artificial Life II, Santa Fe Institute Studies in the Sciences of Complexity, Vol 10, Reading, MA, Addison-Wesley, 41–91, 1992.
15. Marsh DG. Immunogenetic and immunochemical factors determining immune responsiveness to allergens: studies in unrelated subjects. In: Marsh DG, Blumenthal MN (eds), Genetic and Environmental Factors in Clinical Allergy. Minneapolis, University of Minnesota Press, 97–123, 1990.
16. Marsh DG, Neely JD, Breazeale DR, Ghosh B, Freidhoff LR, Ehrlich-Kautzky E, Schou C, Krishnaswamy G, Beaty TH. Linkage analysis of IL4 and other chromosome 5q31.1 markers and total serum IgE concentrations. Science 264:1152–1156, 1994.

17. Meyers DA, Postma DS, Panhuyscn CIM, Xu J, Amelung PJ, Levitt RC, Bleecker ER. Evidence for a locus regulating total serum IgE levels mapping to chromosome 5. Genomics 23:464–470, 1994.

18. Marsh DG. Defining human immune response fingerprints toward ultra-pure allergens: immunochemical and genetic aspects of responsiveness toward the *Amb* V (Ra5) homologues. J Allergy Clin Immunol 78 (Suppl):242–248, 1986.

19. Platts-Mills TAE, Sporik R, Gelber LE, Ward GW. Tracking down the allergens involved in asthma. In: Marsh DG, Lockhart A, Holgate SJ (eds), The Genetics of Asthma, Blackwell Scientific Publ., Oxford, 71–81, 1993.

20. O'Hehir RE, Garman RD, Greenstein JL, Lamb JR. The specificity and regulation of T-cell responsiveness to allergens. Annu Rev Immunol 9:67–95, 1991.

21. Marsh DG, Hsu SH, Roebber M, Kautzky EE, Freidhoff LR, Meyers DA, Pollard MK. Bias WB. HLA-Dw2: a genetic marker for human immune response to short ragweed pollen allergen Ra5. I. Response resulting primarily from natural antigenic exposure. J Exp Med 155:1439–1451, 1982.

22. Marsh DG, Meyers DA, Freidhoff LR, Kautzky EE, Roebber M, Norman PS, Hsu SH, Bias WB. HLA-Dw2: a genetic marker for human immune response to short ragweed pollen allergen Ra5. II. Response after ragweed immunotherapy. J Exp Med 155:1452–1463, 1982.

23. Coulter KM, Yang WH, Dorval GD, Drouin MA, Osterland CK, Goodfriend L. Specific IgE antibody responses to ragweed allergens Ra5S and Ra5G associated with distinct HLA-DR β genes. Mol Immunol 24:1207–1210, 1987.

24. Blumenthal MN, Marcus-Bagley D, Awdeh Z, Johnson B, Yunis EJ, Alper CA. HLA-DR2, [HLA-B7, SC31, DR2], and HLA-B8, SC01, DR3] haplotypes distinguish subjects with asthma from those with rhinitis only in ragweed pollen allergy. J Immunol 148:411–416, 1992.

25. Roebber M, Klapper DG, Goodfriend L, Bias WB, Hsu SH, Marsh DG. Immunochemical and genetic studies of *Amb t* V (Ra5G), an Ra5 homologue from giant ragweed pollen. J Immunol 134:3062–3069, 1985.

26. Goodfriend L, Choudhury AM, Klapper DG, Coulter KM, Dorval G, DelCarpio J, Osterland CK. Ra5G, a homologue of Ra5 in giant ragweed pollen: isolation, HLA-DR-associated activity and amino acid sequence. Mol Immunol 22:899–906, 1985.

27. Marsh DG, Zwollo P, Freidhoff L, Golden DBK, Ansari AA, Kautzky EE, Meyers DA, Holland CL Studies of human immune response to the *Amb* V (Ra5) homologues. J Allergy Clin Immunol 85:201, 1990 (Abs).

28. Marsh DG, Zwollo P, Huang SK, Ghosh B, Ansari AA. Molecular studies of human response to allergens. Cold Spring Harbor Symp Quant Biol 54:459–470, 1990.

29. Zwollo P, Ehrlich-Kautzky E, Ansari AA, Scharf SJ, Erlich HA, Marsh DG. Molecular studies of human immune response genes for the short ragweed allergen, *Amb a* V. Sequencing of HLA-D second exons in responders and non-responders. Immunogenetics 33:141–151, 1991.

30. Huang SK, Zwollo P, Marsh DG. Class II MHC restriction of human T-cell responses to short ragweed allergen, *Amb a* V. Europ J Immunol 21:1469–1473, 1991.

31. Shinomiya N, Kumai M, Marsh DG, Huang SK. Secretion of specific IgE-secreting cells using an enzyme-linked immunospot assay. J Allergy Clin Immunol 92:479–487, 1993.

32. Marsh DG. Genetics of atopy and IgE. In: Frank MM, Austen KF, Claman HN, Unanue ER (eds). Samter's Immunological Diseases, Fifth Edition, Little, Brown and Company, Boston, MA. 1257–1272, 1994.

33. Saltman DL, Dolganov GM, Warrington JA, Wasmuth JJ, Lovett M. A physical map of 15 loci on human chromosome 5q23–q33 by two-color fluorescence *in situ* hybridization. Genomics 16:726–732, 1993.

34. Mossman TR, Coffman RL. Heterogeneity of cytokine secretion patterns and functions of helper T cells. Adv Immunol 46:111–147, 1989.

35. Paul WE, Seder RA. Lymphocyte responses and cytokines. Cell 76:241–251, 1994.

36. Gauchat J-F, Lebman DA, Coffman RL, et al. Structure and expression of germline ε transcripts in human B cells induced by interleukin 4 to switch to IgE production. J Exp Med 172:463–473, 1990.

37. Vercelli D, Geha RS. Regulation of IgE synthesis in humans: a tale of two signals. J Allergy Clin Immunol 88:285–295, 1991.

38. Romagnani S. Human Th1 and Th2 subsets: regulation of differentiation and role in protection and immunopathology. Int Arch Allergy Immunol 98: 279–285, 1992.

39. Turki J, Pak J, Green SA, Martin RJ, Liggett SB. Genetic polymorphisms of the β_2-adrenergic receptor in nocturnal and nonnocturnal asthma: evidence that Gly16 correlates with the nocturnal phenotype. J Clin Invest 95:1635–1641, 1995.

40. Ohe M, Munakata M, Hizawa N, et al. Beta$_2$-adrenergic receptor gene polymorphism and bronchial asthma. Thorax 50:353–359, 1995.

41. Sher ER, Leung DYM, Surs W, et al. Steroid-resistant asthma. J Clin Invest 93:33–39, 1994.

42. Burrows B, Martinez ED, Halonen M, Barbee RA, Cline MG. Association of asthma with serum IgE levels and skin-test reactivity to allergens. New Engl J Med 320:271–277, 1989.

43. Sears MR, Burrows B, Flannery EM, Herbison GP, Hewitt CJ, Holdaway, MD. Relation between airway responsiveness and serum IgE in children with asthma and in apparently normal children. New Engl J Med 325:1067–1071, 1991.

44. Tollerud DJ, O'Connor GT, Sparrow D, Weiss ST. Asthma, hay fever, and phlegm production associated with distinct patterns of allergy skin test reactivity, eosinophilia, and serum IgE levels. Am Rev Resp Dis 144:776–781, 1991.

45. Freidhoff LR, Marsh DG. The relationship among asthma, serum IgE levels and skin-test sensitivity to inhaled allergens. Int Arch Allergy Appl Immunol 100:355–361, 1993.

46. Gauchat J-F, Henchoz S, Mazzel G, et al. Induction of human IgE synthesis in B cells by mast cells and basophils. Nature 365:340–343, 1993.

47. Xu J, Levitt RC, Postma DS, Taylor EW, Amelung PJ, Holroyd KJ, Bleecker ER, Meyers DA. Evidence for two unlinked loci regulating total serum IgE levels. Am J Hum Genet 57:425–430, 1995.

48. Moffatt MF, Sharp PA, Faux JA, Young RP, Cookson WOCM, Hopkin JM. Factors confounding genetic linkage between atopy and chromosome 11q. Clin Exp Allergy 22:1046–1051, 1992.

49. Moffatt MF, Hill MR, Cornélius F, et al. Genetic linkage of T-cell receptor α/δ complex to specific IgE responses. Lancet 343:1597–1600, 1994.

8

GENETIC FACTORS IN ASTHMA

William Cookson[*]

Nuffield Department of Medicine
University of Oxford

INTRODUCTION

The familial aggregation of asthma, rhinitis, and eczema suggests that atopy has a genetic component. Modern molecular genetics now offers the opportunity to characterise the genes predisposing to these illnesses.

Study of the genetics of asthma will increase understanding of the aetiology and patho-physiology of the disease. The early identification of children at genetic risk of asthma may open new approaches to the prevention of disease. The involvement of particular genes may identify a particular clinical course and response to therapy. Eventually genetics may lead to new pharmacological treatments for asthma.

CLINICAL GENETICS

Although most studies of atopic families agree on the presence of major genetic effects, there is no agreement on a model of inheritance, with dominant, recessive, and polygenic models suggested at different times by different authors (1). These differing conclusions to some extent reflect the difficulties in defining exactly what atopy is. Asthma is of at least two varieties: atopic and non-atopic. Although 95% of children suffer from the atopic variety of asthma, the figure is much lower in adults. Atopic asthma and eczema, although sharing many patho-physiological traits, cannot be assumed to arise form identical mechanisms. Atopy can be defined with prick skin tests or the specific IgE (RAST) to common allergens, or with the total serum IgE. However, genes influencing the total IgE are not necessarily the same as those which lead to positive RASTs or skin tests.

Atopy is remarkably common. The prevalence of young adults with a positive prick skin test to house dust or grass pollen has been found to be between 40% and 50% in western populations (2,3,4). It therefore is difficult to consider atopy an abnormal state, and in certain circumstances non-atopy could be considered as abnormal. As a result of

* Wellcome Senior Clinical Research Fellow

New Horizons in Allergy Immunotherapy
edited by Sehon et al. Plenum Press, New York, 1996

55

the high prevalence of atopy, a fifth of marriages may be between two atopics, and many of the population will carry two or more genes predisposing to atopy.

MATERNAL INHERITANCE

Recently there has been increasing awareness that atopy shows a maternal pattern of inheritance. That the risk of asthma is much higher in the children of asthmatic mothers was reported 60 years ago (5), and forgotten, until modern epidemiological studies have shown a maternal inheritance of elevations of the serum IgE (6,7), atopic symptoms (8,9), and prick skin test responses to common allergens (10). This intriguing finding may be due to interactions between the mother and her child through the placenta, or through the breast milk. A genetic mechanism, known as genomic imprinting, in which a paternal "atopy gene" may be suppressed during spermatogenesis, is also possible (11). A maternal inheritance will mean that unaffected mothers may still carry the trait if they have inherited an abnormal gene from their father. The presence of carriers may explain why atopy is sometimes seen in the children of normal parents.

FINDING GENES

Genes which influence atopy can be detected by testing for simple associations with variants of "candidate" genes in samples of affected and unaffected individuals. The candidate approach is limited by the number of known genes with a role in the patho-physiology of atopy.

A second approach, originally called "positional cloning", relies on the localisation of disease genes to particular chromosomal segments by genetic linkage. Genetic linkage is demonstrated in families by the co-transmission of chromosomal markers of known location together with the disease in question. Linkage is followed by strategies to isolate the disease gene from the identified region. Positional cloning has been very successful with single gene disorders, such as Cystic Fibrosis and Huntington's Disease. With complex illnesses, such as Alzheimer's disease or atopy, progress with positional cloning has been difficult, but not impossible.

GENES INFLUENCING ASTHMA AND ATOPY

Many different kind of genes may be involved in atopy and asthma. They can be divided into four classes, as follows:

1. Genes predisposing in general to IgE-mediated inflammation.
2. Genes influencing the specific IgE response to particular allergens.
3. Genes influencing bronchial hyper-responsiveness independently of atopy.
4. Genes influencing non-IgE mediated inflammation.

CLASS 1 ASTHMA GENES

Known genes in the first class include FcεRI-β on chromosome 11 and possibly IL-4 on chromosome 5.

FcεRI-β

Linkage of atopy, defined by IgE responses, to the chromosome 11q13 marker D11S97 was first found in 1989, and the finding replicated by the same group (13), and confirmed by other reputable groups in Japan and Holland (14,15). In each case, linkage was seen in families with severe symptomatic atopy. This distinction may be of importance, as not everyone who has positive skin tests or RASTs suffers from symptoms, and the genes operating in severe or mild forms of atopy may differ. A number of negative linkage studies also been reported in the allergy literature (16,17,18,19): most of these suffered from unrealistic expectations of the power to detect linkage in small sample sizes.

Affected sib pair analysis (which is the most "robust" method of detecting linkage) showed that linkage of atopy to chromosome 11 markers was exclusively maternal (20,21). This is likely to correspond to the maternal effect seen in clinical studies. The recognition of the maternal effect allowed mapping of the atopy gene to the region centromeric to the original D11S97 marker (21), and the demonstration that 60% or less of families with symptomatic atopy can be influenced by the chromosome 11 atopy gene (22). It was also followed by the localisation of the β chain of the high affinity receptor for IgE (*FcεRI*-β) to the same region, in close linkage to atopy (22).

FcεRI-β is an excellent candidate for an atopy gene, as the receptor acts a trigger for the allergic process, and mast cells are now known to release significant amounts of cytokines which can up-regulate the IgE response to allergens. Sequencing of *FcεRI*-β has now detected several variants in addition to the more usual wild type.

The first reported polymophisms were known as *Leu181/Leu183* and *Leu181* (23). *Leu181* has been detected in 10 of 60 (17%) of English families ascertained through an asthmatic proband (23), and *Leu181/Leu183* found in 4.5% of an Australian population sample. Maternal inheritance of both these variants were associated with severe atopy. We have found great difficulty in establishing a reliable assay for these variants, but we have been able to establish that they are in linkage disequilibrium with other polymorphisms, including the microsatellite repeat in intron five of *FcεRI*-β . The presence of linkage disequilibrium makes experimental artifact an unlikely cause of the findings, and it is likely that *FcεRI*-β is the chromosome 11 atopy gene.

We have recently identified a new variant of *FcεRI*-β (Hill MR et al, in preparation) which shows strong associations with atopy and with asthma, without any detectable maternal effect.

IL4 Cytokine Cluster

Linkage of the total serum IgE to markers near the cytokine cluster on chromosome 5q31–33 has been demonstrated by Marsh *et al* (24). Marsh and his colleagues studied Amish pedigrees, selected to contain members with positive skin prick tests. Linkage was however strongest in families with the lowest serum IgE. The result was replicated by Myers *et al* (25) in Dutch asthmatic families. Linkage has not been found in other studies of extended families (Rich S, personal communication). My group have tested 1,500 individuals from 300 nuclear families, and find no evidence for linkage either by sib-pair or by lod score methods. However, in order to test the claim that linkage is predominantly seen with the low IgE phenotype, we have used class D regressive models to account for the specific IgE response. The residual IgE shows evidence of linkage to a microsatellite repeat found in IL4, but not to the other polymorphic markers studied by Marsh or Myers (Dizier *et al*, in preparation). We see no linkage to bronchial hyper-responsiveness or asthmatic phenotypes.

CLASS 2 ASTHMA GENES

Genes in the second class, which restrict the ability to respond to particular allergens, include the class II HLA genes (particularly HLA-DR) and the genes of the T-cell receptor (particularly TCR-α). These genes are of clinical importance, as the risk of asthma in atopic subjects is much higher in those who respond to house dust mite or animal danders than those who react to grass pollens.

HLA-DR

An HLA influence on the IgE response was first noted by Levine *et al* (26), who found an association between HLA class I haplotypes and IgE responses to antigen E derived from ragweed allergen (*Ambrosia artemisifolia*). This association has been subsequently found by Marsh et al to be due to restriction of the response to a component of ragweed antigen (*Amb a* V) by HLA-DR2 (27). To date the association of *Amb a* V (molecular weight 5,000) and HLA-DR2, is the only HLA association to have been consistently confirmed (28). Other results of positive and negative associations have generally been found in small samples, and have not been replicated (28 for review).

We have genotyped for HLA-DR in a large sample of atopic subjects from the British population (28). The subjects were tested for IgE responses to the most common British major allergens. Four hundred and thirty-one subjects from 83 families were studied. Three hundred subjects were used as controls. The subjects and the controls have come from the same relatively homogeneous population. In the United Kingdom and Europe, allergens other than *Bet v* I and those tested for in our study are uncommon causes of sensitisation and IgE-mediated allergy.

The results showed weak associations between HLA-DR allele frequencies and IgE responses to common allergens . A possible excess of HLA-DR1 was found in subjects who were responsive to *Fel d* I compared to those who were not (Odds Ratio (OR)=2, p=0.002), and a possible excess of HLA-DR4 was found in subjects responsive to *Alt a* I (OR=1.9, p=0.006). Increased sharing of HLA-DR/DP haplotypes was seen in sibling pairs responding to both allergens. *Der p* I, *Der p* II, *Phl p* V and *Can f* I were not associated with any definite excess of HLA-DR alleles. No significant correlations were seen with HLA-DP genotype and reactivity to any of the allergens.

TCR-α

In order to examine if the TCR genes influence susceptibility to particular allergens, we have therefore tested for genetic linkage between IgE responses and microsatellites from the TCR-α/δ and TCR-β regions (29). Two independent sets of families, one British and one Australian, were investigated. Because the mode of inheritance was unknown, and because of interactions from the environment and other loci, affected sibling pair methods were used to test for linkage.

No linkage of IgE serotypes to TCR-β was detected, but significant linkage of IgE responses to the house dust mite allergens *Der p* I and *Der p* II, the cat allergen *Fel d* I, and the total serum IgE to TCR-α was seen in both family groups. Replication of positive results of linkage in a second set of subjects is important in interpreting this study.

The results show that a locus in the TCR α/δ region is modulating IgE responses. We have recently found allelic associations with a Vα8.1 polymorphism, and the IgE titre to Der p I: the association is only seen in subjects which are HLA-DR2 positive

(Moffatt MF et al, in preparation). It is likely that other associations exist with other polymorphisms and IgE responses to other major allergens.

CLASS 3 ASTHMA GENES

No genes have yet been identified which predispose to bronchial hyper-responsiveness independently of atopy, although FcεRI-β has been shown to influence both. However, we have recently identified two new chromosomal localisations for bronchial hyper-responsiveness, and it is likely that the genes responsible for these effects will be identified within the next three years.

CLASS 4 ASTHMA GENES

Tumour Necrosis Factor-α is known to be polymorphic, and may influence the severity of asthmatic airway inflammation. It is therefore an excellent candidate for a gene in the fourth class. Associations with TNF-α and asthma have been suggested previously, and we have now confirmed and extended these findings.

REFERENCES

1. Cookson WOCM. The genetics of asthma. in: Burr M. The epidemiology of asthma. Monogr Allergy. S Karger and co. Basel 1993; 31: 171–89.
2. Cline MG & Burrows B. B. Distribution of allergy in a population sample residing in Tuscon, Arizona. Thorax 1989; 44: 425–31.
3. Holford-Strevens V et al. Serum total immunoglobulin E levels in Canadian Adults. J Allergy Clin Immunol 1984; 73: 516–522.
4. Peat JK, Britton WJ, Salome CM & Woolcock AJ. Bronchial Hyperresponsiveness in two populations of Australian school children III. Effect of exposure to environmental allergens. Clin Allergy 1987; 17: 271–81
5. Bray GW. The hereditary factor in hypersensitiveness anaphlaxis and allergy. J Allergy 1931; II: 205–224.
6. Magnusson CG. Cord serum IgE in relation to family history and as predictor of atopic disease in early infancy. Allergy 1988; 43: 241–51.
7. Halonen M, Stern D, Taussig LM, Wright A, Ray CG, Martinez FD. The predictive relationship between serum IgE levels at birth and subsequent incidences of lower respiratory illnesses and eczema in infants. Am Rev Resp Dis 1992; 146: 866–870.
8. Arshad SH, Matthews S, Grant C, Hide DW. Effect of allergen avoidance on development of allergic disorders in infancy. Lancet 1992; 339: 1493–97.
9. Åberg N. Familial occurence of atopic disease: genetic versus environmental factors. Clin Exp Allergy 1994; 23: 829–34.
10. Kuehr J, Karmaus W, Forster J et al. Sensitisation to four common inhalant allergens within 302 nuclear families. Clin Exp Allergy 1993; 23: 600–605.
11. Hall JG. Genomic imprinting. Arch Dis Childhood 1990; 65: 1013–16.
12. Cookson WOCM, Sharp PA, Faux JA, Hopkin JM. Linkage between immunoglobulin E responses underlying asthma and rhinitis and chromosome 11q. Lancet 1989; i : 1292–5.
13. Young RP, Lynch J, Sharp PA, Faux JA, Cookson WOCM, Hopkin JM. Confirmation of genetic linkage between atopic IgE responses and chromosome 11q13. J Med Genet 1992; 29: 236–8.
14. Collée JM, ten Kate LP, de Vries HG, Kliphuis JW, Bouman K, Scheffer H, Gerritsen J. Allele sharing on chromosome 11q13 in sibs with asthma and atopy. Lancet 1993; 342: 936.
15. Shirakawa T, Morimoto K, Hashimoto T, Furuyama J, Yamamoto M, Takai S. Linkage between severe atopy and chromosome 11q in Japanese families. Clinical Genetics: 1994 in press.

16. Lympany P, Welsh K, MacCochrane G, Kemeny DM, Lee TH. Genetic analysis using DNA polymorphism of the linkage between chromosome 11q13 and atopy and bronchial hyperresponsiveness to methacholine. J Allergy Clin Immunol 1982; 80: 619–628.

17. Hizawa N, Yamaguchi E, Ohe M, Itih A, Furuya K, Ohnuma T, Kawakami Y. Lack of linkage between atopy and locus 11q13. Clin Exp Allergy 1992; 22: 1065–69.

18. Rich SS, Roitman-Johnson B, Greenberg B, Roberts S, Blumenthal MN. Genetic analysis of atopy in three large kindreds: no evidence of linkage to D11S97. Clin Exp Allergy 1992; 22: 1070–76.

19. Amelung PJ, Panhuysen CIM, Postma DS, Levitt RC, Koeter GH, Francomano CA, Bleeker ER, Meyers DA. Atopy, asthma and bronchial hyper-responsiveness: exclusion of linkage to markers on chromosomes 11q and 6p. Clin Exp Allergy 1992; 22: 1077–84.

20. Moffatt MF, Sharp PA, Faux JA, Young RP, Cookson WOCM, Hopkin JM. Factors confounding genetic linkage between atopy and chromosome 11q. Clin Exp Allergy 1992; 22: 1046–51.

21. Cookson WOCM, Young RP, Sandford AJ, Moffatt MF, Shirakawa T, Sharp PA, Faux JA, Julier C, le Souef PN, Nakumura Y, Lathrop GM, Hopkin JM. Maternal Inheritance of Atopic IgE Responsiveness on Chromosome 11q. Lancet 1992; 340: 381–84.

22. Sandford AJ, Shirakawa T, Moffatt MF, Daniels SE, Ra C, Faux JA, Young RP, Nakamura Y, Lathrop GM, Cookson WOCM, Hopkin JM. Localisation of atopy and the β subunit of the high affinity IgE receptor (FcεRI) on chromosome 11q. Lancet 1993; 341: 332–4.

23. Shirakawa TS, Li A, Dubowitz M, Dekker JW, Shaw AE, Faux JA, Ra C, Cookson WOCM, Hopkin JM. Association between atopy and variants of the β subunit of the high-affinity immunoglobulin E receptor. Nature Genetics 1994; in press.

24. Marsh DG, Neely JD, Breazeale DR, Ghosh B, Freidhoff LR, Erlich-Kautzky E, Schou C, Krishnaswamy G, Beaty TH. Linkage analysis of IL4 and other chromosome 5q31.1 markers and total serum IgE concentrations. Science 1994; 264: 1152–5.

25. Myers DA, Postma DS, Panhuysen CIM, Xu J, Amelung PJ, Levitt RC, Bleeker ER. Evidence for a locus regulating total serum IgE levels mapping to chromosome 5. Genomics 1994; 23: 464–70.

26. Levine BB, Stember RH, Fontino M. Ragweed hayfever: genetic control and linkage to HL-A haplotypes. Science 1972; 178: 1201–3.

27. Marsh DG, Meyers DA, Bias WB. The epidemiology and genetics of atopic allergy. N Eng J Med 1981; 305: 1551–9.

28. Young RP, Dekker JW, Wordsworth BP, Schou C, Pile KD, Matthiesen F, Rosenberg WMC, Bell JI, Hopkin JM, Cookson WOCM. HLA-DR and HLA-DP genotypes and Immunoglobulin E responses to common major allergens. Clin Exp Allergy 1994: 24: 431–39.

29. Moffatt MF, Hill MR, Cornélis F, Schou C, Faux JA, Young RP, James AL, Ryan G, le Souef P, Musk AW, Hopkin JM, Cookson WOCM. Genetic linkage of the TCR-α/δ region to specific Immunoglobulin E responses. Lancet 1994; 343: 1597–1600.

9

REGULATION OF INTERLEUKIN-12 SIGNALLING DURING T HELPER PHENOTYPE DEVELOPMENT

Nils G. Jacobson, Susanne J. Szabo, Mehmet L. Güler, James D. Gorham, and Kenneth M. Murphy

Department of Pathology
Washington University School of Medicine
St. Louis, Missouri, 63110

1. T HELPER PHENOTYPE DEVELOPMENT AND ATOPY

During antigen activation, helper T cells differentiate to stable phenotypes characterized by production of specific cytokines (1,2). The T helper type 1 (Th1) phenotype is characterized by high levels of interferon-γ (IFNγ) and lymphotoxin production. Th1 development stimulates cell-mediated immune responses, including macrophage activation, and the production of restricted immunoglobulin isotypes such as IgG2a (3). The Th2 phenotype correlates with production of interleukin-4 (IL-4), IL-5, and IL-10, which stimulate humoral responses, including B cell and eosinophil activation, as well as the production of other immunoglobulin isotypes such as IgE (4,5).

The development of T helper phenotype can have dramatic effects on the outcome of both pathogen clearance and immune pathology. In allergic (type I) hypersensitivity, specific antigens react with sensitized mast cells to cause asthma, urticaria, and other atopic responses (6,7). These disease states are mediated by previously synthesized allergen-specific IgE antibodies which are prebound to mast cells and basophils and lead to degranulation of effector molecules when crosslinked by antigen. Production of IgE by B cells requires IL-4 generated by activated Th2 cells and does not occur in Th1-type responses (8). Thus, atopic immune pathology is strongly dependent on the development of a Th2 response in allergen-specific T lymphocytes. We have investigated the feasibility of controlling the atopic state by directing the immune response to the Th1 pole.

Certain cytokines present during the primary activation of naive T cells can affect their development. These include the macrophage-derived cytokine IL-12, which induces stable differentiation toward the Th1 phenotype (9,10). In addition, IL-4, which can be produced by mast cells as well as T cells, causes the differentiation of the Th2 phenotype (11–13). In certain models of T helper phenotype development, IL-4 is required for Th2 development and IL-12 is required for Th1 development (9,13,14). In order to identify the

New Horizons in Allergy Immunotherapy
edited by Sehon et al. Plenum Press, New York, 1996

molecular triggers of atopy, we have addressed the signals responsible for Th1 and Th2 development. We report here our recent findings regarding the molecular responsiveness of T lymphocytes to IL-12.

2. EARLY SIGNALLING EVENTS INDUCED BY IL-12

2.1. Cytokine Signal Transduction by Latent Cytoplasmic Transcription Factors

A variety of cytokines have been shown to activate members of the family of signal transducers and activators of transcription (STATs) (15). In interferon-γ signalling, for example, receptor binding and dimerization causes activation of the Janus family tyrosine kinases Jak-1 and Jak-2, followed by tyrosine phosphorylation of the receptor-associated latent transcription factor Stat1 (16). Tyrosine-phosphorylated Stat1 forms homodimers and rapidly translocates to the nucleus, where it binds to DNA and activates transcription (17). Since the identification of Stat1, a total of five other homologous STAT proteins have been cloned (18). Different cytokine receptors have been shown to exert specificity by recruitment of particular STATs. While several cytokines activate Stat1, 2, 3, 5, and 6, no polypeptide ligand has been previously shown to activate Stat4 (15).

2.2. IL-12-Induced Tyrosine Phosphorylation of Stat3 and Stat4 in Th1 Cells

In order to test if IL-12 uses the Jak-STAT family of signal transduction molecules, we analyzed STAT tyrosine phosphorylation in the Th1 clone 3F6. Total cell extracts of IL-12-

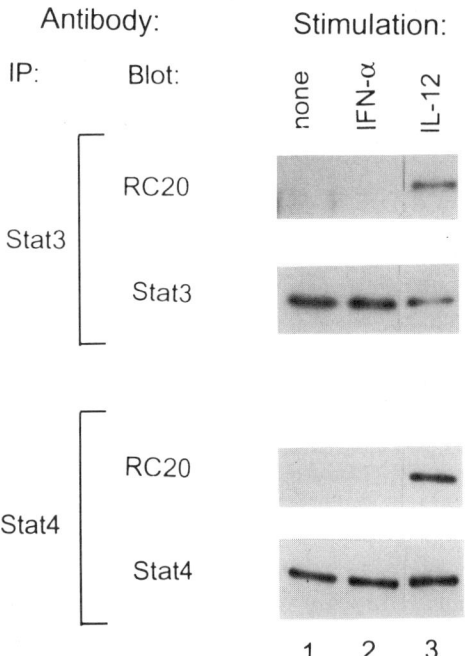

Figure 1. IL-12 induces tyrosine phosphorylation of Stat3 and Stat4 in 3F6 cells. 3F6 cells were stimulated with 10 U/ml IL-12 or 300 U/ml IFNα A/D for 30 minutes. Total cell lysates were then immunoprecipitated with anti-STAT antisera and blotted with the anti-phosphotyrosine reagent RC20 after SDS-PAGE (7% gel). Following stripping, the same blots were reprobed with antisera to Stat3 and Stat4.

treated or untreated 3F6 cells were immunoprecipitated using one of four STAT-specific antisera and examined for phosphotyrosine incorporation by Western blot (Fig. 1). IL-12 stimulation induced tyrosine phosphorylation of both Stat3 and Stat4, whereas IFNα induced tyrosine phosphorylation of neither. We confirmed the presence of non-phosphorylated STATs in unstimulated cells by reprobing stripped blots with antisera to Stat3 and Stat4.

2.3 IL-12 Activates Stat3 and Stat4 for DNA Binding

To determine whether the IL-12-induced STAT factors bind DNA, we performed an electrophoretic mobility shift assay (EMSA) (19) using oligonucleotide probes to which several STAT family members bind. The m67 probe, derived from the serum-inducible element (SIE) of the c-fos promoter, and the FcγRI probe, from the IFNγ response region (GRR) of the high affinity Fcγ receptor promoter, have distinct binding specificity for various STAT family members (20,21). Nuclear extracts from IL-12 treated 3F6 cells generated a gel shift complex containing three bands: a lower band comigrating with the Stat1 homodimer and a closely spaced upper doublet (Fig. 2).

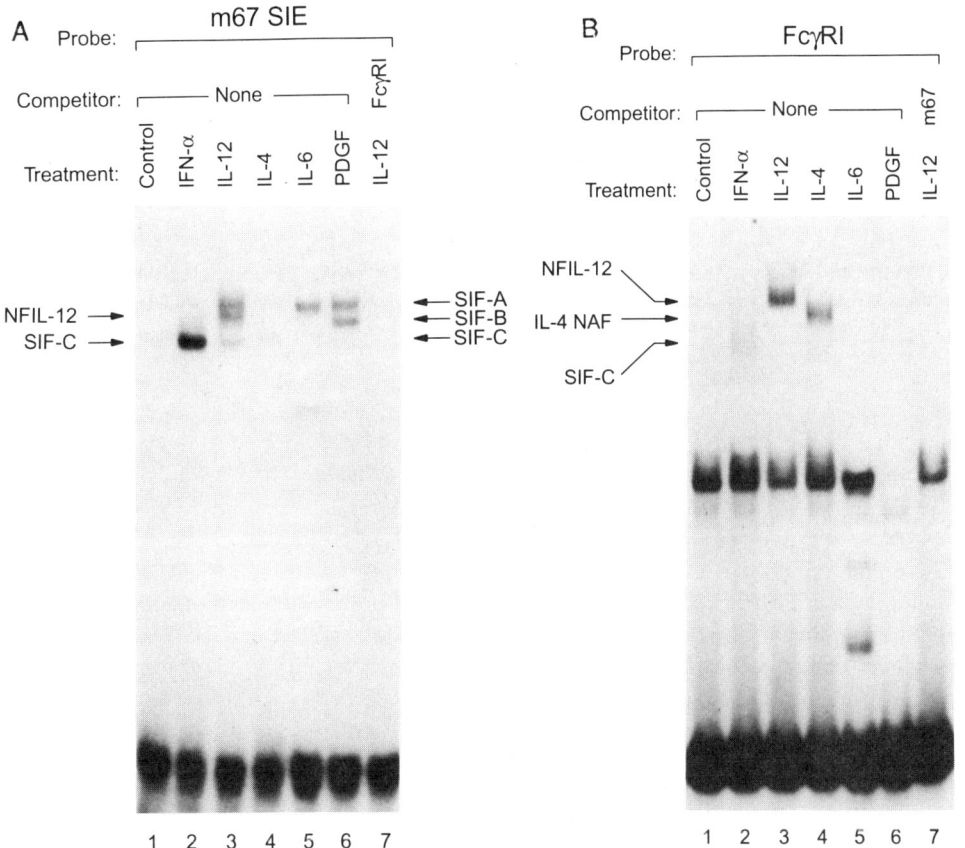

Figure 2. IL-12 induces a unique pattern of bands in a gel shift assay. 3F6 cells were stimulated with IFNα (300 U/ml), IL-12 (10 U/ml), or IL-4 (200 U/ml); HepG2 cells were stimulated with IL-6 (30 ng/ml); and 3T3 cells were stimulated with PDGF-BB (100 ng/ml). Nuclear extracts were prepared and subjected to EMSA using ^{32}P-labeled m67 SIE (A) and Fcγ RI GRR (B) probes. Retarded complexes are labeled with arrows.

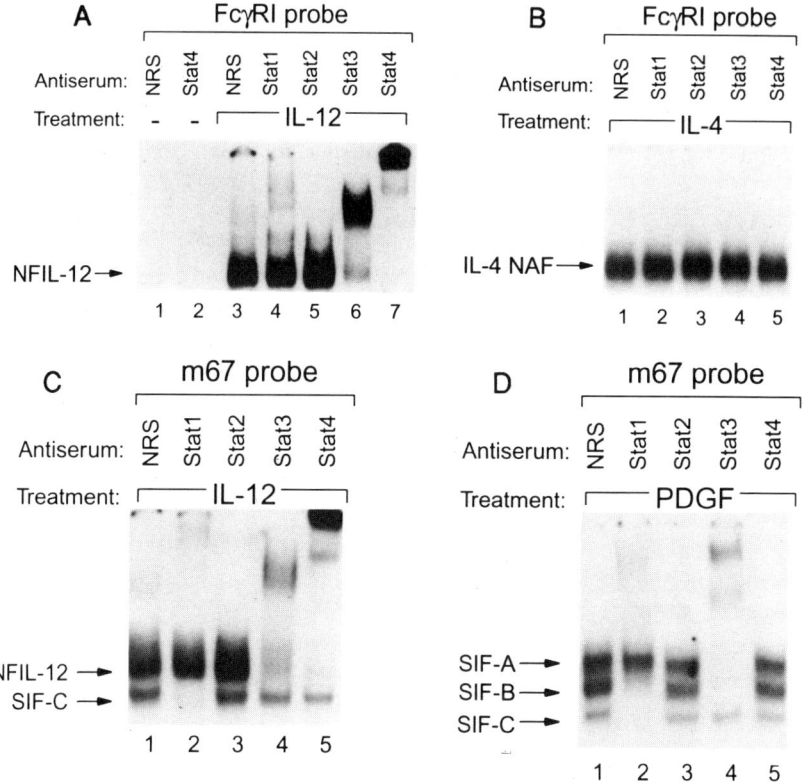

Figure 3. IL-12 induced nuclear complexes contain Stat3 and Stat4. Extracts were prepared from 3T3 cells following (A) IL-12 treatment (10 U/ml) or IL-4 treatment (200 U/ml). EMSA was performed with the FcγRI probe and antisera to Stat1, 2, 3, and 4. (C) IL-12 treated 3F6 nuclear extracts or (D) PDGF-treated 3T3 cell extracts were supershifted using the m67 probe.

We determined the reactivity of the EMSA complexes with anti-STAT antisera using both m67 and FcγRI probes (Fig. 3). With the FcγRI probe, Stat3 and Stat4 antisera removed the majority of the IL-12 induced complexes, whereas Stat1 and Stat2 antisera had no effect. In contrast, the IL-4-induced complex was unaffected by these antisera. With the m67 probe, the IL-12 induced complexes reacted specifically with Stat1, 3, and 4 antisera. The upper doublet shifted completely with Stat4 antiserum and nearly completely with Stat3 antiserum. Control supershifts of PDGF-treated cell extracts yielded the expected shift pattern with Stat1 and Stat3 antisera and showed no effect with Stat4 antiserum. These results indicate that IL-12-induced tyrosine phosphorylation of Stat1, 3, and 4 leads to the formation of DNA-binding complexes containing these STATs.IL-12 induced nuclear complexes contain Stat3 and Stat4. Extracts were prepared from 3T3 cells following (A) IL-12 treatment (10 U/ml) or IL-4 treatment (200 U/ml). EMSA was performed with the FcγRI probe and antisera to Stat1, 2, 3, and 4. (C) IL-12 treated 3F6 nuclear extracts or (D) PDGF-treated 3T3 cell extracts were supershifted using the m67 probe.

3. LOSS OF IL-12 RESPONSIVENESS IN DEVELOPING TH2 CELLS

3.1 Th2 Cells Rapidly Develop Phenotype Irreversibility

To examine the ability of T helper cells to reverse phenotype *in vitro*, we assayed the cytokine production profile of early Th1 and Th2 cells after activation under conditions of phenotype reversal. First, we induced the differentiation of Th1 and Th2 cells by incubating naive T cells from the T cell receptor transgenic DO11.10 mouse (9,22) with antigen and splenic antigen presenting cells, along with phenotype-directing cytokines or antibodies. Th1 cells were generated by the addition of IL-12 and anti-IL-4. Upon restimulation, these cells produced 500 U/ml of IFNγ and undetectable IL-4. Th2 cells were stimulated with IL-4 and anti-IL-12, and produced 300 U/ml of IL-4 and undetectable IFNγ.

To examine the commitment of these cells, we reversed phenotype differentiation by stimulating Th1 and Th2 cells as described in Figure 4. Th1 cells could undergo long-term alterations in phenotype caused by either IL-12 or IL-4 (Fig. 4, Top panel). Addition of IL-4 during the secondary stimulation induced subsequent IL-4 production and reduced IFNγ production. Thus, early Th1 cells respond to both IL-4 and IL-12 for immediate modulation of cytokine production and for T helper phenotype reversal.

We next examined the phenotype commitment of early Th2 cells (Fig. 4, bottom panel). We restimulated Th2 cells in the presence of IL-12, IL-12 plus anti-IL-4, anti-IL-4, IL-4, or without any additions and examined immediate cytokine production and subsequent phenotype development. In contrast with Th1 cells, Th2 cells were unaffected by any condition for both immediate cytokine modulation and phenotype reversal. Despite the addition of high levels of IL-12 or neutralization of IL-4, we detected no IFNγ production either immediately or upon restimulation after 7 days. Furthermore, neither IL-2 nor IFNγ addition restored the ability of IL-12 to induce IFNγ in Th2 cells. IL-4 production remained in the range of 300–450 U/ml regardless of the experimental conditions. Thus, the observed resistance of Th2 cells to phenotype reversal by IL-12 suggested that a loss of IL-12 signaling may accompany early Th2 differentiation.

3.2. Inability of IL-12 to Induce Nuclear Factors in Developing Th2 Cells

The inability of IL-12 to reverse early Th2 differentiation could either be due to a loss of IL-12-mediated signaling or to a dissociation of IL-12 induced signals from effects on differentiation. To distinguish between these possibilities, we examined responses of developing Th1 and Th2 cells to several cytokines by EMSA using m67 and FcγRI oligonucleotide probes. As a control, we also used a probe specific for the ubiquitous and constitutive nuclear factor NF-Y (19). We found a selective difference between early Th1 and Th2 cells for IL-12 signaling (Fig. 5). IL-12 induced EMSA complexes with both the m67 SIE and FcγRI probes in Th1 cells but not in Th2 cells. The inability of Th2 cells to form complexes with these probes was specific to IL-12, since both IL-4 and IFNα induced EMSA complexes with these probes in both Th1 and Th2 cells (Fig. 5).

3.3. Selective Loss of IL-12 Induced Phosphorylation of STAT Proteins in Th2 Cells

Loss of IL-12 induced nuclear factors by early Th2 cells could result either from an absence of STAT proteins or from a defect in their activation. To distinguish between

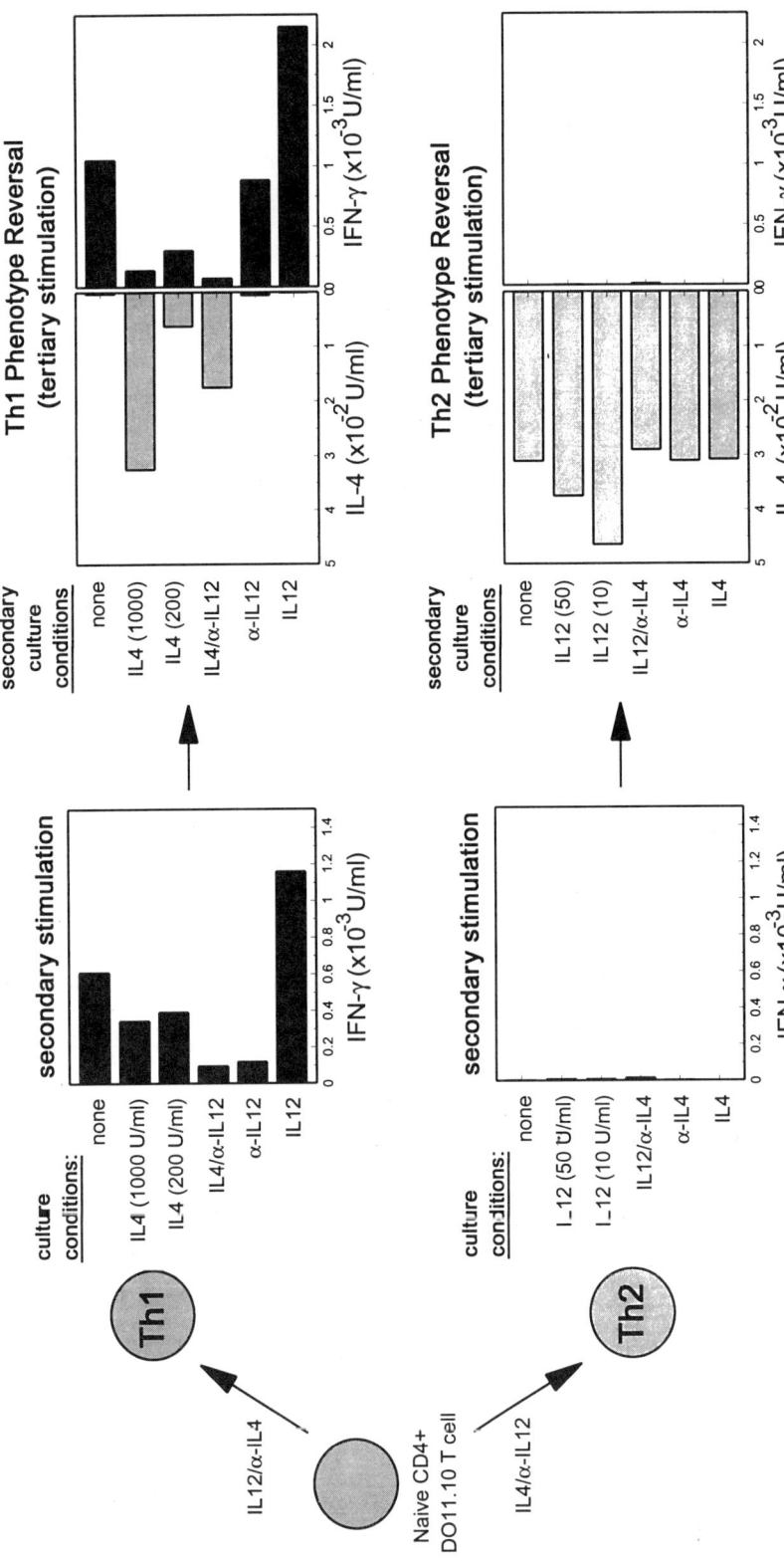

Figure 4. Th2 cells exhibit phenotype irreversibility. FACS-sorted naïve CD4+ DO11.10 T cells were activated with OVA peptide and irradiated APCs with 10 U/ml IL-12 plus 10 μg/ml anti-IL-4 (top panel) or 200 U/ml IL-4 and 3 μg/ml anti-IL-12 (bottom), harvested on day 7 and re-stimulated with indicated conditions for another 7 days, harvested and tested for cytokine production by ELISA.

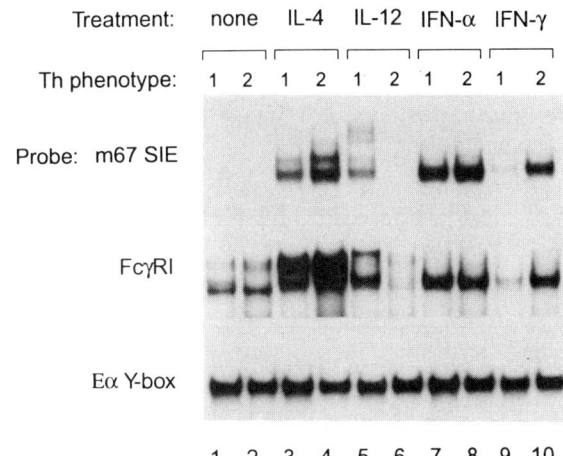

Figure 5. Developing Th2 cells lose IL-12 responsiveness. Nuclear extracts were prepared from Th1 and Th2 cells following incubation with either media, 200 U/ml IL-4 for 20 minutes, 10 U/ml IL-12 for 25 minutes, 300 U/ml IFNα for 30 minutes, or 500 U/ml IFNγ for 10 minutes. EMSA was performed using ^{32}P-labeled m67 SIE, FcγRI, and Eα Y-box oligonucleotide probes.

these possibilities, we examined STAT expression and tyrosine phosphorylation in response to IL-12. Total cellular lysates prepared from IL-12 treated or untreated Th1 and Th2 cells 7 days following primary activation were precipitated using antisera specific for Stat1, Stat3, or Stat4. Precipitated STAT proteins were examined for phosphotyrosine content by Western blot analysis (Fig. 6).

IL-12 treatment led to the selective tyrosine phosphorylation of Stat3 and Stat4 in Th1 cells but not in Th2 cells (Fig. 6). This lack of phosphorylation was not due to the absence of Stat3 and Stat4 expression in Th2 cells, since both Th1 and Th2 cells expressed these proteins as determined by direct Western blotting. IL-12 also increased Stat1 phosphorylation in Th1 cells. In contrast, the level of Stat1 phosphorylation was unchanged in

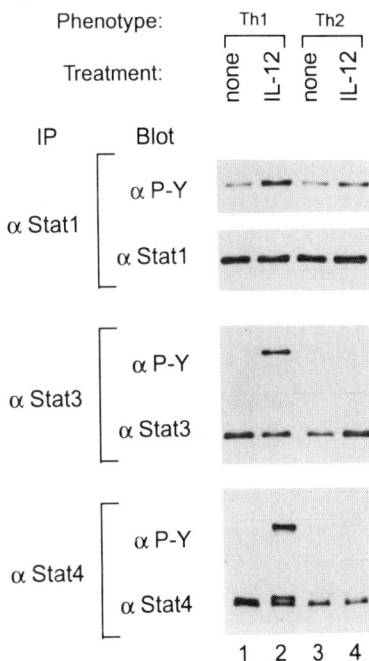

Figure 6. IL-12 induces tyrosine phosphorylation of Stat1, Stat3 and Stat4 in Th1 cells but not in Th2 cells. Whole cell lysates from Th1 and Th2 cells were prepared after treatment for 25 minutes with medium alone or with 10 U/ml IL-12, immunoprecipitated with the indicated anti-STAT antisera, and probed with anti-phosphotyrosine reagent RC20, stripped and reprobed with the indicated STAT antisera.

IL-12 treated Th2 cells. Thus, Th2 cells were selectively unresponsive to IL-12 for tyrosine phosphorylation of Stat1, Stat3, and Stat4. By analyzing populations of T cells at earlier stages of development, we determined that by day 3 Th2 cells begin to lose IL-12 responsiveness. By day 5 post-activation they are completely unresponsive (data not shown) (25).

3.4. Both Th1 and Th2 Cells Express Known Components of the IL-12 Signalling Pathway

Since IL-12 induces the tyrosine phosphorylation of the Jak2 and Tyk2 protein tyrosine kinases (23), we examined the expression and activation of Jak2 and Tyk2 in developing Th1 and Th2 cells. Both proteins were both expressed in Th1 and Th2 cells. IL-12 induced tyrosine phosphorylation of Jak2 in Th1 cells but not in Th2 cells (data not shown) (25).

Since the IL-12 signaling defect in Th2 cells appeared to reside upstream of the Jak2 kinase, we examined the IL-12 receptor itself. The IL-12 receptor consists of at least two separate chains, only one of which (IL-12Rβ) has been cloned. The cloned receptor chain confers nanomolar affinity for IL-12 when expressed in COS cells (24). We examined IL-12 receptor expression on Th1 and Th2 cells by flow cytometry and radioligand binding analysis (data not shown) (25). Both Th1 and Th2 cells have comparable levels and affinity of IL-12-binding sites. Purified CD4[+] naive T cells expressed no detectable IL-12 receptors, which is consistent with the lack of IL-12 receptor expression on resting human peripheral T cells (26,27).

4. GENETIC DIFFERENCES IN IL-12 SIGNALLING IN MICE

In the murine model of *Leishmania major* infection, resistance is strongly correlated with the *in vivo* development of a Th1 response (28). Animals which develop a Th2 response, characterized by high sustained levels of IL-4 production, eventually succumb to infection, whereas animals which develop strong cell-mediated immunity clear the parasite. The observation that different strains of mice are susceptible or resistant to *L. major* infection prompted our analysis of phenotype development in Balb/c (susceptible) and B10.D2 (resistant) animals (29). Our use of TCR-transgenic mice and *in vitro* phenotype assays greatly facilitated these experiments.

4.1. Early IL-12 Receptor Signaling Differs between T Cells from B10.D2 and Balb/C Backgrounds

We activated B10.D2 and Balb/c transgenic T cells with antigen and APCs, with or without the addition of exogenous cytokines. The cytokine profiles of each strain were distinct for T cells allowed to develop under neutral conditions, as previously described (30). We next tested for IL-12 responsiveness by stimulation of these T cell populations *in vitro* (Fig. 7). The default population of B10 T cells remained responsive to exogenous IL-12 upon restimulation on day 7, whereas Balb/c derived default T cells were IL-12 unresponsive (Fig. 7, top panel). As controls, we showed that each strain could become IL-12 unresponsive if induced toward the Th2 phenotype by IL-4 in the primary culture (Fig. 7, middle panel) . Moreover, each strain remained IL-12 responsive when Th1 development

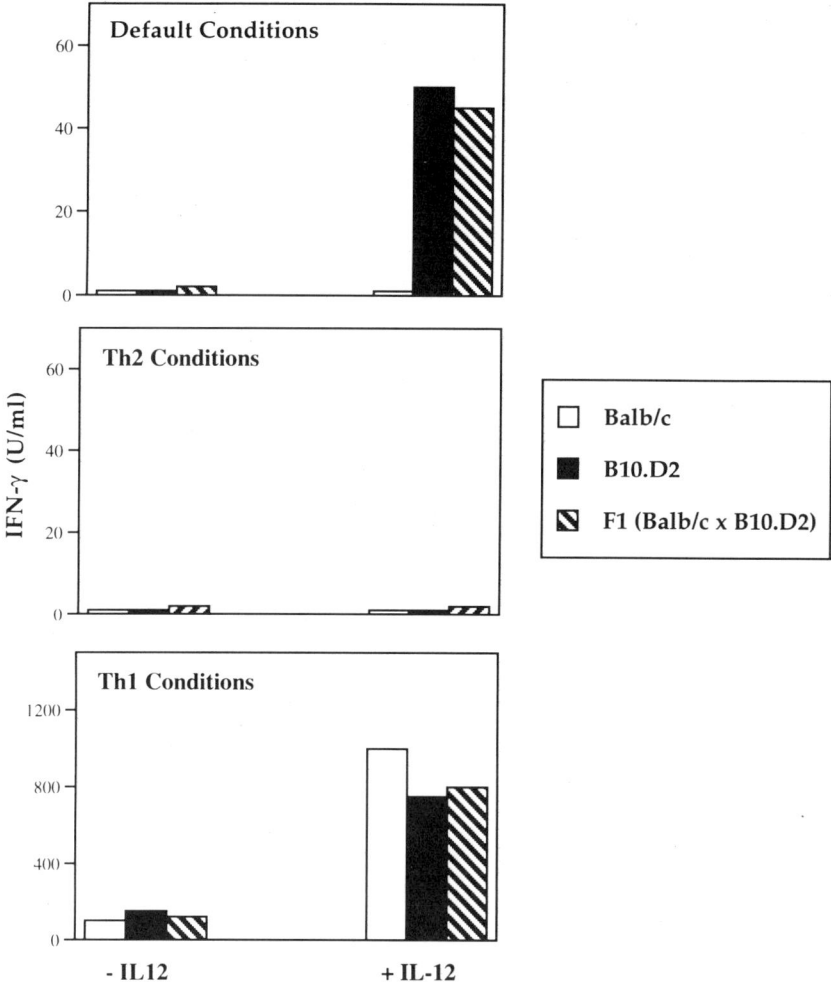

Figure 7. B10.D2 and F1 T cells remain IL-12 responsive under default conditions; Balb/c T cells lose IL-12 responsiveness under default conditions. Balb/c (open bars), B10.D2 (shaded bars), or F1 (B10.D2 x Balb/c, striped bars) T cells were stimulated with OVA peptide under neutral conditions (top panel), Th2 conditions (middle panel,) or Th1 conditions (bottom panel.) Cells were restimulated with OVA and TA3 cells 7 days later in the presence (right side) or absence (left side) of IL-12. IFNγ production was measured in supernatants after 48 hours by ELISA.

was induced by IL-12 in the primary culture (Fig. 7, bottom panel). Thus it appears that default conditions of development lead to distinct phenotypes for B10 and Balb/c T cells with respect to IL-12 responsiveness.

To further characterize the genetic difference between Balb/c and B10.D2 T cells, we examined the F1 (Balb/c x B10.D2) using the *in vitro* development assay (Fig. 7). When tested for IL-12 responsiveness following activation under neutral conditions with APCs, F1 animals produced levels of IFNγ comparable to the B10.D2 controls, significantly more that Balb/c mice. Thus, the genetic effect of B10.D2 on *in vitro* helper T cell development is dominant in F1 crosses with Balb/c mice.

4.2. Segregation in BC1 Generation Suggests That a Single Locus Controls Most of the B10.D2 Dominant Genetic Effect on IL-12 Responsiveness

Since the B10 phenotype is dominant in F1 animals, we produced cohorts of back-crossed (BC1) animals by mating F1 mice with Balb/c in order to test whether the B10.D2 contribution to F1 dominance is polygenic. If only one locus differs between B10.D2 and Balb/c for Th phenotype, we would predict that half of the BC1 mice would be F1-like (IL-12 responsive) and half would be Balb/c-like (IL-12 unresponsive) in the *in vitro* assay. An analysis of T cells derived from 18 BC1 animals activated with IL-12 after a neutral primary stimulation on TA3 cells is shown in Figure 8. About half of the BC1 mice showed F1-like IL-12 responsiveness, and half showed Balb/c-like IL-12 unresponsiveness (Fig. 8). These data are consistent with a single locus controlling *in vitro* T cell development differences between B10.D2 and Balb/c strains.

Further analysis of larger numbers of BC1 mice along with SSLP genetic analysis will allow us to pinpoint the chromosomal location of the gene conferring the B10 phenotype in backcrossed animals (31). Eventually, we hope to use positional cloning the identify the molecular species responsible for strain differences in T helper development.

5. SUMMARY

The experiments described above have allowed us to define the molecular events in IL-12 signalling. Within minutes after IL-12 treatment of responsive cells, Stat1, Stat3,

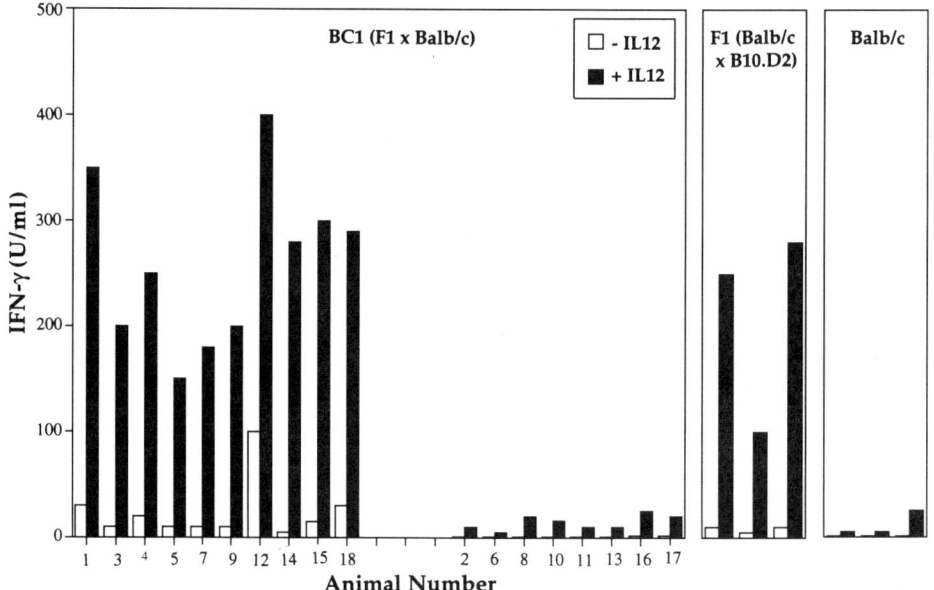

Figure 8. Segregation of IFNγ production in BC1 mice suggests that a single locus controls B10.D2 dominance. BC1 (F1 x Balb/c) T cells (left panel) or control T cells (right panel) stimulated under neutral conditions using TA3 cells as APCs were restimulated 7 days later with OVA peptide in the presence (black bars) or absence (open bars) of IL-12. IFNγ in supernatants was measured 48 hours later by ELISA.

and Stat4 are tyrosine phosphorylated. These molecules form nuclear DNA-binding complexes consisting of homodimeric Stat1 and heterodimeric Stat3-Stat4 complexes. In a murine *in vitro* phenotype development model, T cells rapidly and selectively lose their capacity to respond to IL-12 upon acquisition of the Th2 phenotype. This hyporesponsiveness is manifested by the inability of IL-12 to induce IFNγ production in differentiated Th2 cells, as well as the inability of IL-12 to induce the activation of Stat4. Despite the functional defect of IL-12 signalling in Th2 cells, all known components of the IL-12 signal transduction pathway are present. We speculate that in Th2 cells, the second receptor chain may be absent or one of the other components may be modified.

Genetic experiments in Balb/c and B10.D2 strains of mice have demonstrated several differences in T helper differentiation *in vitro*. Stimulation of T cells under neutral conditions results in a bias of Balb/c T cells toward the Th2 extreme and B10 T cells toward the Th1 extreme of cytokine production. Following stimulation under neutral conditions, B10 T cells retain the ability to respond to IL-12 while Balb/c T cells lose IL-12 responsiveness. Mating experiments have demonstrated that the B10 genetic effect is dominant in F1 mice. Analysis of backcrossed animals has suggested that the ability to respond to IL-12 in the secondary stimulation may be controlled by a single dominant B10 gene.

The results we describe may have profound implications for allergy. Since allergic responses are largely due to the activation of the Th2 subset of T lymphocytes, a better understanding of T cell phenotype development may reveal multiple targets for therapeutic intervention. First, a better understanding of Th1 phenotype induction in response to IL-12 may allow prevention of *in vivo* allergic responses using pharmacological tools which bias allergen-specific responses to the Th1 subset. Second, a molecular explanation of why Th2 cells fail to reverse phenotype in response to IL-12 may allow treatment of atopic individuals to remove the disease-promoting T lymphocyte compartment. Finally, a better understanding of the basis for genetic differences in murine T helper cell differentiation may allow us to identify a causative genetic element in humans, yielding better diagnostic and therapeutic methods.

6. ACKNOWLEDGMENTS

We gratefully acknowledge reagents and advice from Drs. J.E. Darnell Jr., R.D. Schreiber, O. Kanagawa, and E.R. Unanue. This work was supported by NIH grants AI31238 and AI34580.

REFERENCES

1. Mosmann, T. R., H. M. Cherwinski, M. W. Bond, M. A. Giedlin, and R. L. Coffman. 1986. Two types of murine helper T cell clone. I. Definition according to profiles of lymphokine activities and secreted proteins. *J. Immunol.* 136:2348–2357.
2. Kim, J., A. Woods, E. Becker-Dunn, and K. Bottomly. 1985. Distinct functional phenotypes of cloned Ia-restricted helper T cells. *J. Exp. Med.* 162:188–201.
3. Cher, D. J. and T. R. Mosmann. 1987. Two types of murine helper T cell clone. II. Delayed-type hypersensitivity is mediated by Th1 clones. *J. Immunol.* 138:3688–3694.
4. Stevens, T. L., A. Bossie, V. M. Sanders, R. Fernandez-Botran, R. L. Coffman, T. R. Mosmann, and E. S. Vitetta. 1988. Regulation of antibody isotypic secretion by subsets of antigen-specific helper T cells. *Nature* 334:255–258.
5. Snapper, C. M. and W. E. Paul. 1987. Interferon-gamma and B cell stimulatory factor-1 reciprocally regulate Ig isotype production. *Science* 236:944–947.

6. Kline, J. N. and G. W. Hunninghake. 1994. T-lymphocyte dysregulation in asthma. [Review]. *Proceedings of the Society for Experimental Biology & Medicine* 207:243–253.

7. Kay, A. B. 1991. T lymphocytes and their products in atopic allergy and asthma. [Review]. *International Archives of Allergy & Applied Immunology* 94:189–193.

8. Kopf, M., G. Le Gros, M. Bachmann, M. C. Lamers, H. Bluethmann, and G. Kohler. 1993. Disruption of the murine IL-4 gene blocks Th2 cytokine responses. *Nature* 362:245–247.

9. Hsieh, C.-S., S. E. Macatonia, C. S. Tripp, A. O'Garra, and K. M. Murphy. 1993. Development of Th1 CD4+ T cells through IL-12 produced by Listeria-induced macrophages. *Science* 260:547–549.

10. Manetti, R., P. Parronchi, M. G. Giudizi, M.-P. Piccinni, E. Maggi, G. Trinchieri, and S. Romagnani. 1993. Natural killer cell stimulatory factor (interleukin 12 [IL-12]) induces T helper type 1 (Th1)-specific immune responses and inhibits the development of IL-4-producing Th cells. *J. Exp. Med.* 177:1199–1204.

11. Le Gros, G., S. Z. Ben-Sasson, R. A. Seder, F. D. Finkelman, and W. E. Paul. 1990. Generation of interleukin 4 (IL-4)-producing cells *in vivo* and *in vitro*: IL-2 and IL-4 are required for *in vitro* generation of IL-4-producing cells. *J. Exp. Med.* 172:921–929.

12. Swain, S. L., A. D. Weinberg, M. English, and G. Huston. 1990. IL-4 directs the development of Th2-like helper effectors. *J. Immunol.* 145:3796–3806.

13. Hsieh, C.-S., A. B. Heimberger, J. S. Gold, A. O'Garra, and K. M. Murphy. 1992. Differential regulation of T helper phenotype development by interleukins 4 and 10 in an alpha-beta-T-cell-receptor transgenic system. *Proc. Nat. Acad. Sci. USA* 89:6065–6069.

14. Coffman, R. L., K. Varkila, P. Scott, and R. Chatelain. 1991. Role of cytokines in the differentiation of CD4+ T-cell subsets *in vivo*. *Immunol. Rev.* 123:189–207.

15. Darnell, J. E., Jr., I. M. Kerr, and G. R. Stark. 1994. Jak-STAT pathways and transcriptional activation in response to IFNs and other extracellular signaling proteins. [Review]. *Science* 264:1415–1421.

16. Greenlund, A. C., M. A. Farrar, B. L. Viviano, and R. D. Schreiber. 1994. Ligand-induced IFN gamma receptor tyrosine phosphorylation couples the receptor to its signal transduction system (p91). *EMBO* 13:1591–1600.

17. Shuai, K., C. M. Horvath, L. H. Huang, S. A. Qureshi, D. Cowburn, and J. E. Darnell,Jr. 1994. Interferon activation of the transcription factor Stat91 involves dimerization through SH2-phosphotyrosyl peptide interactions. *Cell* 76:821–828.

18. Hou, J., U. Schindler, W. J. Henzel, T. C. Ho, M. Brassuer, and S. L. McKnight. 1994. An interleukin-4-induced transcription factor: IL-4 Stat. *Science* 265:1701–1706.

19. Szabo, S. J., J. S. Gold, T. L. Murphy, and K. M. Murphy. 1993. Identification of cis-acting regulatory elements controlling interleukin-4 gene expression in T cells: roles for NF-Y and NF-ATc. *Mol. Cell. Bio.* 13:4793–4805.

20. Wagner, B. J., T. E. Hayes, C. J. Hoban, and B. H. Cochran. 1990. The SIF binding element confers sis/PDGF inducibility onto the c-fos promoter. *EMBO* 9:4477–4484.

21. Pearse, R. N., R. Feinman, and J. V. Ravetch. 1991. Characterization of the promoter of the human gene encoding the high-affinity IgG receptor: transcriptional induction by gamma-interferon is mediated through common DNA response elements. *Proceedings of the National Academy of Sciences of the United States of America* 88:11305–11309.

22. Murphy, K. M., A. B. Heimberger, and D. Y. Loh. 1990. Induction by antigen of intrathymic apoptosis of CD4+ CD8+ TCR-lo thymocytes *in vivo*. *Science* 250:1720–1723.

23. Bacon, C. M., D. W. McVicar, J. R. Ortaldo, R. C. Rees, J. J. O'Shea, and J. A. Johnston. 1995. Interleukin 12 (IL-12) induces tyrosine phosphorylation of Jak2 andTYK2: Differential use of janus family tyrosine kinases by IL-2 and IL-12. *J. Exp. Med.* 181:399–404.

24. Chua, A. O., R. Chizzonite, B. B. Desai, T. P. Truitt, P. Nunes, L. J. Minetti, R. R. Warrier, D. H. Presky, J. F. Levine, M. K. Gately, and et al. 1994. Expression cloning of a human IL-12 receptor component. A new member of the cytokine receptor superfamily with strong homology to gp130. *J. Immunol.* 153:128–136.

25. Szabo, S. J., N. G. Jacobson, A. S. Dighe, U. Gubler, and K. M. Murphy. 1995. Developmental commitment to the Th2 lineage by extinction of IL-12 signaling. *Immunity*

26. Desai, B. B., P. M. Quinn, A. G. Wolitzky, P. K. A. Mongini, R. Chizzonite, and M. K. Gately. 1992. IL-12 receptor. II. Distribution and regulation of receptor expression. *J. Immunol.* 148:3125–3132.

27. Chizzonite, R., T. Truitt, B. B. Desai, P. Nunes, F. J. Podlaski, A. S. Stern, and M. K. Gately. 1992. IL-12 receptor. I. Characterization of the receptor on phytohemagglutinin activated human lymphoblasts. *J. Immunol.* 148:3117–3124.

28. Locksley, R. M. and P. Scott. 1991. Helper T-cell subsets in mouse leishmaniasis: induction, expansion and effector function. In Immunoparasitol. Today. C. Ash and R. B. Gallagher, editors. Elsevier Trends Journals, UK. a58-a61.

29. Heinzel, F. P., M. D. Sadick, B. J. Holaday, R. L. Coffman, and R. M. Locksley. 1989. Reciprocal expression of interferon gamma or interleukin 4 during the resolution or progression of murine leishmaniasis. *J. Exp. Med.* 169:59–72.

30. Hsieh, C. S., S. E. Macatonia, A. O'Garra, and K. M. Murphy. 1995. T cell genetic background determines default T helper phenotype development *in vitro*. *J. Exp. Med.* 181:713–721.

31. Dietrich, W. F., J. C. Miller, R. G. Steen, M. Merchant, D. Damron, R. Nahf, A. Gross, D. C. Joyce, M. Wessel, R. D. Dredge, and et al. 1994. A genetic map of the mouse with 4,006 simple sequence length polymorphisms [see comments]. *Nature Genetics* 7:220–245.

10

RESPONSIVENESS TO THE MAJOR POLLEN ALLERGEN OF *PARIETARIA OFFICINALIS* IS ASSOCIATED WITH DEFINED HLA-DRB1* ALLELES IN ITALIAN AND SPANISH ALLERGIC PATIENTS

Anna Ruffilli,[1*] Mauro D'Amato,[2] Tonino Menna,[3] Enrico Maggi,[4] Guido Sacerdoti,[1] and Carlos Laho[5]

[1]International Institute of Genetics and Biophysics, CRN, Naples, Italy
[2]Istituto di Biologia Cellulare, CNR, Roma, Italy
[3]Clinica Medica, Policlinico Careggi, Firenze, Italy
[4]Scuola di Allergologia e Immunologia Clinica, Università di Napoli, Italy
[5]Fundaciòn Jimenez Diaz, Madrid, Spain

1. INTRODUCTION

The concept that specific immune responsiveness is genetically controlled was initially developed studying the antibody response of rodent inbred strains to simple synthetic antigens. It became soon clear that among the genes involved (indicated as immune response (Ir) genes), those of the MHC complex played a major role. It was subsequently shown that, in the response to complex proteins, MHC genes in certain experimental models control high/low responder host phenotype and in other influence the repertoire of epitope specificity of antibody and T cell response (5–9, 10). MHC genes participate in the immune response at several level. A major function is "determinant selection": MHC higly polymorphic proteins selectively bind peptides from processed antigens and present the selected peptides for recognition to the appropriate T cell receptor.

In man, the genetics of specific immune responsiveness has been approached investigating the statistical association of genetic markers with responsiveness to specific antigens/epitopes. HLA (human MHC) class II alleles are associated with the response to certain autoantigens (11, 12, 13) , to antigens from *Ascaris* and *Nematodes* (14, 15), and to

* Correspondence: Anna Ruffilli, International Institute of Genetics and Biophysics, CNR, via Marconi 10, 80125 Naples, Italy. Phone: +39 81-7257299; fax: +39 81-5936123; E-mail: Ruffilli@IIGBNA.IIGB.NA.CNR.IT

New Horizons in Allergy Immunotherapy
edited by Sehon et al. Plenum Press, New York, 1996

75

several allergens (16–22). It has also been shown that in the response to certain vaccines the production of protective levels of ab is associated with specific HLA class II haplotypes (23):

We report here the association of HLA DRB1* 1101/04 with the antibody response (IgG and IgE) to Par o 1, the 15KDa major pollen allergen from *Parietaria officinalis,* a weed which represent a major cause of allergy in Mediterranean Europe (24).

2. MATERIAL AND METHODS

The study population consisted of 99 Italian and 40 Spanish allergic patiens. Patient were informed volunteers. Allergy was documented by clinical history and by prick skin test (ST) positivity to at least one of a panel of 18 glycerinated extracts of common inhalant allergens (Hollister-Stier Laboratories). Par o 1 specific IgG and IgE ab levels were determined by the double antibody radioimmunoassay (DARIA) (25). Total IgE level was determined by radioimmunoassay (Pharmacia CAP system, Pharmacia, Upsala, Sweden).

DRB1* typimg was performed by oligotyping and in some cases refined using DNA heteroduplex analysis (26,27).

The associations were investigated by non-parametric (Yates-corrected χ^2) and parametric analysis (stepwise multiple regression).

3. RESULTS AND CONCLUSIONS

Table 1 reports some characteristics of the study population; Table 2 summarized the associations observed.

In the Italians, the alleles HLA-DRB1*1101/04 were positively associated with IgG and IgE antibody (ab) response to Par o 1. The association of DR11 with responsiveness to Par o 1 was confirmed in the Spanish study group (P=0.02, RR=4.0 for IgG ab response and P=0.002, RR=7 for IgE ab response).

In the Italians, DRB1*03 was significantly negatively associated with ab response (Table 2). This negative association was not confirmed in the Spanish. However it is possible that responsiveness was mediated by the codominant alleles as all the DR3 patients who were responders were also DR11 or DR1 (an allele which in the Spanish was significantly positively associated with ab response to *Par o* I), whereas none of the DR3 non responders had these alleles.

Twenty nine Italian patients were monosensitized to *Parietaria.* The proportion of DRB1*1101/04 in Par o 1 responders was higher in these patients than in *Parietaria* allergic patients who had multiple sensitivities (78 and 67% and 81 and 66% for IgG and IgE

Table 1. Study population

	Italians (N=99)		Spanish (N=40)	
	N	%	N	%
ST positive to Parietaria I	76	76	12	30
With IgG ab to *Par o* I	75	75	11	28
With IgE ab to *Par o* I	55	55	8	20

Table 2. Prevalence of HLA- DRB1*-1101/04 and -03 in the Italian study group.
Patients are subdivided in responders and non responders to *Par o* I

	Number of patients with DRB1*1101/04			Number of patients with DRB1*03		
	(%)	P[1]	P[2]	(%)	P[1]	P[2]
IgG ab response						
Responders (N=75)	55 (73)			4 (5)		
Non responders (N=29)	8 (30)			4 (17)	ns	ns
		0.0007	0.003			
IgE ab response						
Responders (N=56)	40 (71)			1 (2)		
Non responders (N=43)	4 (50)			7 (16)		
		ns	0.0012		0.024	0.012

P[1], P[2]: c2 and multiple regression analysis, respectively.

ab response, respectively). The relative risk of monosensitization to *Parietaria* associated with DR 1101/04 was 1.8. Total IgE levels were lower in monosensitized that in multisensitized patients (arithmetic mean 146 and 399 U/ml; respectively) whereas specific IgE levels were comparable (arithmetic means244 and 226 U/ml; respectively) The proportion of DRB1*1101/04 was increased (79%) also in group of 19 subjects who were IgG ab responders to Par o 1 but had undetectable levels of IgE ab and was 100% in a subset of this group consisting of 6 patients who were ST negative to *Parietaria*. It has been reported that the influence of HLA class II genotype on host responsiveness to the chironomid allergen Chi t 1 and to the birch allergen Bet v 1 is increased in monosensitized patients (19, 21). Taken toghether, these observations suggest that genetic abnormalities responsible for allergy in monosensitized patients may differ from those occurring in severe atopy, characterized by multiple sensitization and high total IgE levels: it is possible that in monosensitization the role played by cognate mechanisms in determining susceptibility is more relevant.

Further studies are needed to elucidate the biological mechanisms underlying statistical association. The negative association of responsiveness with HLA-DR3 may help to verify the current paradigmas. In particular, the hypothesis of determinant selection predicts that MHC controlled non responsiveness is genetically recessive; and that antigen presenting cells (APC) from non responders are unable to present the antigen to T cells from MHC-matched responders. Both predictions have been verified in some models (10), but not in others. For example it has been reported that low responsiveness to certain antigens is inherited as a dominant trait (28, 29) and more recently, in studies on the response to hepatitis B virus, it has been shown that APC from non responders can are functional for T lymphocytes from responders (30, 31).

ACKNOWLEDGMENTS

This study was performed in the framework of the multicenter genetic-epidemiological study HLA and Allergy, directed by DG. Marsh and of the HLA and Allergy Network of the European Science Foundation. We thank B. Bjorksten for the determination of total IgE levels and LR. Freidhoff for statistical analyses.

4. REFERENCES

1. Vaz NM., Phillips-Qagliata JM., Levine BR., Vaz EM. H2 linked genetic control of immune responsivenss to ovalbumin and ovomucoid. J. Exp. Med. 134: 1335–48, 1971.
2. Hill SW., Sercarz EE. Fine specificicy of the H2 linked immune response gene for the gallinaceous lysozime. Eur. J. Immunol. 5: 317–234, 1975.
3. Kennedy MW., Fraser EM., Christie JF. MHC classII (I-A) region control of the IgE repertoire to the ABA-1 allergen of the nematode *Ascaris*. Immunology 72: 577–79, 1991.
4. Kagnoff MF. Two genetic loci control the murine immune response to A-gliadin, a wheat protein that activates coeliac sprue. Nature 296: 158–60, 1982.
5. Milich DR., Leroux-Roels G., Louie R., Cisari FC. Genetic regulation of the immunre response to hepatitis B surface antigren (HBsAg). IV. Distinct H2 linked Ir genes control antibody response to different HBs Ag determinants on the same molecule and map to the I-A an I-C subregions. J. Exp. Med. 159: 41–56, 1984.
6. Manca F., Kunkl A., Fenoglio D., Fowler A.,Sercarz E., Celada F. Constraints in T-B cooperatrion related to epitope topology on *E. coli* β–galactosidase. Eur.:J. Immunol. 15: 345–50, 1985.
7. Lozner EC., Sachs DH., Sheare GM. Genetic control of the immune response to Staphylococcal nuclase. I. Control of the antibody response to nuclease by the Ir region of the mouse H-2 complex. J. Exp. Med. 139: 1204–08, 1974.
8. Berzofsky JA. Genetic control of the immune response to mammalian myoglobin in mice. I. More than one I-region gene in H2 control the antibody response. J. Immunol. 120: 360–69, 1979.
9. Riley RL., Wilson LD., German RN., Benjamin D. Immune response to complex protein antigens. I. MHC control of immune response to bovine albumin. J. Immunol. 129: 1553–59, 1982.
10. Berzofsky JA. Ir genes: antigen-specific genetic regulation of the immune response, in: Sela M. eds.: The antigens vol VII, 1987.
11. Shiels DC., Ratatnachiyavong S., McGregor AM., Collins A., Morton NE. Combined segregation and linkage analysis of Graves disease with a thyroid autoimmune diathesis. Am. J. Hum. Gen. 55: 540–44, 1994.
12. Neumuller J., Menzel J., Lillesi H. Prevalence ot HLA-DR3 and autoantibodies to connective tissue components in Dupuytren's contracture. Clin. Immunol. Immunopathol. 71: 142–48,1994.
13. Buyon JP., Slade SG., Reveille JD., Hamel JC., Chan EK. Autoantobody response to the native 52 kDa SS-A/Ro protein in neonatal *lupus erithematosus* and Sjogren's syndrome. J. Immunol. 192: 3679–84, 1994.
14. Tomlison LA., Christie JF., Fraser EM., Mc Laughin D., Mc Intoswh AE., Kennedy MW. MHC restriction of the ab repertoire to the secretory antigens and a major allergen, of the nematode parasite *Ascaris*. J. Immunol. 176: 2349–56, 1989.
15. Kennedy MW., Wassom DL., Mc Intosh AE., Thomas JC. H-2. H2 (I-A) control of the ab repertoire to the secreted antigens of *Trichinella spiralis* in infection and its relevance to resistance and susceptibility. Immunology 73: 36–43, 1991.
16. Marsh. DG. Immunogenetic and immunochemical factors determining immune responsiveness to allergens:studies in unrelated subjects. D.G. Marsh and MN. Blumenthal. Genetic factors in clinical and cnvironmental allergy. University of Minnesota Press, Minneapolis, 1990.
17. Lympany P., Kemeny DM., Welsh KI., Lee TH. An HLA associated non responsiveness to mellitin; a component of bee venom . J. Allergy Clin. Immunol. 86: 160–67, 1990.
18. Cardaba B.,Vilches C., Martin E., de Andres B., del Pozo V., Hernandez D., Gallardo S., Fernandez GC., Villalba M., Rodriguez R,, Basomba A., Kreisler M., Palomino P., Lahoz C. DR7 and DQ2 are positively associated with IgE response to the main allergen of olive pollen (*Ole e* I) in allergic patients. Human Immunol. 38: 2933–38, 1993.
19. Fischer GF., Pickl WF., Fae I., Ebner C., Ferreira F., Breiteneder H., Vikoukal E., Scheiner O., Kraft D.. Association between IgE response against *Bet v* I, the major allergen of birch pollen and HLA-DR alleles. Human Immunol. 33: 259–66, 1992.

20. Reid MJ., William AN., Whisman BA., Goetz DW., Hylander RD., Parker WA., Freeman TM. HLA-DR4 associated non responsiveness to mountain cedar allergen. J. Allergy Clin. Immunol. 89: 593–95, 1991.
21. Tautz C., Rihs H., Thiele A., Zwollo P., Freidhoff LR., Marsh DG., Baur X. Association of class II sequences encoding DR1 and DQ5 specificities with hypersensitivity to chironomid allergen *Chi t* I. J Allergy Clin. Immunol. 93: 918, 1994.
22. Sparholt S., Georgsen J., Madsen HO., Svendsen UG., Schou C. .Association between HLA DR3*0101 and immunoglobulin E responsiveness to *Bet v* I Hum. Immunol. 39:76–78, 1994
23. Grob PJ., Jilg W., Milne A., Townsend TR. Unresolved issues in hepatitis B immunization in: Viral hepatitis and Liver diseases, FB. Hollinger SM.Lemon and HS. Margolis eds. Williams and Wilkins, Baltimore, 1990.
24. Oreste U., Coscia MR., Scotto D'Abusco A., Santonastaso V., Ruffilli A. Purification and characterization of *Par o* I , the major allergen of *Parietaria officinalis* pollen. Int. Arch. Allergy Appl. Imunol. 96: 19–25, 1991.
25. . Platts-Mills TAE., Snajdr MJ., Ishizaka K., Frankland AW. Measurement of IgE antibody by antigen.binding assay; correlation with PK activity and IgG and IgA antibodies to allergens. J. Immunol.120: 1201–12, 1978 .
26. Kimura A., Dong RP., Harada H., Sasazuki T. DNA typing of HLA Class II genes in B-lymphoblastoid cell lines homozygous for HLA specific HLA class II alleles. Tissue Antigens 40: 5–10, 1992.
27. D'Amato M., Sorrentino R. A simple and economical DRB1 typing procedure combining group-specific amplification, DNA heteroduplex and enzyme restriction analysis. Tissue Antigens 43: 295–300, 1994.
28. Salazar M.,Deulofeut H.,Granja C., Deulofeut R., Yunis DE., Marcus-Bagley D., Awdeh Z. Alper CA., Yunis EJ. Normal HBs Ag presentation and T cell defect in the immune response of non responders. Immunogenetics 41:366–74, 1990.
29. Desombere I., Hauser P., Rossau R., Paradijs J., Leroux-Roels G. Non responders to hepatitis B vaccine can present envelope particles to T lymphocytes. J. Immunol. 134: 520–29, 1993.
30. Kanikawaji N., Fujisawa K., Yoshizumi H., Fukunaga M., Yasunami M., Kimura A., Nishimura Y., Sasazuki T. HLA-DQ-restricted T cells specific to streptococcal antigen present in low but not in high responders. J. Immunol. 146: 2560–67, 1991.
31. Haber J., Paradis G., Grinnel CM. Dominant low responsiveness nin the IgG response of mice o the complex protein as type 1 fimbriae from *Actinomyces viscous* T14V. J. Immunol. 146: 1949–54, 1991.

11

HLA-DR3 IS ASSOCIATED WITH THE IgE IMMUNE RESPONSIVENESS TO A RECOMBINANT ALLERGEN FROM *Blomia tropicalis* (BT)

L. Caraballo, B. Martínez, S. Jiménez, and L. Puerta

Institute of Immunological Research
University of Cartagena
Cartagena, Colombia

1. INTRODUCTION

Mite-induced asthma is the commonest form of allergic asthma (AA), being allergens from house dust mites important risk factors for suffering acute attacks. The "IgE-hyperresponsiveness to mite allergens" can be considered as a central phenotype of mite-induced AA. It is easily identifiable (patients' exposure to house dust, skin test (ST), RAST and mite-extract nasal and bronchial provocation) and is determinant of the pathogenesis of atopic asthma, including the generation of the bronchial inflammation that supports airways hyper responsiveness. According to the results of recent genetic linkage studies, overall IgE production in allergic diseases like asthma can be under the influence of genes located at chromosomes five and 11, while specific IgE responsiveness to several environmental allergens is supposed to be controlled by the Human Major Histocompatibility Complex (HLA) and genes coding for TCR. We showed previously that IgE hyper responsiveness to the mite *Dermatophagoides ssp.* in AA patients is HLA-linked (1). We have also found that the gene HLA-DPB1*0401 is remarkably absent (2) and HLA-DR3 is increased among mite-induced AA patients (3). The present work was done to investigate if these results were the same using a recombinant allergen from Bt.

2. SUBJECTS AND METHODS

Patients and controls belonged to the prevalent (mulattos) ethnic group in Cartagena (4). Ninety Five-Bt-induced asthmatics (41 men and 54 women, aged 18–54 years) and 89 non-allergic controls were included in the study. All patients had atopic symptoms related to house dust exposure and were allergic (ST and RAST) to Bt and *Dermatophagoides*

New Horizons in Allergy Immunotherapy
edited by Sehon et al. Plenum Press, New York, 1996

81

pteronyssinus (Dp), demonstrated by ST and RAST. Controls were ST and RAST-negative to these allergens. To ST with Bt an extract containing 0.23 mg/ml of protein in 50% glycerol, 0.125% sodium bicarbonate, 0.25 NaCl and 0.4% phenol was prepared. STs with the other allergens were performed with commercial, standardized allergen extracts (Miles Inc., Pharmaceutical Division). Total levels of IgE (determined using IgE PRIST - Pharmacia) were above 800 KU/L in all AA patients. IgE levels in controls, ranged between 80 and 300 KU/l. RAST for specific IgE to Dp and Df was done with an enzyme-immnunoassay (Phadezym RAST- Pharmacia). RAST for IgE antibodies to Bt was made, as described previously (5). The recombinant allergen (Bt1) was obtained from a cDNA library of Bt, representing at least one epitope of a major allergen (11–13 kD) of Bt (6, 7). IgE binding of sera to Bt1 was detected by plaque immunoassay. HLA was typed by PCR/non-radioactive/sequence specific oligonucleotide (SSO), following the protocol of the 11 International Histocompatibility Workshop. The set of DRB1 SSOs was able to define 45 specificities. Probes for HLA-DRB1were ddUTP-digoxigenine labeled. Autoradiography was done at room temperature with Kodak X-OMAT AR film.

3. RESULTS

Seventy per cent of patients were allergic only to mites. The other 30% showed allergy to only two additional allergens (*Aspergillus* and cockroach). In the group of patients, 40 (42%) had IgE antibodies to the recombinant allergen Bt1. Only 62 sera of the control group could be tested for IgE-binding to Bt1, so they were random selected. Among them, four were positive. When comparing the frequency of HLA-DRB1alleles between the two main groups, a weak positive association of AA with *0301 was found (p=0.05), which disappeared when the p value was corrected by the number of alleles. However, analyzing the distribution of HLA-DRB1*03 (including both *0301 and *0302 alleles) in the forty patients with IgE antibodies to Bt1 and the subgroup of 58 Bt1-IgE-negative controls, a stronger positive association was evident: 45% of patients were HLA-DRB1*03 while only 7% of controls had this allele (p = 0.01).

4. DISCUSSION

This study shows a positive association between HLA-DRB1*03 and the IgE immune responsiveness to a recombinant allergen from Bt, supporting previous works that suggest a relationship between HLA and AA. Both *0301 and *0302 are involved in this association. They seem to be acting like Ir genes, supporting the "IgE-hyperresponsiveness to mite allergen" phenotype. Comparing the polymorphic sequence of these alleles with others at the DRB1 locus, it is possible that residues 71–77 (KRGRVDN), located at the peptide-binding site of HLA-DRB1*03, may be involved in the presentation of peptides derived from the natural Bt allergen represented by the recombinant Bt1 molecule. Several *in vitro* experiments showed that T cell lines or clones are able to recognize mite-allergen-derived peptides in the context of various HLA-DR molecules, which suggest that in vivo, mite-allergen presentation is not restricted to only one HLA-DR allele. Thus, our results, based in the IgE specific immune response to a recombinant allergen, suggest the existence of some kind of hierarchy among HLA-DR molecules for presenting allergenic peptides. In this regard, it has been described recently that HLA-DR3 is also associated with specific IgE to inhaled hapten in acid anhydride workers with respiratory symptoms (8).

Since the IgE responsiveness to mite allergens is critical in the pathogenesis of AA, more studies are required to establish the role of such genes. In this sense, the study of other HLA loci, as well as genes involved in antigen processing is under way in our laboratory. In addition, the use of recombinant allergens to determine the IgE specificity will be very useful to accomplish this work.

5. REFERENCES

1. CARABALLO L, HERNANDEZ M: HLA Haplotype segregation in families with allergic asthma. Tissue Antigens 335:182–186. 1990
2. CARABALLO L, MARRUGO J, JIMENEZ S, ANGELINI G, FERRARA GB: frecuency of DPB1*0401 is significantly decrease in patients with Allergic Asthma in mulatto population. Hum Immunol. 32:157–161. 1991
3. CARABALLO L, PUERTA L, JIMENEZ S, MARTINEZ B, MORENO L. An immunogenetic study of the IgE responsiveness to allergens of Blomia tropicalis (Bt) in patients with allergic asthma. (Abstract) J Allergy Clin Immunol 91:335. 1993
4. CARABALLO L, MARRUGO J, ERLICH H, PASTORIZO M: HLA antigens in the population of Cartagena (Colombia). Tissue Antigens. 39:128–133. 1992
5. PUERTA L, FERNANDEZ-CALDAS E, CARABALLO L, LOCKEY R: Sensitization to Blomia tropicalis and Lepidoglyphus destructor in Dermatophagoides spp. Allergic individuals. J Allergy Clin Immunology. 88:943–950. 1991
6. CARABALLO L, AVJIOUGLU A, MARRUGO J, MARSH D. Sequence and immunological studies on a cDNA clone of Blomia tropicalis. (Abstract) J Allergy Clin Immunol 93:205. 1994
7. CARABALLO L, PUERTA L, MARTINEZ B, MORENO L. Identification of allergens from the mite Blomia tropicalis. Clin Exp Allergy 24:1056–1060. 1994
8. YOUNG RP, BARKER RD, PILE KD, et al. The association of HLA-DR3 with specific IgE to inhaled acid anhydrides. Am J Respir Crit Care Med 151:219–221. 1995

12

RECOMBINANT ALLERGENS FOR IMMUNOTHERAPY

W. R. Thomas

Institute for Child Health Research
GPO Box 855
West Perth
Western Australia 6872
Fax: (61) (9) 388 3414

INTRODUCTION

Starting with Der p 1 (1, 2) from the mite and Dol m 5 (3) from the hornet the u-biquitous allergens are rapidly being cloned. These include Bet v 1, 2 and 3 from birch (4–6) and the allergens from related trees, the group 1 and 5 allergens from timothy (7, 8) and perennial rye (9–11) and group 5/9 from Kentucky blue grass (12, 13). The two chains of the cat Fel d 1 were cloned early (14) and as well as Amb a 1, 2 and 5 from ragweed (15–17). Cockroach (18) and mould allergens (19) are being investigated. Cloning of mite allergens has now been performed in *D. pteronyssinus, D. farinae, Euroglyphus maynei, Blomia tropicalis* and *Lepidoglyphus destructor*. DNA encoding the 7 groups of named mite allergens (20) has now been cloned as well as from further allergens from *D farinae* (21, 22) and *D.pteronyssinus* (23). Allergens have been cloned using data from immunochemical studies or by using IgE-immunoassay to screen phage plaque-libraries. This has identified clones producing both known or previously unrecognised allergens.

The sequence data has provided a precise definition of the allergens and a basis for understanding cross reactivity amongst species. Many allergens have been synthesised as recombinant proteins with much of their natural IgE-binding activity and can be used for evaluating the rank importance of allergens T-cell and antibody-binding activity. It has however been an early ambition that the recombinant allergens will provide a basis for improving immunotherapy using the recombinant allergens or synthetic allergens produced from their sequence information. The scope for using synthetic allergens includes not only their use a substitute for the current extracts where they could provide standardised and effective concentration of the important allergens but also includes novel reagents such as peptides. Because despite some shortcomings immunotherapy is frequently a successful procedure (24) it could be used as one basis for further developments. It should be remem-

New Horizons in Allergy Immunotherapy
edited by Sehon et al. Plenum Press, New York, 1996

bered that improvement in clinical symptoms has no relationship with decreases in serum IgE-antibody levels which may even be elevated and only an approximate association with increased IgG production (25).

NUMBER OF ALLERGENS TO CLONED

Allergic sensitisation judging by IgE-binding is often directed to 1 or 2 components. Thus for birch 97% of allergic patients react with Bet v 1 where it is the only specificity in 60% (26) and absorptions show it accounts for almost the entire antigenic activity. It has been reported that over 60% of anti cat specifities in most sera can be accounted for by anti Fel d 1 (27) and that 90% of binding to ragweed extracts is to Amb a 1 (28). Over 60% of antibodies to timothy grass can be absorbed out by a mixture of Phl p 1 and 5 (7). For the mite it has been recognised that 50–60% of the IgE binding can be accounted for by reactivity to Der p 1 and 2 and that these allergens have reactivity to IgE in 80% of patients (29, 30). Meyer *et al* (31) showed using a pool of sera from 17 Der p 1 and 2 positive patients that absorption with Der p 1 and 2 removed virtually all the IgE binding activity. The allergen Der p 3 which has now been cloned (32) has a similar frequency of reactivity but often to a lower degree (33) and Der p 4, 5 (34, 35) and 7 (36) as well glutathione transferase (23) show reactivity to about 50% of sera. A comparison with the results of IgE Western blotting (37) suggests that these as well as a 95–100 kD component (possibly glucoamylase, Stewart unpublished) constitute all the important specificities. Another aspect is the development of the allergic response. It has been shown by O'Brien and Thomas and by Shibasaki *et al* (38, 39) that children have their predominant response to the major allergens.

The question with respect to immunotherapy is whether or not allergic responses can be altered by changing the type of immune response to only some key allergens or whether reactivity to all specificities needs to decreased. Experiments with animals indicate that immune responses can be suppressed or deviated by lymphokine secretion and hence cross regulation could be achieved without all specificities (40). Thus responses to the entire Fel d 1 molecule can be inhibited by the subcutaneous injection of a peptide containing only some of the T-cell epitopes (41) and the administration of a Der p 1 peptide by the oral or intranasal route inhibits the ability of the whole allergen to immunise mice not only to the epitope on the peptide but also to epitopes elsewhere in the molecule (42, 43). Data has also been obtained to show that mice made unresponsive to Der p 1 by feeding a peptide containing one of the T-cell epitopes will not respond to ovalbumin if it is presented at the same time as Der p 1.

Some studies have not supported this concept. Østerballe who administered a mixture of 3 purified timothy grass allergens for immunotherapy found that the only patients who improved clinically over the 3 years of the study were those whose IgE binding was restricted to the purified allergens (44). Norman *et al* did find clinical improvement with purified Amb a 1 but it was less effective than the whole extract (45). The ineffectiveness of these trials may be because higher doses are required and for the timothy which lacked Phl p 1 that further allergens were necessary. More recent reports on the treatment of cat-allergic patients with peptides based on Fel d 1, communicated at the 1994 meeting of the American Academy of Allergy and Immunology did show that clinical improvement despite the fact that patients typically recognise components other than the Fel d 1. Perhaps significantly it was the higher dose groups which gave improvement.

T-CELL REACTIVITY TO PEPTIDES AND MODIFIED ALLERGENS FOR IMMUNOTHERAPY

The mechanism of current immunotherapy is not known. Although it may be accomplished without altering IgE, these antibodies do mediate the immediate release of vasoactive amines and lipid mediators from mast cells and basophils as well as help to initiate later reactions via the cytokine cascade. Peptides or modified allergens which lack serological activity but can alter immune responses by interactions with T cells are likely candidates for immunotherapeutics. It may not only be possible to achieve high doses with few side effects but they may also be presented different types of antigen presenting cells and be accompanied by different bystander and regulatory signals.

Many recombinant allergens are synthesised by bacteria as polypeptides with high IgE-binding activity but as shown for studies with Der p 1 and 2 often only very large peptides have appreciable serological reactivity (46, 47). Some IgE binding has been found for synthetic peptides from these molecules but as documented for it Der p 2 is small (48) and if the peptides do not aggregate would be monovalent and unable to cross-link IgE. Rogers *et al* have successfully produced unresponsiveness in mice using a large recombinant peptide of Fel d 1 made by shuffling the T-cell epitopes (49).

The thinking to date has been to screen patients usually using T-cell clones or lines for reactivity to an overlapping panel of peptides in order to locate the immunodominant CD4 T-cell epitopes and to use these for immunotherapy. The experiments with Fel d 1 and Der p 1 in mice show that these epitopes can indeed induce unresponsive and in the case of intranasal Der p 1 peptide, a peptide with a single epitope inhibited responses to reimmunisation of primed mice with the whole allergen. The clinical trial with the Fel d 1 peptides indicates that this may also occur in humans. A strategy for the outbred humans would therefore be to identify a mixture of peptides designed so each patient responds to at least one epitope. The data published for Der p 2 shows this can be done with peptides from 2 or 3 regions (50) and Der p 1 shows a very interesting concentration of T-cell epitopes in the region 105–133. This was first noted from T-cell clones in two laboratories (51, 52). Several clones reacted to peptides mapped to this region and in the study of Higgins *et al* this was despite the fact that the peptides were recognised by different restriction elements, either DP or DR (53).

We have investigated the human T-cell epitopes of Der p 1 using polyclonal proliferative assays. The lymphocyte culture has been performed in serum free medium, initially to avoid variations associated with different batches of serum but then because it was recognised that enhanced responses could be obtained (54) including large responses to peptides in both normal and mite-allergic people. The statistical difference between T-cell stimulation of allergic and non-allergic patients was not noted as found in previous studies (55, 56). Variations in the efficiency of culture may be important because O'Brien *et al* found 30% of the allergic patients did not respond to Der p 1 or Der p 2 and there was considerable overlap between allergic and non-allergic. Also the later study by O'Brien and Thomas which compared anti Der p 1 and 2 antibodies with T-cell stimulation the purified allergen found that patients not infrequently had large T-cell stimulation in the absence of detectable IgE antibody (39). Using the serum free medium it has been possible to reliably measure polyclonal T-cell proliferations to series of 19-mer peptides overlapping by 5 residues. To date 5/8 have had major reactivities to peptides in the region 105–133 and 4/8 to peptide 60–88. The 105–133 central region of Der p 1 by analogy to the X-ray crystallographic structure of the homologues papain and actinidin and by recent molecular modelling is known to form a flexible loop connecting the 2 globular domains of the molecule (57, 58). It is therefore may have a selective advantage in binding to MHC molecules before processing. It is also an area of high sequence variation and antigenicity amongst mite species (59–61).

The strategies above concentrate on the immunodominant CD4 epitopes. Experimental studies have shown that immunoregulation is , especially in the case of oral an inhalation tolerance, mediated by CD 8+ T cells which are presumable class I restricted (62–64). It has been reported that people undergoing immunotherapy for hay fever have CD8+ T cells which inhibit proliferative responses and IgE production *in vitro*. More recently it has been reported that T cells with γ δ T cell receptors can mediate inhalation tolerance (65) and could provide another avenue of immunotherapy particularly since at least in some cases they are restricted by nonpolymorphic antigen presenting molecules. The T-cell epitopes which are revealed by studying responses to peptides of people exposed to allergens or immunised animals is a measure of the immunodominant epitopes not the complete number of epitopes that can be recognised. By way of illustration we have found 2 cryptic or sub-dominant epitopes for the response of mice to both Der p 1 and 2 (43, 66) by immunising mice with individual peptides. Mice immunised with these epitopes produce T cells which respond not only to the peptide but also to the whole allergen. It was then shown that oral tolerance to the whole allergen could be induced by feeding fusion peptides containing the cryptic epitopes (43). Studies on oral tolerance in experimental autoimmune encephalomyelitis have shown a discrepancy between peptides which induce tolerance and those which induce autoimmunity (67).

ALLERGEN POLYMORPHISMS

The sequence information from cloning allergens quickly revealed that most allergens consisted of mixtures of products from gene families or products of allelic variation. The Amb a 1 for example consists of 4 isoallergens with 73–89% homology apparently from different genes and each isoallergen consists of several variants (68). The Amb a 2 allergen is in fact an isoallergen of Amb a 1 sharing 70% homology. The grass group allergens also have multiple members with about 70% homology in the group 5/9 family (8, 13) and minor variants have been found for the group 1 (10, 11). Some variants of tree allergen has been found (69–71). The Fel d 1 chain 1 has been found to have minor variations and the chain two has more frequent polymorphism with one clone showing 7 variant out of the 92 amino acids (72). The protein sequence of the cat allergen isolated from dust and pelts however corresponds to the major sequence found by cloning. For the house dust mite each clone described to date for the group 1 (73) and 2 (74, 75) has had minor differences with each differing by 1–4 residues. The relationship of the variants to the allergen predominant in extracts and in environment is not well known but Nishiyama *et al* were able to detect a variant in extracts by HPLC and peptide analysis (76). For Der p 1 clones from commercial mites 6 positions have shown to vary with one substitution for each variant, in 5 of the cases to a residue known to be in Der f 1. There does not as yet appear to any association between the presence of any of the substitution so it feasible that all possible combinations of the substitutions may exist. Species variations or cross reactivities are well known for most allergens including trees, grass, different species of ragweed and mites. They pose two questions. Can immunotherapy be effective with a single formulation for the cross reacting allergens and if not are the diagnostic methods available to distinguish the different allergies. The mite allergens provide a good example because several species can coexist in the same locality or house. The allergens group 1 allergens of *D. pteronyssinus, D. farinae* and *E. maynei* (57, 60, 61) are about 80% homologous while the group 2 from *D. pteronyssinus* and *D. farinae* are 88% (57, 75, 77). Homologies for the group 3 and 7 are 80% and 86% (unpublished). Although they cross react serologically it is not clear if this is reflected at the T-cell level. Our studies with Der p 1 and Der p 2 have shown T-cell proliferation to both allergens in polyclonal assays although to lesser degree with Der f 1 reflecting the fact that the place of the study Western Australia does not have *D. farinae* (78). The responses to Der p 2 and Der f 2 were indistinguishable correlating with the closer homology of these 2 allergens. To look at cross reactivity more closely, proliferations were performed with a set of overlapping peptides from Der p 1 and from Eur m 1 because this species is found in Western Australia often at-risk levels (78). It was reasoned that the pattern of peptide recognition would give a clearer idea of which species was giving the primary sensitisation and which structures were cross reactive. In the results so far show that 2/8 people responded preferentially to peptides of Eur m 1. One allergic person responded to 170–188 of Eur m 1 with no response to the Der p 1 equivalent and to the 105–133 peptides with only a small response to the Der p 1 equivalents although peptide 65–83 of the two allergens were recognised equally well. There is notable only a single amino acid difference in the last peptides but these are multiple changes in the others. The second patient responded only to 2 Eur m 1 peptides and not Der p 1 peptides but curiously responded well to affinity purified Der p 1 suggesting the presence of unknown polymorphisms or possibly that the 19 mer peptides were not detecting all epitopes. The 6 other responders recognised Der p 1 peptides with a small but detectable response to the Eur m 1 equivalent. Clearly clonal studies would be of interest. Finally one individual responded strongly to the peptide 45–60 when it had tyrosine in position 50 but had no response to the same region when it contained the alternate histidine residue found in several cDNA clones. This person also responded to other epitopes not known to contain polymorphic residues.

ACKNOWLEDGMENTS

This work was supported by the National Health and Medical Research Council, The Asthma Foundation of Western Australia and ImmuLogic Pharmaceutical Corporation.

REFERENCES

1. Thomas, W.R., G.A. Stewart, R.J. Simpson, K.Y. Chua, T.M. Plozza, R.J. Dilworth, A. Nisbet, and K.J. Turner. 1988. Cloning and expression of DNA coding for the major house dust mite allergen *Der p* I in Escherichia coli. *Int Arch Allergy Appl Immunol.* 85:127–9.
2. Chua, K.Y., G.A. Stewart, W.R. Thomas, R.J. Simpson, R.J. Dilworth, T.M. Plozza, and K.J. Turner. 1988. Sequence analysis of cDNA coding for a major house dust mite allergen, *Der p* I. Homology with cysteine proteases. *J Exp Med.* 167:175–82.
3. Fang, K.S.F., M. Vitale, P. Fehlner, and T.P. King. 1988. cDNA cloning and primary structure of a white-faced hornet venom allergen. *Proc Natl Acad Sci.* 85:895–899.
4. Seiberler, S., O. Scheiner, D. Kraft, D. Lonsdale, and R. Valenta. 1994. Characterization of a birch pollen allergen, Bet v III, representing a novel class of Ca2+ binding proteins: specific expression in mature pollen and dependence of patients' IgE binding on protein-bound Ca2+. *EMBO.* 13:3481–6.
5. Valenta, R., M. Duchene, K. Pettenburger, C. Sillaber, P. Valent, P. Bettelheim, M. Breitenbach, H. Rumpold, D. Kraft, and O. Scheiner. 1991. Identification of profilin as a novel pollen allergen; IgE-autoreactivity in sensitized individuals. *Science.* 253:557–58.

6. Breiteneder, H., K. Pettenburger, A. Bito, R. Valenta, D. Kraft, H. Rumpold, O. Scheiner, and M. Breitenbach. 1989. The gene coding for the major birch pollen allergen *Bet v*1, is highly homologous to a pea disease resistance response gene. *Embo J.* 8:1935–8.

7. Laffer, S., S. Vrtala, M. Duchene, R. van Ree, D. Kraft, O. Scheiner, and R. Valenta. 1994. IgE-binding capacity of recombinant timothy grass (Phleum pratense) pollen allergens. *J Allergy Clin Immunol.* 94:88–94.

8. Vrtala, S., W.R. Sperr, I. Reimitzer, R. van Ree, S. Laffer, W.D. Muller, P. Valent, K. Lechner, H. Rumpold, and D. Kraft. 1993. cDNA cloning of a major allergen from timothy grass (Phleum pratense) pollen; characterization of the recombinant Phl pV allergen. *J Immunol.* 151:4773–81.

9. Singh, M.B., T. Hough, P. Theerakulpisut, A. Avjioglu, S. Davies, P.M. Smith, P. Taylor, R.J. Simpson, L.D. Ward, J. McCluskey, R. Puy, and R.B. Knox. 1991. Isolation of cDNA encoding a newly identified major allergenic protein of rye-grass pollen: Intracellular targeting to the amyloplast. *Proc Natl Acad Sci USA.* 88:1384–8.

10. Perez, M., G.Y. Ishioka, L.E. Walker, and R.W. Chesnut. 1990. cDNA cloning and immunological charaterisation of the rye grass allergen *Lol p I*. *J. Biol. Chem.* 265:16210–15.

11. Griffith, I.J., P.M. Smith, J. Pollock, P. Theerakulpisut, A. Avjioglu, S. Davis, T. Hough, M.B. Singh, R.J. Simpson, L.D. Ward, and R.B. Knox. 1991. Cloning and sequencing of *Lol p* I, the major allergenic protein of rye-grass pollen. *FEBS Letters.* 279:210–15.

12. Mohapatra, S.S., R. Hill, J. Astwood, A.K. Ekramoddoullah, E. Olsen, A. Silvanovitch, T. Hatton, F.T. Kisil, and A.H. Sehon. 1990. Isolation and characterization of a cDNA clone encoding an IgE-binding protein from Kentucky bluegrass (Poa pratensis) pollen. *Int Arch Allergy Appl Immunol.* 91:362–8.

13. Silvanovitch, A., J. Astwood, L. Zang, E. Olsen, F. Kisil, A. Sehon, S.S. Mohapatra, and R.D. Hill. 1991. Nucleotide sequence analysis of three *Poa p IX* isoallergens of Kentucky bluegrass pollen. *J. Biol. Chem.* 266:1204–10.

14. Morgenstern, J.P., I.J. Griffith, A.W. Brauer, B.L. Rogers, J.F. Bond, M.D. Chapman, and M.C. Kuo. 1991. Amino acid sequence of *Fel d* I, the major allergen of the domestic cat: Protein sequence analysis and cDNA cloning. *Poc Natl Acad Sci USA.* 88:9690–94.

15. Rafnar, T., I.J. Griffith, M. Kuo, J.F. Bond, B.L. Rogers, and D.G. Klapper. 1991. Cloning of *Amb a I* (Antigen E), the major allergen family of short Ragweed pollen. *J Biol Chem.* 266:1229–36.

16. Rogers, B.L., J.P. Morgenstern, I.J. Griffith, X. Yu, C.M. Counsell, A.W. Brauer, T.P. King, R.D. Garman, and M. Kuo. 1991. Complete sequence of the allergen *Amb a* II. Recombinant expression and reactivity with T cells from Ragweed allergic patients. *J Immunol.* 147:2547–52.

17. Ghosh, B., M.P. Perry, and D.G. Marsh. 1991. Cloning the cDNA encoding the *Amb t* V allergen from giant ragweed (*Ambrosia tridida*). *Gene.* 101:231–8.

18. Chapman, M.D. 1993. Dissecting cockroach allergens. *Clin Exp Allergy.* 23:459–61.

19. Vijay, H.M., in *Recent Trends in Aerobiology, Allergy and Immunology* S.N. Agashe, Eds. (Oxford and IBH Publishing Co, New Dehli, 1994) pp. 247–77.

20. King, T.P., D. Hoffman, H. Løwenstein, D.G. Marsh, T.A.E. Platts-Mills, and W.R. Thomas. 1994. Allergen nomenclature. *Int Arch Allergy Immunol.* 105:224–233.

21. Aki, T., K. Ono, P. Soon-Young, T. Wada, T. Jyo, S. Shigeta, Y. Murooka, and S. Oka. 1994. Cloning and characterization of cDNA coding for a new allergen from the house dust mite, *Dermatophagoides farinae.* *Int Arch Allergy Immunol.* 103:349–56.

22. Aki, T., A. Fujikawa, T. Wada, T. Jyo, S. Shigeta, Y. Murooka, S. Oka, and K. Ono. 1994. Cloning and expression of cDNA coding for a new allergen from the house dust mite, *Dermatophagoides farinae*: homology with human heat shock cognate proteins in the heat shock protein 70 family. *J Biochem.* 115:435–40.

23. O'Neill, G., G.R. Donovan, and B.A. Baldo. 1994. Identification of a major allergen of the house dust mite, Dermatophagoides pteronyssinus, homologous with glutathione-S-transferase. *Biochim Biophys Acta.* 1219:521–524.

24. Bousquet, J. 1994. Specific immunotherapy in asthma: Is it effective? *J Allergy Clin immunol.* 94:1–11.

25. Norman, P.S. 1980. An overview of immunotherapy: Implications for the future. *J Allergy Clin Immunol.* 65:87–96.

26. Ipsen, H., and H. Løwenstein. 1983. Isolation and immunochemical charaterisation of the major allergen of birch pollen (*Betula verrucosa*). *J Allergy Clin Immunol.* 72:150–159.

27. Schou, C. 1993. Defining allergens of mammalian origin. *Clin Exp Allergy.* 23:7–14.

28. King, T.P. 1976. Chemical and biological properties of atopic allergens. *Adv Immunol.* 23:77–105.

29. Chapman, M.D., and T.A.E. Platts-Mills. 1980. Purification and characterization of the major allergen from *Dermatophagoides pteronyssinus*-antigen P_1. *J Immunol.* 125:587–92.

30. Van der Zee, J.S., P. van Swieten, H.M. Jansen, and R.C. Aalberse. 1988. Skin tests and histamine release with P1-depleted Dermatophagoides pteronyssinus body extracts and purified P1. *J Allergy Clin Immunol.* 81:884–95.

31. Meyer, C.H., J.F. Bond, M. Chen, and M.T. Kasaian. 1994. Comparison of the levels of the major allergens *Der p I* and *Der p II* in standardised extract of the house dust mite, *Dermatophagoides pteronyssinus*. *Clin Exp Allergy.* 24:1041–48.

32. Smith, P.M., M.B. Singh, and R.B. Knox, in *Molecular biology and immunology of allergens* D. Kraft, A. Sehon, Eds. (CRC Press, Boca Raton, 1993) pp. 157–160.

33. Stewart, G.A., L.D. Ward, R.J. Simpson, and P.J. Thompson. 1992. The group III allergen from the house dust mite *Dermatophagoides pteronyssinus* is a trypsin-like enzyme. *Immunology.* 75:29–35.

34. Tovey, E.R., M.C. Johnson, A.L. Roche, G.S. Cobon, and B.A. Baldo. 1989. Cloning and sequencing of a cDNA expressing a recombinant house dust mite protein that binds human IgE and corresponds to an important low molecular weight allergen :published erratum appears in J Exp Med 1990 Apr 1;171(4):1387:. *J Exp Med.* 170:1457–62.

35. Lin, K.L., K.Y. Chua, W.R. Thomas, B.L. Chiang, and K.H. Hsieh. 1994. Characterisation of *Der p V* allergen. cDNA analysis and IgE-mediated reactivity to the recombinant protein. *J Allergy Clin Immunol.* 94:989–996.

36. Shen, H.D., K.Y. Chua, K.L. Lin, K.H. Hsieh, and W.R. Thomas. 1993. Molecular cloning of a house dust mite allergen with common antibody binding specificities with multiple components in mite extracts. *Clin Exp Allergy.* 23:934–40.

37. Tovey, E.R., and B.A. Baldo. 1987. Comparison by electroblotting of IgE-binding components in extracts of house dust mite bodies and spent mite culture. *J Allergy Clin Immunol.* 79:93–102.

38. Shibasaki, M., S. Isoyama, and H. Takita. 1994. Influence of age on IgE responsiveness to *Dermatophagoides farinae*: An immunoblot study. *Int Arch Allergy Immunol.* 103:53–58.

39. O'Brien, R.M., and W.R. Thomas. 1994. Immune reactivity to *Der p* I and *Der p* II in house dust mite sensitive patients attending paediatric and adult allergy clinics. *Clin Exp Allergy.* 24:737–42.

40. Miller, A., O. Lider, and H.L. Weiner. 1991. Antigen-driven bystander suppression after oral administration of antigens. *J Exp Med.* 174:791–98.

41. Briner, T.J., M.C. Kuo, K.M. Keating, B.L. Rogers, and J.L. Greenstein. 1993. Peripheral T cell tolerance reduced in naive and primed mice by subcutaneous injection of peptides from the major□ cat allergen, Fel d I. *Proc Nat Acad Sci.* 90:7609–12.

42. Hoyne, G.F., R.E. O'Hehir, D.C. Wraith, W.R. Thomas, and J.R. Lamb. 1993. Inhibition of T-cell and antibody responses to house dust mite allergen by inhalation or the dominant epitope in naive and sensitised mice. *J Exp Med.* 178:1783–88.

43. Hoyne, G.F., Callow, M.G., Kuo, M-C. & Thomas, W.R. 1994. Inhibition of T-cell responses by feeding peptides containing major and cryptic epitopes: studies with the *Der p I* allergen. *Immunology.* 83:190–95.

44. Osterballe, O. 1982. Immunotherapy with grass pollen major allergens. Clinical results from a prospective 3-year double blind study. *Allergy.* 37:379–388.

45. Norman, P.S., W.L. Winkenwerder, and L.M. Lichtenstein. 1968. Immunotherapy of hayfever with ragweed antigen E: Comparison with whole pollen extract and placebos. *J Allergy.* 42:93–108.

46. Greene, W.K., J.G. Cyster, K.Y. Chua, R.M. O'Brien, and W.R. Thomas. 1991. IgE and IgG binding of peptides expressed from fragments of cDNA encoding the major house dust mite allergen Der p I. *J Immunol.* 147:3768–73.

47. Chua, K.Y., W.K. Greene, P. Kehal, and W.R. Thomas. 1991. IgE binding studies with large peptides expressed from *Der p* II cDNA constructs. *Clin Exp Allergy.* 21:161–166.

48. Van't Hof, W., P.C. Driedijk, M. Van den Berg, A.G. Beck-Sickinger, G. Jung, and R.C. Aalberse. 1991. Epitope mapping of the Dermatophagoides pteronyssinus house dust mite major allergen Der p II using overlapping synthetic peptides. *Mol Immunol.* 28:1225–32.

49. Rogers, B.L., J.L. Bond, S.J. Craig, A.K. Nault, D.B. Segal, J.P. Morgenstern, M. Chen, C.B. Bizinkauskas, C.M. Counsell, A.M. Lussier, T. Luby, M. Kuo, T.J. Briner, and R.D. Garman. 1994. Potential therapeutic recombinant proteins comprised of peptides containing recombined T cell epitoopes. Mol Immunol. 31:955–66.

50. O'Hehir, R.E., A. Verhoef, E. Panagiotopoulou, S. Keswani, J.D. Hayball, W.R. Thomas, and J.R. Lamb. 1993. Analysis of human T cell responses to the group II allergen of *Dermatophagoides* species : Localisation of major antigenic sites. *J Allergy Clin Immunol.* 92:105–33.

51. Yssel, H., K.E. Johnson, P.V. Schneider, J. Wideman, A. Terr, R. Kastelein, and J.E. De Vries. 1992. T cell activation inducing epitopes of the house dust mite allergen Der p I. Proliferation and lymphokine production patterns by Der p I-specific CD4+ T cell clones. *J Immunol.* 148:738–45.

52. O'Hehir, R.E., G.F. Hoyne, W.R. Thomas, and J.R. Lamb. 1993. House dust mite allergy:from T cell epitopes to immunotherapy. *Europ J Clin Invest.* 23:763–72.

53. Higgins, J.E., C.J. Thorpe, R.E. Hayball, J.R.J.D. Lamb, and O'Hehir. 1994. Overlapping T-cell epiopes in the group I allergen of *Dermatophagoides* species restricted by HLA-DP and HLA-DR class II molecules. *J Allergy Clin Immunol.* 93:891–99.

54. Upham, J.W., B.J. Holt, M.J. Baron-Hay, A. Yabuhara, B.J. Hales, W.R. Thomas, R.K.S. Loh, P. O'Keefe, L. Palmer, P. Le Souef, P.D. Sly, P.R. Burton, B.W.S. Robinson, and P.G. Holt. 1995. Allergen-specific T-cell reactivity is detecable in close to 100% of atopic and normal individuals: covert responses are unmasked by serum-free medium. *Clin Exp Allergy.*

55. O'Brien, R.M., W.R. Thomas, and A.M. Wootton. 1992. T cell responses to the purified major allergens from the house dust mite Dermatophagoides pteronyssinus. *J Allergy Clin Immunol.* 89:1021–31.

56. Rawle, F.C., E.B. Mitchell, and T.A.E. Platts-Mills. 1984. T-cell response to the major allergen from the house dust mite, *Dermatophagoides pteronyssinus*, antigen P1: comparison of patients with asthma, atopic dermatitis and perennial rhinitis. *J Immunol.* 133:195–201.

57. Thomas, W.R., and K.Y. Chua, in *Molecular Biology and Immunology of Allergens* D. Kraft, Eds. (CRC Press, Boca Raton, 1992) pp. 21–29.

58. Topham, C.M., N. Srinivasan, C.J. Thorpe, H. Overington, and N.A. Kalsheker. 1994. Comparative modelling of major house dust mite allergen *Der p* I: structure validation using an extended environmental amino acid propensity table. *Protein Engineering.* 7:869–94.

59. Greene, W.K., K.Y. Chua, G.A. Stewart, and W.R. Thomas. 1990. Antigenic analysis of group I house dust mite allergens using random fragments of Der p I expressed by recombinant DNA libraries. *Int Arch Allergy Appl Immunol.* 92:30–8.

60. Dilworth, R.J., K.Y. Chua, and W.R. Thomas. 1991. Sequence analysis of cDNA coding for a major house dust mite allergen, Der f I. *Clin Exp Allergy.* 21:25–32.

61. Kent, N.A., M.R. Hill, J.N. Keen, P.W.H. Holland, and B.J. Hart. 1992. Molecular characterisation of group I allergen Eur m I from house dust mite Euroglyphus maynei. *Int Arch Allergy Appl Immunol.* 99:150–152.

62. Kemeny, D.M., and D. Diaz-Sanchez. 1993. The role of CD8+ T cells in the regulation of IgE. *Clin Exp Allergy.* 23:466–470.

63. McMenamin, C., and P.G. Holt. 1993. The natural immune response to inhaled soluble protein antigens involves major histocompatibility (MHC) class I resticted CD8+ T cell mediated butMHC class II dependent immune deviation resulting in selective suppression of immunoglobulain E production. *J Exp Med.* 178:889–99.

64. Renz, H., G. Lack, J. Saloga, R. Schwinzer, K. Bradley, J. Loader, A. Kupfer, G.L. Larsen, and E.W. Gelfand. 1994. Inhibition of IgE production and normaalisation of airways responsiveness by sensitized CD8 T cells in a mouse model of allergen sensitization. *J Immunol.* 152.

65. McMenamin, C., C. Pim, M. McKellar, and P.G. Holt. 1994. Regulation of IgE responses to inhaled antigen by antigen specific gamma delta T cells. *Science.* 265:1869–71.

66. Hoyne, G.F., M.G. Callow, M.-C. Kuo, and W.R. Thomas. 1993. Characterisation of T cell responses to the house dust mite allergen Der p II in mice. Evidence for major and cryptic epitopes. *Immunology.* 78:65–73.

67. Higgins, P.J., and H.L. Weiner. 1988. Suppression of experimental autoimmune encephalomyelitis by oral administration of myelin basic protein and its fragments. *J Immunol.* 144:441–45.

68. Griffith, I.J., J. Pollock, D.G. Klapper, B.L. Rogers, and A.K. Nault. 1991. Sequence polymorphism of *Amb a* I and *Amb a* II, the major allergens in *Ambrosia artemisiifolia* (Short Ragweed). *Int Arch Allergy Appl Immunol.* 96:296–304.

69. Laemmli, U.K. 1970. Cleavage of structural proteins during the assembly of the head of bacteriophage T4. *Nature.* 227:680–82.

70. Larsen, J.N., P. Stroman, and H. Ipsen. 1992. PCR based cloning and sequencing of isogenes encoding the tree pollen major allergen *Car b* I from *Carpinus betulis*, Hornbeam. *Mol Immunol.* 29:703–11.

71. Breiteneder, H., F. Ferreira, K. Hoffmann-Sommergruber, C. Ebner, M. Breitenbach, H. Rumpold, D. Kraft, and O. Scheiner. 1993. Four recombinant isoforms of *Cor a* I, the major allergen of hazel pollen, show different IgE-binding properties. *Eur J Biochem.* 212:355–62.

72. Griffith, I.J., S. Craig, J. Pollock, X. Yu, J.P. Morgenstern, and B.L. Rogers. 1992. Expression and genomic structure of the genes encoding *Fel d* I, the major allergen from the domestic cat. *Gene.* 113:263–68.

73. Chua, K.Y., P.K. Kehal, and W.R. Thomas. 1993. Sequence polymorphisms of cDNA clones encoding the mite allergen *Der p* I. *Int Arch Allergy Appl Immunol.* 101:364–68.

74. Thomas, W.□., K.Y. Chua, and W.A. Smith. 1992. Molecular polymorphisms of house dust mite allergens. *Exp Appl Acarology.* 16:153–64.

75. Yuuki, T., Y. Okumura, T. Ando, H. Yamakawa, M. Suko, M. Haida, and H. Okudaira. 1990. Cloning and sequencing of cDNAs corresponding to mite major allergen *Der f* II. *Arerugi.* 39:557–61.

76. Nishiyama, C., T. Yuuki, Y. Usui, N. Iwamoto, Y. Okumura, and H. Okudaira. 1994. Effects of amino acid variations in recombinant *Der f* II on its human IgE and mouse IgG recognition. *Int Arch Allergy Immunol.* 105:62–9.

77. Trudinger, M., K.Y. Chua, and W.R. Thomas. 1991. cDNA encoding the major mite allergen *Der f* II. *Clin Exp Allergy.* 21:33–7.

78. Colloff, M.J., G.A. Stewart, and P.J. Thompson. 1991. House dust mite acarofauna and Der p I equivalent in Australia: the relative importance of Dermatophagoides pteronyssinus and Euroglyphus maynei. *Clin Exp Allergy.* 21;225–30.

13

STRUCTURAL AND ANTIGENIC STUDIES OF COCKROACH ALLERGENS AND THEIR RELEVANCE TO ASTHMA

Martin D. Chapman,[1*] Lisa D. Vailes,[1] Mary Lou Hayden,[1]
David C. Benjamin,[2] Thomas A. E. Platts-Mills,[1] and L. Karla Arruda[1]

Asthma and Allergic Diseases Center
[1]Department of Internal Medicine and
[2]Department of Microbiology
University of Virginia Health Sciences Center
Charlottesville, Virginia

1. INTRODUCTION

Allergic reactions to cockroach (CR) were first described over 30 years ago by Bernton and Brown, amongst patients presenting to their allergy clinic in New York (1). These observations were followed up by several groups, notably by Dr. Kang and colleagues in Chicago in the 1970's, and it is now well established that CR cause IgE antibody responses; that these responses are often associated with asthma; and that the prevalence of CR asthma in some populations in the U.S. is comparable to that of other common aeroallergens, such as dust mite, cat, and pollens (2, 3). Atopic individuals who live in CR infested housing become sensitized by inhalation of potent CR allergens and produce vigorous IgE antibody (ab) responses. There is a strong association between the development of IgE ab to CR and asthma. In some towns and cities in the U.S., up to 60% of house dust allergic, asthmatic patients become sensitized to CR (2–6). Allergic reactions to CR are not confined to urban or inner city populations, but occur wherever housing conditions sustain extensive cockroach infestation. For example, in Louisville, Kentucky, no differences were found between the prevalence of CR allergy in patients living in inner city or rural areas, with ~40% prevalence of positive skin test reactivity in both groups being reported in a 10 year retrospective study (7). IgE ab to CR is an important risk factor for Emergency Room admission with asthma and is most commonly found among lower socio economic groups living in sub-standard housing, which in the U.S.

---

* To whom corespondence and reprint requests should be addressed at: Asthma and Allergic Diseases Center, Box 225, University of Virginia HSC, Charlottesville, VA 22908, USA. Tel 804–982–3324, FAX 804–924–5779.

New Horizons in Allergy Immunotherapy
edited by Sehon et al. Plenum Press, New York, 1996

often comprise a high proportion of minority groups (African Americans and Hispanics) (8–9).

"Cockroach asthma" has been reported in several other parts of the world, including South East Asia, Europe, and Central America (reviewed in Ref. 3). In the U.S., the principal domicilliary CR species are *Blattella germanica* and *Periplaneta americana*, whereas in Taiwan and Japan, *P. americana* and *P. fuliginosa* appear to predominate. Until recently, the molecular nature of allergens produced by either CR species had not been defined. Immunochemical studies had identified a series of protein allergens, MW 10–70kd, but there was no sequence data on these allergens and it was difficult to establish the relationships between allergens identified by different research groups (10–15). Two allergens, Bla g 1 and Bla g 2, had been purified using monoclonal antibodies and protein purification techniques, and immunoassays for these allergens have been widely used for monitoring environmental CR allergen exposure (16, 17). Over the past few years, several groups have applied molecular cloning techniques to identify and sequence allergens from either *B. germanica* or *P. americana*. The aims of these studies are to establish the allergen structures, physical properties and biologic function; to develop expression systems for producing recombinant allergens; and to use the sequence information to study the immune response to CR allergens in patients with asthma.

2. MOLECULAR BIOLOGY

2.1. *Blattella germanica*

Two allergens were initially purified from *B. germanica:* Bla g 1, a 20–25kd, highly acidic protein, also produced by *P. americana*; and Bla g 2, a 36kd protein, found primarily in *Blattella* spp. (16, 17). The prevalence of IgE ab to Bla g 1 and Bla g 2, assessed by skin testing or serum IgE ab assay was 30–50-% and 60–80%, respectively, and some patients were strongly sensitive to one allergen, but not to the other. More importantly, ~20% of CR allergic patients did not have IgE ab to either protein, suggesting that CR produce other important allergens. To investigate this possibility, a unidirectional cDNA library was prepared from *B. germanica* mRNA and screened by plaque immunoassay with IgE ab in a CR allergic serum pool, with a large panel of individual sera from CR allergic patients, and with hyperimmune mouse polyclonal IgG ab to Bla g 2.

Screening the *B.germanica* cDNA library identified six clones which reacted with IgE ab. We initially focused on a clone which reacted strongly with IgE antibody in 46–64% of sera and sequence analysis showed that the cDNA encoded a ligand binding protein or calycin (18). This allergen was designated Bla g 4 in the WHO/IUIS nomenclature. Sequence homology searches showed that the calycin protein family also included other major allergens, including mouse and rat urinary proteins, β-lactoglobulin from cows milk, and dog allergens. Since X-ray crystal coordinates were available for α_{2u}-globulin and bilin binding protein (a butterfly calycin), three dimensional models of the tertiary structure of Bla g 4 were obtained, which predicted two possible structures differing at a loop region between the α-helix and C-terminal β strand (18).

Five other CR allergen clones were obtained from the *B.germanica* cDNA library by IgE ab screening and two clones were fully sequenced. Bla g 5 showed sequence homology to Glutathione-S-transferase enzymes (GST's) and elicited IgE antibody responses in ~70% of CR allergic patients (19). Bla g 6 showed up to 70% homology with troponins and gave positive IgE antibody plaques in 50% of patients. The sequence homology between Bla g 5 and GST's ranged from 27% with *D. pteronyssinus* GST (which has also been shown to be an allergen) up to 51% with GST from the mosquito, *Anopheles gambiense* (19). Sequence comparisons showed that 13/18 residues that are conserved in GST's were present in Bla g 5, and that 3/4 residues that have been shown to be involved in binding glutathione by X-ray crystallography were conserved in Bla g 5. In keeping with these structural observations, GST enzyme activity was detected in *B. germanica* frass extracts and natural Bla g 5 was purified from these extracts by glutathione affinity chromatography. The N-terminal sequence (39 residues) of affinity purified Bla g 5 was identical to that predicted from the cDNA sequence, except that there were three additional amino acids at the N-terminus. Thus the complete amino acid sequence was obtained from the cDNA and the additional residues obtained by protein sequencing.

Although sera were selected for the CR allergic serum pool based on their reactivity with Bla g 1 and Bla g 2, IgE antibody screening of the library was not successful in identifying cDNA encoding these allergens. However, a full length cDNA encoding Bla g 2 was obtained by screening the library with polyclonal mouse IgG ab. This cDNA encoded a 24 amino acid signal peptide and a 328 amino acid mature protein, which showed sequence homology to aspartic proteases (Figure 1). Partial amino acid sequence of Bla g 2 protein showed >90% concordance with the deduced cDNA sequence. The degree of sequence homology between Bla g 2 and aspartic proteases ranged from 25–30%: the active aspartic acid residues involved in catalytic activity of the enzyme were conserved (at positions 31 and 215 in Bla g 2), as well as the surrounding amino acids (Figure 1) (20).

2.2. *Periplaneta americana*

Immunochemical studies by Wu, Lan and colleagues have identified a 72kd protein allergen produced by *P. americana*, which is an important cause of IgE responses in patients presenting with asthma in Taiwan (14, 21). The allergen was identified by immunoblotting and, subsequently, a panel of monoclonal antibodies to this allergen were produced (22). The 72kd allergen, originally described as Cr-PI, has been designated Per a 3 in the WHO/IUIS nomenclature. Recently, Wu *et al* screened a *P. americana* cDNA library with IgE antibodies and obtained several cDNA clones which encode 45–80kd IgE binding proteins (23). One of these clones encodes Per a 3 and the full sequence of this cDNA is now being determined.

	28- - - - - - - - - - - - -41	211 - - - - 217
Bla g 2	TVFDSTSCNVVVAS	QAIIDTS
Mosquito AP	VVFDTGSSNLWVPS	EAIADTG
Human Cathepsin D	VVFDTGSSNLWVPS	EAIVDTG
Human Cathepsin E	VIFDTGSSNLWVPS	QAIVDTG
Human Renin	VVFDTGSSNVWVPS	LALVDTG
Human Pepsin	VVFDTGSSNLWVPS	QAIVDTG
Bovine Chymosin	VLFDTGSSDFWVPS	QAILDTG
Barley AP	VIFDTGSSNLWVPS	AAIADSG

Figure 1. Homology between Bla g 2 and Aspartic Proteases at the active-site aspartyl residues. (Szecsi, *Scand J Clin Invest* 1992, 52:5; Cho Raikhel, *J Biol Chem* 1992, 267:21823; Faust *et al., Proc Natl Acad Sci* 1985, 82:4910).

Table 1. Molecular properties of cockroach allergens

Species	Allergen*	Prevalence of IgE ab	MW	Function	Sequence
Blattella	Bla g 1	30-50%	20-25 kd	Unknown	None
germanica	Bla g 2	60%	36 kd	Aspartic protease	cDNA/P
	Bla g 4	40-60%	18 kd	Calycin	cDNA
	Bla g 5	70%	23 kd	Glutathione transferase	cDNA/P
	Bla g 6	50%	18 kd	Troponin C	cDNA
Periplaneta	Per a 1	~50%	20-25 kd	Unknown	None
americana	Per a 3	"100%"	72-78 kd	Unknown	cDNA (pending)

2.3. Allergen Expression in Different CR Species

The production of monoclonal antibodies to CR allergens and the isolation of cDNA clones has facilitated comparisons of antigenic cross-reactivity and allergen expression among CR species, especially *B. germanica* and *P. americana*. Monoclonal antibodies generally recognize species specific epitopes on CR allergens. Thus mAb based immunoassays for Bla g 2 do not detect *P. americana* and, conversely, the ELISA for Per a 3 does not react with *B. germanica* extracts (17, 22, 24, 25). The only cross-reactive CR allergen identified to date is the Bla g 1/Per a 1 homologue, which has been purified from both CR species. However, while *P. americana* extracts react in a mAb based ELISA for Bla g 1, this assay appears to underestimate the allergen present in *P. americana* extracts, suggesting that the affinity of the mAb (raised against Bla g 1) is lower for Per a 1 (17).

Immunoassays using high titer polyclonal antibodies to Bla g 2 could not be inhibited by *P. americana* extracts, providing further evidence that Bla g 2 was a species specific allergen. However, experiments using antibodies as probes may simply reflect the specificity of the antibodies, rather than differences in protein expression, therefore, it is important to use hybridization techniques to compare mRNA and DNA expression between species. Expression of Bla g 2 and Bla g 4 in *B. germanica* and *P. americana* was compared by Northern blotting or PCR based techniques. Northern analysis showed a 1.3kb mRNA for Bla g 2 which was only present in *B. germanica*. Further, a 1kb PCR fragment could be amplified from genomic DNA from *B. germanica*, but not from *P. americana*. These results strongly suggest that Bla g 2 is only expressed in *B. germanica* (20). The 0.65kb mRNA for Bla g 4 was also only detected in *B. germanica*. However, PCR analysis followed by Southern hybridization revealed that DNA encoding Bla g 4 was present in both CR species. These results suggest that the DNA encoding Bla g 4 is not transcribed into mRNA in *P. americana*.

2.4. Biologic Activity of Cloned CR Allergens

2.4.1. Functional Activity. Predictions of biologic function based on sequence comparisons enable the protein families to which allergens belong to be established and stimulate further research on whether the protein function is relevant to its ability to cause IgE responses. Our results show that two important *B. germanica* allergens are enzymes. The aspartic protease (Bla g 2) is found in high concentration in CR digestive organs (gut, oesophagus and proventriculus) and is most likely a digestive enzyme that is secreted with CR feces. This is in keeping with earlier evidence that CR fecal extracts have potent activity in RAST inhibition assays, and with immunofluorescence studies demonstrating staining of CR allergens in intestinal epithelial cells and in Malpighian tubules (CR excretory organs) (26, 27). Cockroaches are known to produce high levels of GST for detoxification purposes and we assume that this enzyme is also eliminated in feces or other secretions. CR washes are a potent source of both Bla g 1 and Bla g 2 and may contain other allergens including the calycin allergen, Bla g 4. Rodent calycin allergens are pheromone binding proteins and we have speculated the CR calycin, Bla g 4, could also bind one of several pheromones that CR are known to secrete. The source and tissue distribution of Bla g 4 and Bla g 5 is as yet unknown, but should become established once the relevant immunoassays are developed, or by application of *in situ* nucleic acid hybridization techniques.

2.4.2. In Vivo Reactivity. Quantitative intradermal skin tests have been used to assess the allergenic activity of natural and recombinant CR allergens. Natural Bla g 1 and Bla g 2 elicit positive immediate skin tests at concentrations down to $10^{-4}\mu g/ml$ in CR allergic patients, whereas non-allergic controls show no response at $10\mu g/ml$ (20). Bla g 4 has been expressed in the pGEX expression system and the recombinant allergen shows skin test reactivity at concentrations from 10^{-1} to $10^{-5}\mu g/ml$ (18). Because of difficulties in maintaining supplies of recombinant allergens, Bla g 2 and Bla g 5 are now being expressed in pGEX and other vectors with the aim of producing a panel of recombinant CR allergens for research and diagnostic use. Current evidence, based on both serologic and *in vivo* data, suggests that it should be possible to diagnose *B. germanica* sensitivity using a cocktail of recombinant Bla g 2, Bla g 4 and Bla g 5.

3. FUTURE DIRECTIONS

It is now established that CR allergens are an important cause of asthma and the cloning of allergens from both *B. germanica* and *P. americana* opens up a variety of fields for further investigation. These include expression of recombinant allergens and analysis of their structural properties; use of mutagenesis techniques to identify antigenic sites and functional amino acid residues; and detailed studies of the immune response, particularly T cell responses and the identification of T cell epitopes. As noted above, expression systems for recombinant CR allergens have been developed and the next phase of these studies will be to carry out multi-center clinical trials to compare the *in vitro* and *in vivo* properties of the recombinants and to establish their specificity and sensitivity for diagnostic use. Expressed allergens will be essential for three dimensional structural studies by NMR or X-ray crystallography. Since the crystal structures of calycins, aspartic proteases and GST's are known, it will be possible to generate mutants at the ligand binding sites or enzyme catalytic sites to analyse the biologic activity of these allergens, and also to predict surface residues that may be involved in IgE recognition. Using mutagenesis of mite allergen, Der p 2, we have demonstrated dramatic differences in IgE antibody binding by mutation of single cysteine residues involved in formation of small disulfide loops, and this approach can be directly applied to CR allergens (28).

Preliminary experiments have shown that T cells from allergic patients proliferate to natural Bla g 2 (29) and the next phase of these studies is to make quantitative comparisons of T cell responses to recombinant CR allergens in panels of patients with CR asthma. These studies require purified natural allergens or recombinant allergens, because CR extracts are heterogeneous and are known to contain proteolytic enzymes. The identification of T cell epitopes will be essential if new approaches to immunotherapy are to be developed, similar to those now undergoing clinical trial for cat allergy and ragweed allergy (see Wallner, Chapter 32).

It should not be forgotten that there is a huge industry directed towards the production an development of CR management and control procedures, though few of these programs have been tested for their effects on CR allergenic activity. Immunoassays for CR allergens clearly provide the means by which to assess the efficacy of pest management programs. Furthermore, it is possible that studies on the molecular biology of CR proteins, including allergens, could identify targets for improved biologic or chemical control of CR populations e.g. through affecting pheromone activity or enzyme function.

All these approaches offer exciting prospects for improving the diagnosis and treatment of CR allergic asthma and no doubt there will be considerable progress in these areas before the next International Workshop!

ACKNOWLEDGMENTS

This work was supported by National Institutes of Health Grants AI 32557 and AI 34607. Dr. L. Karla Arruda is recipient of an Underrepresented Minority Research Award from the American Academy of Allergy and Immunology and the National Institute of Allergy and Infectious Disease.

REFERENCES

1. Bernton HS, McMahon TF, Brown H. Cockroach asthma. Brit J Dis Chest 1972;66:61–66.
2. Kang B, Vellody D, Homburger H, Yunginger JW. Cockroach as a cause of allergic asthma. Its specificity and immunologic profile. J Allergy Clin Immunol 1979;63:80–86.
3. Chapman MD, Vailes LD, Hayden ML, Platts-Mills TAE, Arruda LK. Cockroach allergens and their role in asthma. *In* "Allergy and Allergic Diseases", Ed. A.B. Kay, Blackwells Scientific Publ., Oxford, U.K. 1996, In Press.
4. Mendoza J, Snyder FD. Cockroach sensitivity in children with bronchial asthma. Ann Allergy 1970;28:159–163.
5. Hulett AC, Dockhorn RJ. House dust mite (*D. farinae*) and cockroach allergy in a midwestern population. Ann Allergy 1979;42:160–165.
6. Kang B. Study on cockroach antigen as a probably causative agent in bronchial asthma. J Allergy Clin Immunol 1976;58:357–365.
7. Garcia DP, Corbett ML, Sublett JL, Pollard SJ, Meiners JF, Karibo JM, Pence HL, Petrosko JM. Cockroahc
8. Call RS, Smith TF, Morris E, Chapman MD, Platts-Mills TAE. Risk factors for asthma in inner city children. J Peds 1992;121:862–866.
9. Gelber LE, Seltzer L, Bouzoukis JK, Pollart SM, Chapman MD, Platts-Mills TAE. Sensitization and exposure to indoor allergens (dust mite, cat and cockroach) as risk factors for asthma among patients presenting to hospital. Amer Rev Resp Dis 1993;147:573–578.
10. Twarog FJ, Picone FJ, Strunk RS, So J, Colten HR. Immediate hypersensitivity to cockroach: isolation and purification of the major antigens. J Allergy Clin Immunol 1976;59:154–160.
11. Stankus RP, O'Neil CE. Antigenic/allergenic characterization of American and German cockroach extracts. J Allergy Clin Immunol 1988;81:563–570.
12. Helm RM, Bandele EO, Swanson MC, Campbell AR, Wynn, SR. Identification of a German cockroach-specific allergen by human IgE and rabbit IgG. Int Arch Allergy appl Immunol 1988;87:230–238.
13. Kang BC, Chang JL, Johnson J. Characterization and partial purification of the cockroach antigen in relation to house dust and house dust mite (D. f.) antigens. Ann Allergy 1989;63:207–212.
14. Wu CH, Lan JL. Cockroach hypersensitivity: Isolation and partial characterization of major allergens. J Allergy Clin Immunol 1988;82:727–735.
15. Musmand JJ, Horner WE, Lopez M, Lehrer SB. Identification of important allergens in German cockroach extract by sodium dodecylsulphate-polyacrylamide gel electrophoresis and Western blot analysis. J Allergy Clin Immunol 1995;95:877–885.

16. Schou C, Lind P, Fernandez-Caldas E, Lockey RF, Lowenstein H. Identification and purification of an cross-reacting, acidic allergen from American (*Periplaneta americana*) and German (*Blattella germanica*) cockroach. J Allergy Clin Immunol 1990;86:935–946.

17. Pollart SM, Vailes LD, Mullins DE, Hayden ML, Platts-Mills TAE, Sutherland WM, Chapman MD. Identification, quantitation and purification of cockroach allergens using monoclonal antibodies. J Allergy Clin Immunol 1991;87:511–521.

18. Arruda LK, Vailes LD, Hayden ML, Benjamin DC, Chapman MD. Molecular cloning of cockroach (*Blattella germanica*) allergen, Bla g 4: Identification of calycins as a cause of IgE antibody responses. Submitted.

19. Vailes LD, Chapman MD, Arruda LK. Molecular cloning of german cockroach allergens: glutathione transferase and troponin. J Allergy Clin Immunol 1995;95:347

20. Arruda LK, Vailes LD, Mann BJ, Shannon J, Fox JW, Vedvick TS, Hayden ML, Chapman MD. Molecular cloning of a major cockroach (*Blattella germanica*) allergen, Bla g 2: Sequence homology to the aspartic proteases. J Biol Chem 1995;270:19563–19568.

21. Lan JL, Lee DT, Wu CH, Chang CP, Yeh CL. Cockroach hypersensitivity: Preliminary study of allergic cockroach asthma in Taiwan. J Allergy Clin Immunol 1988;82:736–740.

22. Wu CH, Chang BT, Fann MC, Lan JL. Production and characterization of monoclonal antibodies against major allergens of American cockroach. Clin Exp Allergy 1990; 20:675–682.

23. Wu CH, Lee MF, Liao SC. Cloning of cDNA coding for Cr-PI allergens of American cockroach. J Allergy Clin Immunol 1995; In Press.

24. Pollart SM, Smith TF, Morris E, Gelber LE, Platts-Mills TAE, Chapman MD. Environmental exposure to cockroach allergens: analysis using a monoclonal antibody based enzyme immunoassay. J Allergy Clin Immunol 1991;87:505–510.

25. Schou C, Fernandez-Caldas E, Lockey RF, Lowenstein H. Environmental assay for cockroach allergens. J Allergy Clin Immunol 1991;550–510.

26. Lehrer S, Horner WE, Menon P, Stankus RP. Comparison of cockroach allergenic activity in whole body and fecal extracts. J Allergy Clin Immunol 1991;87:574–580.

27. Zwick H, Popp W, Sertl K, Rausher H, Wanke T. Allergenic structures in cockroach hypersensitivity. J Allergy Clin Immunol 1991;87:626–629.

28. Smith AM, Chapman MD. Reduction in IgE binding to allergen variants generated by site directed mutagenesis: Contribution of disulphide bonds to the antigenic structure of the major house dust mite allergen, Der p 2. Submitted.

29. Slunt JB, Hayden ML, Chapman MD. Humoral and cellular immune response to cockroach and cat allergens in patients with asthma. J Allergy Clin Immunol 93:288.

14

PJUFO: A PHAGEMID FOR DISPLAY OF cDNA LIBRARIES ON PHAGE SURFACE SUITABLE FOR SELECTIVE ISOLATION OF CLONES EXPRESSING ALLERGENS

Reto Crameri,[*] Stefanie Hemmann, and Kurt Blaser

Swiss Institute of Allergy and Asthma Research (SIAF)
CH-7270 Davos, Switzerland

1. ABSTRACT

We have developed a phagemid vector (pJuFo) for the selective isolation of genes encoding proteins for which a ligand is available. The physical linkage of cDNA-encoded proteins to the genetic information required for their production was achieved by exploiting the high affinity interaction of the Jun and Fos leucine zippers. The gene encoding Jun preceeded by the *pelB* leader sequence placed under control of a *lac* promoter/operator element was cloned as N-terminal fusion to the minor viral coat protein gIII. The Jun/gIII fusion protein become structurally incorporated into phage particles during infection with helper phage. The gene encoding Fos, proceeded by the *pelB* leader sequence was coexpressed from a second *lac* promoter/operator as N-terminal fusion peptide to cDNA encoded proteins. The resulting Fos-fusions secreted into the periplasmic space of *E. coli* could become associated with Jun-decorated phage particles and thus displayed on phage surface. To avoid dissociation of the Jun/Fos heterodimeres cysteines were engineered at the N- and C-termini of both leucine zippers providing a covalent link of the cDNA gene products to the genetic information required for their production. The vector allows the construction of phage display cDNA expression libraries which can be screened by biopanning in microtiter plates coated with a ligand exhibiting affinity to the gene products of interest. The expression products from a cDNA library from *Aspergillus fumigatus*, a mold known to produce more than 40 IgE binding proteins, have been displayed on the surface of phage M13 using pJuFo. Phage displaying IgE-binding proteins were selectively enriched over non-specific phage by consecutive rounds of growth and selection in a microtiter plate coated with serum IgE from allergic individuals. A vast variety of phage

[*] Correspondence to R. Crameri, Swiss Institute of Allergy and Asthma Research, Obere Strasse 22, CH-7270 Davos, Switzerland. Fax: (+ 41) 81 43 16 07.

New Horizons in Allergy Immunotherapy
edited by Sehon et al. Plenum Press, New York, 1996

103

encoding and displaying different IgE-binding proteins with an apparent molecular mass ranging from 20 to > 40 kDa were isolated from this library.

2. INTRODUCTION

Recently, recombinant DNA-technology has been successfully applied to clone, characterise and produce an impressive list of allergens from different sources [1]. The majority of cDNAs encoding allergenic proteins has been isolated using λ-phage vectors such as λgt11 [2] or similar phage vectors like vectors of the λ-ZAP series [3] which allow *in vivo* excision of the cloned inserts. The λ-expression vectors provide a great ease in screening cDNA libraries for clones expressing antigens by screening immobilised plaques with antigen-specific antibodies [4]. Allergens can be detected visualising clones able to bind IgE antibodies from serum of allergic individuals [5, 6]. However, cloning in λ-vectors does not allow a direct selection of genes encoding proteins of interest due to the immobilisation of the libraries on solid supports which is required for screening. Other disadvantages of these systems are the limited number of plaques screenable with a reasonable effort which may hamper the detection of products from rare mRNA species [7] or the loss of antigenicity of expressed proteins due to conformational and functional changes occurring during the adsorption to nicrocellulose membranes [8].

The polymerase chain reaction (PCR) is an incomparably sensitive method to amplify genes even if they are expressed at low level [9]. A prerequisite which strongly limits the use of PCR to clone genes lies in the need to determine the N-terminal amino acid sequence of the gene product of interest, in order to design degenerated primers for PCR amplification of gene-specific cDNA [9]. However, PCR has proved to be a fast and reliable method for the amplification of allergens from different isolates of the same species [10] or to clone isogenes or allergens sharing philogenetically conserved N-terminal sequences [11, 12].

In contrast to conventional cloning and PCR technology, filamentous phage display cloning links physically each gene product to the genetic material that encodes it by fusion of the genes of interest to a phage gene coding for a phage coat protein [13, 14]. This strategy allows specific enrichment of phage displaying a polypeptide for which a ligand is available and due to the physical linkage between gene and gene product, the selective isolation of the gene [15, 16].

The use of filamentous phage to display peptide libraries as fusion with the minor coat protein (gIII) of phage M13 was first described by Smith and co-workers [17–19]. Surface-expression systems based on filamentous phage or phagemid vectors have recently been extended to display proteins [20, 21], to select DNA binding proteins with altered recognition sequences [21, 22] and for the isolation of antibody fragments from combinatorial libraries [13, 14, 23–25]. The isolation of biologically active antibody fragments from combinatorial libraries displayed on phage surface demonstrates that filamentous phage allows expression and assembly of functional heterodimeric molecules which can be selected by powerful enrichment procedures [25].

Unfortunately, these systems do not allow the construction of cDNA libraries. Translational stop codons at the 3' end of non-translated regions of eukaryotic mRNA [26] prevent the construction of fusion proteins N-terminal to the gIII phage coat protein, while fusion to the membrane-bound C-terminus of gIII would hamper the incorporation of the fusion protein into the phage coat [27, Figure 1]. We have extended the ease of use and efficiency of the phage surface display technology by covalently linking the expressed products from cDNA libraries to the phage surface exploiting the intrinsic property of the leucine zippers Jun and

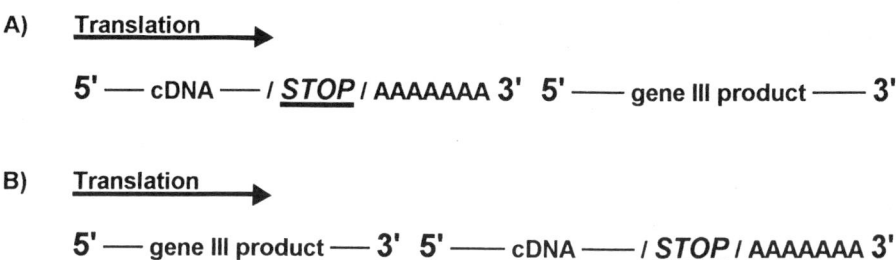

Figure 1. cDNAs can not be fused to the 5'-end of the gene III product of filamentous phage due to translational stop codons present in poly (A)$^+$-selected mRNA (A). Fusions to the 3'-end of gIII are possible but block the incorporation of the fusion products into the phage coat (B).

Fos to form heterodimeres [28] combined with the ability of the pComb3 phagemid [25] to promote assembly of functional heterodimeric molecules within the periplasmic space of *E. coli*. The resulting phagemid, pJuFo, allows the expression and display of cDNA libraries on phage surface. The physical linkage between gene product displayed on phage surface and the genetic information responsible for its production readily provide protein for functional studies and the cDNA of the insert for nucleotide sequence determination. Thus, pJuFo provides a rational cloning approach for the isolation of allergen-specific cDNAs from large phage surface display libraries generated from mRNA of complex allergenic systems l16].

3. RESULTS AND DISCUSSION

3.1. The pJuFo Vector

The pJuFo vector has been described in detail [15] and was originally designed to physically link expression products from cDNA libraries to the genetic information required for their production. In this way, products displayed on phage surface become available for specific gene-product/ligand interactions [15,16] and could be used for selective isolation of genes encoding proteins of interest (Figure 2). This strategy allows access to very large libraries (> 10^{11} clones) screenable in a single well of a microtiter plate with a powerful enrichment technique [16, 25, 29]. Digestion of pJuFo, encoding a selected insert, with *Spe* I and *Nhe* I allows the removal of the gIII fragment [25]. After religation of the compatible cohesive ends, a phagemid that produces secreted proteins is obtained. For the purification of the secreted proteins by Ni^{2+}-chelate affinity chromatography [30] a construct was developed by fusing a [His]$_6$ polypeptide tag at the N-terminus of the Fos leucine zipper [29]. The tagged recombinant proteins could be rapidly purified by standard methods from periplasmic space of *E. coli* cells induced with isopropyl-β-D-thiogalacto-pyranoside during the exponential phase of growth [31].

3.2. Construction of a cDNA Expression Library in pJuFo and Screening of Products Diaplayed on Phage Surface

Basically all methods used for the construction of cDNA libraries in other systems, particuralrly plasmids [32, 33] and filamentous phage [25] can be applied to pJuFo. An

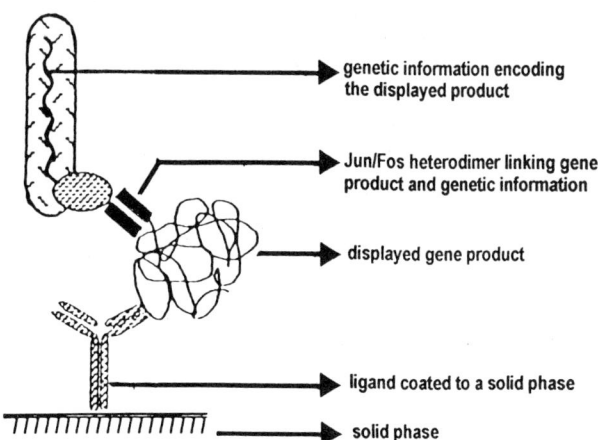

genetic information encoding
the displayed product

Jun/Fos heterodimer linking gene-
product and genetic information

displayed gene product

ligand coated to a solid phase

solid phase

Figure 2. The physical linkage of the gene product displayed on phage surface to the genetic information required for its production achieved by heterodiemrisation of the Jun and Fos leucine zippers allows specific isolation of genes by gene-product/ligand interaction.

important issue considered during the design of pJuFo was to choose the restriction sites of the multiple cloning site in a way, that commercially available libraries constructed in λ-phage (preferentially of the λ-Zap series [3]), could easily be subcloned into pJuFo after restriction with *Xba* I and *Kpn* I [15, 16]. The size and complexity of the generated phage surface display library predominantly depend from the size of the pre-made library used, from the ligation efficiency and from the efficiency of the transformation procedure [32]. We use routinely electrocompetent *E. coli* XL1-Blue cells [34] and an electroporation procedure which is currently the most efficient transformation method described [35]. After transformation phage surface expression libraries are generated by helper phage superinfection as published previously [16, 25]. Since the first half of the gIII protein is obligatory for infectivity, phage harbouring solely fusion proteins will not be infective. For propagation of the recombinant phagemid a helper phage is needed to provide all other proteins required for replication and packaging of the phagemid. The helper phage will also provide native gIII protein which will compete with the Jun/gIII fusion for incorporation into the virion and render the packaged phagemid infective [25]. Alternatively, unidirectional cDNA libraries can be constructed into *Xba* I/*Kpn* I digested pJuFo using Poly (A)+-selected mRNA [36] reverse transcribed with a poly-T primer containing a *Kpn* I restriction site and followed by the addition of *Xba* I adapters [32].

To minimise problems arising from proteolytic degradation of phage-displayed proteins, phage used in screening experiments should be from a freshly amplified stock or from frozen aliquots of freshly prepared libraries precipitated with polyethylene glycol [37]. For the enrichment of phage displaying proteins with affinity to human serum IgE, a specific IgE-ligand surface can be obtained adding serum from allergic patients to microtiter plate wells pr-coated with anti-human IgE [16]. This system has proved to be very efficient for the isolation of different clones from an *A. fumigatus* library constructed into pJuFo (Table 1). In general, no major problems are encountered if polyclonal or monoclonal antibodies directly adsorbed to a solid phase or captured with solid phase adsorbed isotype specific antibodies are used to enrich antigen-specific phage [16, 29]. The use of pJuFo to select genes encoding proteins with affinity to different ligands needs some theoretical considerations of the interaction between displayed protein and ligand (see 3. 3.). Single phage displaying allergens can be amplified, purified by PEG-precipitation [37] and used to assess the IgE binding capacity of the displayed protein in ELISA and Western blots [15, 16]. Moreover, DNA isolated from the phagemid harbouring clone can be used for the determination of the length and nucleotide sequence of the insert.

Table 1. Main characteristics of phage displaying IgE-binding proteins which were isolated from an *A. fumigatus* phage surface display library by selective enrichment. After 6 rounds of selection in a microtiter plate coated with IgE from serum of *A. fumigatus* allergic individuals [16], all selected clones yielded phage recognised by human IgE

Phage No	Insert length[a] (bp)	MW of the protein[b](kDa)	Expression level[c] (mg/l culture)	IgE-binding properties[d]
2	1080	40	36	++++
7	860	10	65	++
19	760	28	220	++
28	630	21	45	++++
32	870	38	140	++++
38	920	43	120	++++
46	690	18	140	++++
48	1270	42	45	++++

[a] Estimated from agarose gels.

[b] Estimated from polyacrylamide gels.

[c] Produced as inclusion body protein after subcloning of the fragments into pDS76/RBSII, 6 x His [31]. The yields represent mg of Ni^{2+}-chelate affinity purified proteins per litre culture [30].

[d] Sera from 30 patients with ABPA [59] were tested for the ability to bind to recombinant proteins in an IgE-specific ELISA [41]. Proteins recognised by > 50% of the sera (++++), proteins recognised by < 50 % of the sera (++).

3.3. Considerations for the Screening of Phage Displaying Proteins and for the Identification of the Gene Products

One of the advantages of pJuFo surface display compared to conventional solid-phase based screening systems is the possibility to select genes physically linked to their gene product as secreted proteins. Secreted proteins are believed to assume a native like structure [38] and phage enrichment in a liquid phase avoids denaturation of the recombinant proteins which may occur during adsorption to nitrocellulose membranes or other solid phases [8, 39]. However, the phage-display screening strategy requires the immobilisation of the ligand used for product/ligand based enrichment of phage [16]. It is therefore mandatory to immobilise the ligand used to screen a phage display library in such a way that allows conservation of the functional biophysical properties of the ligand [29]. Thus, before screening of a phage surface display library it should be tested if the immobilised ligand is still able to interact with the target. A potential limitation of the pJuFo system might be related to the affinity between ligand and gene product. Systematic studies to elucidate the required affinity to allow a specific enrichment of binding phage have not been carried out at present, however DNA-binding proteins with a Kd as low as 5×10^{-7} have been successfully enriched from phage display libraries [21, 22].

3.4. High Level Expression of Gene Products

The depletion of the gIII fragment from the pJuFo construct allows the expression of secreted recombinant protein from the weak *lac*-promoter of the phagemid (see 3.1.). However, secreted proteins are produced at low yields [40] and still contain the Fos leucine zipper as fusion partner. In the case of allergens, high yields of recombinant proteins are desired in order to be able to perform clinical studies [41–44] and to develop reagents for the routine assessment of allergic conditions [45]. A *Bgl* II restriction site engineered at the 3'-end of the Fos leucine zipper allows directional subcloning of the inserts as *Bgl* II/*Puv* II fragment into high level expression vectors of the pDS-series [31]. We have used this approach to produce inclusion bodies proteins from the inserts of affinity-enriched phage (Table 1). In particular, r*Asp f* I/a, a major allergen of *A. fumigatus* has been produced at industrial scale, showing the feasibility of this approach [46, 47]. The disadvantage of producing inclusion body protein is, that an *in vitro* refolding protocol needs to be worked out. The successful refolding of allergens in vitro, which is a requirement for IgE-binding [48,49], might be laborious [50] or even unsuccessful in the case of cysteine-rich proteins. However, our knowledge of protein folding is rapidly increasing [51] and the use of cloned genes involved in the process of folding may help to increase the fraction of protein that can be produced in a soluble form in *E. coli* [52,53].

3.5. Concluding Comments

Although classical cloning systems have proved to be extremely successful for the isolation of allergens, they are labour intensive to approach cloning of several components from complex systems such as *A. fumigatus*, a mold known to produce more than 40 different allergenic molecules [54] or ragweed pollen reported to be composed of at least 52 antigens [55] of which 22 have been shown to bind to human serum IgE [56]. A rational cloning approach to isolate genes encoding proteins which share common functional properties would implicate the selective enrichment of clones expressing gene products being able to bind selectively to the common ligand, which for allergens corresponds to human serum IgE. The described pJuFo cloning system fulfils this requirement and has been successfully used to isolate cDNAs encoding allergens from an *A. fumigatus* phage surface display library (Table 1). The demonstration that proteins encoded in a cDNA library can be displayed on the surfaces of phage and screened by ligand/product interaction has implications beyond the isolation of allergenic proteins. Recently, the vector has been modified to allow direct functional selection of cDNA clones from libraries [57] and to select proteins interacting with the large subunit of HIV-1 reverse transcriptase [58]. The fact that the pJuFo system is about 10^{10} times more sensitive than other cDNA cloning systems [29] makes it attractive for cloning of any cDNA. pJuFo is presently used in different laboratories and the goals are moving fast from the original aim of improving cDNA cloning [15, 16] to fundamental questions regarding protein/protein and protein/DNA interactions. In principle pJuFo can be used to isolate the gene encoding any protein for which a ligand or a receptor is available and thus also to increase or decrease the binding affinity of these proteins by random mutagenesis and selection. It represents a versatile tool for the discovery of functionalimportant proteins or targets of potential industrial interest.

4. ACKNOWLEDGMENTS

We are grateful to Dr. R. A. Lerner (the Scripps Research Institute, La Jolla, CA, USA) for providing the pComb3 phagemid and for fruitful discussions, to Dr. D. Stüber (Hoffmann La Roche, Basel, CH) for the supply of expression vectors and unpublished information and to Dr. T. Curran (Roche Research Center, NJ, USA) for the Jun and Fos cDNAs. We are indebted to Dr. G. Menz (Hochgebirgsklinik, Davos, CH) for the supply of human sera from *A. fumigatus* allergic individuals. We thank Dr. A. Faith for careful reading of the manuscript.This work was supported in part by a Swiss National Science Foundation Grant (31–30185.90 to R. Crameri) and from the Ciba-Geigy Jubiläumstiftung.

5. REFERENCES

1. WHO/IUIS (1994) Allergen nomenclature. *ACI News* 6, 38–44.
2. Mierendorf, R. C., Percy, C. & Young, R. A. 1987) *Meth. Enzymol.* 152, 458–469.
3. Short, J. M., Fernandez, J. M., Sorge, J. A. & Huse, W. D. (1988) *Nucleic Acids Res.* 16, 7583–7600.
4. Helfman, D. M., Feramisco, J. R., Fiddes, J. C., Thomas, R. G. & Hughes, S. H. (1983) *Proc. Natl. Acad. Sci. USA* 80, 31–35.
5. Valenta, R., Duchêne, M., Pettenburger, K., Sillaber, C., Valent, P., Bettelheim, P., Breitenbach, M., Rumpold, H., Kraft, D. & Scheiner, O. (1991) *Science* 253, 557- 560.
6. Sieberler, S., Scheiner, O., Kraft, D., Lonsdale, D. & Valenta, R. (1994) *EMBO J.* 13, 3481–3486.
7. Mohapatra, S. D., Nicodemus, C. F., Schou, C. & Valenta, R. (1994) *ACI News* 6, 45–48.
8. Hollander, Z. & Katchalski-Katzir, E. (1986) *Mol. Immunol.* 23, 927–933.
9. McPerson, M. J., Quirke, R. & Taylor, G. R. (eds.) *PCR: a practical approach.* IRL Press, Oxford, 1993.
10. Moser, M., Crameri, R., Menz, G. & Suter, M. (1993). *Agents and Actions* 43, 131–137.
11. Larsen, J. N., Stomary, R. & Ipsen, H. (1992) *Mol. Immunol.* 29, 703–711.
12. Lu, G., Villalba, M., Coscia, M. R., Hoffman, D. R. & King, T. P. (1993) *J. Immunol.* 150, 2823–2830.
13. Kang, A. S., Barbas III, C. F., Janda, K. D., Bencovic, S. J. & Lerner, R. A. (1991) *Proc. Natl. Acad. Sci. USA* 88, 4363–4366.
14. Barbas III, C. F., Kang, A. S., Lerner, R. A. & Bencovic, S. J. (1991) *Proc. Natl. Acad. Sci. USA* 88, 7978–7982.
15. Crameri, R. & Suter, M. (1993) *Gene* 137, 69–75.
16. Crameri, R., Jaussi, R., Menz, G. & Blaser, K. (1994) *Eur. J. Biochem.* 226, 53–58.
17. Smith, G. P. (1985) *Science* 228, 1315–1317.
18. Parmley, S. F. & Smith, G. P. (1988) *Gene* 73, 305–318.
19. Scott, J. K. & Smith, G. P. (1990) *Science* 249, 386–390.
20. Bass, S., Greene, R. & Wells, J. A. (1990) *Protein* 8, 309–314.
21. Rebar, E. J. & Pabo, C. O. (1994) *Science* 263, 671–673.
22. Wu, H., Yang, W-P. & Barbas III, C. F. (1995) *Proc. Natl. Acad. Sci. USA* 92, 344–348.
23. Clackson, T., Hoogenboom, H. R., Griffiths, A. D. & Winter, G. (1991) *Nature* 352, 624–628.
24. Burton, D. R., Barbas III, C. F., Persson, M. A. A., Koenig, S., Chanock, R. M. & Lerner, R. A. (1991) *Proc. Natl. Acad. Sci. USA* 88, 10134–10137.
25. Barbas III, C. F. & Lerner, R. A. (1991) *Methods Comp. Methods Enzymol.* 2, 119–124.
26. Abelson, J. & Butz, W. (1980) *Science* 214, 1317–1484.
27. Boeke, J. D., Model, P. & Zinder, N. D. (1982) *Mol. Gen. Genet.* 186, 185–192.
28. Pernelle, C., Clerc, F. F., Dureuil, C., Bracco, L. & Tocque, B. (1993) *Biochemistry* 32, 11682–11687.
29. Suter, M., Foti, M., Ackermann, M. & Crameri R. (1995) *In: Phage display of peptides and proteins*, Kay, B. K. (ed.) Academic Press, New York (in press).
30. Hochuli, E., Bannwerth, W., Döbeli, H., Genz, R. & Stüber, D. (1988) *Bio/Technology* 6, 1321–1325
31. Stüber, D., Matile, H. & Garotta, G. *In: Immunological methods*, Lefkovits, I. & Pernis, B. (eds.) pp. 121–152, Academic Press, New York.
32. Sambrook, J., Fritsch, E. F. & Maniatis, T. (1989) *Molecular cloning: a laboratory manual*, 2nd edn, Cold Spring Harbor Laboratory, Cold Spring Harbor, NY.
33. Glover, D. M. (ed) *DNA cloning: a practical approach.* IRL-Press, Oxford, 1985.
34. Bullock, W. O., Fernandez, J. M. & Short, J. M. (1987) *Biotechniques* 5, 276–381.
35. Dower, W. J., Miller, J. F. & Ragsdale, C. W. (1988) *Nucleic Acids Res.* 16, 6127–6145.
36. Huse, W. D. & Hansen, C. (1988) *Strategies* 1, 1–3.
37. Cwirla, S. E., Peters, E. A., Barrett, R. W. & Dower, W. J. (1990) *Proc. Natl. Acad. Sci. USA* 87, 6378–6382.
38. Skerra, A. & Plückthun, A. (1988) *Science* 240, 1038–1041.
39. Butler, J. E. (1992) *In: Structure of antigens*, van Regenmortel, M. H. H. (ed.) pp 209–259, CRC Press, Boca Raton.
40. Blight, M. A. & Holland, B. (1994) *Tibtech.* 12, 450–455.
41. Moser, M., Crameri, R., Brust, E., Suter, M. & Menz, G. (1994) *J. Allergy Clin. Immunol.* 93, 1–11.
42. Nikolaizik, W. H., Moser, M., Crameri, R., Little, S., Warner, J. O., Blaser, K. & Schöni, M. H. (1995) *Am. J. Respir. Crit. Care Med.* (in press).
43. Müller, U. R., Dudler, T., Schneider, T., Crameri, R., Fischer, H., Skrbic, D., Maibach, R., Blaser, K. & Suter, M. (1995) *J. Allergy Clin. Immunol.* (in press).
44. Disch, R., Menz, G., Blaser, K. & Crameri, R. (1995) *Int. Arch. Allergy Immunol.* (in press).

45. Crameri, R., Lidholm, J., Grönlund, H., Blaser, K. & Menz, G. (1995) this volume.
46. Suter, M., Moser, M., Menz, G., Blaser, K. & Crameri, R. (1993) *In: Molecular biology and immunology of allergens*, Kraft, D. & Sehon, A. (eds.) pp. 267–269, CRC Press, Boca Raton.
47. Moser, M., Crameri, R., Menz, G., Schneider, T., Dudler, T., Virchow, C., Gmachl, M., Blaser, K. & Suter, M. (1992) *J. Immunol.* 149, 454–460.
48. Dudler, T., Schneider, T., Annand, R. R., Gelb, M. H. & Suter, M. (1994) *J. Immunol.* 152, 5514–5522.
49. Laver, W. G., Air, G. M., Webster, R. G. & Smith-Gill, S. J. (1990) *Cell* 61, 553–556.
50. Dudler, T., Chen, W-Q., Wang, S., Schneider, T., Annand, R. R., Dempcy, R. O., Crameri, R., Gmachl, M., Suter, M. & Gelb, M. H. (1992) *Biochim. Biophys. Acta* 1165, 201–210.
51. Gething, M. J. & Sambrook, J. (1992) *Nature* 355, 33–45.
52. Dale, G. E., Schönfeld, H. J., Langen, H. & Stieger, M. (1994) *Protein Eng.* 7, 933–939.
53. Amrein, K. E., Takacs, B., Stieger, M., Molons, J., Flint, N. A. & Burn, P. (1995) *Proc. Natl. Acad. Sci. USA* 92, 1048–1052.
54. Borga, A. (1990) PhD Thesis, Carolinska Institute, Repro Print AB, Stockholm.
55. Lowenstein, H. & Marsh, D. G. (1981) *J. Immunol.* 126, 943–948.
56. Lowenstein, H., & Marsh, D. G. (1983) *J. Immnol.* 130, 727–731.
57. Gramatikoff, K., Georgiev, O. & Schaffner, W. (1994) *Nucleic Acids Res.* 22, 5761–5762.
58. Hottiger, M., Gramatikoff, K., Gregoriev, O., Chaponnier, Chr., Schaffner, W. & Hübscher, U. (1995) *Nucleic Acids Res.* (in press.)
59. Leser, C., Kauffman, H. F., Virchow, C. & Menz, G. (1992) *J. Allergy Clin. Immunol.* 90, 589–599.

15

AUTOMATED SEROLOGY WITH RECOMBINANT ALLERGENS

A Feasibility Study

Reto Crameri,[1*] Jonas Lidholm,[2] Günter Menz,[3] Hans Grönlund,[2] and Kurt Blaser[1]

[1]Swiss Institute of Allergy and Asthma Research (SIAF)
CH-7270 Davos, Switzerland
[2]Pharmacia Diagnostics AB
S-751 82 Uppsala, Sweden
[3]Hochgebirgsklinik
CH-7275 Davos, Switzerland

1. ABSTRACT

Diagnosis of allergic conditions is based on skin prick- and/or intradermal tests and on serology. Both methods make use of allergenic preparations and the results mainly depend on the quality of the substances applied and on the reactivity of the subjects. Recombinant allergens can be produced as highly pure proteins. They may contribute to a significant improvement of the diagnosis of allergic diseases provided that the allergens became available in a pure, fully antigenic form suitable for routine assessments. We have studied the diagnostic properties of recombinant *Aspergillus fumigatus* allergen I (r*Asp f* I/a), a major allergen recognised by about 60 % of the *A. fumigatus* allergic individuals, to test the feasibility of using recombinant allergens for automated serology in the Pharmacia CAP System, a new solid-phase immunoassay. ImmunoCAPs carrying immobilised r*Asp f* I/a were produced and evaluated using sera from well characterised patients with allergic bronchopulmonary aspergillosis (ABPA), allergic asthmatics with or without *A. fumigatus* sensitisation, and healthy control persons. The clinical parameters used for the diagnosis of allergy to *A. fumigatus* were RAST and skin test reactivity to commercial *A. fumigatus* extracts. IgE antibodies recognising r*Asp f* I/a were determined by a direct antigen-specific ELISA and with the newly developed r*Asp f* I/a ImmunoCAPs. Quantitative results

---

* Correspondence to: R. Crameri, Swiss Institute of Allergy and Asthma Research, Obere Strasse 22, CH-7270 Davos, Switzerland. Fax : (+ 41) 81 43 16 07.

New Horizons in Allergy Immunotherapy
edited by Sehon et al. Plenum Press, New York, 1996

111

from the two r*Asp f* I/a detection systems correlated closely, indicating that this recombinant allergen can be incorporated in the Pharmacia CAP System with unaltered antigenic activity. The behaviour of a panel of recombinant *A. fumigatus* allergens in the Pharmacia CAP System will be evaluated in the near future to assess the potential of recombinant allergens for the automated diagnosis of allergic conditions.

2. INTRODUCTION

The ability to mount an IgE-mediated response to allergens is a prerequisite for the development of a positive type I skin reaction towards allergenic substances [1]. Thus, in clinical practice, the diagnosis of a specific allergy is usually based on the clinical history supplemented by diagnostic tests. A clinical history leading to a suspicion of allergy is the basis for testing type I hypersensitivity, while diagnostic serology is used to show the presence of IgE antibodies [2]. Elevated total serum IgE has been an important immunologic finding to confirm the suspicion of allergy [3]. However, the diagnostic value of this parameter is limited by the fact that many patients with asthma or atopic dermatitis may show high levels of total serum IgE in the absence of allergy [4]. The detection of antibodies of the IgE isotype specific to allergen preparations in sera of allergic subjects determined by radioimmunosorbent tests (RAST) or enzyme-linked immunosorbent assays (ELISA) has substantially contributed to a better serologic diagnosis of allergic conditions [5–7]. Skin testing and allergen-specific serology are reliable diagnostic methods when defined antigens/allergens are applied [1, 8], but often a lack of correlation between skin test results and serology is reported [9, 10]. In fact, results from antigen-specific ELISA against allergen extracts do not correlate with skin test data due to immunochemical perturbations within the enzymatic assays [11, 12]. In contrast, reliable serologic data correlating fairly well with skin test results can be obtained using highly pure recombinant allergens [11, 13, 17]. The application of recombinant DNA technology to produce allergenic proteins offers the possibility to generate highly pure, perfectly standardised allergens of known biologic activity [14, 15]. Although more then 100 allergens have been completely or partly sequenced [16], only few publications dealing with clinical applications of recombinant allergens are reported [11, 13, 17, 18], probably because commercial recombinant allergen preparations are not available. In this report we evaluate the performance of r*Asp f* I/a, a major allergen of *A. fumigatus* [11] in the Pharmacia CAP-System, a solid-phase immunoassay calibrated against the WHO standard for IgE [19] which has the advantage of being fully automated [20].

3. MATERIALS AND METHODS

3.1. Subjects

Allergic asthmatics with or without *A. fumigatus* sensitisation, patients with ABPA [21, 22] and healthy control individuals entered this study. None of the subjects participating had taken medication that might interfere with the performance of the test at the time of the study. All the allergic individuals had asthma and met the guidelines for the diagnosis and management of asthma [23], patients with ABPA had asthma and fulfilled at least six of the seven diagnostic criteria proposed by Rosenberg et al. [21] and Patterson et al. [22]. The healthy controls had no history of atopy, allergy or asthma and had normal serum IgE levels.

3.2. Production of r*Asp f* I/a and r*Asp f* I/a ImmunoCAPs

r*Asp f* I/a was expressed as hexahistidine-tagged fusion protein in *E. coli* and purified by Ni^{2+}-chelate affinity chromatography as described [24, 25]. Purity was assessed by SDS-PAGE (4–20%) and samples of 1 mg r*Asp f* I/a were lyophilised for long term storage.

CAP is a new laboratory system representing a further development of Phadebas RAST. The system is build around a new type of solid-phase hydrophilic carrier which consists of a CNBr-activated cellulose derivative. Instrumentation and information software management allow the automated measurement of total and specific IgE in undiluted serum or plasma [19, 20]. r*Asp f* I/a-ImmunoCAPs were produced at the Pharmacia Specific Allergen Service Departement using highly pure recombinant *Asp f* I/a protein.

3.3. r*Asp f* I/a-Specific ELISA and r*Asp f* I/a ImmunoCAP Determinations

Anti-r*Asp f* I/a antibodies of the IgE isotype in sera of healthy controls, allergic asthmatics and patients with ABPA were determined by an antigen-specific ELISA and results expressed as arbitrary ELISA-units (EU ml^{-1}) calibrated against an in house reference standard [11]. r*Asp f* I/a ImmunoCAP assays were run with the fluoroimunoassay version and the results expressed quantitatively in kU l^{-1} of specific anti-r*Asp f* I/a IgE.

3.4. Skin Tests with Commercial *A. fumigatus* Extracts

Sera for serologic analyses were obtained immediately before skin testing and stored at -20 °C until use. For intradermal tests two commercial *A. fumigatus* extracts obtained from Allergopharma (Hamburg, Germany) and Bencard (Smithkline Beecham, Neuss, Germany) were used as recommended by the suppliers. Histamine dihydrochloride (0.001%) and physiologic saline solution (0.9%) served as positive and negative control, respectively. Patients were regarded as being sensitised to *A. fumigatus* if the wheal had at least half the size of the skin reaction induced by the histamine control.

3.5. Analysis of the Results

Correlation coefficients between ELISA and ImmunoCAP results were determined with Pearson's linear regression analysis.

4. RESULTS AND DISCUSSION

The main objective of this study was to evaluate the performance of a major allergen from *A. fumigatus* produced as recombinant protein in the Parmacia CAP system to evaluate the feasibility of producing reagents for automated diagnosis using recombinant allergens.

4.1. Characterisation of the Patient and Control Groups

A group of allergic asthmatics with (n = 10) or without *A. fumigatus* sensitisation (n = 9), patients with ABPA (n = 30) and a group of healthy controls (n = 10) entered this study. All subjects showed a positive histamine response and were negative to physiologic saline solution in intradermal test. The negative control group of healthy subjects and asthmatics without *A. fumigatus* sensitisation showed no sensitisation to commercial *A. fumigatus* extracts in intradermal skin test. *A. fumigatus*-specific IgE was not detectable in sera of these individuals (RAST class 0). In agreement with these findings, specific IgE against r*Asp f* I/a was not detectable in an r*Asp f* I/a-specific ELISA or with r*Asp f* I/a ImmunoCAPs. All patients with ABPA showed a positive skin reaction to both commercial *A. fumigatus* extracts in intradermal test, the subjects with allergic asthma and *A. fumigatus* sensitisation reacted at least to one of the commercial extracts. Patients with ABPA and subjects allergic to the fungus had an *A. fumigatus* specific RAST of > 1. Sera from these two groups were analysed for r*Asp f* I/a-specific serum IgE in ELISA and with the newly developed r*Asp f* I/a ImmunoCAPs. The ELISA determinations showed the presence of r*Asp f* I/a-specific IgE in 73 % of the individuals which is in agreement with earlier reports [11, 26]. r*Asp f* I/a elicited immediate typ I reaction in skin test of all patients with a serum titre > 10 EU ml^{-1} whereas the 11 patients with IgE values below the detection level (10 EU ml^{-1}) did not reacted to intradermally applied r*Asp f* I/a (data not shown). The results obtained with the r*Asp f* I/a ImmunoCap System were in perfect accordance with the ELISA results. All sera of subject with < 10 EU ml^{-1} r*Asp f* I/a-specific IgE scored below the cut off value of the ImmunoCAP System of < 0.35 kU l^{-1}. The Immuno-CAP determination of sera from individuals with > 10 EU l^{-1} specific IgE varied from 0.5 kU l^{-1} to 45 kU l^{-1} (Figure 1). The close correlation between the two r*Asp f* I/a-specific IgE detection methods demonstrates that this recombinant allergen can be incorporated in the Pharmacia CAP System with unaltered antigenic activity. Moreover, skin test data and serologic data with r*Asp f* I/a [11, 17] showed an excellent correlation suggesting the possibility of relying on serologic data to diagnose allergic diseases. The results of this study

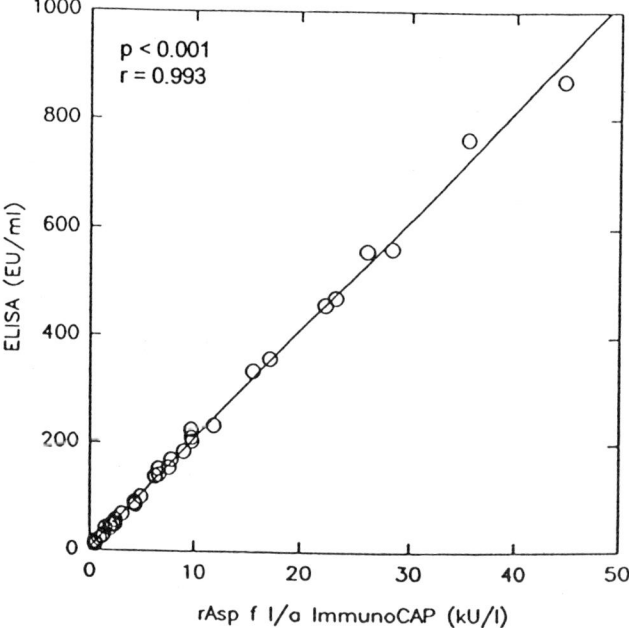

Figure 1. Correlation between the IgE results obtained with an r*Asp f* I/a-specific ELISA and with r*Asp f* I/a ImmunoCAP determinations in a sample of 50 sera from *A. fumigatus* allergic individuals.

corroborate earlier findings [11, 17, 18] and indicates that recombinant allergens are suitable to develop reagents for a fully automated diagnosis of allergic conditions. r*Asp f* I/a, although a major allergen, is not sufficient to recognise all *A. fumigatus* allergic individuals. However, a new panel of recombinant *A. fumigatus* allergens recently reported [27, 28] will allow testing the feasibility of using only recombinant allergens to diagnose an allergy to this mold. We assume that recombinant allergens commercially available in a form suitable for routine assessment will have a broad impact in the diagnosis of allergy in the near future providing the long awaited perfectly standardised allergenic preparations.

5. ACKNOWLEDGMENTS

We are grateful to Dr. D. Stüber (Hoffmann LaRoche, Basel, CH) for the supply of expression vectors and unpublished information and to Dr. C. H. Heusser (Ciba-Geigy, Basel, CH) for providing TN-142 anti-human IgE monoclonal antibody. We thank Dr. A. Faith for careful reading of the manuscript. This study was supported in part by a Swiss National Science Foundation Grant (31–30185.90 to R. Crameri).

6. REFERENCES

1. Dreborg, S. & Frew, A. (1993) *Allergy* 48, 49–54.
2. Henderson, L. L., Swedlund, H. A., Van Dellen, R. G., Marcoux, J. P., Carryer, H. M., Peters, G. A. & Gleich, G. J. (1971) *J. Allergy Clin. Immunol.* 48, 361–365.
3. Spitz, E., Gelfand, W. W., Sheffer, A. L. & Austen, K. F. (1972) *J. Allergy Clin. Immunol.* 49, 337–347.
4. Heiner, D. D. & Rose, B. (1970) *J. Allergy* 45, 30–41.
5. Gleich, G. J. & Jones, R. T. (1975) *J. Allergy Clin. Immunol.* 53, 346–351.
6. Schellenberg, R. R. & Adkinson, N. F. (1975) *J. Immunol.* 115, 1577–1583.
7. Urbanek, R., Kemeny, D. M. & Samuel, D. (1985) *J. Immunol. Meth.* 79, 123–131.
8. Dreborg, S., Backman, A., Basomba, A., Bousquet, J., Dieges, P. & Malling, H. J. (1989) *Allergy* 44, 1–59.
9. Vijay, H. M., Perelmutter, L. & Bernstein, I. L. (1978) *Int. Arch. Allergy. Appl. Immunol.* 56, 517–522.
10. van der Zee, J. S., de Groot, H., van Swieten, P., Jansen, H. M. & Aalberse, R. C. (1988) *J. Allergy Clin. Immunol.* 82, 270–281.
11. Moser, M., Crameri, R., Brust, E., Suter, M. & Menz, G. (1994) *J. Allergy Clin. Immunol.* 93, 1–11.
12. Butler, J. E. & Hamilton, R. G. In: Butler, J. E. (ed.) *Immunochemistry of solid-phase immunoassays.* Boca Raton: CRC Press, 1991, 173–198.
13. Müller, U. R., Dudler, T., Schneider, T., Crameri, R., Fischer, H., Skrbic, D., Maibach, R., Blaser, K. & Suter, M. (1995) *J. Allergy Clin. Immunol.* (in press).
14. Scheiner, O. (1992) *Int. Arch. Allergy Immunol.* (1992) 98, 93–96.
15. Bousquet, J. & Valenta, R. (1994) *ACI News* 6, 54–59.
16. WHO/IUIS (1994) Allergen nomenclatue. *ACI News* 6, 38–44.
17. Disch, R., Menz, G., Blaser, K. & Crameri, R. (1995) *Int. Arch. Allergy Immunol.* (in press).
18. Nicolaizik, W. H., Moser, M., Crameri, R., Little, S., Warner, J. O., Blaser, K. & Schöni, M. H. (1995) *Am. J. Crit. Care Med.* (in press).
19. Axen, R., Drevin, H., Kober, A. & Yman, L. In: Johansson, S. G. O. (ed.) *IgE antibodies and the Pharmacia CAP system in allergy diagnosis.* Parmacia Publication, 1988, 3–5.
20. Bousquet, J., Chanez, P., Chanal, I. & Michel, F. B. J. Allergy Clin. Immunol. (1990) 85, 1039–1043.
21. Rosenberg, M., Patterson, R., Mintzer, R., Cooper, J., Roberts, M. & Harris, K. E. (1977) *Ann. Intern. Med.* 86, 405–414.
22. Patterson, R., Greenberger, P. A., Radin, R. C. & Roberts, M. (1982) *Ann. Intern. Med.* 96, 286–291.
23. Scheffer, A. L. (ed.) Guidelines for the diagnosis and management of asthma. (1991) *J. Allergy Clin. Immunol.* 88, 425–534.
24. Moser, M., Crameri, R., Menz, G., Schneider, T., Dudler, T., Virchow, C., Gmachl, M., Blaser, K. & Suter, M. (1992) *J. Immunol.* 149, 454–460.

25. Suter, M., Moser, M., Menz, G., Blaser, K. & Crameri, R. (1993) In: Kraft, D. & Sehon, A. (eds.) *Molecular biology and immunology of Allergens.* Boca Raton: CRC Press, 1993, 267–279.

26. Arruda, K. L., Platts-Mills, T. A. E., Fox, J. W. & Chapman, M. D. (1990) *J. Exp. Med.* 172, 1529–1532.

27. Crameri, R., Jaussi, R., Menz, G. & Blaser, K. (1994) *Eur. J. Biochem.* 226, 53–58.

28. Crameri, R., Hemmann, S. & Blaser, K. *This volume.*

16

BIOLOGICAL AND IMMUNOLOGICAL IMPORTANCE OF BET v 1 ISOFORMS

M. Breitenbach,[1] F. Ferreira,[1] A. Jilek,[1] I. Swoboda,[2] C. Ebner,[2] K. Hoffmann-Sommergruber,[2] P. Briza,[1] O. Scheiner,[2] and D. Kraft[2]

[1]Institut für Genetik und Allgemeine Biologie
Universität Salzburg, Austria
[2]Institut für Allgemeine und Experimentelle Pathologie
Universität Wien, Austria

SUMMARY

In 2D-PAGE analysis of Bet v 1, the major birch pollen allergen, up to 12 isoforms can be demonstrated that differ in their isoelectric points from about pH 4.9 to pH 5.9. The molecular weights of these isoforms seem to be rather similar, but minor variations can also be seen. Preliminary experiments with birch leaves seem to indicate that in aging leaves some isoforms can be found that do not occur in pollen. In birch cells cultured in vitro, Bet v 1 isoforms can be induced by bacterial infection that do not occur in pollen (Swoboda et al. (1995), *Pant, Cell and Environment* 18, 865–874). In a recent paper (Swoboda et al (1995)., *J. Biol. Chem.* 270, 2607–2613) we show that in natural Bet v 1 from pollen the isoforms are due to different protein sequences. The derived protein sequences of 10 different isoforms (corresponding to 13 different cDNAs) were determined and confirmed by plasma desorption mass spectrometry of purified natural Bet v 1 after trypsin and endoproteinase Glu-C digestion. These experiments also showed that pollen Bet v 1 isoforms were reactive to patients' sera to different degrees and that common post-synthetic modifications (besides N-terminal methionine cleavage) did not occur on Bet v 1.

Recombinant isoforms were produced in E. coli, purified and tested with selected patients allergic to birch pollen (Ferreira et al., *J. Exp. Med.*, in the press). The pattern of IgE binding to Bet v 1 isoforms widely differs. Also, T-cell clones from individual patients in some cases are specific to peptides occurring only in certain isoforms. It was of particular interest that three of the naturally occurring pollen Bet v 1 isoforms do not or hardly bind IgE of untreated patients allergic to Bet v 1. However, a comparison of IgE reactivity in patients before and after conventional immunotherapy with natural pollen extract clearly showed that this form of immunotherapy induced IgE to the isoforms that had been unreactive in untreated patients. One of these, Bet v 1d, showed a particularly strong

New Horizons in Allergy Immunotherapy
edited by Sehon et al. Plenum Press, New York, 1996

117

potency towards T-cell stimulation. The isoform(s) that do not bind IgE in untreated patients but still show T-cell reactivity could be potentially utilized for a new form of immunotherapy that avoids the risk of anaphylaxis.

INTRODUCTION

Bet v 1, the major allergen of the birch, Betula verrucosa, has been the subject of many investigations in several European laboratories. On two-dimensional polyacrylamide gel electrophoresis the allergen showed a marked microheterogeneity (even after immune-affinity purification) that was noted early on and attributed to the fact that the allergen might consist of several isoforms (1). Undoubtedly, the most important advance in our knowledge about this allergen was the determination of the complete cDNA sequence of the major isoform in 1989 (ref.2). The amino acid sequence derived from this cDNA sequence was in agreement with a previously determined partial N-terminal sequence (ref. 2 and publications cited therein) and a recombinant non-fusion protein produced in E. coli showed identical reactivity to patients' IgE when compared with the natural mixture of isoforms in quantitative immunological tests (3). This clearly showed that a relevant sequence had been cloned. Computer-aided sequence comparisons showed that this major tree allergen was rather highly conserved in evolution and belonged to a family of proteins inducible in plant somatic tissues by pathogens (so-called PR proteins, of which several families are known, see ref. 4 for review). However, many questions remained to be answered. Among them are the following: What is the biological (enzymatic?) function of the Bet v 1 family of proteins? Do proteins belonging to this family occur in all (dicotyledonous and monocotyledonous) pollens? If yes, why are the proteins major allergens only in the Fagaceae? What is the chemical basis of the up to 12 isoforms constituting the allergen? If these isoforms are due to different amino acid sequences, what is the relevance of the isoforms for the patient with respect to IgE binding and T-cell stimulation? Finally, what is the biological function of the isoforms and do the isoforms occurring in pollen and in somatic tissues after infection with pathogens differ from each other? We have investigated here the last three of these questions.

MATERIALS AND METHODS

Protein Methods

Natural Bet v 1 was prepared from commercially available birch pollen (Allergon AB, Engelholm, Sweden) by extraction with dilute buffer, affinity chromatography on immobilized monoclonal antibody, Bip1, and reversed phase HPLC on a Hypersil WP300-C8 column, as described previously (3, 5, 6). Recombinant non-fusion (rnf) Bet v 1a from E. coli harboring the appropriate expression construct was purified by chromatofocusing on a PBE-94 ion exchanger column followed by reversed phase HPLC (3). The purified protein preparations were digested with trypsin or endoproteinase Glu-C (both enzymes were of sequencing grade and supplied by Böhringer, Mannheim, FRG) and the resulting peptides were either analyzed directly by PDMS (plasma desorption mass spectrometry) or purified by reversed phase HPLC on a microBondapak-C18 column prior to mass spectrometry as described previously (7). Two-dimensional protein gels were run by isoelectric focusing in the first dimension and SDS-PAGE in the second dimension and immunoblotted as described previously (1).

Mass Spectrometry

The peptide mixtures or HPLC-purified peptides were adsorbed on nitrocellulose-layered targets, spin-dried and mass spectra were obtained on a Bio-Ion 20K time of flight mass spectrometer (Uppsala, Sweden) using accelerating voltages 18 kV and -15 kV as described previously (7).

Cloning and Sequencing of Bet v 1 Isoform-Encoding cDNAs

Most of the Bet v 1 isoform-encoding cDNAs presented here were obtained by PCR using an oligonucleotide, Cora1, containing an oligodT tract, a spacer sequence and a HindIII recognition site for the 3'-end and an oligonucleotide, Cora2, containing an EcoRI recognition site followed by the first 19 nucleotides of the Bet v 1a coding region, as described previously (7). The PCR products were cloned into a pUCBM20 plasmid for sequencing and recloned into pMW175 or 172 for expression (8). A birch pollen cDNA library was constructed in the phage expression vector, lambda-ZAP (Stratagene, La Jolla, CA, USA) and screened with serum IgE from a patient displaying RAST class >3.5, as described previously (2). Bet v 1 isoform clones obtained by either method were sequenced on both strands according to the dideoxy chain termination method (9).

Immunological Methods

For immunoblot analysis of rnfBet v 1 isoforms, proteins were separated by 15% SDS-PAGE, electroblotted, and bound IgE was detected using I125-labeled rabbit anti-human-IgE (Pharmacia) as described previously (3). A similar method was used for the detection of bound human IgG (10).

RESULTS

Microheterogeneity of Pollen Bet v 1

It was noted early on that in conventional two-dimensional separations of Bet v 1, the major allergen of birch pollen, a number of isoforms could be seen (1). The isoforms differ in charge (pI ranges from about 4.9 to 5.9) and also in molecular weight, but they all seem to be recognized about equally well by the monoclonal antibody, Bip1. About 12 isoforms could be separated (Fig. 1, upper panel). After affinity chromatography on immobilized Bip1, two-dimensional separation and, again, immunoblotting with Bip1, the pattern of isoforms remains unchanged (Fig. 1, middle panel), however, contaminating proteins of the pollen exudate are now absent, as an identical pattern is obtained by Coomassie Brilliant Blue R-250 or silver staining (data not shown). The major Bet v 1 isoform (2), now called Bet v 1a, was expressed as a recombinant non-fusion (rnf) protein in E. coli using the pMW vector system (11,12), purified, and tested for its immunological equivalence with natural Bet v 1. In solution competition experiments employing a sandwich ELISA for Bet v 1, titration of rnfBet v 1a against natural Bet v 1 showed complete equivalence on a weight basis (3). rnfBet v 1a is a single species of polypeptide with no postsynthetic modifications (besides cleavage of the start methionine) as shown by mass spectrometry (next paragraph). Apparently, renaturation from 8M urea leads to a conformer (or group of conformers) that is equivalent to natural Bet v 1. Nevertheless, two-

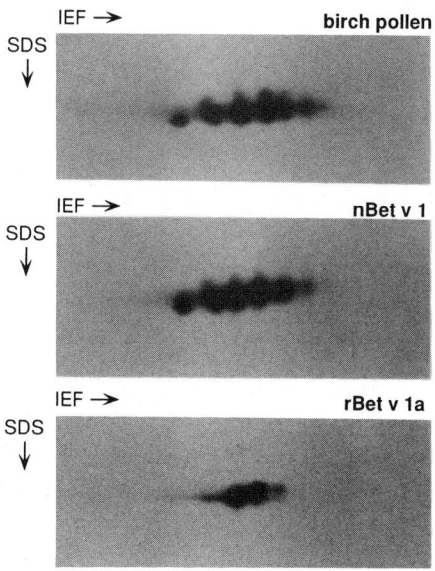

Figure 1. Autoradiographs of two-dimensional separations of Bet v 1 detected with monoclonal antibody Bip1 as described in ref. (1). IEF: direction of isoelectric focusing; SDS: direction of SDS-PAGE. In the upper two panels, the isoelectric points of the isoforms span the pH range from 4.9 (left) to 5.9 (right). The molecular weight is about 17 kD. Upper panel: unpurified birch pollen extract; middle panel: affinity purified natural Bet v 1; lower panel: recombinant non-fusion Bet v 1a purified from E. coli.

dimensional analysis of rnfBet v 1a yields four (two major and two minor) spots that seem to coincide with four of the spots seen in natural Bet v 1 (Fig. 1, lower panel). While we have no convincing explanantion for the apparent heterogeneity of rnfBet v 1a, it clearly means that, although 10 different isoform protein sequences have been found on a cDNA basis and have been confirmed by mass spectrometry (ref.7 and next paragraph), there is no one-to-one correlation between a particular isoform protein sequence and a spot in the two-dimensional pattern.

Pollen Bet v 1 Isoform Sequences

The Bet v 1 preparation shown above (Fig.1, middle panel) was analyzed by PDMS after digestion with trypsin and endoproteinase Glu-C (7). For comparison, the affinity-purified rnfBet v 1a was analyzed in a similar fashion. The molecular masses of all peptides obtained in this way (either in a complex mixture or after HPLC purification) were carefully compared in a computer-aided search with all peptide fragments predicted from the cDNA sequences of isoforms (Fig.2). These were obtained either by immunological screening of a birch pollen epression cDNA library in lambda-ZAP or by PCR using primers complementary to the highly conserved N terminus of Bet v 1a and to the polyA tail of the mRNA. In the comparison, an exhaustive search for all possible known postsynthetic modifications on the peptides was performed. Especially, phosphopeptides (phosphorylation would explain the large charge heterogeneity on the isoforms) and glycopeptides were searched. It is well known that phosphopeptides would survive the conditions during purification, proteolysis and PDMS used by us (7). The results of this investigation can be summarised as follows: All of the isoform sequences found as cDNAs were confirmed by PDMS. In some cases, very closely related sequences could be confirmed only as a group (7). Bet v 1a seems to comprise more than half of the natural Bet v 1 in pollen. No other isoforms reactive to Bip1 seem to exist in birch pollen above the detection limit of the PDMS method used. Please note that natural Bet v 1 as well as the

```
                  ▬▬▬▬▬▬▬▬▬▬▬▬▬▬▬▬▬▬    ▬▬▬▬▬▬▬▬▬▬▬▬▬▬▬▬    ▬▬▬▬▬▬▬
                  ▬▬▬▬▬▬▬▬▬▬▬▬▬▬▬▬▬   ▬▬▬▬▬▬▬▬▬▬▬▬▬▬    ▬▬▬▬▬▬▬▬▬▬▬▬▬▬▬▬
Bet v 1 a    MGVFNYETETTSVIPAARLFKAFILDGDNLFPKVAPQAISSVENIEGNGGPGTIKKISFPEGFPFKYVKDRVDEVDHTNF
Bet v 1 j    .........A......................................................................
Bet v 1 f/i  .......I.A......................................................................
Bet v 1 d/h  .......I..................V.......................N..............................
Bet v 1 g    .......S.................E....I...................N..............................
Bet v 1 e    .........A...........................................I......G...................
Bet v 1 l    .........A........M.........K.V...................N..............................
Bet v 1 b    ....................E..T.I........................T....S......E.......A..
Bet v 1 k    .......S............E..T.I........................T....S......E.......A..
Bet v 1 c    .......S............E..T.I........................T....S......E.......A..


                  ▬▬▬▬▬▬▬▬▬▬▬▬    ▬▬▬▬▬▬▬▬▬▬▬▬▬▬    ▬▬▬▬▬▬▬▬▬▬▬▬
                                ▬▬▬▬▬▬▬▬▬▬▬▬▬▬▬▬    ▬▬▬▬▬▬▬▬▬▬
Bet v 1 a    KYNYSVIEGGPIGDTLEKISNEIKIVATPDGGSILKISNKYHTKGDHEVKAEQVKASKEMGETLLRAVESYLLAHSDAYN
Bet v 1 j    ..S........V...................N.......N..............I..........................
Bet v 1 f/i  ..S........V...................N.......N..............I..........................
Bet v 1 d/h  ...........V.................CV.........N........................................
Bet v 1 g    ...........V.................CV.........N........................................
Bet v 1 e    ..S........V...................N.......N..............I..........................
Bet v 1 l    ...........V.................CV.........N........................................
Bet v 1 b    ..S..M...AL.......C..............................M...HM..I..K..A.................
Bet v 1 k    ..S..M...AL.......C..............................M...HM..I..K..A.................
Bet v 1 c    ..S..M...AL.......C..............................Q.M...HM..I..K..A...............
```

Figure 2. Derived amino acid sequences of 10 different Bet v 1 isoforms occurring in birch pollen. Isoforms f and i as well as isoforms d and h differ at the nucleotide level but code for the same protein. Dots indicate amino acid identities with Bet v 1a, letters indicate amino acid sequence differences with respect to Bet v 1a. The single letter code is used. Bars above the sequence of Bet v 1a indicate T-cell epitopes of Bet v 1a as determined with overlapping synthetic peptides (14).

cDNA library were prepared from the same commmercially available birch pollen. Both in the rnfBet v 1a and in natural Bet v 1, the N-terminal methionine is cleaved off, but no other postsynthetic modifications could be detected, in particular, no glycosylation or phosphorylation.

Immunological Reactivity of Pollen Bet v 1 Isoforms

We have investigated both the IgE-binding properties and the ability to stimulate T-cells to proliferate of a selection of the isoforms described here. To this end, 9 isoforms (Bet v 1a,b,c,d,e,f,g,j,and l) were expressed as rnf proteins in E. coli (13) and tested for IgE binding (refs. 8, 13 and this paper) and five of them (Bet v 1 a,b,d, e, and l) were tested with T-cell clones from 8 patients (8). Fig. 3 shows immunoblots of five randomly chosen untreated patients allergic to birch pollen (RAST class >3.5). Extracts from E. coli cells expressing the nine Bet v 1 isoforms mentioned above as rnf proteins were electroblotted and decorated with the patients_sera. Equal amounts of the isoforms were applied to each lane as monitored by Coomassie Brilliant Blue R-250 staining (upper panel). It is immediately obvious that in untreated patients isoforms d, g, and l do not bind IgE, while all other isoforms tested do bind IgE. This pattern held true for all further patients tested.

Next, it seemed interesting to us to compare the IgE reactivity of the same untreated patients with their IgG reactivity towards Bet v 1 isoforms before and after immunotherapy (Fig. 4). Before conventional immunotherapy with unpurified birch pollen extracts, most patients display no IgG reactivity towards the Bet v 1 isoforms tested. However, some patients show weak reactivity towards the isoforms not recognized by IgE (for instance, patient 2, isoform l) that is more prominent on longer exposure (not shown).

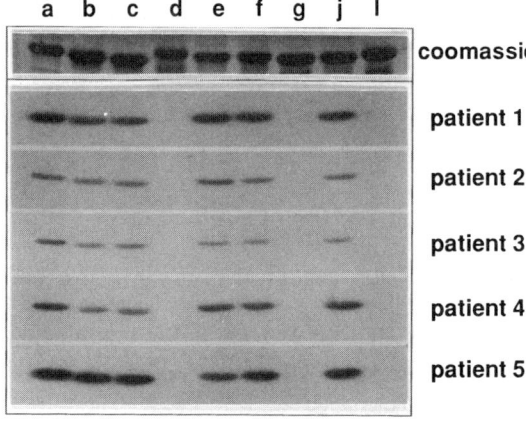

Figure 3. Autoradiographs of one-dimensional IgE immunoblots of 9 different rnfBet v 1 isoforms. On the top of the Figure the isoform designations are shown. The top panel shows the staining of the 17 kD region of the SDS-PAGE stained with Coomassie Brilliant Blue R-250. The following panels show five randomly chosen untreated patients allergic to Bet v 1.

In one patient (Fig. 5) we saw strong IgG reactivity towards isoforms g and l, which are both not recognized by IgE of untreated patients. The bottom panel shows that equal amounts of protein were applied to each lane. The sera tested after immunotherapy (Fig. 4) invariably show that IgG directed against all nine isoforms are induced by immunotherapy, although the amount of IgG directed against the isoforms maybe somewhat lower in certain patients. In some patients (1 and 4), immunotherapy induces IgE directed against isoforms d, g and l, while in some others the induction is weak or not present at all (patients 2 and 3). As we showed previously (10), other antigens or allergens present in unpurified birch pollen extracts in some patients also strongly induce IgE which may be detrimental for the patient.

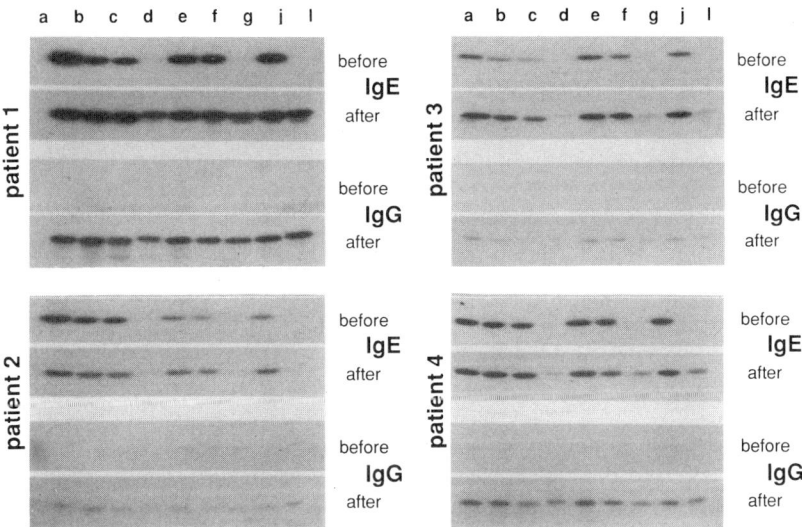

Figure 4. Autoradiographs of one-dimensional IgE and IgG immunoblots of 9 different rnfBet v 1 isoforms. On the top of the Figure the isoform designations are shown. Sera of four randomly chosen patients allergic to Bet v 1 were drawn before and after conventional immunotherapy. Equal amounts of the rnfBet v 1 isoforms were applied to each lane. IgE and IgG immunoblots were performed as described in refs. (3) and (10).

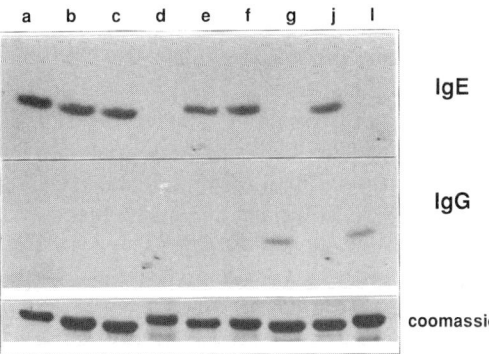

Figure 5. Autoradiographs of one-dimensional IgE and IgG immunoblots of 9 different rnfBet v 1 isoforms. On the top of the Figure the isoform designations are shown. Results with serum of the singular patient is shown that showed relatively strong IgG reactivity to Bet v 1 even before conventional immunotherapy. The bottom panel shows the staining of the 17 kD region of the SDS-PAGE stained with Coomassie Brilliant Blue R-250. Conditions are as in Fig. 4.

We now wanted to compare the IgE-binding properties of Bet v 1 isoforms with their activity in skin prick tests and their potency towards stimulating proliferation of T-cell clones derived from the same untreated patients whose sera were used for the IgE-binding studies (ref. 8, data not shown in detail). The skin prick test reactivity of purified isoforms d and l was very low as compared to Bet v 1b (intermediate) and Bet v 1 a and e (high), meaning that IgE-binding and skin prick test activity correlated very well. Surprisingly, isoform d that was nearly inactive in skin prick tests and IgE binding, was the most potent isoform (even more than Bet v 1a) in terms of T-cell stimulation (8). This must mean that on processing in antigen-presenting cells isoform d can produce potent linear T-cell epitopes that are not present in Bet v 1a. A comparison of the linear T-cell epitopes of Bet v 1a as determined with synthetic peptides (14) with the sequence of Bet v 1d (Fig.2) reveals that this is indeed possible. This suggests the use of isoform d or of mutant forms of Bet v 1 derived thereof, for a new kind of therapy (see Discussion).

Other Isoforms

In order to test the hypothesis that birch members of the Bet v 1 protein family are indeed PR proteins, a birch suspension cell culture was established and it was tried to induce the synthesis of Bet v 1 by pathogens and by several kinds of stress conditions. Infection of the cell culture with several species of bacteria and fungi including species non-pathogenic for birch led to induction of (a) 17 kD protein(s) immunologically cross-reacting with Bet v 1. Various kinds of stress conditions and chemical elicitors had no effect (ref. 15, data not shown in detail). Three different cDNAs coding for Bet v 1 isoforms were cloned and sequenced from the infected cell culture and shown to be closely related to but different from the pollen isoforms of Bet v 1 (ref.16). Finally, two-dimensional immune blots of birch leaves harvested in September or October, but not of birch leaves at the beginning of the vegetation period, contained Bet v 1 but showed a pattern of Bet v 1 isoforms different from that of pollen (unpublished observations). However, no sequence information as to these possible new isoforms is yet available.

DISCUSSION

Sequence Comparisons

Comparing the isoform sequences presented here (Fig.2 and ref.16) with all of the presently known sequences of members of the Bet v 1 protein family (to be published elsewhere), it is obvious that the 10 birch pollen isoforms and the three inducible isoforms are more closely related among each other than with any Bet v 1 family sequences belonging to different species. This would indicate that probably in higher plants only one Bet v 1 protein family exists and not two families (pollen family and PR family), although the pollen proteins are constitutive while the PR proteins are induced by pathogens. However, the known birch isoforms clearly are divided in subgroups according to sequence similarity. For instance, the group of three isoforms (d, g, and l) that do not bind IgE of untreated patients, harbors four amino acid exchanges (S57N; S112C; I113V; D125N) with respect to Bet v 1a that do not occur in any other isoform. Only four more amino acid exchanges in this group are shared with one or more other isoforms. The epitopes on Bet v 1 that are recognized by IgE are conformational in nature (8). We speculate that the four amino acid exchanges unique to the d,g,l isoform group must strongly influence the epitope(s) recognized by IgE. The isoforms induced by pathogen infection (Sc1, 2, and 3 in ref. 16) form a group that is more distantly related to the pollen isoforms. The group is separated by 24 to 43 amino acid exchanges from Bet v 1a and is also more heterogeneous in itself as Sc1 and 2 are separated by only 2 amino acid exchanges while both Sc1 and 2 are separated by 42 (43) exchanges from Sc3. However, even this group is closer to Bet v 1a than Aln g 1 (ref. 17), the major allergen from alder, the species most closely related to but different from birch.

It is noteworthy that the 10 isoform sequences discussed here and confirmed by mass spectrometry are not in complete agreement with isoform sequences presented at the same meeting by the Danish group (Larsen, J.N., et al., this volume).

Biological Importance of Bet v 1 Isoforms

Unfortunately, the amino acid sequences of members of the Bet v 1 protein family give no clue to a possible biological (enzymatic?) function of these proteins. It is well established that proteins of the Bet v 1 family are induced by infection with pathogens. However, all attempts to show a possible antibacterial or antimicrobial function of Bet v 1 so far failed (15 and Ferreira, F. et al., unpublished results). Recently, two groups (unpublished results of Heberle-Bors, E. et al. and Bufe, A. et al.) favored an RNAse function for Bet v 1. A weak RNAse activity was shown for natural Bet v 1 but not for purified rnfBet v 1. Our own attempts to reproduce these results revealed several interesting RNAses in the birch pollen exudate which were not identical with Bet v 1 while rnfBet v 1 showed no such activity and we think it is at least an open question whether Bet v 1 is indeed an RNAse.

However, the molecular properties of birch pollen and leaf Bet v 1 give us some hints about possible functions. The subcellular localization of Bet v 1 coinciding with cytoplasmic ribosomes (18) is in good agreement with our finding presented here that N- or O-glycosylation is totally absent from natural Bet v 1 (cytoplasmic proteins have never been observed to be glycosylated). In spite of its cytoplasmic localization, Bet v 1 is very quickly (within seconds to minutes) released upon wetting of pollen. As has been mentioned above, some isoforms of Bet v 1 are accumulated in old leaves. One hypothesis that would be in accordance with these observations, is that Bet v 1 might be an inhibitor of plant cell metabolism that is needed in resting tissues of the plant (pollen, old leaves of deciduous trees). Such a role as an inhibitor of plant cell metabolism could also be instrumental in defense against pathogens without Bet v 1 being an antimicrobial substance in itself. Finally, Bet v 1 could be a signalling molecule of pollen that is recognized by the stigma and would serve for the biochemical coordination between pollen and stigma in fertilization. Specific receptor(s) for Bet v 1 on the stigma should be expected in this case.

Possible Therapeutic Uses of Bet v 1 Isoforms

Allergen-specific immunotherapy of type I allergic diseases with unpurified allergen extracts (conventional immunotherapy) is partly or completely successful in about 85% of the patients. The success rate increases with increasing maintenance dose of the allergen extract, however the risk of anaphylactic side effects is also increasing in this case (8). Conventional immunotherapy may in some cases sensitize the patient to new proteins (ref. 10 and the present paper). In patients treated successfully by conventional immunotherapy, no correlation is obvious between level of the induction of IgG to the allergens in question and therapeutic success. Rather, an influence on Th2-cells producing IL-4 is more probable which depends on the allergen dose (19). Considering these findings, we are proposing here a new form of allergen-specific immune therapy that is based on the application of isoforms (like Bet v 1d) or recombinant full length mutant forms of Bet v 1 derived thereof that stimulate T-cell clones efficiently but do not bind serum IgE. This form of immunotherapy would combine two advantages: The immune system of the patient would be reacting to most of the relevant T-cell epitopes and the risk of anaphylaxis would be negligible.

ACKNOWLEDGMENTS

This work was supported by grant P10019-MOB (to F.F. and M.B.) of the Austrian Fonds zur Förderung der Wissenschaftlichen Forschung and by a grant of the Austrian Ministry of Science and Education (to M.B.).

REFERENCES

1. Rohac, M., Birkner, T., Reimitzer, I., Bohle, B., Steiner, R., Breitenbach, M., Kraft, D., Scheiner, O., Gabl, G., Rumpold, H. (1991) *Mol. Immunol.* 28, 887–906
2. Breiteneder, H., Pettenburger, K., Bito, A., Valenta, R., Kraft, D., Rumpold, H., Scheiner, O., Breitenbach, M. (1989) *EMBO J.* 8, 1935–1938
3. Ferreira, F., Hoffmann-Sommergruber, K., Breiteneder, H., Pettenburger, K., Ebner, C., Sommergruber, W., Steiner, R., Bohle, B., Sperr, W.R., Valent, P., Kungl, A.J., Breitenbach, M., Kraft, D., Scheiner, O. (1993) *J. Biol. Chem.* 268, 19574–19580
4. Carr, J.P., Klessig, D.F. (1989) In: *Genetic engineering: principles and methods*, vol. 11 (ed. J.K. Setlow), pp. 65–100. Plenum Press, New York.
5. Jarolim, E., Rumpold, H., Endler, A.T., Ebner, H., Breitenbach, M., Scheiner, O., Kraft, D. (1989a) *Allergy* 44, 385–395
6. Jarolim, E., Tejkl, M., Rohac, M., Schlerka, G., Scheiner, O., Kraft, D., Breitenbach, M., Rumpold, H. (1989b) *Int. Arch. Allerg. Appl. Immunol.* 90, 54–60
7. Swoboda, I., Jilek, A., Ferreira, F., Engel, E., Hoffmann-Sommergruber, K., Scheiner, O., Kraft, D., Breiteneder, H., Pittenauer, E., Schmid, E., Vicente, O., Heberle-Bors, E., Ahorn, H., Breitenbach, M. (1995) *J. Biol. Chem.*, 270, 2607–2613
8. Ferreira, F.; Hirtenlehner, K.; Jilek, A.; Godnik-Cvar, J.; Breiteneder, H.; Grimm, R.; Hoffmann-Sommergruber, K.; Scheiner, O.; Kraft, D.; Breitenbach, M.; Rheinberger, H.J.; Ebner, C. (1996) *J. Exp. Med.*, (in press)
9. Sanger, F., Nicklen, S., Coulson, A.R. (1977) *Proc. Natl. Acad. Sci. U.S.A.* 74, 5463–5467
10. Birkner, T., Rumpold, H., Jarolim, E., Ebner, H., Breitenbach, M., Skvaril, F., Scheiner, O., Kraft, D. (1990) *Allergy* 45, 418 - 426
11. Way, M., Pope, B., Gooch, J., Hawkins, M., Weeds, A.G. (1990) *EMBO J.* 9, 4103–4109
12. Studier, F.W., Rosenberg, A.H., Dunn, J.J., Dubendorff, J.W. (1990) *Meths. Enzymol.* 185, 60–89
13. Weiss, C., Kramer, B., Ebner, C., Susani, M., Briza, P., Hoffmann-Sommergruber, K., Breiteneder, H., Kraft, D., Scheiner, O., Breitenbach, M., Ferreira, F. (1996) *Int. Arch. Allerg. immunol.*, (in press)

14. Ebner, C., Szepfalusi, Z., Ferreira, F., Jilek, A., Valenta, R., Parronchi, P., Maggi, E., Romagnani, S., Scheiner, O., Kraft, D. (1993) *J. Immunol.* 150: 1047–1054

15. Swoboda, I., Scheiner, O., Kraft, D., Breitenbach, M., Heberle-Bors, E., Vicente, O. (1994) *Biochim. Biophys. Acta* 1219, 457–464

16. Swoboda, I., Scheiner, O., Heberle-Bors, E., Vicente, O. (1995) *Plant, Cell and Environment* 18, 865–874

17. Breiteneder, H., Ferreira F., Reikerstorfer A., Duchene M., Valenta R., Hoffmann- Sommergruber K., Ebner C., Breitenbach M., Kraft D., Scheiner O. (1992) *J. Allergy Clin. Immunol.* 90, 909 - 917

18. Grote, M. (1991) *J. Histochem. Cytochem.* 39, 1395–1401

19. Secrist, H., DeKruyff, R.H., Umetsu, D.T. (1995) *J. Exp. Med.* 181, 1081–1090

17

MODULATION OF IgE-BINDING PROPERTIES OF TREE POLLEN ALLERGENS BY SITE-DIRECTED MUTAGENESIS

Fátima Ferreira,[1] Angelika Rohlfs,[1] Karin Hoffmann-Sommergruber,[2] Siegfried Schenk,[2] Christof Ebner,[1] Peter Briza,[1] Alexander Jilek,[1] Dietrich Kraft,[2] Michael Breitenbach,[1] and Otto Scheiner[2]

[1]Inst. f. Genetik u. Allg. Biologie
Universität Salzburg
A-5020 Salzburg, Austria
[2]Inst. f. Allg. u. Exp. Pathologie
Universität Wien
A-1090 Vienna, Austria

1.INTRODUCTION

In the last few years, the use of recombinant DNA techniques for the characterization of atopic allergens offered new aspects for diagnosis and therapy of Type I allergies (1). It has made it possible to produce large quantities of well characterized "wild-type" recombinant allergens, or first-generation recombinant products, and many of them are now being developed for diagnosis and possibly therapy of Type I allergies. For instance, recombinant Asp f 1 expressed in *E. coli* was successfully used for serologic and clinical diagnosis of A. fumigatus allergy (2). It has been demonstrated that the use of two recombinant birch pollen allergens, Bet v 1 and Bet v 2 (profilin), allows accurate *in vitro* (ELISA, immunoblots) and *in vivo* (skin prick test, intradermal test) diagnosis of birch pollen allergy (3,4). In addition, recombinant Bet v 1 could be efficiently used for identifying food cross-sensitization induced by Bet v 1-related proteins (4). These studies demonstrate that recombinant allergens are adequate tools for in vivo and in vitro allergen-specific diagnosis, which might be considered as an important step towards allergen-specific therapy. Presently, specific-immunotherapy is performed using natural allergen extracts that may contain, besides the desired allergen, other unwanted components.

In addition to their use for characterization of allergens, recombinant DNA techniques also offered the unique possibility of arbitrarily altering the nucleotide sequence of a gene and, subsequently, the sequence of the encoded protein in order to produce novel "mutant" proteins, or second generation recombinant products, displaying altered proper-

New Horizons in Allergy Immunotherapy
edited by Sehon et al. Plenum Press, New York, 1996

ties. Previously we have shown that isoforms of Cor a 1, the major hazel pollen allergen, displayed striking differences in their ability to bind IgE from allergic patients (5). Since these isoforms showed high amino acid sequence similarity, we speculated that the differences in IgE-binding was a result of sequence dissimilarities. In particular, the exchange at position 10 from a threonine in Bet v 1a and Cor a 1/11 isoform to proline in Cor a 1/16 isoform seemed to correlate to its lower IgE-binding capacity. In this study, we have tested this hypothesis using a PCR-based site-directed mutagenesis approach to produce a single amino acid exchange in the Cor a 1/16 isoallergen.

2. MATERIALS AND METHODS

2.1. DNA Constructs

The cDNAs coding for Bet v 1a (6) and Cor a 1/16 (5) were cloned in the pMW175 expression vector (7). The amino acid exchange at position 10 (Pro→Thr) in Cor a 1/16 was engineered by PCR-mediated mutagenesis using the following primers:

NcoI mutagenic primer 5'-GGGCCATGGGTGTTTTCAATTACGAGGTT-GA-GACCACCTCCGTT-3', base exchanged indicated in bold; NcoI site is underlined.

EcoRI primer 5'-CCCGAATTCTTAGTTGTATTCAGCAGAGTGTGCGAA-3', EcoRI site is underlined.

The PCR was performed with 1 ng template (pMW175/Cor a 1/16 construct) and 1 μM of each primer, using 30 cycles of 1 min denaturation at 95°C, 1 min annealing at 42°C, and 1 min extension at 72°C. The PCR product was digested with NcoI and EcoRI and subcloned in the pMW175 expression vector. The resulting plasmids were used to transform competent *E. coli* BL21 cells. All PCR amplified products were sequenced according to the dideoxi chain termination method (8).

2.2. Expression of Cor a 1/16, Cor a 1/16T10, and Bet v 1a

E. coli BL21 cells containing the pMW175/Bet v 1a, pMW175/Cor a 1/16, and pMW175/Cor a 1/16T10 plasmids were grown and expression of the recombinant allergens induced by adding IPTG to a final concentration of 1 mM. After incubation at 37°C for 6 h, cells were harvested by centrifugation and lysed by repeated freeze-thaw cycles.

2.3. SDS-Page and Immunoblots

E. coli lysates of recombinant Cor a 1/16, Cor a 1/16T10, and Bet v 1a or purified proteins were analyzed by SDS-PAGE according to the method of Laemmli (9), using 15% acrylamide gels. Proteins were visualized by staining with Coomassie Brilliant Blue R-250. For immunoblot analysis, proteins were separated by 15% SDS-PAGE and electroblotted onto nitrocellulose membranes. Immunoblots using a monoclonal anti-Bet v 1, BIP 1, were performed as described previously (10). IgE immunoblots were carried out using sera from birch pollen allergic patients. Bound IgE was detected using ^{125}I-rabbit anti-human IgE. *E. coli* lysates harboring the plasmid without insert were used as a control. In all experiments, reagents, and cell lysates were from identical batches and were used in the same concentrations. Autoradiography was performed at -70°C for 12–48 h with intensifying screens.

2.4. Purification of Recombinant Allergens

rBet v 1a, rCor a 1/16, and rCor a 1/16T10 proteins were purified from crude bacterial lysates by chromatofocusing and reversed-phase HPLC (10). Purified proteins were analysed by SDS-PAGE according to the method of Laemmli (9) and visualized by staining with Coomassie Brilliant Blue R-250.

2.5. Trypsin Treatment, and Matrix-Assisted Laser Desorption/ Ionization Mass Spectrometry (MALDI-MS) of Cor a 1/16 and Cor a 1/16T10 Proteolytic Fragments

Purified Cor a 1 proteins (100 µg in distilled water) were heated for 20 min at 95°C and diluted with an equal volume of 0.2 M NH_4HCO_3. One microgram of trypsin was added and the mixture incubated at 37°C for 2 h. Afterwards, trypsin was added again, and incubation continued for an additional 4-h period. The reaction was stopped by adding 1/10 vol of trifluoracetic acid and dried *in vacuo*. The resulting peptide mixtures were subjected to MALDI-MS analysis using the HP G2025A system equipped with a nitrogen laser.

2.6. T-Cell Proliferation Assays

Isolation of Bet v 1-specific T-cell clones from the peripheral blood of birch pollen allergic patients (as indicated by typical case history, positive skin tests, and positive RAST) and proliferation assays were done as previously described (11).

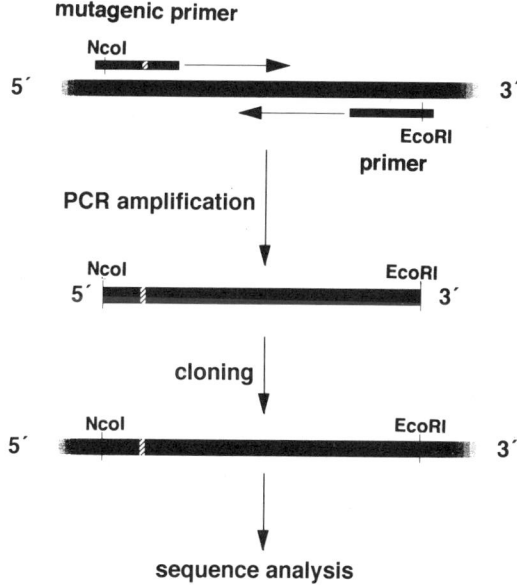

Figure 1. PCR mutagenesis of the Cor a 1/16 cDNA. The 5' Nco mutagenic primer and the 3' EcoRI primer were used in a PCR with the Cor a 1/16 cDNA.

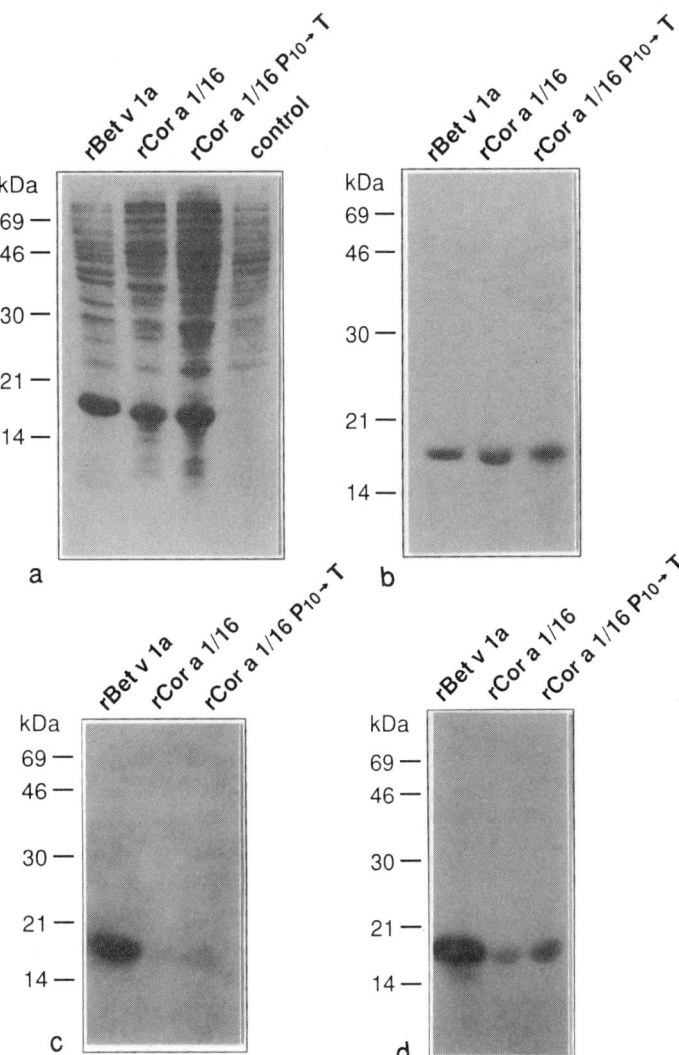

Figure 2. Expression, purification and immunoblot analysis of Cor a 1/16T10 mutant protein. (a), Coomassie-stained 15% SDS-polyacrylamide gel of lysates of *E. coli* BL21 host strain containing Cor a 1/16, Cor a 1/16T10, and Bet v 1a pMW175 expression plasmids. Control, host strain BL21 lysate containing the pMW175 expression vector without an insert. (b), Coomassie-stained 15% SDS-polyacrylamide gel of purified rCor a 1/16, rCor a 1/16T10 and rBet v 1a. (c) and (d), Immunoblots of purified rCor a 1/16, rCor a 1/16T10, and rBet v 1a probed with BIP 1, a monoclonal anti-Bet v 1, and with a polyclonal anti-rBet v 1a, respectively.

3. RESULTS AND DISCUSSION

3.1. Expression, Purification, and Mass Spectrometry Analysis of Cor a 1/16 Proteins

In this study, we have used PCR-mediated mutagenesis to generate a mutant of the Cor a 1/16 allergen. A mutant primer was used that had the proline codon at amino acid position 10 replaced by a threonine codon. The strategy for the construction of this Cor a 1/16 mutant (Cor a 1/16T10) is outlined in Figure 1.

The cDNAs coding for Bet v 1a, Cor a 1/16 and Cor a 1/16T10 were subcloned in the pMW175 expression vector and high-levels of recombinant non-fusion proteins were produced by induction with IPTG. Figure 2A shows a Coomassie-stained gel of expressed Bet v 1a, Cor a 1/16, and Cor a 1/16T10 proteins.

The recombinant proteins were purified from crude bacterial lysates using chromato-focusing and reversed-phase HPLC. The proteins appeared homogeneous as determined by SDS-PAGE and Coomassie-staining (Figure 2B).

In order to confirm at the protein level the sequence of the Cor a 1/16T10 mutant allergen, purified rCor a 1/16 and rCor a 1/16T10 were digested with trypsin and the proteolytic fragments subjected to MALDI-MS. Nine peptides were detected for both Cor a 1/16 and Cor a 1/16T10, and their molecular weights were determined from the obtained spectra (Table 1). The observed mass signals could be easily matched with the molecular weight of peptides predicted from the amino acid sequence deduced from the published Cor a 1/16 sequence (T1, T4-T6, T9–10, T12, T18–19). These peptides covered about 70% of the Cor a 1/16 sequence. All peptides detected by MALDI-MS of rCor a 1/16 digests were also detected in rCor a

Table 1. Mass determination of tryptic fragments T1-T19 of rCor a 1/16T10. Theoretical m/z values give the calculated masses of the peptides plus one proton $[M+H]^+$

Fragment	Sequence	m/z theor.	m/z observed
T1	GVFNYEVETPSVISAAR	1840.03	1839.6
T1 P10 → T	GVFNYEVETSVISAAR	1844.02	1843.2
T2	LFK	407.53	-
T3	SYVLDGDK	896.96	-
T4	LIPK	470.62	470.3
T5	VAPQAITSVENVGGNGGPGTIK	2067.29	2067.3
T6	NITFGEGSR	981.04	981.2
T7	YK	310.36	-
T8	YVK	409 49	-
T9	ERVDEVDNTNFK	1466.54	1466.6
T10	YSYTVIEGDVLGDKLEK	1929.96	1929.4
T11	VCSELK	678.81	-
T12	IVAAPGGGSTLK	1071.25	1071.2
T13	ISSK	434.50	-
T14	FHAK	502.58	-
T15	GDHEINAEEMK	1273.35	-
T16	GAK	275.32	-
T17	EMAEK	607.69	-
T18	LLR	401.52	401.5
T19	AVETYLLAHSAEYN	1581.71	1581.7

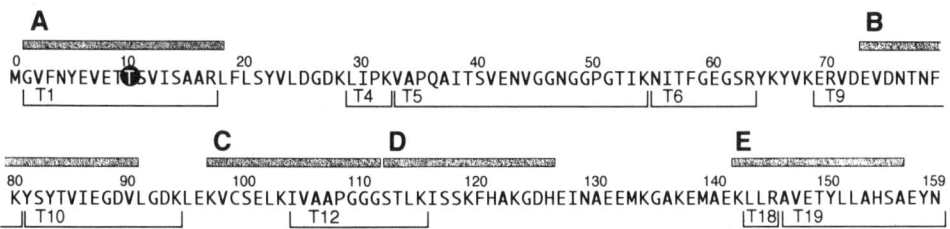

Figure 3. Tryptic peptides of rCor a 1/16T10 (T1-T19) identified by MALDI-MS. The positions of peptides stimulating specific T cell clones (A-E) are indicated by boxes above the sequence.

1/16T10 digests, except for the signal at m/z 1839 corresponding to the N-terminal peptide T1 (Table 1). According to the Cor a 1/16T10 cDNA sequence, peptide T1 should contain the single amino acid exchange (Pro → Thr) when compared to Cor a 1/16. In tryptic digests of rCor a 1/16T10 a signal at m/z 1843 (T-P10 → T) corresponded exactly to the expected mass of T1 with an exchange of proline for a threonine (Table 1). Figure 3 shows the recorded mass signals of rCor a 1/16T10 proteolytic digests mapped onto the cDNA-derived Cor a 1/16T10 sequence according to their molecular mass and enzyme specificity. Thus, the single amino acid substitution engineered in the Cor a 1/16 cDNA to produce Cor a 1/16T10 was also confirmed at the protein level by mass spectrometry analysis of proteolytic digests of rCor a 1/16T10 mutant protein.

3.2 Immunological Properties of Cor a 1/16T10

To evaluate the antibody-binding properties of purified rCor a 1/16T10 mutant protein in comparison to rCor a 1/16 and rBet v 1a, we performed immunoblotting experiments.

Figures 2C and 2D show immunoblots of the purified proteins using a monoclonal anti-Bet v 1 antibody, BIP 1, (Fig. 2C) and a rabbit anti-rBet v 1a serum (Fig. 2D). Both antibodies showed strong reactivity to rBet v 1a. In contrast, BIP 1 did not react with rCor a 1/16 or with rCor a 1/16T10, and the polyclonal anti-Bet v 1a showed a weak reactivity to both rCor a 1/16 and rCor a 1/16T10 proteins.

Immunoblots experiments using sera from birch pollen allergic patients showed remarkable differences in the IgE-binding properties of rCor a 1/16 and rCor a 1/16T10. Figure 4 shows the IgE-binding patterns of rBet v 1a, rCor a 1/16, and rCor a 1/16T10 using sera from five birch pollen allergic patients. All patients showed a marked increase in IgE-binding to rCor a 1/16T10 mutant protein compared to wild type rCor a 1/16, except patient 2. For patients 1, 4, and 5, the replacement of proline at position 10 by a threonine resulted in a change of the antibody-binding pattern from "no-binding" to strong IgE-binding. Interestingly, rCor a 1/16T10 mutant protein in some cases displayed higher IgE-binding activity than rBet v 1a (patients 1, 2, 3, and 5).

Presently, there are no data available on the 3D-structure of Bet v 1 or homologous proteins. Also, there are no precise informations available about IgE-binding motif(s) on the Bet v 1 or Bet v 1-related allergens. However, there are indications that IgE-binding structures on the Bet v 1 molecule might be determined by the protein conformation (10).

Among all standard amino acids, proline seems to occupy a unique position. Proline imposes strong conformational constraints on the peptide chain because the side-chain is cyclized back onto the backbone amide position. When present inside an alpha-helix, the possibility of making hydrogen bonds to the preceding turn is hindered and a kink of 20°

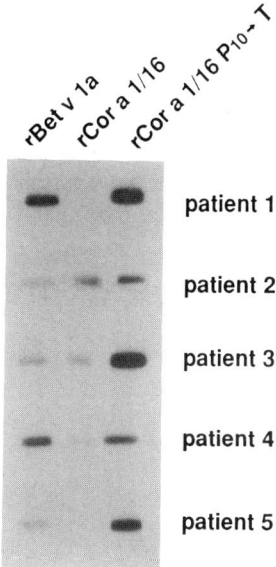

Figure 4. IgE-binding to rCor a 1/16T10, rCor a 1/16, and rBet v 1a. Immunoblot experiments showing serum IgE-reactivity of 5 birch pollen allergic patients.

or more will be introduced in the alpha-helix. In addition, proline can introduce structural heterogeneity since the X-proline (X being any amino acid) bond can assume either the stereoisomeric cis or trans conformation (for a review see 12).

Taking into consideration the exceptional properties of proline, it is possible that the substitution in Cor a 1/16 of proline-10 for a threonine residue might cause conformational changes with the result of a dramatic increase in its IgE-binding activity. This correlates well with the fact that Bet v 1a, which displays high IgE-binding activity, has a threonine at position 10. It will be interesting to test whether the substitution of threonine-10 in Bet v 1a for a proline will lower its IgE-binding activity.

3.3 Activation of Allergen-Specific T Cell Clones

The ability of rCor a 1/16T10 to activate allergen-specific T cell clones was evaluated using Bet v 1a-specific T cell clones. We tested fourteen clones that were established from the peripheral blood of birch pollen allergic patients and were shown to recognize distinct epitopes (A-E) scattered over the whole Bet v 1a molecule (Fig. 5) (ref. 11). Seven of these Bet v 1a-specific T cell clones also recognize the corresponding sequence on Cor a 1/16. The epitope recognized by the clone RR9 comprises the amino acid substitution on rCor a 1/16T10. This clone reacted with both rCor a 1/16 and rCor a 1/16T10 mutant protein. Except for the clone WD25, all other clones reacting with rCor a 1/16 also reacted with rCor a 1/16T10. It is not clear why this clone failed to proliferate in response to rCor a 1/16T10. As shown in Fig. 5, this clone recognizes an epitope (epitope E) corresponding to the C-terminal region (142–156) of Bet v 1a and Cor a 1/16. The possibility of a mutation in the peptide epitope recognized by this clone can be ruled out since MALDI-MS analysis of proteolytic fragments of rCor a 1/16T10 confirmed the structural integrity of the region corresponding to epitope E (see Fig. 3 and Table 1). It is conceiv-

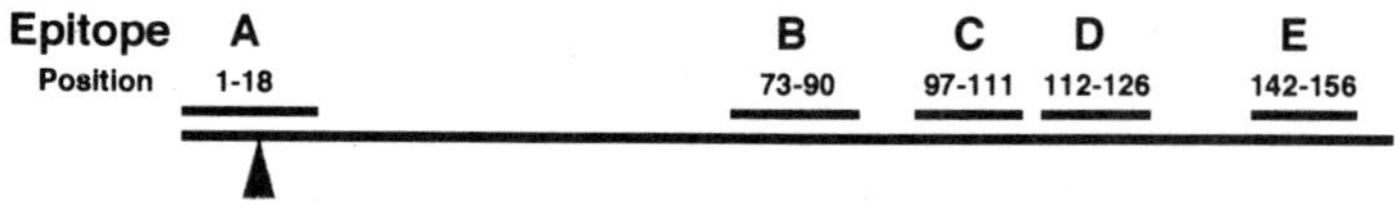

Epitope	A		B	C	D	E
Position	1-18		73-90	97-111	112-126	142-156

TCC	EPITOPE	rBet v 1a	rCor a 1/16	rCor a 1/16 $P_{10} \rightarrow T$
BE6	A	+	-	-
WD27		+	-	-
RR9		+	+	+
MH23	B	+	-	-
WF22		+	++	++
WF20		+	-	-
MS2	C	+	-	-
WF17		+	-	-
TF1		+	-	-
WF38	D	+	+	+
RR4	E	+	+	+
WD24		+	+	+
TF10		+	+	+
WD25		+	+	-

Figure 5. Proliferative responses of human Bet v 1-specific T cell clones (TCC) to rCor a 1/16, rCor a 1/16T10, and rBet v 1a. On top, the black bar represents the Bet v 1a amino acid sequence. The positions of the epitopes (A-E) recognized by the TCC are indicated by boxes above the Bet v 1a sequence.

able that the single amino acid exchange at position 10 in Cor a 1/16T10 can affect the conformation of the protein to an extent that the processing by antigen presenting cells is different and a non-reactive peptide is created or that the epitope is destroyed. In this respect, Finnegan and Amburgey (13) showed that a single amino acid change in the staphylococcal nuclease protein affects the structure of the processed peptides in such a manner that stimulatory determinants are no longer presented to certain T cell clones.

4. CONCLUSIONS

The results presented here suggest that it is possible to modulate the IgE-binding properties of tree pollen allergens by single amino acid substitutions at crucial positions. This finding makes it possible to develop second-generation of recombinant allergens with antibody-binding properties specifically modulated for diagnosis and for therapy.

Following this line, we are presently testing the effect of single amino acid exchanges on the IgE-binding properties of Bet v 1a, which were based on the patterns of amino acid substitutions of Bet v 1 isoforms displaying low IgE-binding properties.

The identification of positions crucial for IgE binding might be facilitated by cloning and sequencing isoforms of a particular allergen and determining their IgE-binding properties. In addition, isoforms with low or no IgE-binding activity could be useful tools for defining IgE-binding structures on allergens.

ACKNOWLEDGMENTS

This work was supported by grants P10019-MOB (to F.F. and M.B.), S06704-MED (to C.E.), and S06707-MED (to O.S.).

5. REFERENCES

1. Scheiner, O., Bohle, B., Breitenbach, M., Breiteneder, H., Duchene, M., Ebner, C., Ferreira, F., Hoffmann-Sommergruber, K., Pettenburger, K., Rumpold, H., Steiner, R., Tejkl, M., Valenta, R., Kraft, D. (1992) Recombinant allergens: production and possible clinical applications. In: Godard P., Bousquet J., Michel F.B.,eds. Advances in Allergology and Clinical Immunology, Carnforth, Park Ridge:Parthenon Publishing Group, pp.115–127.

2. Moser, M., Crameri, r., Menz, G., Schneider, T., Dudler, t., Virchow, C., Gmachl, M., Blaser, K., Suter, M. (1992) Cloning and expression of recombinant Aspergillus fumigatus allergen I/a (rAsp fI/a) with IgE binding and Type I skin test activity. J. Immunol. 149, 454–460.

3. Menz, G., Dolocek, C., Schönheit-Kenn, U., Ferreira, F., Moser, M., Schneider, T., Suter, M., Boltz-Nitulescu, G., Ebner, C., Kraft, D., Valenta, R. Serological and skin test diagnosis of birch pollen allergy with recombinant Bet v 1, the major birch pollen allergen. Clin. Exp. Allergy (in press).

4. Pauli, G., Oster, J.P., Deviller, P., Heiss, S., Bessot, J.C., Susani, M., Ferreira F., Kraft, D., Valenta, R. Skin testing with recombinant allergens rBet v 1 and rBet v 2: Diagnostic value for birch pollen and associated allergies. J. Allergy Clin. Immunol. (in press).

5. Breiteneder, H., Ferreira, F., Hoffmann-Sommergruber, K., Ebner, C., Breitenbach, M., Rumpold, H., Kraft, D., Scheiner, O. (1993) Four recombinant isoforms of Cor a I, the major allergen of hazel pollen, show different IgE-binding properties. Eur. J. Biochem. 212, 355–362.

6. Breiteneder, H., Pettenburger, K., Bito, A., Valenta, R., Kraft, D., Rumpold, H., Scheiner, O., Breitenbach, M. (1989) The gene coding for the major birch pollen allergen Bet v 1, is highly homologous to a pea disease resistance response gene. EMBO J. 8, 1935–1938.

7. Studier, F.W., Rosenberg, A.H., Dunn, J.J., Dubendorff, J.W. (1990) Use of T7 RNA polymerase to direct expression of cloned genes. Methods Enzymol. 185, 60–89.

8. Sanger, F., Nicklen, S., Coulson, A.R. (1977) DNA sequencing with chain termination inhibitors. Proc. Natl. Acad. Sci. USA 74, 5463–5467.

9. Laemmli, U.K. (1970) Cleavage of structural proteins during assembly of the head of bacteriophage T4. Nature 227, 680–685.

10. Ferreira, F., Hoffmann-Sommergruber, K., Breiteneder, H., Pettenburger, K., Ebner, C., Sommergruber, W., Steiner, R., Bohle, B., Sperr, W., Valent, P., Kungl, A., Breitenbach, M., Kraft, D., Scheiner, O. (1993) Purification and characterization of recombinant Bet v 1, the major birch pollen allergen. Immunological equivalence to natural Bet v 1. J. Biol. Chem. 268, 19574–19580.

11. Ebner, C., Szepfalusi, Z., Ferreira, F., Jilek, A., Valenta, R., Parronchi, P., Maggi, E., Romagnani, S., Scheiner, O., Kraft, D. (1993) Identification of multiple T cell epitopes of Bet v 1, the major birch pollen allergen, using allergen-specific T cell clones and overlapping peptides. J. Immunol. 150, 1047–1054.

12. Vanhoof, G., Goossens, F., De Meester, I., Hendriks, D., Scharpe, S. (1995) Proline motifs in peptides and their biological processing. FASEB J. 9, 736–744.

13. Finnegan, A. and Amburgey, C.F. (1989) A single amino acid mutation in a protein antigen abrogates presentation of certain T cell determinants. J. Exp. Med. 170, 2171–2176.

18

ADVANTAGES AND DISADVANTAGES OF RECOMBINANT ALLERGENS AND PEPTIDES FOR SPECIFIC IMMUNOTHERAPY

Carsten Schou[*]

ALK-Abelló Group
Bøge Alle 10–12
DK-2970 Hørsholm, Denmark

INTRODUCTION

The only causal treatment for allergic diseases currently available is hyposenzitization alias specific immunotherapy (SIT). The treatment is basically the injection of the causative agent i.e. an aqueous extract of the allergen source in question.

The exact mechanism underlying succesful SIT is still relatively obscure and the only rational progress that this way of curing allergic disease has undergone during its long life time has been due to the increasing knowledge of the allergens in the extracts used.

At the present it is debated wether SIT downregulates an ongoing allergen specific Th2-like immune response or upregulates a Th1-like response directed to the disease causing allergen molecules. Evidence for the first mechanism has been provided by Secrist et al. (1) for grass and house dust mite allergy. This matter is still under debate and the outcome is likely to influence the rational design of future allergy vaccines including the potential use of recombinant allergens or peptides derived from the amino acid sequences of major allergens.

ALLERGENS

The majority of allergies are due to relatively few sources. Approximately half a dozen grasses, a few local trees and weeds, the ubiquitous house dust mites, mammalian pets, molds and some insects including stinging hymenopterans. A total of about 30 sources will cover 99% of all Type 1 allergies.

* Research Manager

New Horizons in Allergy Immunotherapy
edited by Sehon et al. Plenum Press, New York, 1996

137

Extracts of each source will contain 20–50 readily dissolvable proteins that are all potential allergens. Just a few of these are responsible for most of the allergic immune response for the individual patient as well as for the allergic population in general. The various sources contain from 1 to 4 of such major allergens.

Most of the allergens characterized so far have an apparent MW between 10 and 40 kD i.e. they exhibit a large array of determinants for antibody binding (B-cell epitopes) and T-cell receptor engaging (T-cell epitopes).

Recently it has been realized that each of the major allergens are present in a number of forms that varies with respect to their amino acid sequences (2–6). These are named isoallergens and although the variations are not very large it has been shown to influence the interaction with the immune system (5, and Dr. S. Sparholt pers. comm.).

The isoallergenic variation is likely to have implications for the potential use of recombinant allergens and peptides derived from allergens.

Not only does each source have several major allergens but each allergen occurs in several variations.

Anecdotic information floats, about patients that react primarily to one birch tree and not so strongly to others. The has inspired studies of genomic DNA of individual birch trees by Southern blotting with probes derived from the sequence of Bet v 1, the major allergen of white birch *Betula verrucosa* (C. Cvitanich pers. comm.). This technique has revealed that each tree displays a limited number of isovariants and that the complement of variants differs from one tree to the next. These results lend some credence to the patients' impressions. The influence of this exposure difference on the ensuing allergic immune response is currently not understood, but it may play a role if selected isoallergens should be used for future treatment strategies.

EPITOPES

The availibility of B-cell epitopes is largely dependent on the appropriate three dimensional structure of the allergen molecule. If future causal treatment of allergy will exploit antigen presentation in the classical way by means of antigen presenting cells (APC) it is likely that B-cell epitopes on the allergen used for treatment will play an important role. Is has recently been demonstrated that antibody binding to allergen molecules greatly enhances antigen presentation to allergen specific T-cells in-vitro and it is highly possible that the same phenomenon is encountered in-vivo (7). Depending on the allergen and the expression system used, B-cell epitope availability has varied extensively on allergens produced by means of recombinant DNA techiques. The *Fagales* allergens e.g. Bet v 1 readily folds up properly and house dust mite group 1 allergens e.g. Der p 1 expressed in *E. coli* are at the other extreme. Furthermore it has been demonstrated that B-cell epitopes presented by isovariants differ quite extensively.

T-cell epitopes do not have the same 3-D constraints as B-cell epitopes and the availability of these should not present the same problems as with B-cell epitopes. Recombinant allergens are powerful T-cell stimulators. Thus for future vaccination purposes it is likely that recombinant allergens could regulate ongoing immune responses or elicit de-novo reactions that could potentially override ongoing ones. Since the immune mechanisms of current SIT are poorly understood it is at present impossible to construct "rational" vaccines as replacement for the ones used now. Many studies have demonstrated that each allergen molecule displays a large array of T-cell epitopes that are scattered along the entire polypeptide chain (8–11). If recombinant allergens will be exploited one will furthermore have to consider the variation with respect to T-cell epitopes seen among different isovariants of each major allergen. Another point is that the major allergens as defined by IgE-binding studies are not necessarily the only allergens of importance for the T-cell response of allergic patients as demonstrated by van Neerven et al. (11) for cat allergy.

The use of synthetic peptides for anergizing ongoing T-cell responses of the allergic immune response directly exploits T-cell epitopes. The mechanism adressed probably bypasses the classical antigen presenting pathways by bombarding the system with high concentrations of peptide. Relatively little is known about this approach at the present, but if properly selected the peptides will not provide IgE binding and thus should theortically preclude the IgE-mediated side effects of immunotherapy.

CONCLUSION

The novel insight into the diversity of the allergic immune response of patients holds a promise of a rational design of future allergy vaccines. At the same time however it raises concern about the possibility of covering the whole array of variability with just a limited number of components derived from each allergen source. These vaccines should optimally be suitable for all or most patients reactive with the source in question and be as effective as current SIT and have fewer side effects. Although SIT is a very safe and effective treatment if properly performed the possible side effects are still considered troublesome.

The diverse genetics of the outbred human population will no doubt pose problems for the "designers" of allergy vaccines of the future especially as neither the influence of HLA class II restriction nor that of TCR engagement has been worked out in detail (12,13).

An issue of a completely different nature is the economics involved, at government as well as manufacturer levels. The production and subsequent registration of products based on recombinant techniques are very resource consuming and will have to be taken into account. In this respect synthetic peptides could probably be treated as chemicals and would therefore be more easily handled.

No matter which way we go we are likely to encounter difficulties, but the development in recent years in the understanding of the interaction between allergens and the human immune system will no doubt benefit the future management of allergic disease.

REFERENCES

1. Secrist H, Chelen CJ, Wen Y, Marshall JD, Umetsu DT. Allergen immunotherapy decreases interleukin-4 production in CD4+ T cells from allergic individuals. J Exp Med 1993;178:2123
2. Rafnar T, Griffith IJ, Kuo M, Bond JF, Rogers BL, Klapper DG. Cloning of Amb a I (Antigen E), the major allergen family of short ragweed pollen. J Biol Chem 1991;266:1229–1236.
3. Breiteneder H, Ferreira F, Reikerstorfer A, Duchene M, Valenta R, Hoffmann-Sommergruber K, Ebner C, Beritenbach M, Kraft D, Scheiner O. Complementary DNA cloning and expression in E. coli of Aln g I, the major allergen of alder (Alnus glutinosa). J Allergy Clin Immunol 1992;90:909–917.
4. Breiteneder H, Pettenburger K, Bito A, Valenta R, Kraft D, Rumpold H, Scheiner O, Breitenbach M. The gene coding for the major birch pollen allergen Bet v I is highly homologous to a pea disease resistance gene. EMBO J 1989;8:1935–1938.
5. Breiteneder H, Ferreira F, Hoffmann-Sommergruber K, Ebne C, Breitenbach M, Rumpold H, Kraft D, Scheiner O. Four recombinant isoforms of Cor a I, the major allergen of hazel pollen show different IgE-binding properties. Eur J Biochem 1993;212:355–362.

6. Larsen JN, Strøman P, Ipsen H. PCR based cloning and sequencing of genes encoding the tree pollen major allergen Car b I from *Carpinus betulus* (hornbeam). Mol Immunol 1992;29:730–711.

7. van der Heijden FL, van Neerven RJJ, van Katwijk M, Bos JB, Kapsenberg ML. Serum IgE-facilitated allergen presentation in atopic disease. J Immunol 1993;150:3643–3650.

8. Yssel H, Johnson KE, Schneider PV, Wideman J, Terr A, Kastelein, De Vries JE. T cell activation including epitopes of the house dust mite allergen Der p I. J Immunol 1992;148:738–745.

9. O'Brien MR, Thomas W, Tait DB. An immunogenetic analyses of T-cell reactive regions of the major allergen from the house dust mite, Der p I, with recombinent truncated fragments. J Allergy Clin Immunol 1994;93:628–634.

10. Higgins AJ, Thorpe JC, Hayball DJ, O'Hehir ER, Lamb RJ. Overlapping T-cell epitopes in the group I allergen of *Dermatophagoides* species restricted by HLA-DP and HLA-DR class II molecules. J Allergy Clin Immunol 1994;93:891–899.

11. van Neerven RJJ, van de Pol MM, van Milligen FJ, Jansen HM, Aalberse RC, Kapsenberg ML. Characterization of cat dander-specific T lymphocytes from atopic patients. J Immunol 1994;224:717–722.

12. Moffat MF, Hill MR, Cornelis F, Schou C, Faux JA, Young RP, James AL, Ryan G, le Souef P, Musk AW, Hopkin JM, Cookson WOCM. Genetic linkage of T-cell receptor afpha/delta complex to specific IgE responses. Lancet 1994;343:1597–1600.

13. Young RP, Dekker JW, Wordsworth BP, Schou C, Pile KD, Matthiesen F, Rosenberg WMC, Bell JI, Hopkin JM, Cookson WOMC. HLA-DR and HLA-DP genotypes and immunoglobulin E responses to common major allergens. Clin Exp Allergy 1994;24:431–439.

19

T CELL EPITOPES OF Phl p 1, MAJOR POLLEN ALLERGEN OF TIMOTHY GRASS (*Phleum pratense*)

Crossreactivity with Group I Allergens of Different Grasses

Siegfried Schenk,[1] Heimo Breiteneder,[1] Markus Susani,[2]
Nader Najafian,[1] Sylvia Laffer,[1] Michael Duchêne,[1]
Rudolf Valenta,[1] Gottfried Fischer,[3] Otto Scheiner,[1]
Dietrich Kraft,[1] and Christof Ebner[1]

[1]Institute of General and Experimental Pathology
University of Vienna, Austria
[2]Institute of Molecular Biology
Academy of Science, Salzburg, Austria
[3]Institute of Blood Group Serology
General Hospital, Vienna, Austria

1. INTRODUCTION

Recently several group I grass pollen allergens, such as Phl p 1 from timothy grass (*Phleum pratense*), some isoforms of Lol p 1 from rye-grass *(Lolium perenne)*, and Sec c 1 from rye (*Secale cereale;* S. Laffler, unpublished results) have been characterized by molecular cloning techniques[1–3] and were found to display a high degree of amino acid (AA) sequence-similiarity. T lymphocytes play an important role in the induction of IgE-synthesis, and therefore in the development of Type I allergy[4–6]. In this study humoral and cellular responses to recombinant Phl p 1 (from timothy grass) were analyzed. T cell lines (TCL) and T cell clones (TCC) were established to determine T cell epitopes of this aller-gen. IgE-crossreactivity among pollen allergens of different grass species has been ob-served on the IgE-level[1]. We investigated T cell-crossreactivity among grass group I allergens. The knowledge of major and/or crossreacting T cell epitopes of grass pollen al-lergens[2,7] is important for the development of vaccines for immunotherapy (IT) in the fu-ture.

New Horizons in Allergy Immunotherapy
edited by Sehon et al. Plenum Press, New York, 1996

2. MATERIAL AND METHODS

2.1. Patients

Nine patients (EC, GZ, HER, HN, KH, LV, NO, PS, RH) allergic to grass pollen (typical case history, positive skin tests, and positive RAST [RAST class 3–6]) were selected for this study. HLA (MHC class II) typing[8] was performed as described.

2.2. Grass-Pollen Extracts

Pollens from *Phleum pratense* (timothy grass), *Dactylis glomerata* (cock's foot grass), *Poa pratensis* (Kentucky blue grass), *Lolium perenne* (rye grass) and *Secale cereale* (rye) were purchased from Allergon AB (Engelholm, Sweden). Aqueous extracts were prepared and used for cell culture as described[9].

2.3. Expression and Purification of Recombinant Non-Fusion Phl p 1

r Phl p 1 protein expressed in *E. coli* was purified by ion exchange chromatography (M. Susani, unpublished results).

2.4. Overlapping Peptides

76 dodecapeptides overlapping for three residues (neighbours share 9 AA) were synthesized (Cambridge Research Biochemicals Limited, Cambridge, U.K.) according to the sequence of Phl p 1[1]. Epitope mapping of TCL and TCC was performed as described[10,11].

2.5. IgE-Immunoblots

Plasma samples were tested for IgE-binding to r Phl p 1 and to aqueous extracts of *Phleum pratense, Dactylis glomerata, Poa pratensis, Lolium perenne* and *Secale cereale* in immunoblots as described[9].

2.6. Allergen-specific T cell lines (TCL) and T cell clones (TCC)

Allergen-specific TCL and TCC were established according to methods described[10,11].

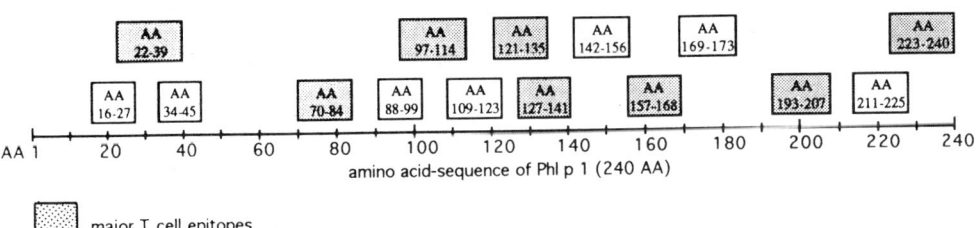

Figure 1. T cell epitopes of Phl p 1. Bars indicate T cell stimulating fragments of the AA sequence of Phl p 1.

2.7. Characterization of TCL and TCC

Proliferation assays, characterization of TCC phenotype and cytokine production pattern were performed as described[10,11]. Definition of TCR Vβ and HLA-restriction are described in this volume (H. Breiteneder et al).

3. RESULTS

3.1. IgE-Immunoblots

All patients displayed IgE-binding to natural *Phleum, Dactylis, Poa, Lolium* and *Secale* extract. Moreover, IgE-binding to recombinant Phl p 1 could be observed (not shown).

3.2. Allergen-Specific T Cell Lines and Clones

TCL were established from the peripheral blood; 40 Phl p 1-specific TCC could be isolated.

3.3. Epitope Mapping of TCL and TCC

Proliferation assays performed with overlapping peptides revealed 15 T cell epitopes on Phl p 1 (Figure 1). Eight T cell epitopes were found to stimulate T cells of several donors. Individual patients recognized 1–7 T cell specificities on the molecule.

3.4. Crossreactivity with Other Grass Species

Seven TCC reacting with two major epitopes on Phl p 1 (AA 70–84: "GSCFEIKCTKPE/ACS" and AA 97–114: "EEPIAPYHFDLS/GHA/FGA") were tested for reactivity with pollen extracts of several grasses in order to compare T cell epitopes of Phl p 1 with T cell epitopes of group I pollen allergens of other grass species. Results are summarized in Table 1.

Table 1. Proliferation of Phl p 1-specific T cell clones in response to stimulation with aqueous pollen extracts of five different grass species. +: stimulation index >10; (+): stimulation index 3–10; −: no proliferation

	T cell clone	KH27	GZ53	PS8	NO32	EC29	NO14	NO29
	T cell epitope (AA on Phl p 1)		——70-84——				—97-114—	
	TCR Vβ	17	13.1	1	17	5.1	13.1	4
grass pollen extracts	*Phleum pratense*	+	+	+	+	+	+	+
	Dactylis glomerata	+	+	+	−	+	+	+
	Poa pratensis	+	+	+	(+)	+	+	−
	Lolium perenne	+	+	+	(+)	+	+	+
	Secale cereale	(+)	−	(+)	−	(+)	+	+

Table 2. Cytokine-production of Phl p 1-specific T cell clones

T cell clone	Cytokine production			Th-subset
	IL-4 (pg/ml)	IL-2 (U/ml)	IFN-γ (pg/ml)	
EC 2	114	<0.1	<1.5	2
EC 26	<3	5	100	1
EC 27	100	2.8	150	0
EC 29	725	6	110	0
EC 55	290	<0.1	100	0
GZ 3	937	<0.1	50	2
GZ 52	>4000	27	70	2
GZ 53	2157	0.2	<1.5	2
GZ 69	3843	18	<1.5	2
HER 30	2130	1.2	200	2
HER 32	<3	<0.1	3300	1
HER 38	742	<0.1	400	—
HER 47	<3	0.6	3000	1
HER 81	1502	21	210	0
HN 6	28	<0.1	120	0
KH 8	<3	8	<1.5	1
KH 27	860	12	2400	0
LV 24	2876	<0.1	180	2
LV 32	456	<0.1	<1.5	2
NO 5	>4000	>60	170	2
NO 6	2600	0.5	<1.5	2
NO 9	>4000	<0.1	<1.5	2
NO 14	1320	1.5	800	0
NO 20	>4000	48	160	2
NO 21	130	<0.1	100	0
NO 24	150	<0.1	120	0
NO 29	>4000	48	140	2
NO 31	314	<0.1	170	0
NO 32	584	4	200	0
NO 34	58	< 0.1	< 1.5	2
NO 37	818	0.5	1300	0
NO 54	1334	3.8	300	0
NO 55	880	13	<1.5	2
PS 8	2600	2.6	80	2
PS 10	394	<0.1	<1.5	2
PS 11	574	16	160	0
PS 15	62	<0.1	<1.5	2
PS 16	26	<0.1	<1.5	2
RH 5	1700	<0.1	150	2
RH 18	425	6	300	0

3.5. Phenotype and Cytokine Production of Phl p 1-Specific TCC

39/40 TCC displayed the T helper cell (Th) phenotype (CD 3+, CD 4+, CD 8-). One clone (HER 38) was found to express CD 8. The TCR was identified as TCR α/β in all cases. Upon specific stimulation, 20/39 TCC revealed a high IL-4/IFN-γ ratio (Th2-like type of cytokine production), 15/39 TCC secreted both IL-4 and IFN-γ (Th0-cells). In supernatants of 4/39 TCC IFN-γ, but no IL-4 could be measured (Th1-clones; Table 2).

3.6. T Cell Receptor Analysis and HLA Restriction

TCC used for crossreactivity experiments were analyzed for TCR Vβ gene usage (Table 1). Blocking studies performed with these TCC indicated peptide presentation by HLA-DR molecules.

4. DISCUSSION

Multiple T cell epitopes were indentified on Phl p 1, some of which were relevant in several patients (Fig.1) and can therefore be designated "major epitopes"[11,12,13]. Cross-reacting T cell epitopes were found within group I allergens of different grass species (Tab.I). TCR and MHC analysis of TCC was performed to ensure specificity of the cross-reactivity experiments (as discussed by Heimo Breiteneder in this volume).

IL-4, produced by T helper cells, is the crucial cytokine in the induction of IgE synthesis[4-6,14]. In this study, a large proportion of the T cell clones investigated (20/39) produced high IL-4 levels and low amounts of IFN γ (Th2-cells; Tab.II), indicating their importance in the pathogenesis of the disease. Specific IT is a well established method in treatment of patients suffering from Type I-allergy to airborne allergens[15,16]. Recently it could be shown that the cytokine production pattern of allergen-specific T lymphocytes is influenced by successful IT[17]. The use of peptides representing T cell epitopes could improve the efficacy of IT, as they might modulate the T cell response to allergens[13,18-20]. These peptides are not capable of binding IgE antibodies[10], therefore the risk of anaphylactic side effects during IT would be eliminated and higher doses could be applied. Recently it was shown that treatment with single peptides (representing immunodominant T cell epitopes) is able to suppress the immune response to a complete allergenic protein[13,18,19]. Concerning type I-allergy to grass pollens, crossreacting major T cell epitopes might represent tools for IT in the future.

5. ACKNOWLEDGMENT

This work was supported by *Fonds zur Förderung der wissenschaftlichen Forschung* (FWF) Project S 06700-MED, Subprojects S 06703-MED, S 06704-MED, S 06707-MED and by *Grant of Pharmacia Diagnostics*.

6. REFERENCES

1. Laffer S, Valenta R, Vrtala S et al. Recombinant major allergen *Phl p* I from timothy grass (*Phleum pratense*) inhibits IgE-binding to multiple isoforms of group I grass pollen allergens from eight different grass species. J Allergy Clin Immunol 1994 (in press).

2. Perez M, Isihoka GY, Walker LE, Chestnut RW. cDNA cloning and Immunological Characterization of the Rye Grass Allergen *Lol p* I. J Biol Chem 1990;265:16210–5.

3. Griffith IJ, Smith PM, Pollock J, Theerakalpisut P, et al. Cloning and sequencing of *Lol p* I, the major allergenic protein of rye-grass pollen. FEBS Lett 1991;279:210–5.

4. Mosmann TR, Coffman RL. Heterogeneity of cytokine secretion patterns and function of T helper cells. Adv Immunol 1989;46:111–47.

5. Wierenga AE, Snoek M, DeGroot C et al. Evidence for compartmentalization of functional subsets of CD4+ T lymphocytes in atopic patients. J Immunol 1990;144:4651–6.

6. Romagnani S. Human Th1 and Th2: Doubt no more. Immunol Today 1991;12:256–7.

7. Spiegelberg HL, Beck L, Stevenson D, Ishioka GY. Recognition of T Cell Epitopes and Lymphokine Secretion by Rye Grass Allergen *Lolium perenne* I-Specific Human T Cell Clones. J Immunol 1994;152:4706–11.

8. Fischer GF, Pickl WF, Faé I, et al. Association between IgE-response against Bet v 1, the major allergen of birch pollen, and HLA-DRB alleles. Hum Immunol 1991;33:259–65.

9. Jarolim E, Rumpold H, Endler AT, Ebner H, Breitenbach M, Scheiner O, Kraft D. IgE and IgG antibodies of patients with allergy to birch pollen as tools to define the allergen profile of *Betula verrucosa* . Allergy 1989;44:385–95.

10. Ebner C, Szépfalusi Z., Ferreira F, et al. Identification of multiple T cell epitopes on Bet v I, the major birch pollen allergen, using specific T cell clones and overlapping peptides. J Immunol 1993;150:1047–54.

11. Ebner C, Schenk, S, Szépfalusi, Z, et al. Multiple T cell specificities for *Bet v* I, the major birch pollen allergen, within single individuals. Studies using specific T cell clones and overlapping peptides. Eur J Immunol 1993;23:1523–7.

12. Van Neerven RJJ, Van de Pol MM, Van Milligen FJ, Jansen HM, Aalberse RC, Kapsenberg M. Characterization of Cat Dander-Specific T Lymphocytes from Atopic Patients. J Immunol 1994;152:4203–10.

13. Hoyne GF, O´Hehir RE, Wraith DC, Thomas WR, Lamb JR. Inhibition of T cell and antibody response to the house dust mite allergen by inhalation of the dominant T cell epitope in naive and sensitized mice. J Exp Med 1993;178:1783–8.

14. Del Prete GF, Maggi E, Parronchi P, et al. IL-4 is an essential factor for the IgE-synthesis induced in vitro by human T cell clones and their supernatants. J Immunol 1988;140:4193–8.

15. Norman PS, Winkenwerder WL, Lichtenstein LM. Immunotherapy of hay fever with antigen E: comparison with whole pollen extracts and placebos. J Allergy 1968;42:93–99.

16. Bousquet J, Becker WM, Hejjaoudi A, et al. Differences in clinical and immunological reactivity of patients allergic to grass pollen and to multiple-pollen species. II. Efficacy of a double blind, placebo controlled, specific immunotherapy with standardized extracts. J Allergy Clin Immunol 1991;88:43–53.

17. Secrist H, Chelen CJ, Wen Y, Marshall JD, Umetsu DT. Allergen immunotherapy decreases interleukin 4 production in CD4+ T cells from allergic individuals. J Exp Med 1993;178:2123–30.

18. Litwin A, Pesce AJ, Fischer T, Michael M, Michael JG. Regulation of the human response to ragweed pollen by immunotherapy. A controlled trial compasring the effect of immunosuppressive peptic fragments of short ragweed with standard treatment. Clin Exp Allergy 1991;21:457–65.

19. Briner TJ, Kuo MC, Keating, KM, Rogers BL, Greenstein JL. Peripheral T cell tolerance induced in naive mice and primed mice by subcutaneous injection of peptides from the cat major allergen Fel d 1. Proc Natl Acad Sci USA 1993;90:7608–12.

20. Wallner BP, Gefter M.L. Immunotherapy with T-cell-reactive peptides derived from allergens. Allergy 1994;49:302–8.

RECOMBINANT EXPRESSION AND EPITOPE MAPPING OF GRASS POLLEN ALLERGENS

Cenk Suphioglu, Penelope M. Smith, Eng K. Ong, R. Bruce Knox, and
Mohan B. Singh

School of Botany
The University of Melbourne
Parkville, Vic. 3052, Australia

SUMMARY

We have studied the expression of recombinant forms of Group 1 allergens from
rye-grass and Bermuda grass pollens. Recombinant Lol p 1 expressed in bacteria bound
serum IgE from allergic patients. Based on analysis of fragments of the Lol p 1 cDNA
clone, the major IgE-reactive epitope has been mapped to the C-terminus. However, although SDS-denatured natural Cyn d 1 (from Bermuda grass) bound IgE, the full or partial recombinant proteins expressed in bacteria did not bind IgE. We have since expressed
Cyn d 1 in the yeast *Pichia pastoris* and restored IgE binding.

cDNA clones encoding two isoforms of Lol p 5, Lol p 5A and Lol p 5B, have been
expressed in bacteria and resulting polypeptides show IgE-binding. Random fragments of
these clones have been generated and when expressed as partial recombinant proteins in
bacteria, allowed us to identify the major IgE-binding epitopes. The allergenic epitopes
were localised towards the C-terminal half of the molecule. Although both isoforms
shared similar IgE-reactive epitopes, Lol p 5B did not recognise the Lol p 5A-specific
monoclonal antibody A7. At sequence level, there appear to be several amino acid differences between the antigenic epitopes of these two isoallergens. These results aid in the design of diagnostics and in grass pollen immunotherapy.

INTRODUCTION

Grass pollen is the major source of allergens found in the outdoor environment (1).
The most important pollen sources are common agricultural pasture grasses that have been
widely introduced throughout the world, but vary between temperate and tropical climates. The best characterised are those from cool temperate climates, including Bermuda
grass, canary grass, cocksfoot, Kentucky blue-grass, perennial rye-grass, sweet vernal

New Horizons in Allergy Immunotherapy
edited by Sehon et al. Plenum Press, New York, 1996

147

grass, timothy and Yorkshire fog (2). Apart from Bermuda grass, all these grasses belong to a single sub-family Pooideae (3).

The most comprehensive studies have been made of proteins from rye-grass pollen, Kentucky blue, timothy and Bermuda grass. Perennial rye-grass, *Lolium perenne*, pollen extracts contain more than 17 proteins that bind IgE from sera of grass pollen-allergic patients (4). Although the pattern of allergens appears complex, the immunochemical picture is actually simpler as many of these allergens share cross-reactive epitopes. Out of the 17 IgE-binding proteins shown by 2-dimensional Western analysis, 12 belong to variants of either of two major allergens, Lol p 1 and Lol p 5, which together account for nearly all the IgE binding reactivity of crude rye-grass pollen extract (5).

We and others reported the molecular cloning of Lol p 1 (6–7). The second allergen, Lol p 5, has been identified only as a result of molecular cloning (8). Moreover, cloning of an isoform of Lol p 5, designated Lol p 5B, has been recently reported (9).

Compared with rye-grass, Bermuda grass (*Cynodon dactylon*) pollen appears to contain fewer IgE-binding proteins. While grass pollen allergens are frequently antigenically and allergenically cross-reactive with allergens of other grasses, the allergens of Bermuda grass appear to be distinct (10–13) and individuals allergic to Bermuda grass require separate diagnosis and therapy (14). We have recently cloned Cyn d 1, the major allergen of Bermuda grass pollen (15) which at both amino acid and nucleotide sequence level, differs from Group 1 homologues of closely related grasses.

Recombinant allergens offer a number of advantages compared with their natural counterparts. First, the technology permits the production of defined allergens in large quantities, permitting the development of new diagnostic assays that are of far greater specificity than previously possible and provide the potential for international standards (16). Second, determination of the structure and identification of allergenic epitopes is feasible, providing a new understanding of the molecular basis of IgE interactions. Third, there is the exciting possibility offered by modified allergens or peptides as effective therapeutic modalities (17–18). Since we have cloned the major allergens of rye and Bermuda grass pollens, we should now facilitate their expression in bacterial and yeast cells in order to evaluate their IgE-reactivity, and therefore their diagnostic potential, and determine their B-cell epitopes, and thus their therapeutic value, which may lead to a more effective disease management for grass pollen allergic individuals.

MATERIALS AND METHODS

Plant Material

Grass pollen was either collected fresh from Melbourne gardens or obtained from Greer laboratories (NC, USA) as a dry, non-defatted pollen and stored at -20 °C until required.

Monoclonal Antibodies

Monoclonal antibody (mAb) 3A2 was produced as described in Smith *et al.*, (15). Lol p 5A-specific mAb FMC-A7 and Lol p 1-specific mAb FMC-A1 were produced at the Flinders Medical Centre (Adelaide, South Australia) and were a gift from Prof. H. Zola. Details of production and specificity have been published earlier by Smart *et al.*, (19) and its specificity has been further studied by Singh *et al.*, (8).

Human Sera

Sera were collected from subjects with a previous clinical record of spring hay fever symptoms, who had not earlier undergone hyposensitization treatment, positive skin-prick test and radioallergosorbent test (RAST) towards crude grass pollen extracts. The RAST scores for all sera was four. Sera were also obtained from subjects who were not atopic when assessed by RAST, and used as negative controls. All sera were stored at -20°C in 0.5–1 ml aliquots. Skin-prick and RAST tests were performed according to methods described elsewhere (20).

cDNA Fragments of Lol P 5

Construction of random cDNA fragment libraries of Lol p 5 in λgt11.
Random cDNA fragments were generated and analysed as reported previously (21–22). Briefly, the full length EcoRl cDNA insert of the λgt11 clone 12R (encoding Lol p 5A) and clone 19R (encoding Lol p 5B) were isolated and self-ligated and the circularised cDNA were then sonicated using a Branson sonifer 450 (Branson Sonic Power, Danbury, USA) to produce random cDNA fragments. EcoRl-linkered fragments were ligated to alkaline phosphatase treated λgt11 arms (Promega Biotec, Madison, Wisc., USA), the ligated DNA was packaged, plaques were grown in E. *coli* Y1090 and screened with mAb and serum IgE from grass pollen allergic individuals.

Immunological Screening of Fusion Proteins from λgt11 Clones. Immunological screening was essentially the same as that reported previuosly (8). Protein plaque lifts were either screened with serum IgE from grass pollen allergic individuals (diluted 1:4 in phosphate buffered saline [PBS] with 0.5% bovine serum albumin [BSA]) or with monoclonal antibodies (diluted 1:1000 in PBS/BSA). The bound antibodies were detected using rabbit immunoglobulins to human IgE (Dakopatts, CA, USA; diluted 1:200 in PBS/BSA) followed by incubation in peroxidase-conjugated anti-rabbit Ig (Promega, WI, USA; diluted 1:2500 in PBS/BSA) for the detection of human IgE antibodies, and peroxidase-conjugated anti-mouse Ig (Silenus, Vic, Australia; diluted 1:500 in PBS/BSA) for the detection of mouse antibodies. Colour was developed using standard chromogenic methods (20). Once identified , single positive clones were purified and stored at 4°C.

Isolation of λ DNA and Direct Sequencing. Lambda-lysates were made as previuosly reported by Singh et al. λ DNA was isolated from liquid lysates using the method of Messe et al., (23) or by Qiagen-tip 20 (Qiagen, Germany) according to the manufacturers instructions. DNA was digested with restriction endonucleases and separated on 1% agarose gels. Pure λ DNA was used for direct sequencing employing the $[\gamma-^{32}P]ATP$ end-labelled primer protocol of the *fmol*™, PCR-based, DNA Sequencing System (Promega, WI, USA) according to the manufacturers instructions.

Nucleotide Sequencing

cDNA inserts isolated from λ clones were sub-cloned into the plasmid vector pBluescript for sequencing as reported elsewhere (8). DNA sequences were determined by the dideoxy chain termination method (24) using T7 DNA polymerase (T7 DNA sequencing kit; Pharmacia LKB, Sweden) following the manufacturer's instructions.

Expression of Allergens in *E. Coli*

Clones encoding Lol p 1, Lol p 5 and Cyn d 1 were subcloned into the expression vector p*Trc* 99A. Soluble bacterial proteins were isolated from cultures after recombinant protein production was induced with 1 mM IPTG according to the method of Amman *et al.* (1988) (25). The proteins were separated by sodium dodecylsulfate-polyacrylamide gel electrophoresis (SDS-PAGE), the proteins transferred to nitrocellulose and the Western blot probed with mAbs and IgE as described elsewhere (20).

Expression of Cyn d 1 in the yeast *Pichia pastoris*

Clone CD1 (encoding Cyn d 1) was inserted into the multiple cloning site of the yeast expression vector pHIL-S1 (Invitrogen, CA, USA). The constructs were sequenced to confirm that the open reading frame (ORF) of the cloned insert was in the same reading frame of the vector's secretion signal sequence. This is needed for effective secretion of the recombinant CD1 protein. Constructs were then linearized with the restriction enzyme (RE) *Bgl* II and used to transform yeast spheroplasts (26–27). Since the transformants will not be producing alcohol oxidase (the product of the *AOX*1 gene) as the *AOX*1 gene has been disrupted with the cloned insert, they can not efficiently metabolise methanol as a carbon source and therefore grow poorly on media supplemented with methanol as the sole carbon source (28–29). The transformant cells were then grown to saturation for 2 days at 30°C in buffered minimal glycerol-complex medium and the secretion of the re-combinant CD1 protein was induced with methanol (30). After 2 days of expression the cells were pelleted and the supernatant analysed for the product with SDS-PAGE and Western blotting. Western blots were probed with Cyn d 1-specific mAb 3A2 and IgE from a panel of sera from individuals allergic to Bermuda grass pollen followed by horse-radish-peroxidase labelled anti mouse Ig (for detection of mAb-binding) and ^{125}I-labelled anti-human IgE (for detection of IgE-binding), as described previously (20).

RESULTS AND DISCUSSION

Recombinant Fragments of Lol p 1

We have previously reported the cloning of Lol p 1, the major allergen of rye-grass pollen (6). At the time of cloning of Lol p 1, partial cDNA fragments encoding the same allergen, were isolated and sequenced from the same library. Fusion proteins encoded by four such clones, namely cDNA clones 3R, 5R, 7R and 13R, were used to delineate the re-gions of Lol p 1 protein which bind antibodies. A diagramatic representation of the over-lapping regions expressed by the cDNA clones is shown in Figure 1. When the entire coding region of Lol p 1 is expressed in bacteria the recombinant fusion protein recog-nises both the Lol p 1-specific mAb FMC A1 as well as serum IgE from grass pollen aller-gic individuals. Since all cDNA clones encode amino acid residue numbers 96 to 221, the mAb A1 binding epitope can be localised to this region. Indeed, in reality, the epitope may be much shorter then this region and further work needs to be carried out to resolve this epitope further; perhaps with synthetic peptides. On the other hand, only one clone (eg. 13R) encodes an IgE binding protein which possesses the amino acid residues 221–240. Consequently, this amino acid sequence has been designated as the IgE-binding epitope of Lol p 1. This result is very interesting since Esch and Klapper (31) localised

Clone

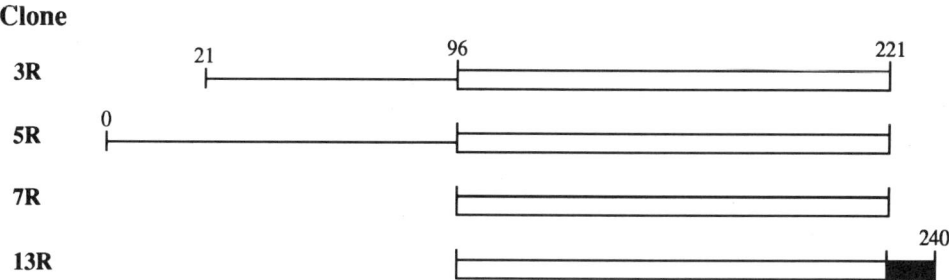

Figure 1. Diagramatic representation of antibody binding to recombinant fragments of Lol p 1. Empty bars represents the area shared by the fusion protein of all clones to which mAb FMC A1 binds. Solid bar represents the region which is unique to clone 13R fusion protein that is responsible for IgE binding from sera of grass pollen allergic sera.

this epitope to a 28 amino acid fragment of Lol p 1, since identified to be the C-terminal of the allergen. However, since the other cDNA clones encoding Lol p 1 do not bind IgE and only encode the first nine amino acid residues of this region, it is unlikely that these amino acids compose the IgE-binding site of the allergen but may form part of the epitope. The comparison of C-terminal amino acid sequences of Group 1 allergens (Table 1) reveals a high degree of similarity, especially with those of meadow fescue and Kentucky bluegrass, all belonging to the same sub-family Pooideae, highlighting the possible basis of allergenic cross-reactivity observed among Group 1 allergens.

Recombinant Fragments of Cyn d 1

We have previously identified cDNA clones encoding Cyn d 1, the major allergen of Bermuda grass pollen (15). In comparison to the recombinant proteins of Lol p 1, none of the clones encoding partial or full-length Cyn d 1 that were expressed in bacteria bound to IgE. However, natural Cyn d 1 appears to bind human IgE relatively strongly (Figure 2A). This suggests that the IgE-binding epitope(s) of Cyn d 1 may be comformational in nature. Bacteria also do not possess the post-translational modifications of the higher eukaryotes

Table 1. Comparison of *C*-terminal amino acid sequences of Group 1 Allergens. Amino acids which do not differ from Lol p 1 are indicated by an asterisk. Underlined amino acids indicate that the amino acid is similar to that of Lol p 1. Amino acids said to be similar are: A, S, T; D, E; N, Q; R, K; I, L, M, V; F, Y, W. [a] deduced from cDNA clone 13R[6]; [b] determined by protein microsequencing[31]; [c] deduced from cDNA clone 3B[15]; [d] deduced from cDNA clone 18B[15]

Grass	Allergen	Amino Acid Sequence	IgE binding
Lolium perenne	Lol p 1[a,b]	YTTEGGTKSEVEDVIPEGWKADTSYSAK	+
Lolium perenne	Lol p 1[b]	**********F***************	+
Festuca elatior	Fes e 1[b]	**********A******	+
Festuca elatior	Fes e 1[b]	******************	+
Poa pratensis	Poa p 1[b]	********A*A*********V****E	+
Agrostis alba	Agr a 1[b]	********A*A************E	+
Anthoxanthum odoratum	Ant o 1[b]	******K*V*A*********V****E	+
Cynodon dactylon	Cyn d 1[c]	L*S*S*GHV*Q******D**P**V*KS*IQF	−
Cynodon dactylon	Cyn d 1[d]	L*S***AHLVQD****AN**P**V*TS*LQFGA	−

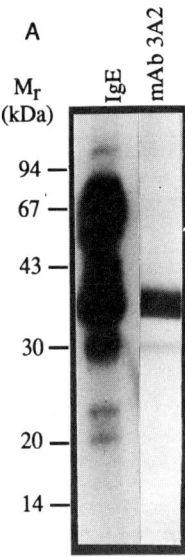

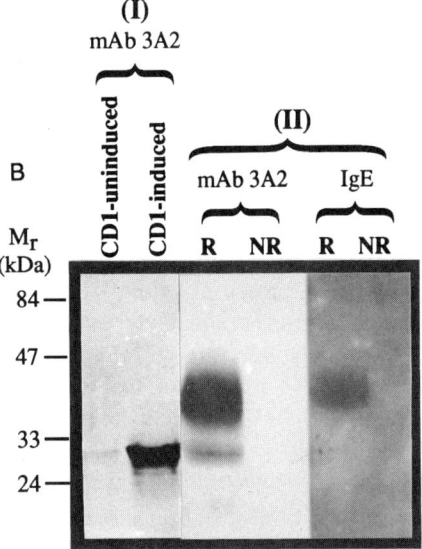

Figure 2. Specificity of mAbs and IgE for recombinant and natural Cyn d 1. **A.** Total Bermuda grass pollen proteins were separated by SDS-PAGE and transferred to nitrocellulose. The Western blots were then probed with **IgE** or mAb **3A2**, followed by ^{125}I-labelled anti-human IgE (for detection of IgE-binding) and horse-radish-peroxidase labelled anti mouse Ig (for detection of mAb-binding). **B.** cDNA encoding the complete coding region of Cyn d 1 (CD1) was expressed in *E. coli* (**I**) and yeast (**II**). Bacterial proteins from cultures which had not been induced with IPTG (**CD1-uninduced**) and those which had been induced (**CD1-induced**) were then separated by SDS-PAGE and transferred to nitrocellulose. Yeast proteins secreted into the media from recombinant cells (**R**) and non-recombinant cells (**NR**) were also seperated by SDS-PAGE and transferred to nitrocellulose. Western blots were then probed with mAbs **3A2** or **IgE** from sera of Bermuda grass pollen allergic individuals.

and as a result, bacterially expressed Cyn d 1 shows monoclonal antibody binding but lacks IgE-reactivity.

By comparing the Cyn d 1 C-terminal sequence with those known to bind IgE, it may be possible to predict positions which are important for IgE binding. However, comparison of C-terminal amino acid sequences of Cyn d 1 with those of other Group 1 aller gens shows little similarity (Table 1). However, this lack of amino acid similarity and different botanical classification of Cyn d 1 with other Group 1 allergens may explain the absence of allergenic cross-reactivity among Cyn d 1 and other grasses. This lack of allergenic cross-reactivity may be a consequence of novel and conformational IgE-binding epitopes that are present only in Cyn d 1 and not in other Group 1 allergens and vice-versa.

Yeast Expression of Cyn d 1

The lack of IgE reactivity in the C terminus of Cyn d 1 cannot account for the lack of IgE reactivity of the complete Cyn d 1 recombinant protein encoded by clone CD1. Natural Cyn d 1 shows high IgE reactivity on Western blots although recombinant Cyn d 1 expressed as a bacterial fusion or a non-fusion protein shows no reactivity (Fig. 2). On the other hand, the IgE-binding capacity is restored when Cyn d 1 is expressed in the yeast *Pichia pastoris*. Moreover, mAb 3A2 binding is maintained and no antibody binding is detected with non-recombinant yeast vector constructs, used as negative controls (Fig. 2B). Unlike bacteria, yeast has many of the advantages of higher eukaryotic expression systems such as protein processing, protein folding and post-translational modifications. Moreover, N-linked glycosylation of the high-mannose type is a feature of the secreted proteins from *Pichia*. Since Cyn d 1 contains a single N-glycosylation site, it may be possible that either glycosylation is required for correct conformation of the protein for IgE-binding or oligosaccharide chains may be indirectly responsible for the IgE-binding capacity of Cyn d 1. Indeed, the recombinant Cyn d 1 expressed in yeast is approximately 8 kDa larger in molecular mass than the natural allergen (~32 kDa), which suggests that the yeast protein may possess N-linked glycosylation of the high-mannose type. However, the length of the oligosaccharide chains added post-translationally to proteins in *Pichia* (average 8–14 mannose residues per side chain) is much shorter than the chains in the yeast *S. cerevisiae* (50–150 mannose residues) (32–33).

Another attractive feature of *Pichia* in this study is that high expression levels (~1.5g per litre of media) of Cyn d 1 were obtained. Secreted recombinant Cyn d 1 comprises the vast majority of the total protein in the culture medium. Since *Pichia* is known to secrete only very low levels of natural proteins, and there there are only very low amounts of protein in minimal *Pichia* growth medium (29) means that minimal downstream processing is necessary.

Recombinant Random Fragments of Lol p 5

cDNA clones encoding two isoforms of Lol p 5, Lol p 5A and Lol p 5B, have been previously cloned in our laboratory (8–9). In an attempt to map their antigenic and allergenic epitopes we have taken the approach of generating random fragments of the cDNA clone encoding the full-length allergens and screening replicate fusion-protein lifts with either Lol p 5A-specific mAb A7 or serum IgE from grass pollen allergic individuals. As a result, many fragments in the size range of 72–118 and 118–310 base pairs were identified as either mAb A7-reactive, IgE-reactive or both. None of the fragments of clone 19R encoding Lol p 5B bound mAb A7 but bound IgE. IgE-reactive fragments of Lol p 5B occurred predominantly in the C-terminal half of the allergen. On the other hand, fragments of Lol p 5B indicated mAb A7 binding towards the N-terminal end of the allergen and this epitope was resolved down to 35 amino acids. There appears to be several amino acid differences between the two allergens in this region, which may be responsible for the mAb A7-reactivity of Lol p 5A. The IgE-reactivity pattern of Lol p 5A was similar to that of Lol p 5B, with IgE-reactive fragments corresponding to the C-terminal half of the allergen. Although epitopes were resolved down to a minimum of 35 amino acid residues, these should now be further dissected by using synthetic peptide mapping. Moreover, the antigenicity of Lol p 5B should be further investigated for mAb A7 binding with synthetic peptides based on the amino acid sequence of Lol p 5B and corresponding to the mAb A7-binding epitope of Lol p 5A.

CONCLUSIONS

Taken together, these results suggest that the IgE-binding epitopes of Cyn d 1 may depend upon the conformation of the molecule, where glycosylation of the protein may play a critical role. In contrast, there is little difference in binding of IgE by natural and recombinant Lol p 1, Lol p 5A and Lol p 5B indicating that most epitopes present on natural Lol p 1, 5A and 5B are also present on the recombinant molecules and that the major IgE-binding epitopes may not be dependent on conformation. Thus, Cyn d 1 and Lol p 1 may have distinct IgE-binding epitopes, in spite of their high sequence identity (64 % amino acid identity). This would explain the limited mutual cross-inhibition of IgE binding by Bermuda grass and rye-grass pollen extracts (12–13). Similar findings have been reported for the ragweed allergens Amb a 1 and Amb a 2. Both the natural allergens bind IgE from ragweed allergic individuals to a similar extent but although they show 65% amino acid identity, recombinant Amb a 2 does not bind IgE, while recombinant Amb a 1 does bind IgE (34). It is anticipated that hyposensitization treatment with recombinant allergens, or their IgE-reactive epitopes, can be used as a therapeutic modality for alleviation of the allergic response. For example, the non-IgE-reactive form of Cyn d 1, as expressed in *E. coli*, could be one such candidate for evaluation as a therapeutic agent. On the other hand, since IgE-reactive recombinant Cyn d 1 can be readily produced in large amounts in yeast, its potential as an important diagnostic tool in grass pollen allergy, along with others such as bacterially expressed Lol p 1 and Lol p 5A/5B, can now be seriously evaluated.

ACKNOWLEDGMENTS

We thank the Australian National Health and Medical Research Council for financial support of this research.

REFERENCES

1. Allergy Principles and Practice; Volumes I & II. Middleton E, Reed CE, Ellis EF, Adkinson NF, Yunginger JW (Eds). The CV Mosby Company, St.Louis, 1988.
2. King TP, Hoffman D, Lowenstein H et al. Allergen Nomenclature. Int Arch Allergy Immunol 1994;105:224–233.
3. Watson L. World grass genera. In: Reproductive versatility in the grasses. Chapman, G.P. (Ed) Cambridge University Press. 1990:258–265.
4. Smith PM, Ong EK, Avjioglu A et al. Analysis of ryegrass pollen allergens using two dimensional electrophoresis and immunoblotting. In: Kraft D, Sehon A, eds. Molecular biology and immunology of allergens.Boca Raton:CRC Press, 1993:141–143.
5. Bond JF, Segal DB, Yu X-B et al. Human IgE reactivity to purified recombinant and native grass allergens. J. Allergy Clin Immunol 1993;91:339.
6. Griffith IJ, Smith PM, Pollock J et al. Cloning and sequencing of *Lol p* I, the major allergenic protein of ryegrass pollen. FEBS Lett 1991;279:210–215.
7. Perez M, Ishioka GY, Walker LE et al. cDNA cloning and immunological characterization of the ryegrass allergen *Lol p* I. J Biol Chem 1990;265:16210–16215.
8. Singh MB, Hough T, Theerakulpisut P et al. Isolation of cDNA encoding a newly identified major allergenic protein of ryegrass pollen: Intracellular targetting to the amyloplast. Proc Natl Acad Sci USA 1991;88:1384–1388.
9. Ong EK, Griffith IJ, Singh MB et al. Cloning of a cDNA encoding a group-V (group-IX) allergen isoform from rye-grass pollen that demonstrates specific antigenic immunoreactivity. Gene 1993;134:235–240.

10. Marsh DG, Haddad ZH, Campbell PH. A new method for determining the distribution of allergenic fractions in biological materials: its application to grass pollen extracts. J Allergy 1970;46:107–121.

11. Bernstein IL, Perera M, Gallagher J et al. *In vitro* cross-allergenicity of major aeroallergenic pollens by the radioallergosorbent technique. J Allergy Clin Immunol 1976;57:141–152.

12. Martin BG, Mansfield LE, Nelson HS. Cross-allergenicity among the grasses. Ann Allergy 1985;54:99–104.

13. Schumacher MJ, Grabowski J, Wagner CM. Anti-Bermuda grass RAST binding is minimally inhibited by pollen extracts from 10 other grasses. Ann Allergy 1985;55:584–587.

14. Bush RK. Aerobiology of pollen and fungal allergens. J Allergy Clin Immunol 1989;84:1120–1124.

15. Smith PM, Singh MB, Knox RB. Characterization and cloning of the major allergen of Berrnuda grass, *Cyn d* I. In: Molecular Biology and Immunology of Allergens. Kraft, D. (ed) CRC Press, USA;1994.

16. Yang M, Olsen E, Dolovich J et al. Immunologic characterization of a recombinant Kentucky bluegrass (*Poa pratensis*) allergenic peptide. J Allergy Clin Immunol 1991;87:1096–1104.

17. Scheiner O. Recombinant allergens: biological, immunological and practical aspects. Int Archs Allergy Immunol 1992;98:93–96.

18. Bousquet J, Breitenbach M, Dreborg S, et al. Diagnosis of allergy and specific immunotherapy using recombinant allergens and epitopes. In: Kraft D, Sehon A, eds. Molecular biology and immunology of allergens.Boca Raton:CRC Press, 1993:311–320.

19. Smart IJ, Heddle RJ, Zola H et al. Development of monoclonal mouse antibodies specific for allergenic components of ryegrass (*Lolium perenne*) pollen. Int Arch Allergy Appl Immunol 1983;72:243–248.

20. Suphioglu C, Singh MB, Simpson RJ et al. Identification of canary grass (*Phalaris aquatica*) pollen allergens by immunoblotting: IgE and IgG antibody-binding studies. Allergy 1993;48:273–281.

21. Greene WK, Cyster JG, Chua KY et al. IgE and IgG binding of peptides expressed from fragments of cDNA encoding the major house dust mites allergen *Der p* I. J Immunol 1991;147:3768–3773.

22. Greene WK, Thomas WR. IgE binding structures of the major house dust mite allergen *Der p* I. Mol Immunol 1992;29:257–262.

23. Messe E, Olson S, Leis L et al. A quick method for high yeilds of lambda bacteriophage DNA. Nucl Acid Res 1990;18:1923.

24. Sanger F, Nicklen S, Coulson AR. DNA sequencing with chain terminating inhibitors. Proc Natl Acad Sci USA 1977;74:5463–5467.

25. Amman E, Ochs B, Abel KJ. Tightly regulated *tac* promoter vectors useful for the expression of unfused and fused proteins in *Escherichia coli.* Gene 1988;69:301–315.

26. Cregg JM, Tschopp JF, Stillman C et al. High-level expression and efficient assembly of Hepatitis b surface antigen in the methylotrophic yeast *pichia pastoris*. Bio/Technology 1987;5:479–485.

27. Sreekkrishna K, Potenz RHB, Cruze JA et al. High level expression of heterologous proteins in methylotrophic yeast *Pichia pastoris*. J Basic Microbiol 1988;28:265–278.

28. Cregg JM, Madden KR, Barringer KJ et al. Functional characterization of two alcohol oxidase genes from the yeast, *Pichia pastoris*. Mol Cell Biol 1989;9:1316–1323.

29. Koutz PJ, Davis GR, Stillman CA et al. Structural comparison of the *Pichia pastoris* alcohol oxidase genes. Yeast 1989;5:167–177.

30. Barr KA, Hopkins SA, Sreekrishna K. Protocol for efficient secretion of HSA developed from *Pichia pastoris*. Pharm Eng 1992;12:48–51.

31. Esch RE, Klapper DG. Isolation and characterization of a major cross-reactive grass group I allergenic determinant. Mol Immunol 1989;26:557–561.

32. Grinna LS, Tschopp JF. Size distribution and general structural features of N-linked oligosaccharides from methylotrophic yeast *Pichia pastoris*. Yeast 1989;5:107–115.

33. Tschopp JF, Sverlow G, Kosson R et al. High level secretion of glycosylated invertase in the methylotrophic yeast *Pichia pastoris*. Bio/Technology 1987;5:1305–1308.

34. Kuo M-C, Zhu X-J, Koury R et al. Purification and immunochemical characterization of recombinant and native ragweed allergen *Amb a* II. Mol Immunol 1993;30:1077–1087.

21

MOLECULAR CHARACTERIZATION OF ALTERNARIA ALTERNATA AND CLADOSPORIUM HERBARUM ALLERGENS

Gernot Achatz,[1] Hannes Oberkofler,[1] Erich Lechenauer,[1] Birgit Simon,[1] Andrea Unger,[1] Doris Kandler,[1] Christoph Ebner,[2] Hansjörg Prillinger,[3] Dietrich Kraft,[2] and Michael Breitenbach[1]

[1]Institute of Genetics and General Biology
University of Salzburg, Austria
[2]Institute of General and Experimental Pathology
AKH, University of Vienna, Austria
[3]Institute of Applied Microbiology
University of Bodenkultur, Vienna, Austria

1. INTRODUCTION

Investigations of fungal air spora have demonstrated that conidium-forming fungi usually predominate over other fungal groups. Cladosporium herbarum, Alternaria alternata, Penicillium sp.and Aspergillus sp., listed in decreasing frequency of occurrence, are most consistently associated with the highest mean percentages of total fungal spore catches. In addition to daily variations in meteorologic conditions and seasonal changes, both of which have enormous impact on the concentration of air spora, the amount and type of vegetation of a region or microenvironment may be important factors in determining the composition of the airborne fungal population. Over the past two decades most allergologists have recognized a need for more information on fungal allergy because of increased awareness of the problem and the greater number of patients suffering from asthma and rhinitis due to fungi. Seasonal variation in regard to fungi in the air or to those in homes, and their detection and monitoring but also the biological relevance of the allergenic protein in the fungal organism are new fields of studies (1, 2). In the environment, Cladosporium herbarum is the most frequently encountered mould in the air. The dry conidia are carried easily through the air and can be detected in extremely large numbers e.g. a concentration of 35000 conidia/cubic meter can often be measured. The indoor counts to a large extent reflect the outdoor concentration. Depending on climate conditions the conidia may begin to appear in the atmosphere in spring and rise to a peak in either late summer or early autumn. Cladosporium herbarum is one of the most common colonizer of dying and dead plants and also occurs in various soil types and on food. It can

New Horizons in Allergy Immunotherapy
edited by Sehon et al. Plenum Press, New York, 1996

157

frequently be found in uncleaned refrigerators, foodstuff, on wet window frames, in houses with poor ventilation and houses with straw roofs (3, 4, 5).

Spores of Alternaria alternata are the most important mould allergens in the United states. Alternaria is found predominantly on the East coast, in the upper Midwest and in southern California, probably ranking third only to ragweed and grass pollens as a natural cause of allergy. Known habitats of Alternaria alternata are soils, corn silage, rotten wood, composts and various forest plants. It is frequently found on wet window frames. It is considered an outdoor mould and appears when the weather is warm (3, 4, 5).

One of the most notable properties of fungal antigens is their complexity, which makes great problems for diagnosis. Skin testing is often said to be more sensitive than in vitro testing. At least in the case of mould allergens, such statements can be questioned. It is also a major clinical problem to identify the extent to which symptoms of a mould atopic patient can be attributed to mould allergy. This is because exposure to moulds is a continuum without definite seasonal end-points. Given the importance of the two moulds mentioned above and the unclear situation with respect to classical allergen characterization, it seemed highly desirable to us to clone and sequence cDNAs coding for the major and minor allergens of the two moulds. Cloning, sequencing, and recombinant production of allergens seems to be a prerequisite to improvements in both diagnosis and therapy. We are reporting here ten complete sequences of cDNAs coding for major and minor allergens of Cladosporium herbarum and Alternaria alternata.

2. METHODS

2.1. Biological Materials

Sera from 194 patients allergic to moulds were selected for this study. About 60% of them had positively tested to Alternaria or Cladosporium in RAST, the others had positively tested to a mould allergen mixed RAST (Pharmacia, Uppsala, Sweden). The sera were supplied by three Austrian allergy clinics: i) Allergieambulatorium Reumannplatz, Vienna: 133 sera; ii) Lungenambulanz Krankenhaus Lainz, Vienna: 38 sera; iii) Allergieambulanz Landeskrankenhaus Salzburg: 23 sera. None of the patients had received hyposensitization treatment before testing was performed.

Cladosporium herbarum (strain collection number: 28–0202) was obtained from the microbiological strain collection of the Institute of Botany, University of Regensburg, FRG (courtesy Prof. Helmuth Bezel).

Alternaria alternata was obtained from the Institut für Gärungsgewerbe, Technical University of Berlin (strain collection number: 08–0203, courtesy Prof. Ulf Stahl).

Cultivation of the two moulds was done as described previously (6).

2.2. Procedures

cDNA libraries from Cladosporium herbarum and Alternaria alternata were constructed as described (6). Using serum IgE from Alternaria and Cladosporium allergic patients a series of IgE-binding clones were obtained. Recombinant allergens were then tested as fusion and non-fusion proteins for their IgE reactivity. cDNA clones encoding major and minor allergens were subjected to DNA sequence analysis and the deduced amino acid sequences were compared with the SWISS PROT protein data-base.

Table 1. Summary of major and minor allergens of Alternaria alternata and Cladosporium herbarum recognized by our patients' collective

kD (biological function)	Alternaria alternata			Cladosporium herbarum		
	Allergen	% of patients	Cloned	Allergen	% of patients	Cloned
110 red.	-		-	Cla h 8	11	-
100 red.	-		-	Cla h 9	6	-
85 red.	Alt a 3	42	-	-		-
63 red. (PDI)	Alt a 4	37	+	-		-
53 red. (ALDH)	Alt a 10	2	+	Cla h 6	20	+
48 red. (enolase)	-		-	Cla h 3	40	+
45 red.	Alt a 2	47	-	Cla h 2	43	-
42 red.	Alt a 9	5	-	Cla h 7	17	-
39 red.	Alt a 8	7	-	-		-
30 non-red	Alt a 1	80	-	-		-
30 red.	Alt a 5	33	-	Cla h 1	61	-
22 red. (homolog to YCP4 yeast protein)	Alt a 7	30	+	Cla h 5	22	+
11 red. (P1 ribosomal protein)	Alt a 11		+	Cla h 10	20	+
11 red. (P2 ribosomal protein)	Alt a 6	25	+	Cla h 4	22	+

Summary of all allergens of Alternaria alternata and Cladosporium herbarum that are recognized by our patients. With the exception of Alt a 1, all allergens can be detected in an immune blot under reducing conditions. In total, ten IgE-reactive proteins could be detected in Alternaria, five of which have been cloned. Nine IgE-reactive proteins could be detected in Cladosporium, five of which have been cloned. Five allergens co-migrate and could be closely related in both moulds. Four of them (ALDH, YCP4, P1 and P2) not only co-migrate in Alternaria and Cladosporium, but could be shown by cDNA cloning and sequencing to be very probably functionally closely related.

3. RESULTS

3.1. Analysis of the cDNA Inserts

A total of about 150 positive clones were identified by screening each of the two libraries with a serum mixture of two patients. In the case of Cladosporium herbarum as well as in the case of Alternaria alternata 5 different types of inserts could be detected. In order to confirm that the recombinant phages isolated in this way indeed expressed fusion proteins reactive with the IgE used for screening of the libraries, the fusion proteins were induced, separated by SDS-PAGE and tested in immune blots again. According to our sequencing data one could see that the cloned allergens of Cladosporium herbarum and Alternaria alternata belong to 5 groups of homologous proteins (Table 1): Allergen Alt a 10 (Mr=53 kDa, EMBL accession number: X78227) of Alternaria alternata and Cla h 6 (Mr=53 kDa, EMBL accession number: X78228) of Cladosporium herbarum by comparison with the protein data base were identified as aldehyde dehydrogenases (ALDHs). Aspergillus fumigatus ALDH yielded the highest score of identity and homology.

Allergen Alt a 6 (Mr=11 kDa, EMBL accession number: X78222) of Alternaria alternata, allergen Alt a 11 (Mr=11 kDa, EMBL accession number: X84216) of Alternaria alternata, Cla h 4 (Mr=11 kDa, EMBL accession number: X78223) of Cladosporium herbarum and Cla h 10 (Mr=11 kDa, EMBL accession number: X85180) of Cladosporium herbarum were identified as ribosomal proteins (P1 and P2). P1 and P2 are members of a family of three eukaryotic acidic ribosomal phosphoproteins (P-proteins), P0, P1 and P2, which are well known lupus erythematodes antigens (7).

Allergens Alt a 7 (Mr=22 kDa , EMBL accession number: X78225) of Alternaria alternata and Cla h 5 (Mr= 22 kDa, EMBL accession number: X78224) of Cladosporium herbarum show significant homologies to the YCP4 gene of Saccharomyces cerevisiae. YCP4 in Saccharomyces cerevisiae was identified by genome sequencing and has no known function. It is a non-essential yeast gene (8). A possible function for the YCP4 gene is indicated by the recent finding that the Schizosaccharomyces pombe homolog of YCP4 confers resistance to brefeldin A. This protein shares 58% homology with Alt a 7 and Cla h 5 (14).

Allergen Alt a 4 (Mr=63kD, EMBL accession number:X84217) of Alternaria alternata shows high homology to PDI (protein disulfide isomerase), a well known enzyme responsible for the proper folding of proteins to their 3-dimensional structure (9).

Allergen Cla h 6 (Mr=47 kDa, EMBL accession number: X78226) of Cladosporium herbarum is an enolase. In Saccharomyces cerevisiae, two very closely related enolases exist, one of which (enolase 1) is a heat shock protein (10). It is impossible to decide by sequence comparison alone whether Cla h 6 is also a heat shock protein. Further experiments are clearly needed to clarify this point .

3.2. Comparison of the Recombinant Allergens with the Native Allergens

The fusion part of the recombinant allergens made it hard to correlate the bands in the Westernblot with the natural allergens. Therefore we cloned all ten cDNAs as recombinant non-fusion allergens in the expression vector pMW172, transformed the recombinant plasmids in the E. coli strain BL21 and induced recombinant allergen synthesis with IPTG. Two interesting questions could be answered by these experiments. First, by alignment with Coomassie-stained SDS-PAGE gels of Alternaria and Cladosporium extracts we could show that the ten cloned allergens are not prominent protein bands in the extracts. Second, exact co-migration and similar IgE binding of recombinant and natural allergens was observed (6). The co-migration indicates the correspondence between cloned allergens and bands in immune blots of fungal raw extracts and very probably means, that the nine allergens we are dealing with here are not postsynthetically modified.

4. DISCUSSION

We are presenting here our successful attempt to characterize the allergens of Alternaria alternata and Cladosporium herbarum by cDNA cloning, sequencing, and expression in E. coli of recombinant non-fusion proteins. This approach seems to be the only one that leads to a reproducible well characterized and pure source of allergens for diagnosis and therapy (2).

The ten new mould allergens presented here represent six new allergenic proteins: ALDH, Enolase, YCP4, PDI and the acidic ribosomal proteins P1 and P2. Four of them (ALDH, YCP4 and P1 as well as P2) were found to be allergens in both fungi, Alternaria and Cladosporium. A comparison of these allergens with the known allergens of pollens, house dust mites and foodstuffs allows for a few generalizations to be made:

1. None of the mould allergens that are now known with respect to sequence and/or enzymatic function corresponds to a previously known non-fungal allergen, although many of the known fungal allergens do occur as homologous allergens in more than one fungal species.

2. We notice that all the newly sequenced fungal allergens presented here are soluble cytoplasmatic proteins (as judged from their function). For comparison, both, soluble cytoplasmatic proteins (11, 12) and secreted proteins have been found among cloned and sequenced pollen allergens. The cytoplasmatic allergens are very probably non-glycosylated. Indeed, the ten allergens presented here were produced as recombinant non-fusion proteins and exhibited exactly the same electrophoretic mobility and IgE-binding properties in Western blots as the natural allergens of the mould extracts.

3. All the allergens presented here are rather highly conserved proteins. At least one of them, enolase, has been shown to be an important allergen of Candida albicans (13). The human P1 and P2 ribosomal proteins are well known lupus erythematodes antigens, the relevant epitope for LE being the highly conserved C-terminal sequence KEESEESDD/EDMGFGLFD. Deletions of the C-terminal part of the P2 sequence showed, that the KEESEE-epitope is not the only IgE binding epitope in the P2 protein.

4. Most of the ten allergens presented here are "household" proteins needed for basic metabolism like glycolysis or protein synthesis. This fact makes it unlikely that these allergenic proteins be spore-specific. However, the fungal material used for the present study contained vegetative cells as well as conidiospores and cells and conidiospores were not separated prior to allergen extraction. Further investigations will show whether some of the not yet cloned and sequenced allergens of Alternaria and Cladosporium are indeed spore-specific.

5. REFERENCES

1. Karlsson-Borgå Å., Jonsson P., Rolfsen W. Annals of Allergy 63, 521 (1989).
2. Kraft D., Sehon A. Molecular Biology and Immunology of Allergens (Edited by Kraft D. and Sehon A.) CRC Press Boca Raton, Ann Arbor, London, Tokyo (1993).
3. Ainsworth G.C. Dictionary of fungi. 6th edition (Commonwealth Mycological Institute) (1971).
4. Al-Doory Y., Domson J.F. Mould Allergy (Lea & Febiger, Philadelphia 1984) ISBN 0–8121–0897–3 (1984).
5. Webster J. Introduction to fungi. Cambridge University Press (London, New York, New Rochelle, Melbourne, Sydney) (1986) .
6. Achatz, G., Oberkofler, H., Lechenauer, E., Simon, B., Unger, A., Kandler, D., Ebner, C., Prillinger, H., Kraft, D., Breitenbach, M. Mol. Immunol. 32, 213 (1995).
7. Rich B.E. and Steitz J.A. Mol. Cell. Biol. 7, 4065 (1987).
8. Biteau N., Fremaux C., Hebrard S., Menara A., Aigle M., Crouzet M. Yeast 8, 61(1992).
9. Freedman, R.B., Hirst, T.R., Tuite, M.F. TIBS, 19, 331 (1994).
10. Iida H., Yahara I. Nature 315, 688 (1984).
11. Breiteneder H., Pettenburger K., Bito A., Valenta R., Kraft D., Rumpold H., Scheiner O., Breitenbach M. EMBO 8, 1935 (1989).
12. Valenta R., Duchene M., Pettenburger K., Sillaber C., Valent P., Bettelheim P., Breitenbach M., Rumpold H., Kraft D., Scheiner O. Science 253, 557 (1991).
13. Franklyn K.M., Warmington J.R., Ott A.K., Ashman R,B. Immunol. Cell. Biol. 68, 173 (1990) .
14. Toda, T., Shimanuki, M., Saka, Y., Yamano, H., Adachi, Y., Shirakawa, M., Kyogoku, Y., Yanagida, M. Mol. Cell. Biol. 12, 5474 (1992).

22

PRODUCTION OF RECOMBINANT ALLERGENS AND THEIR APPLICATION FOR IMMUNOTHERAPY

Yasushi Okumura

Central Research Laboratory
Asahi Breweries, Ltd.
2–13–1 Ohmori-kita, Ohta-ku
Tokyo 143, Japan

INTRODUCTION

In this decade, various allergic diseases, especially atopic asthma and atopic dermatitis caused by house dust mite, greatly increase in Japan. Although the correct reasons are still unknown, it is thought that house dust mites increase in Japanese housing environments. There are many kinds of good therapeutic agents for the diseases, but there are no drugs without side effects. For example, steroids and immunosuppressors such as cyclosporin[1] and FK-506[2] are the most effective drugs but they inhibit all immune responses of the patients. On the other hand, so-called immunotherapy seems the most attractive therapy for the diseases because it is highly specific against the corresponding allergen. In other words, the therapy does not seem to affect total immune system of the patients except the allergic response. Although the therapy should be the most desirable therapy for the atopic diseases, it does not become a major therapy. The reasons are as follows: The mode of action of the therapy is unknown, large amounts of the corresponding purified allergens are not available and there is no precise diagnosis for the therapy. Recently, new approach for the immunotherapy has started. That is, Wallner et al. reported that peptide (derived from cat allergen, *Fel d* I) based immunotherapy for cat allergy was effective (in this symposium).

We attempted to clarify the mode of action and establish the therapy. At first, we tried to obtain large amounts of *Der f* I and II as pure forms, because both allergens seem to be the most important allergens for atopic asthma and atopic dermatitis. Large amounts of the allergens purified must be necessary not only for the therapy but for the study and the diagnosis. However, it is very difficult to prepare the purified allergens in large from the mite bodies, because the contents are very small. Therefore, we developed a large scale production system for major mite allergens, *Der f* I and II using gene technology[3,4]. Of course, recombinant allergens should have the same physicochemical and immunologi-

New Horizons in Allergy Immunotherapy
edited by Sehon et al. Plenum Press, New York, 1996

163

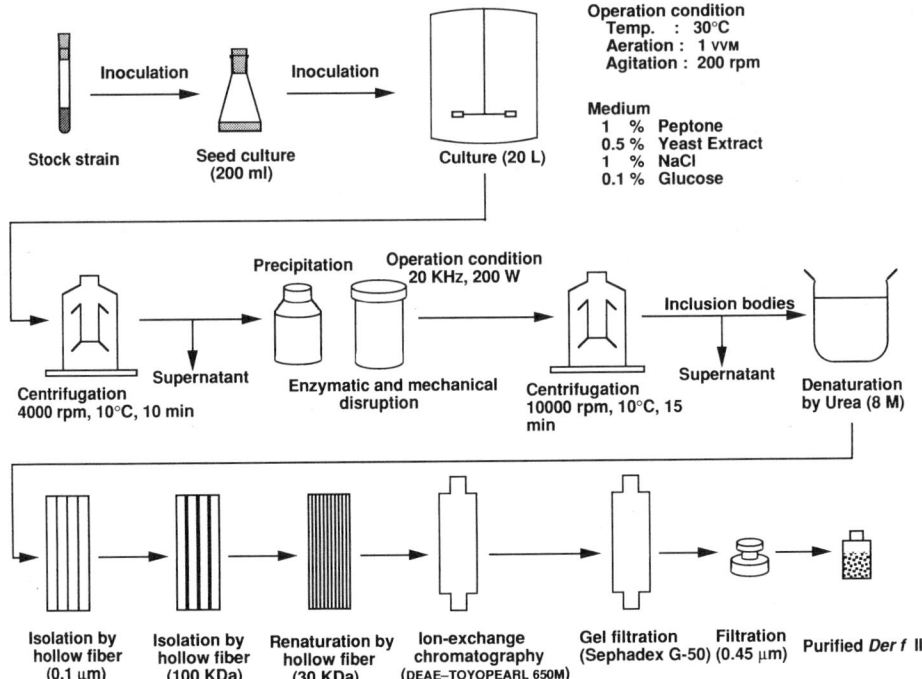

Figure 1. Production scheme of rDer f II.

cal characteristics as those of the native allergens. Fortunately, the recombinant Der f I and II were identical with native Der f I and II purified from mite bodies, respectively[3,5].

Since the purified mite allergens have been available in large, immunotherapy using the recombinant Der f II was attempted on mouse experimental asthma model. In the recombinant Der f II-fed mice, the bronchoconstriction significantly reduced on the allergen inhalation challenge, while the bronchia of control mouse was constricted. This result

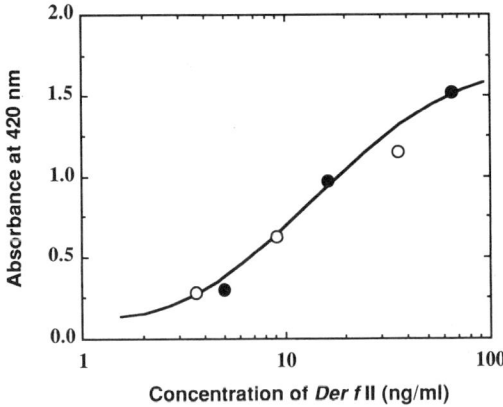

Figure 2. Comparison of human IgE binding activity of rDer f II with that of native Der f II. The activities were measured with RAST-EIA kit (Kabi Pharmacia Diagnostics AB). ○ rDer f II; ● native Der f II.

showed that the recombinant mite allergen, *Der f* II, seemed to be effective for immunotherapy in the mouse model. Now, we have studied mode of action of the therapy.

PRODUCTION OF RECOMBINANT *Der f* II (r*Der f* II) AND ITS PROPERTIES

r*Der f* II was directly expressed in *Escherichia coli* JM109 as previously described (3). The preparation scheme is shown in Fig. 1. The transformant of *E. coli* carrying *Der f*

```
   1   TTTTTTTTTTTTTTTTTTTCCATCAAAATTAAAAATTCATCAAAA ATG AAA TTC GTT TTG GCC ATT GCC TCT    70
                                                    1 Met Lys Phe Val Leu Ala Ile Ala Ser     9

  71   TTG TTG GTA TTG AGC ACT GTT TAT GCT CGT CCA GCT TCA ATC AAA ACT TTT GAA GAA TTC   130
  10   Leu Leu Val Leu Ser Thr Val Tyr Ala Arg Pro Ala Ser Ile Lys Thr Phe Glu Glu Phe    29
                                               pro ➡

 131   AAA AAA GCC TTC AAC AAA AAC TAT GCC ACC GTT GAA GAG GAA GAA GTT GCC CGT AAA AAC   190
  30   Lys Lys Ala Phe Asn Lys Asn Tyr Ala Thr Val Glu Glu Glu Glu Val Ala Arg Lys Asn    49

 191   TTT TTG GAA TCA TTG AAA TAT GTT GAA GCT AAC AAA GGT GCC ATC AAC CAT TTG TCC GAT   250
  50   Phe Leu Glu Ser Leu Lys Tyr Val Glu Ala Asn Lys Gly Ala Ile Asn His Leu Ser Asp    69

 251   TTG TCA TTG GAT GAA TTC AAA AAC CGT TAT TTG ATG AGT GCT GAA GCT TTT GAA CAA CTC   310
  70   Leu Ser Leu Asp Glu Phe Lys Asn Arg Tyr Leu Met Ser Ala Glu Ala Phe Glu Gln Leu    89

 311   AAA ACT CAA TTC GAT TTG AAT GCC GAA ACA AGC GCT TGC CGT ATC AAT TCG GTT AAC GTT   370
  90   Lys Thr Gln Phe Asp Leu Asn Ala Glu Thr Ser Ala Cys Arg Ile Asn Ser Val Asn Val   109
                                         mature ➡

 371   CCA TCG GAA TTG GAT TTA CGA TCA CTG CGA ACT GTC ACT CCA ATC CGT ATG CAA GGA GGC   430
 110   Pro Ser Glu Leu Asp Leu Arg Ser Leu Arg Thr Val Thr Pro Ile Arg Met Gln Gly Gly   129

 431   TGT GGT TCA TGT TGG GCT TTC TCT GGT GTC GCC GCA ACT GAA TCA GCT TAT TTG GCC TAC   490
 130   Cys Gly Ser Cys Trp Ala Phe Ser Gly Val Ala Ala Thr Glu Ser Ala Tyr Leu Ala Tyr   149

 491   CGT AAC ACG TCT TTG GAT CTT TCT GAA CAG GAA CTC GTC GAT TGC GCA TCT CAA CAC GGA   550
 150   Arg Asn Thr Ser Leu Asp Leu Ser Glu Gln Glu Leu Val Asp Cys Ala Ser Gln His Gly   169
           N-glycosylasion site
 551   TGT CAC GGC GAT ACA ATA CCA AGA GGC ATC GAA TAC ATC CAA CAA AAT GGT GTC GTT GAA   610
 170   Cys His Gly Asp Thr Ile Pro Arg Gly Ile Glu Tyr Ile Gln Gln Asn Gly Val Val Glu   189

 611   GAA AGA AGC TAT CCA TAC GTT GCA CGA GAA CAA CAA TGC CGA CGA CCA AAT TCG CAA CAT   670
 190   Glu Arg Ser Tyr Pro Tyr Val Ala Arg Glu Gln Gln Cys Arg Arg Pro Asn Ser Gln His   209

 671   TAC GGT ATC TCA AAC TAC TGC CAA ATT TAT CCA CCA GAT GTG AAA CAA ATC CGT GAA GCT   730
 210   Tyr Gly Ile Ser Asn Tyr Cys Gln Ile Tyr Pro Pro Asp Val Lys Gln Ile Arg Glu Ala   229

 731   TTG ACT CAA ACA CAC ACA GCT ATT GCC GTC ATT ATT GGC ATT AAA GAT TTG AGA GCT TTT   790
 230   Leu Thr Gln Thr His Thr Ala Ile Ala Val Ile Ile Gly Ile Lys Asp Leu Arg Ala Phe   249

 791   CAA CAT TAT GAT GGA CGA ACA ATC ATT CAA CAT GAC AAT GGT TAT CAA CCA AAC TAT CAT   850
 250   Gln His Tyr Asp Gly Arg Thr Ile Ile Gln His Asp Asn Gly Tyr Gln Pro Asn Tyr His   269

 851   GCC GTC AAC ATT GTC GGT TAC GGA AGT ACA CAA GGC GTC GAT TAT TGG ATC GTA CGA AAC   910
 270   Ala Val Asn Ile Val Gly Tyr Gly Ser Thr Gln Gly Val Asp Tyr Trp Ile Val Arg Asn   289

 911   AGT TGG GAT ACT ACC TGG GGT GAT AGC GGA TAC GGA TAT TTC CAA GCC GGA AAC AAC CTC   970
 290   Ser Trp Asp Thr Thr Trp Gly Asp Ser Gly Tyr Gly Tyr Phe Gln Ala Gly Asn Asn Leu   309

 971   ATG ATG ATC GAA CAA TAT CCA TAT GTT GTA ATC ATG TGA ACATTTGAAATTGAATATATTTATTTG 1036
 310   Met Met Ile Glu Gln Tyr Pro Tyr Val Val Ile Met ***                              322

1037   TTTTCAAAATAAAAACAACTACTCTTGCGAGTATTTTTTACTTTT  1081
```

Figure 3. Nucleotide sequence of *Der f* I gene and deduced amino acid sequence.

II expression plasmids was cultivated in a 30-liter jar fermentor containing 20 liter of L-broth under the following operation conditions: temperature 30°C, aeration 20 liter/min and agitation 200 rpm. After 3hr cultivation, IPTG (isopropyl β-D-thiogalactoside) was added to 0.1mM for induction of the *Der f* II gene expression. The cultivation was continued for further 10 hr. r*Der f* II produced as inclusion bodies were extracted, dissolved with 8M urea and then refolded by removing urea using hollow fiber systems. After the refolding process, the recombinant allergen was purified by ion-exchange column chromatography followed by gel filtration.

The physicochemical and immunological properties of the finally purified r*Der f* II were compared with those of native *Der f* II derived from mite bodies. r*Der f* II different from the native had one additional methionine at the N-terminus derived from initiation

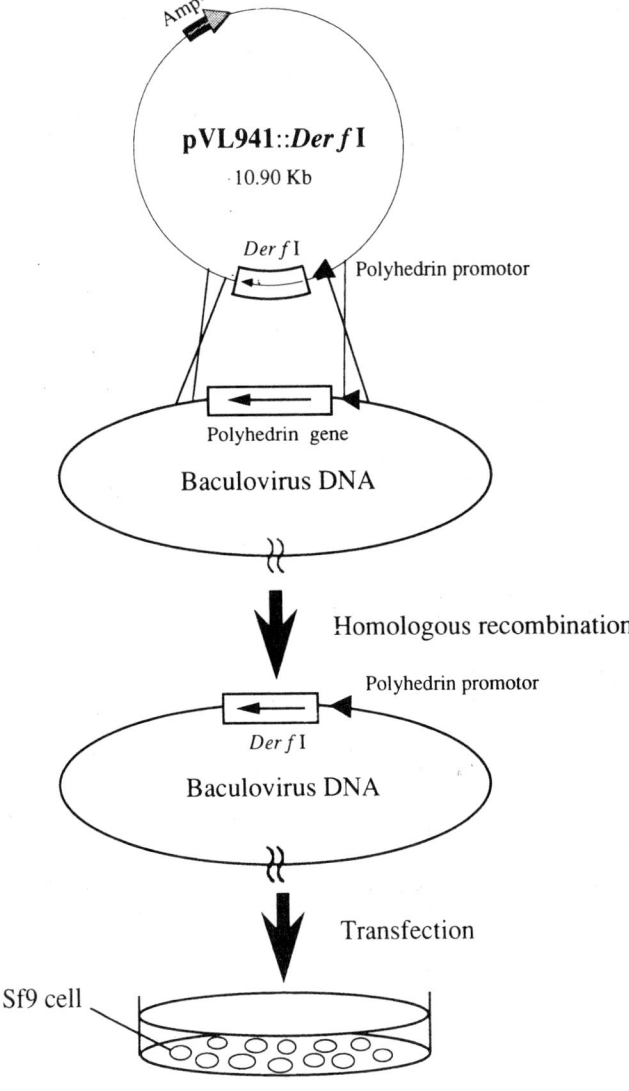

Figure 4. Construction scheme of r*Der f* I expression virus.

codon ATG. The other characteristics were identical with those of the native one. As shown in Fig.2, it is clear that the binding activities of both allergens to mite allergic patients' sera IgE antibodies are completely identical each other. The skin test also showed that r*Der f* II had the same allergenicity as the native (data not shown).

PRODUCTION OF r*Der f* I AND ITS PROPERTIES

Although *Der f* I cDNA had been isolated[6], we also attempted the isolation and independently obtained the cDNA from gene library of *Dermatophagoides farinae* constructed previously. The sequence shown in Fig. 3. In our gene, there were slight differences from the sequence reported by Dilworth *et al.*[6], but both genes seemed to be same. It is clear from Fig. 3 that the *Der f* I gene had prepro-form and one N-glycosylation site.

At first, we tried the production of r*Der f* I using *E. coli* system. We tried various refolding conditions, nevertheless we could not obtain the active form. It is thought that the sugar moiety of *Der f* I should be necessary for the correct refolding. If that t is right, *E. coli* system should be unsuitable for the production of active form of *Der f* I because *E. coli* system cannot attach sugar chain to expressed proteins. Therefore, we selected an eukaryote system, insect cell/baculovirus system, which has glycosylation ability of proteins.

Fig. 4 shows the scheme of construction of recombinant baculovirus containing *Der f* I gene and Fig. 5 shows the production scheme of r*Der f* I. In this system, r*Der f* I was secreted to the medium as a pro-form that had less IgE binding activity than the native. The precursor was purified by column chromatography and subjected to acid treatment for making the mature form. Under acidic conditions, the precursor changed to the mature form by autocatalysis. The IgE binding activities of native *Der f* I, pro-form and mature form of r*Der f* I are shown in Fig.6. It is clear that the mature form of r*Der f* I has the

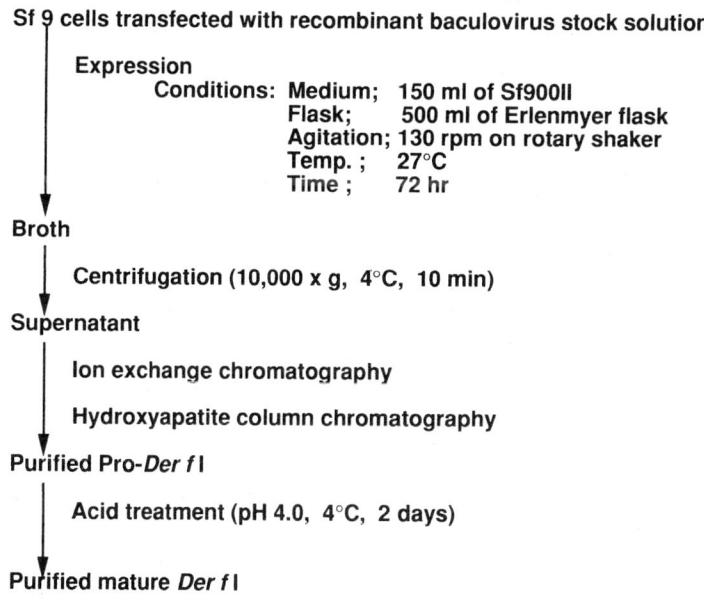

Figure 5. Production scheme of r*Der f* I.

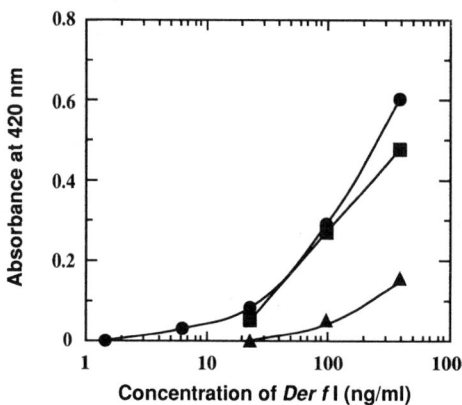

Figure 6. Human IgE binding activities of native *Der f* I, pro- and mature r*Der f* I. The activities were measured with RAST-EIA kit (Kabi Pharmacia Diagnostics AB). ● native *Der f* I; ▲ pro-r*Der f* I; ■ mature r*Der f* I.

same IgE binding activity as that of the native one. Additionally, we compared amino acid sequence of the mature r*Der f* I to that of the native using a protein sequencer (Applied Biosystems, model 473A). The sequence data showed that r*Der f* I had the same amino acid sequence as that of the native allergen (data not shown).

IMMUNOTHERAPY OF MOUSE EXPERIMENTAL ASTHMA MODEL USING r*Der f* II

Since we have been able to prepare large amounts of purified major house dust mite allergens, *Der f* I and II, by gene technology, we applied the r*Der f* II to immunotherapy on mouse experimental asthma model. Fig. 7 shows the experimental protocol. Male A/J mice at 7 weeks of age were intranasaly immunized with 25µl of 4 mg/ml of r*Der f* II once a week. The immunization was continued for 11 weeks. After that, the mice were orally administered for 4 weeks with r*Der f* II or with PBS as control once a day. After this treat-

Antigen : r*Der f* II
Animals : male A/J mice, 7 weeks of age
Experimental groups:
    a) control (n=9)
    b) r*Der f* II 0.1mg/day (n=8)
    c) r*Der f* II   1mg/day (n=9)

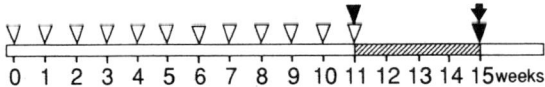

0 1 2 3 4 5 6 7 8 9 10 11 12 13 14 15weeks

▽ : Immunization = 100µg r*Der f* II, intranasally
▼ : Measurement of plasma IgE levels
⬇ : Determination of airway constriction
▨ : Oral administration of PBS or r*Der f* II solution

Figure 7. Sensitization and immunotherapy schedule.

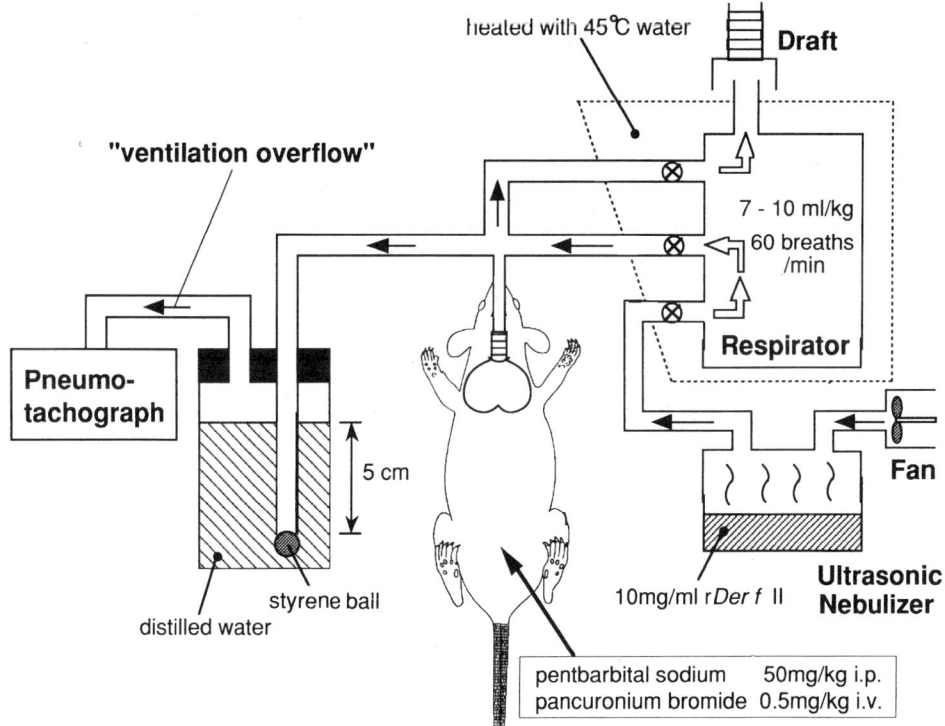

Figure 8. Determination of airway constriction.

ment, the mice were subjected to the allergen inhalation test. The immunotherapy of r*Der f* II on the experimental asthma model was evaluated as shown in Fig. 8. Depending on contraction of trachea, amount of the overflowed air increased and was measured with a pneumotachograph. A small tube was directly inserted to the mouse's trachea for the measurement of the real contraction of trachea. Therefore, this system avoided to measure the nasal inflammation.

The distribution of the ventilation overflowed air of the individual mouse at 5, 6 and 7 min after the allergen challenge is shown in Fig.9. The mean value of the overflowed air decreased and the contraction began later according to the dose of r*Der f* II. From the results, it is suggested that oral administration of r*Der f* II was effective therapy for mouse experimental asthma model.

We have been studying the mechanism of the therapy, but the mechanism is still unknown. IgE titers of the mice were measured before and after the immunotherapy. There was no difference of the titer observed between control mice and r*Der f* II administered mice (data not shown).

CONCLUSION

We established the production procedures for major house dust mite allergens, *Der f* I and II in a large scale, respectively. The recombinant allergens produced by gene technology had the advantages of quality and quantity to the native allergens from natural sources. It seems to be substantially impossible to prepare large amounts of the purified allergens from natural sources, while the recombinant allergens are easily prepared as pure

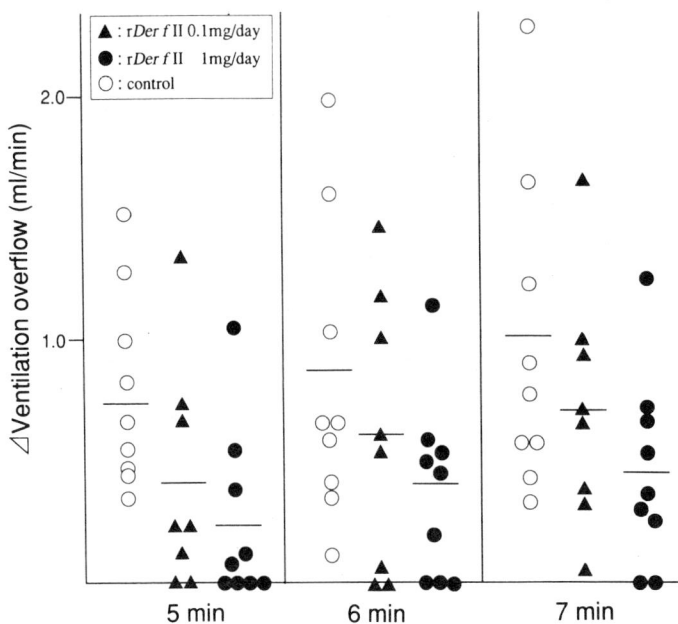

Figure 9. Distribution of ventilation overflow at 5, 6 and 7 min. Short horizontal line shows mean value of the overflowed air in each group.

forms. In other words, since the recombinant allergens can be supplied by request, they seem to be suitable not only for standard compounds but for basic research, diagnosis and immunotherapy. Additionally, rDer f I is absolutely free from contamination of Der f II and *vice versa*. This seems to be one of the most advanced properties in the recombinant allergens.

We also established mouse experimental asthma model. We used intranasal route for sensitization because atopic patients against house dust mite allergens seem to be sensitized through nose, larynx or throat. Therefore, we selected the nasal sensitization route. In our animal model, it was clarified that immunotherapy using rDer f II was effective against the experimental asthma model.

We are studying the mode of action but the mechanism of immunotherapy is still unknown.

REFERENCES

1. Pederson, C., et al.: Inhibitory effect of cyclosporin A on histamine release from human leukocytes and rat mast cells. Allergy 40: 103–107, 1985
2. Schreiber, S. L. and Crabtree, G. R.: The mechanism of action of cyclosporin A and FK506. Immunol. Today 13: 136–142, 1992
3. Shouji, H., et al.: Activation of recombinant mite allergen Der f I expressed in insect cells. Abstracts of XV International Congress of Allergology and Clinical Immunology 1994, 102

4. Yuuki, T., et al.: Cloning and expression of cDNA coding for the major house dust mite allergen Der f II in Escherichia coli. Biosci. Biotech. Biochem. 55:1223–1238, 1991

5. Nishiyama, C., et al.: Effects of amino acid variations in recombinant *Der f* II on its human IgE and mouse IgG recognition. Int. Arch. Allergy Immunol. 105:62–69, 1994

6. Dilworth, R. J., et al.: Sequence analysis of cDNA coding for a major house dust mite allergen, *Der f* I. Clin. Exp. Allergy 21:25–32, 1991

23

USE OF RECOMBINANT GROUP 5 ALLERGENS TO INVESTIGATE IgE-MEDIATED SENSITIZATION TO BLOMIA TROPICALIS AND DERMATOPHAGOIDES PTERONYSSINUS

L. Karla Arruda,[1] Lisa D. Vailes,[1] Enrique Fernandez-Caldas,[2]
Charles K. Naspitz,[3] Federico Montealegre,[4] and Martin D. Chapman[1]

[1]Asthma and Allergic Diseases Center
Department of Internal Medicine
University of Virginia, Charlottesville, Virginia
[2]University of South Florida College of Medicine
Tampa, Florida
[3]Paulista School of Medicine
São Paulo, SP, Brazil
[4]Ponce School of Medicine
Ponce, Puerto Rico

1. INTRODUCTION

In tropical and subtropical areas of the world, mites of the genus *Blomia* have been recognized as important cause of sensitization and development of asthma. These non-pyroglyphidae mites belong to the *Glycyphagidae* family, and are currently classified among the "domestic mites"[1]. IgE antibody responses to *Blomia*, including *B. tropicalis* and *B. kulagini*, have been documented by skin testing and serologic studies[2-7]. Exposure to *B. tropicalis* has been reported in houses from different geographic areas, including Hong Kong, Brazil, Colombia, Venezuela, India, Taiwan, Spain, Egypt and other countries[1, 8]. In the United States, *B. tropicalis* has been found in significant numbers in homes from Tampa FL, New Orleans LA, Memphis TN, Galveston TX, Delray Beach and San Diego CA[9,10]. In these areas, *B. tropicalis* was the fourth most frequent mite species found in house dust, in addition to *Dermatophagoides pteronyssinus*, *D. farinae* and *Euroglyphus maynei*.

The antigenic cross-reactivity between *B. tropicalis* and *D. pteronyssinus* has been extensively investigated by several groups[2,3,5,6,11]. The results of these studies using different techniques revealed that *B. tropicalis* is a source of multiple allergens and that the majority of the *B. tropicalis* allergens are species-specific; however a small proportion may

New Horizons in Allergy Immunotherapy
edited by Sehon et al. Plenum Press, New York, 1996

173

be cross-reactive with *D. pteronyssinus*. In addition, analysis of *B. tropicalis* mite body or whole culture extracts has shown undetectable levels of Group 1 and Group 2 *Dermatophagoides* allergens, suggesting that the crossreactivity is associated with antigens other than these *Dermatophagoides* major allergens[11]. Since both mites are commonly found in house dust samples from such environments, establishing the antigenic relationship between the mite species is fundamental for allergy diagnosis and treatment, as well as for understanding the role of mite allergens in the development of allergic diseases. At present, no purified *B. tropicalis* allergens have been reported. The purpose of this investigation was to use molecular cloning techniques to further identify, characterize and determine the sequence of *B. tropicalis* allergens.

2. METHODS AND RESULTS

To further investigate the antigenic crossreactivity between *B. tropicalis* and *D. pteronyssinus*, we performed RAST analysis in a large panel of sera from mite allergic patients living in different areas of the world. IgE antibody responses to *B. tropicalis* were measured in a panel of sera of asthmatic patients from Brazil, Puerto Rico and Florida (n=83), and compared to patients with asthma or atopic dermatitis from Charlottesville, VA and England (n=56)[12], allergic to *D. pteronyssinus*, but unlikely to have been exposed to *B. tropicalis*. In the first group, 83% of *B. tropicalis* RAST positive patients had a positive RAST to *D. pteronyssinus*. The ratio *D. pteronyssinus* /*B. tropicalis* RAST was >10 in only 22% of the patients, suggesting that this group has been exposed to both mite species. On the other hand, the ratio *D. pteronyssinus* /*B. tropicalis* RAST among the group from VA/England was >10 in 68% of patients (p<0.001), and 50% or the VA/England patients had detectable IgE to *B. tropicalis* by RAST. In keeping with previous observations, our results suggested that only 20–30% of *B. tropicalis* allergens may be cross-reactive with D. pteronyssinus.

Identification of *B. tropicalis* allergens was accomplished using molecular cloning techniques. A cDNA library was constructed from whole body *B. tropicalis* mRNA, and screened with IgE antibodies. A serum pool was prepared using sera from mite allergic asthmatic patients with high titers of IgE antibody to *B. tropicalis* (RAST to *B. tropicalis* 600–4,700 units/ml), and used to probe nitrocellulose filters blotted with clones expressing recombinant proteins. Although eight positive cDNA clones were isolated, partial sequence revealed that 7/8 shared the same nucleotide sequence. The complete sequence of a representative 522bp-cDNA clone, containing a 432 open reading frame, was determined. The predicted amino acid sequence of the protein encoded by the 522bp cDNA clone showed sequence homology to Der p 5, a 14kd *D. pteronyssinus* allergen described by Tovey *et al.*[13,14] In addition, the cDNA clone was further analyzed by plaque immunoassay using individual sera from the complete panel (n=139). The results showed that among patients from Brazil, Puerto Rico and Florida (exposed to both *B. tropicalis* and *D. pteronyssinus*), 57/83 (69%) had IgE to the cloned protein. On the other hand, among patients from Charlottesville and England (unlikely to have been exposed to *B. tropicalis*), only 13/56 (23%) had detectable IgE to this protein (p<0.005). In keeping with the allergen nomenclature, the *B. tropicalis* allergen has been designated as Blo t 5[15].

Recombinant Blo t 5 was expressed in *E. coli*. Blo t 5 cDNA was subcloned into the pGEX-4T1 vector and expressed as a fusion protein with Glutathione-S-transferase (GST). Purification of Blo t 5-GST from bacterial lysates was accomplished by chromatography over glutathione sepharose. Digestion of the fusion protein with thrombin released Blo t 5 from the fusion partner, and subsequent purification was carried out over the glutathione column. Purified Blo t 5 was recovered in the flow-through, and appeared as a single 14kd band on silver-stained SDS-PAGE gel. Blo t 5 was radiolabeled with ^{125}I and used in an antigen-binding radioimmunoassay to measure anti-Blo t 5 IgE antibodies in sera from *B. tropicalis* allergic patients . The prevalence of IgE to Blo t 5 was 45% among patients from Brazil, Puerto Rico and Florida. In addition, recombinant Blo t 5 induced positive immediate skin tests in selected *B. tropicalis* allergic patients. These results showed that recombinant Blo t 5 expressed in bacteria retains IgE binding capacity, demonstrated by serologic experiments and by skin testing for immediate hypersensitivity.

3. CONCLUSIONS

We have identified a major *B. tropicalis* allergen Blo t 5 by cDNA cloning, and produced recombinant allergen in *E. coli*. IgE antibodies to Blo t 5 can be identified in 45–69% of sera of *B. tropicalis* allergic patients, using antigen-binding RIA and plaque immunoassay, respectively. The difference in prevalence probably reflects the higher sensitivity of the plaque immunoassay. Blo t 5 shows sequence homology to Der p 5, a 14kd *D. pteronyssinus* allergen, however the function of both allergens remains unknown and no homologies have been found with other proteins. In keeping with previous studies, our results on serologic analysis of a large panel of sera suggested that the majority of *B. tropicalis* allergens are species-specific. Recombinant Blo t 5 and Der p 5 produced in bacteria retain IgE-binding activity [14], and are currently being used for detailed studies on the antigenic cross-reactivity between the two proteins. These studies are very important for a better understanding of the development of the allergic response to mites, particularly in the tropical and subtropical areas of the world, where exposure to *B. tropicalis* may be as high as to *D. pteronyssinus*.

4. ACKNOWLEDGMENTS

This work was supported by National Institutes of Health Grants AI 34607 and AI 20565.

5. REFERENCES

1. Arruda LK and Chapman MD: A review of recent immunochemical studies of *Blomia tropicalis* and *Euroglyphus maynei* allergens. *Exp Appl Acarol* 1992;16:129–140.
2. Van Hage-Hamsten M, Machado I, Barros MT, Johansson SGO. Immune response to *Blomia kulagini* and *Dermatophagoides pteronyssinus* in Sweden and Brazil. *Int Arch Allergy Appl Immunol* 1990;91:186–91.
3. Llerena LP, Fernandez-Caldas E, Gracia LRC, Lockey RF. Sensitization to *Blomia tropicalis* and *Lepidoglyphus destructor* in *Dermatophagoides* spp-allergic individuals. *J Allergy Clin Immunol* 1991; 88:943–950.
4. Rizzo MC, Arruda LK, Chapman MD, Fernandez-Caldas E, Baggio D, Platts-Mills TAE, Naspitz CK. IgG and IgE antibody responses to dust mite allergens among children with asthma in Brazil. *Ann Allergy* 1993; 71:152–158.
5. Arlian LG, Vyszenski-Moher DL, Fernandez-Caldas E: Allergenicity of the mite, *Blomia tropicalis*. *J Allergy Clin Immunol* 1993;91:1042–50.
6. Stanaland BE, Fernandez-Caldas E, Jacinto CM, Trudeau WL, Lockey RF. Sensitization to *Blomia tropicalis*: Skin test and cross-reactivity studies. *J Allergy Clin Immunol* 1994;94:452–7.

7. Caraballo L, Puerta L, Martinez B, Moreno L. Identification of allergens from the mite *Blomia tropicalis*. *Clin Exp Allergy* 1994; 24:1056–1060.

8. Fernandez-Caldas E, Puerta L, Mercado D, Lockey RF, Caraballo LR. Mite fauna, Der p I, Der f1 and *Blomia tropicalis* allergen levels in a tropical environment. *Clin Exp Allergy* 1993;23:292–297.

9. Fernandez-Caldas E, Fox RW, Bucholtz GA, Trudeau WL, Ledford DK, Lockey RF. House dust mite allergy in Florida. Mite survey in households of mite-sensitive individuals in Tampa, Florida. *Allergy Proc* 1988; 11:263–267.

10. Arlian LG, Bernstein D, Bernstein IL, Friedman S, Grant A, Lieberman P, Lopez M, Metzger J, Platts-Mills TAE, Shatz M, Spector S, Wasserman SI, Zeiger RS. Prevalence of dust mites in the homes of people with asthma living in eight different geographic areas of the United States. *J Allergy Clin Immunol* 1992; 90:292–300.

11. Arruda LK, Rizzo MC, Chapman MD, Fernandez-Caldas E, Baggio D, Platts- Mills TAE, Naspitz CK. Exposure and sensitization to dust mite allergens among asthmatic children in Sao Paulo, Brazil. *Clin Exp Allergy* 1991;21:433–439.

12. Sporik R, Holgate ST, Platts-Mills TAE, Cogswell J. House dust mite allergen (*Der p* I) exposure and the development of sensitization and asthma in childhood: A prospective study. *N Engl J Med* 1990; 323:502–507.

13. Tovey ER, Johnson MC, Roche AL, Cobon GS, Baldo BA. Cloning and sequencing of a cDNA expressing a recombinant house dust mite protein that binds human IgE and corresponds to an important low molecular weight allergen. *J Exp Med* 1989; 170:1457–1462.

14. Lin K-L, Hsieh K-H, Thomas WR, Chiang B-L, Chua K-Y. Characterization of *Der p* V allergen, cDNA analysis, and IgE-mediated reactivity to the recombinant protein. *J Allergy Clin Immunol* 1994; 94:989–996.

15. King TP, Hoffman D, Lowenstein H, Marsh DG, Platts-Mills TAE, Thomas W. Allergen Nomenclature. *Int Arch Allergy Immunol* 1994; 105:224–233.

24

DUAL EFFECTS OF ALLERGEN-mPEG CONJUGATES

Induction of Immunological Suppression and Inactivation of Sensitized Mast Cells

A. H. Sehon, S. Bitoh, and G. Lang

Department of Immunology
Faculty of Medicine
University of Manitoba
Winnipeg, MB, Canada, R3E 0W3

1. ATTEMPTS TO SUPPRESS IGE ANTIBODY RESPONSES IN ALLERGIC INDIVIDUALS

Since the early 1970s the research in this laboratory has been directed toward the development of methods for the specific suppression of IgE antibodies (1,2). Among the more recent strategies used, the administration of tolerogenic conjugates — consisting of different allergens/antigens coupled to optimal numbers of molecules of monomethoxy-polyethylene glycol (mPEG) — proved to be the most effective method for the specific long-term suppression of the induction of antibody responses in mice and rats to the corresponding immunogenic compounds (3,4). This method involves two steps:

Step I. *Injection of tolerogenic conjugates of the appropriate immunogenic allergen (AL), i.e., AL(mPEG)$_n$,*

Step II. *Administration of the unmodified AL 7 days after injection of the immunosuppressive AL(mPEG)$_n$.*

Thereafter, without further administration of AL(mPEG)$_n$ and in spite of repeated injections of the unmodified AL over extended periods (of up to 300–500 days) no anti-AL antibody response is induced.

The interval of 7 days between Steps I and II was shown to be necessary so as to allow the propagation of AL-specific CD8$^+$ suppressor T (Ts) cells which are activated by AL(mPEG)$_n$; additional injections of the unmodified AL maintain the proliferation of these cells, which suppress the specific T helper cells that recognize also the epitopes of the same AL, though not necessarily the same epitopes as those recognized by the Ts cells. The above proposed mechanism is based on the following experimental evidence:

New Horizons in Allergy Immunotherapy
edited by Sehon et al. Plenum Press, New York, 1996

177

(a) The Ts cells were cloned in our laboratory from single cells which had been isolated from spleens of immunosuppressed mice (5).
(b) The transfer of the cloned Ts cells, or of the corresponding Ag-specific monoclonal suppressor factor (TsF) (which was released from these cells), into intact naive mice resulted in the downregulation of their immune response to the Ag in question (6). This TsF has the properties of the $\alpha\beta$ heterodimer of the cell receptors of the corresponding Ts cells (7).
(c) Mice pretolerized to a given protein antigen, Ag_A, by treatment with $Ag_A(mPEG)_n$ were also immunologically unresponsive to an unrelated Ag_B, on condition that Ag_B was injected into these tolerized mice in the form of a covalent adduct with Ag_A, i.e., as Ag_A-Ag_B, but not as a mixture with Ag_A. This *"linked immunological suppression"* was also achieved in naive mice by treating them first with TsF_A and administering thereafter the Ag_A-Ag_B adduct, on condition that these mice had not been depleted of normal $CD8^+$ T cells (8).

Obviously, any clone of Ts cells recognize only one epitope (i.e., one immunogenic determinant) of the respective multideterminant protein. A possible mechanism underlying this *"cognate phenomenon of linked immunological suppression"* was postulated on the basis of an extensive experimental study (8).

In clinical trials — involving close to 300 patients suffering from IgE-mediated allergies — designed to validate the possible efficacy of immunotherapy with mPEG conjugates of diverse ALs, *it was established that whereas this treatment did not affect markedly the pre-existing IgE levels, the patients' AL-specific IgG levels were significantly and rapidly increased.* The results of these clinical trials, which were conducted under the aegis of Pharmacia AB of Uppsala in a number of medical centres in different countries, are documented in a comprehensive review article (9). The main conclusions of these clinical studies are : (i) In comparison with conventional immunotherapeutic preparations containing unmodified pollen ALs, substantially higher doses of the essentially nonallergenic $AL(mPEG)_n$ conjugates could be tolerated by allergic patients and did not lead to untoward physiological effects; this loss in allergenicity is attributable to the masking of some of the epitopes of the allergenic molecules by the mPEG chains grafted onto the AL molecule, and/or to the conformational distortion of these epitopes as a result of this coupling reaction. (ii) The beneficial effects of a short course of injections with $AL(mPEG)_n$ were similar to those obtained with conventional allergenic extracts over many years, i.e., most of these patients showed fewer symptoms of rhinoconjunctivitis and required less medication during the pollination season.

In spite of the fact that treatment of allergic patients over a relatively short period of time with $AL(mPEG)_n$ did not result in the anticipated drop in IgE antibodies, but led to an increase in AL-specific IgG antibodies, we believe that these mPEG conjugates may still prove to be useful agents for immunotherapy of IgE-mediated allergies since they are essentially nonallergenic and, most importantly, since the increase in IgG antibodies is still regarded as one of the principal parameters of successful hyposensitization regimens (10). It may also be appropriate to point out that way back, in the 1950s and in the early 1960s, it had been shown (11) that *sera of allergic patients contained even prior to initiation of immunotherapy not only "reaginic" but also "blocking" antibodies, which correspond in modern terms to IgE and IgG antibodies, respectively.* Therefore, it may be suggested that the discrepancy between the enhancement of IgG responses in allergic patients and the induction of tolerance in mice, brought about by the administration of mPEG conjugates of the same AL, may be attributable to (i) the much higher dose of the conjugates, on a weight basis, which was administered to mice, and (ii) the difference in the immunological status of these two types of recipients, i.e., whereas the mice in our original experiments (12) had not been stimulated by AL prior to administration of the tolerogenic AL(mPEG)$_n$, the immunological system of the patients had been stimulated repeatedly by exposures to the AL prior to beginning their immunotherapy.

In essence, the results of these clinical trials confirmed the fundamental rule of immune responsiveness, viz., that it is much more difficult to inactivate or eliminate long-lived memory cells of an established ongoing immune response (which have been expanded in response to repeated exposures to a given antigen) than the precursor cells prior to induction of the immune response. The discrepancy of the effect of AL(mPEG) conjugates on presensitized allergic patients and naive rodents demonstrated that mPEG conjugates may up-regulate or down-regulate the immune response depending on the immunological status of the recipient. Indeed, the plausibility of this interpretation was supported by the results of experiments simulating the immunological status in mice to that of allergic patients, i.e., for these experiments the mice were sensitized to produce anti-OVA IgE antibodies prior to receiving injections of the tolerogenic OVA(mPEG)$_{10}$ conjugates. Under these conditions, there was no apparent difference between the reactivities of the two species to AL(mPEG); thus, although the IgE responses of these mice were markedly reduced at relatively high doses of the conjugate, their IgG responses were enhanced after secondary immunization with OVA (12,13). *However, the mechanism, underlying the diverging effects of tolerogenic mPEG conjugates on different isotypes (i.e. IgE versus IgG) depending on the immunological status of the recipient (i.e. naive versus presensitized) and on the doses of the conjugates, remains to be elucidated.*

It is important to point out that the different allergenic preparations available at the time of these exploratory clinical trials contained multiple molecular components and, therefore, the resulting conjugates were complex mixtures of chemically ill-defined mPEG derivatives. However, in recent years, as a result of the application of recombinant DNA technology, the principal AL responsible for some of the common IgE-mediated allergies which afflict masses of people around the world have been isolated, characterized and synthesized as chemically well-defined and pure molecules, and even some of their main B and T cell epitopes have been delineated in molecular terms (14,15). Hence, it is suggested that mPEG conjugates of recombinant allergens may prove to be effective agents for the downregulation of IgE Abs.

2. ALLERGEN-SPECIFIC INHIBITION OF THE EFFECTOR PHASE OF IgE-MEDIATED ALLERGIES BY AL(mPEG) CONJUGATES

As stated earlier, for induction of *specific Ts cells* by administration of Ag(mPEG) conjugates, one or more of the T cell epitopes of the Ag in the conjugate must be accessible to the progenitors of the Ts cells. In other words, the Ts cell progenitors must be able to recognize some of the epitopes shared by both the unmodified and PEGylated Ag. Indeed, we showed that about 5% of the Ag(mPEG)$_n$ conjugates could bind to reverse immunosorbents consisting of immobilized polyspecific Abs to the Ag in question, and that this fraction of the Ag(mPEG) conjugate could inactivate naive B cells; this finding supports the additional conclusion that not only Ts cell epitopes, but also some B cell epitopes of the Ag incorporated in the conjugate remain accessible to homologous antibodies (unpublished studies).

Table 1. Reduced allergenicity of OVA(mPEG)$_{11}$ in
Prausnitz-Küstner (P-K) reactions*

Dose injected into each sensitized site	P-K titers in three rats		
OVA			
100 ng/site	320	320	640
1 µg/site	320	640	640
OVA(mPEG)$_{11}$			
1 µg/site	<10	<10	<10
10 µg/site	<10	<10	<10
100 µg/site	<10	20	<10
500 µg/site	160	320	640
1 mg/site	640	640	1280

* Skin sites on the backs of 3 S-D rats were sensitized with 100 µl of the 2-fold serially diluted pooled antiserum containing murine anti-OVA IgE antibodies; the diluent was PBS containing 0.1% normal mouse serum. Forty-eight hours after sensitization each skin site was injected with 50 µl containing different doses of OVA or OVA(mPEG)$_{11}$ in PBS, and immediately thereafter the rats were given intravenously 1 ml of 1% Evans Blue dye in PBS. The P-K titers represent the reciprocals of the maximum dilutions of the antiserum, at which skin reactions were readily discernable, i.e., >5 mm in diameter. Titers <10 indicate that no significant P-K reaction was observed at the lowest dilution of 1/10 of the serum.

On the basis of this finding and of the observation that mPEG conjugates were essentially nonallergenic, we turned recently our attention to the possibility of the direct interaction of these mPEG conjugates with mast cells sensitized with IgE Abs to (some of) the epitopes of the Ag in question, and to studying the effect of this interaction if it actually occurred. As reviewed below, *to our surprise we established that a conjugate of OVA and mPEG was capable of inactivating both in vivo and ex vivo mast cells sensitized with murine anti-OVA IgE Abs.*

The results listed in Table 1 demonstrate that, utilizing a modified Prausnitz-Küstner (P-K) system, OVA(mPEG)$_{10}$ had greatly reduced allergenicity (<1%) by comparison with that of the original unmodified OVA. In spite of this considerable reduction in allergenicity, injection of 10 µg of OVA(mPEG)$_{11}$ (i.e., at a dose which was too low to induce skin reactions) into rat skin sites — which had been sensitized with a polyspecific murine anti-OVA IgE serum — resulted in inhibition of skin reactions as revealed on subsequent i.v. challenge with 1 mg of OVA (see Table 2).

Moreover, injection of OVA-mPEG into skin sites which had been sensitized conjointly with a mixture of a polyspecific anti-OVA IgE serum and murine monoclonal anti-DNP IgE Abs in different ratios prevented PCA reactions on challenge with OVA, or DNP$_6$-BSA, or DNP$_9$-OVA (see Table 3) (16). These results also support the view that AL(mPEG) conjugates of a single AL may be capable of inactivating mast cells sensitized with IgE antibodies to a mosaic of allergens, as long as a membrane-fixed IgE antibody — which is directed against one of the epitopes of the AL in question — can combine with the appropriate epitope when the latter is presented as an integral constituent of the appropriate nonallergenic AL(mPEG) conjugate.

Furthermore, as illustrated in Table 4, treatment of OVA-sensitive mice with OVA(mPEG)$_{10}$ by either the i.v. or the respiratory route protected the mice from systemic anaphylaxis on challenge with OVA (16). *These results further support the inference that an essentially nonallergenic mPEG conjugate of a given allergen may have the*

Table 2. Inhibition by OVA(mPEG)$_{11}$ of anti-OVA IgE-mediated PCA*

Injection of skin sites sensitized with anti-OVA IgE with	PCA titers after intervals of 24, 12 or 1 hour(s) between injection of OVA(mPEG)$_{11}$ into the sensitized skin sites and iv injection of OVA.		
	24-hours	12-hours	1-hour
Nil	320, 640, 320		
PBS	320, 640, 320	320, 640, 640	320, 640, 640
OVA(mPEG)$_{11}$ 1 µg/site	80, 40, 20	80, 20, 40	40, 20, 20
OVA(mPEG)$_{11}$ 10 µg/site	<10, 20, <10	<10, 20, <10	<10, <10, <10

* Skin sites on the backs of nine S-D rats were sensitized by id injection with 100 µl of a 2-fold serially diluted pooled murine antiserum containing anti-OVA IgE Abs. Twenty-four, 36 or 47 hours later 50 µl containing PBS, or 1 or 10 µg of OVA(mPEG)$_{11}$, was injected into each site. Forty-eight hours after sensitization, each rat was challenged iv with 1 mg of OVA in PBS supplemented with Evans Blue. The results represent individual PCA titers.

therapeutic potential for reducing or abrogating the symptoms of common allergies and asthma. It is planned to extend these in vivo studies to asthmatic dogs, which are sensitized from birth to a given allergen(s) by methods developed in Dr. Becker's laboratory (17).

The above *in vivo* results were confirmed in an *ex vivo* system which consisted of rat basophilic leukemia (RBL) cells that had been passively sensitized with murine anti-OVA IgE Abs. As illustrated in Fig. 1 treatment of these cells with OVA(mPEG)$_{10}$ led to a dose-related inhibition of the release of serotonin on subsequent challenge with OVA.

Table 3. Inhibition by OVA(mPEG)$_{11}$ of PCA reactions to unrelated IgE Abs

Sensitization of skin sites with a mixture of IgE Abs to OVA and DNP*		Ag used for challenge	PCA reactions in skin sites pretreated with**		
			NIL	PBS	OVA(mPEG)$_{11}$
[A]	1/320:NIL	OVA	+	+	—
	1/320:1/1,280		+	+	—
	1/320:1/640		+	+	—
	1/320:1/320		+	+	—
[B]	1/320:1/1,280	DNP$_6$-BSA	+	+	—
	1/320:1/640		+	+	—
	1/320:1/320		+	+	±
	NIL:1/160		+	+	+
[C]	1/320:NIL	DNP$_3$-OVA	+	+	—
	1/320:1/1,280		+	+	—
	1/320:1/640		+	+	—
	1/320:1/320		+	+	+
	NIL:1/160		+	+	+

* Each skin site on backs of 3 SD rats was sensitized with 100 µl of a mixture consisting of (i) the pooled anti-OVA IgE Abs, and (ii) the supernatant of the culture of clone 26.82 producing anti-DNP IgE monoclonal Ab (the respective dilutions of the pool of IgE Abs and of the culture supernatant are indicated in the first column). Twenty four hours later, one set of skin sites was left untouched, and the second and third sets received, respectively, 50 µl of PBS and 50 µl PBS containing 1 µg of OVA(mPEG)$_{11}$.
** After a further interval of 24 hours, each rat was given an i.v. injection of 1 mg OVA, or of DNP$_6$-BSA, or of DNP$_9$-OVA with 1% Evans Blue solution in PBS. The symbols (+), (−) and (±) refer, respectively, to PCA reactions exceeding 5 mm in diameter, no detectable PCA reactions, and faint reactions.

Table 4. Protective effect of OVA(mPEG)$_{11}$ on
systemic anaphylaxis*

Injection on day 32	Mortality	
	Exp. 1	Exp. 2
PBS	4/4	3/4
OVA(mPEG)$_{11}$		
ip	3/4	3/4
sc	4/4	4/4
iv	0/4	0/4
Inhalation	0/4	1/4

* BDF1 mice were immunized twice with 1 μg of OVA adsorbed on
Al(OH)$_3$ on days 1 and 28. On day 28 the mice were also injected
with *Pertussis toxin* in order to enhance histamine releasing factor.
Four days later, on day 32, the mice received an injection of 1 mg
of OVA(mPEG)$_{11}$ in saline by the ip, iv, or sc route or an aerosol of
0.1% (w/v) of the conjugate in saline for 20 min. On day 33, all
mice were given an iv injection of 1 mg of OVA to induce systemic
anaphylaxis.

In vitro inactivation by OVA(mPEG)$_{11}$ of sensitized rat mast cells

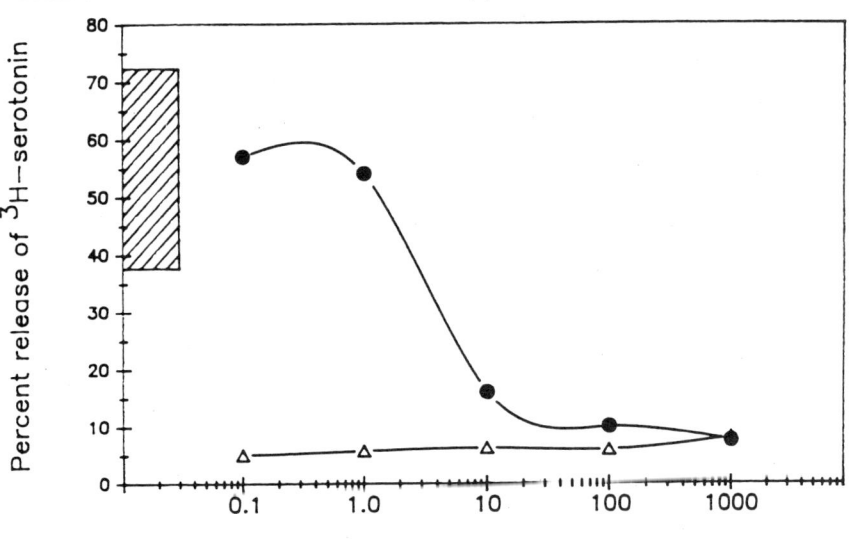

Addition of mPEG conjugate of OVA (ng/ml)

Figure 1. Rat basophilic leukemia cells (10^5) of the 2H3 line were sensitized with 10 μg/ml of partially purified
mouse anti-OVA IgE Abs in the presence of 100 nci ^{3}H-5HT. No release of ^{3}H-5HT from sensitized cells was detected without addition of OVA; the range of release of ^{3}H-5HT from the sensitized cells on addition of 1 μg/ml of
OVA only is indicated by the shaded area. The triangles represent the percent release of ^{3}H-5HT from sensitized
mast cells by OVA(mPEG)$_{11}$ [over the range of 100 pg/ml - 1 μg/ml], without addition of OVA. The filled circles
indicate the percent release of ^{3}H-5HT from cells that had been incubated for one hour with OVA(mPEG)$_{11}$ at various concentrations, washed thrice and then treated with OVA for 30 minutes. These data points represent the mean
of three independent experiments.

Hypothetical Mechanism Underlying Inactivation of Mast Cells by AL(mPEG)$_n$ Conjugates

The weak allergenicity of the OVA(mPEG)$_{10}$ preparation observed at high doses may be envisaged to be due to (i) some minute polyvalent under-PEGylated contaminant(s) present in the conjugate preparation, or (ii) the interaction of the multiple mPEG molecules of one conjugate molecule, which is fixed to a cell-bound IgE Ab, with the mPEG molecules of an adjacent conjugate anchored on another IgE Ab on the same mast cell; the intertwining of mPEG molecules fixed to two IgE molecules would lead essentially to the cross-linking of the Fcε receptors and to subsequent degranulation. Clearly both effects would occur more readily at higher doses of the conjugate.

We believe that the following mechanism may plausibly explain the observed inactivation of IgE Ab-carrying mast cells by allergen-mPEG conjugates. As generally accepted, following cellular stimulation by receptor-mediator signalling, the receptor and its ligand are endocytosed. However, in this particular case, the mPEG component of the conjugates is resistant to breakdown by intracellular enzymes and would, therefore, remain internalized in the cell for an extended period of time. It may, therefore, be expected that these molecules could have an inhibitory effect on the metabolism of the cell and lead to its "paralysis" and to the consequent inhibition of the release of inflammatory mediators and cytokines. This as yet hypothetical mechanism is supported by the above demonstration that mast cells sensitized with IgE Abs to two distinct specificities can be inactivated with respect to their responsiveness to both Ags by treatment with mPEG conjugates of a single allergen. Experiments are planned to establish if this phenomenon applies also to mast cells sensitized with IgE Abs specific to three or more epitopes of different allergens. In principle, this hypothesis may be extended to include even a chemically precisely defined conjugate consisting of a single Bε epitope of a given allergen and a linear or a branched mPEG molecule; this possibility is in the process of being tested.

ACKNOWLEDGMENTS

These studies were supported by grants from the Thorlakson Foundation of Winnipeg and the Medical Research Council of Canada.

REFERENCES

1. Lee, W.Y. and Sehon, A.H. 1978. Suppression of reaginic antibodies. Immunol. Reviews, *41*:200–247.
2. Filion, L.G., Lee. W.Y. and Sehon, A.H. 1980. Suppression of the IgE antibody response to ovalbumin in mice with a conjugate of ovalbumin and isologous gamma-globulins. Cell. Immunol. *54*:115–128.
3. Wilkinson, I., Jackson, C-J.C., Lang, G.M., Holford-Strevens, V. and Sehon, A.H. 1987. Tolerance induction in mice by conjugates of monoclonal immunoglobulins and monomethoxypolyethylene glycol. Transfer of tolerance by T cells and T cell extracts. J. Immunol. *139*:326–331.
4. Sehon, A.H. 1991. Suppression of antibody responses by chemically modified antigens, Carl Prausnitz Memorial Lecture, XVIII Symposium Collegium Internationale Allergologicum, Int. Arch. Allergy appl. Immunol. 94:11–20.
5. Takata, M., Maiti, P.K., Kubo, R.T., Chen, Y-H. Holford-Strevens, V., Rector, E.S. and Sehon, A.H. 1990. Cloned suppressor T cells derived from mice tolerized with conjugates of antigen and monomethoxypolyethylene glycol. J. Immunol. *145*:2846–2853.
6. Takata, M., Maiti, P.K., Bitoh, S., Holford-Strevens, V., Kierek-Jaszczuk, D., Chen, Y., Lang, G.M. and Sehon, A.H. 1991. Downregulation of helper T cells by an antigen-specific monoclonal Ts factor. Cell. Immunol. *137*:139–149.

7. Chen, Y., Takata, M., Maiti, P.K., Mohapatra, S., Mohapatra, S.S. and Sehon, A.H. 1994. The suppressor factor of Ts cells induced by tolerogenic conjugates of OVA and mPEG is serologically and physicochemically related to the $\alpha\beta$ heterodimer of the TCR. J. Immunol. *152*:3–11.
8. Bitoh, S., Takata, M., Maiti, P.K., Holford-Strevens, V., Kierek-Jaszczuk, D. and Sehon, A.H. 1993. Antigen-specific suppressor factors of noncytotoxic $CD8^+$ suppressor T cells downregulate antibody responses also to unrelated antigens when the latter are presented as covalently linked adducts with the specific antigen. Cell. Immunol. *150*:168–193.
9. Dreborg, S. and Åkerblom, E. 1990. Immunotherapy with monomethoxypolyethylene glycol modified allergens. In: S.D. Bruck (Ed.), CRC Crit. Rev. Therap. Drug Carrier Syst. *6*:315–365.
10. Bousquet, J., Breitenbach, M., Dreborg, S., Kenimer, J., Løwenstein, H. and Norman, P.S. 1993. "Round Table Discussion on Diagnosis of allergy and specific immunotherapy using recombinant allergens and epitopes." In: Molecular Biology and Immunology of Allergens (Eds. Kraft, D. and Sehon, A.), CRC Press, Inc., pp 311–320.
11. Sehon, A.H. and Gyenes, L. 1964. Physiochemical and immunochemical principles applied to the common forms of allergy. In: Sensitivity Chest Diseases (Eds. Harris, M.C. and Shure, N.) Philadelphia, Davis, pp 1–35.
12. Sehon, A.H. 1983. Downregulation of IgE antibodies by suppressogenic conjugates. In: Progress In Immunology V (Eds. T. Tada and Y Yamamura), New York, Academic Press, pp 483–491.
13. Sehon, A.H. and Lang, G.M. 1986. The use of nonionic, water soluble polymers for the synthesis of tolerogenic conjugates of antigens. In: Mediators of Immune Regulation and Immunotherapy (Eds. Singhal, S.K. and Delovitch, T.L.) New York, Elsevier, pp 190–203.
14. Molecular Biology and Immunology of Allergens. 1993. (Eds. Kraft, D. and Sehon, A.H.) Boca Raton, CRC Press.
15. Molecular Biology of Allergens and the Atopic Immune Response (Eds. Sehon, A.H., Kraft, D. and Hay-Glass, K.); this volume.
16. Bitoh, S., Wakefield, R., Lang, G. and Sehon, A.H. 1995. Inhibition of the effector phase of IgE-mediated allergies by tolerogenic conjugates of allergens and monomethoxypolyethylene glycol. Int. Arch. Allergy Immunol. *107*:316–318.
17. Becker, A.B., Hershkovich, J., Simons, F.E.R., Simons, K.J., Lilley, M.K. and Kepron, M.W. 1989. Development of chronic airway hyperresponsiveness in ragweed-sensitized dogs. J. Appl. Physiol. *66*:2691–2697.

25

RECOMBINANT ALLERGENS

Steps on the Way to Diagnosis and Therapy of Type I Allergy

Rudolf Valenta,[1*] Sylvia Laffer,[1] Susanne Vrtala,[1] Hans Grönlund,[2]
Lena Elfman,[2] Wolfgang R. Sperr,[3] Peter Valent,[3] Fatima Ferreira,[4]
Peter Mayer,[5] Ekke Liehl,[5] Susanne Heiss,[1] Renate Steiner,[1]
Hans Georg Eichler,[6] Markus Susani,[7] and Dietrich Kraft[1]

[1]Institute of General and Experimental Pathology
 AKH, University of Vienna, Austria
[2]Pharmacia Diagnostics
 Uppsala, Sweden
[3]Department of Internal Medicine I, Division of Hematology
 AKH, University of Vienna, Austria
[4]Institute of Genetics and Developmental Biology
 University of Salzburg, Austria
[5]Sandoz Research Center
 Vienna, Austria
[6]Department of Clinical Pharmacology
 AKH, University of Vienna, Austria
[7]Advanced Biological Systems
 Academy of Sciences, Salzburg, Austria

1. INTRODUCTION

Several groups have started to characterize cDNAs coding for allergens to obtain information regarding the nature of allergenic proteins as well as to use recombinant allergens as tools to study their interaction with the immune system (1). It is now that an increasing number of recombinant allergens has become available and unexpectedly it has turned out, that due to structural and immunological similarities among them, it may be possible to define a limited number of model allergens (epitopes) for diagnosis and perhaps specific therapy of Type I allergic diseases (1–3). Before certain recombinant allergens can be used for diagnosis and therapy they need to be extensively characterized *in vitro* and *in vivo*. In the present chapter the development of recombinant tree (4) and grass pollen allergens (5) and their way to diagnosis and therapy of Type I allergy is summarized.

* Correspondence: Rudolf Valenta, MD., Inst. of General and Experimental Pathology, AKH, University of Vienna, Währinger Gürtel 18–20, A-1090 Vienna, Austria. Tel: +43–1–40400–5108; Fax: +43–1–40400–5130.

New Horizons in Allergy Immunotherapy
edited by Sehon et al. Plenum Press, New York, 1996

185

2. *IN VITRO* CHARACTERIZATION OF RECOMBINANT ALLERGENS

2.1. Qualitative and Quantitative Measurement of Specific IgE Using Recombinant Allergens

So far specific IgE responses were measured by using allergen extracts prepared from natural sources. Depending on the allergen source, the method of extraction and the storage, such extracts consisted of a difficult to standardize mixture of allergenic and non-allergenic components. Positive serum IgE reactivity or a positive skin prick test with a traditional extract indicated at best that patients were sensitized against one of the components (allergens) present in the extract. Allergen extracts should therefore be refered to as extracts but not as "allergens" because they consist of a mixture of many different components. In contrast to natural allergen extracts, recombinant allergens represent defined components which for the first time allowed to determine the patients reactivity profile (allergogram) (6). One of the unexpected findings was that panels of only a few recombinant tree and grass pollen allergens could almost substitute natural allergen extracts regarding *in vitro* diagnostic sensitivity (4, 5). It needs however to be emphasized that the major advantage of recombinant allergens lies in the possbility of measuring specific IgE directed against defined components (7). While the first IgE binding tests with recombinant allergens were done only on a qualitative basis, the availability of purified recombinant allergens also allowed to quantitate specific IgE levels (8, 9). As an example Figure 1 and Table 1 show that recombinant timothy grass pollen allergens can be used for diagnosis of grass pollen allergy in different populations. It is hence expected that qualitative and quantitative *in vitro* IgE measurements can be performed with recombinant allergens regardless what population is tested (9).

2.2. Cross-Reactivity Among Allergens to Reduce the Number of Epitopes Needed for Diagnosis and Therapy

Concerns have been raised whether certain recombinant allergens share IgE-epitopes with isoallergenic variants or homologous allergens present in other species. Isoallergenic variants have been described for many relevant allergens as derivatives, which differ in their amino acid composition (10). On a clonal level (monoclonal antibodies, T-cell clones) it could be demonstrated that the immune system may be able to discriminate such isoallergens (11, 12). For diagnosis and therapeutical purposes it is therefore desirable to select isoallergens which harbour the majority of the IgE-epitopes and T-cell determinants. One way of selecting the relevant isoforms is shown in Figure 2. A single recombinant Phl p 1 isoallergen could be used to inhibit IgE binding to the natural occuring Phl p 1 isovariants as demonstrated by a two-D-IgE-inhibition experiment. IgE binding to group 2/3 timothy grass pollen allergens which contain different IgE epitopes was not affected.

This experiment clearly indicates that recombinant allergens can be defined which share IgE epitopes with most isoallergenic variants. Moreover recombinant Phl p 1 was shown to share IgE epitopes with group 1 isoallergens from other grass species and it was demonstrated that certain recombinant timothy grass pollen allergens are able to bind a high percentage of IgE-antibodies directed against natural grass pollen extracts (13, 14, 15). The selection of recombinant allergens should therefore be based on evaluating their IgE-binding capacity using as many sera as possible. This concept may be also relevant to determine whether recombinant allergens comprise the relevant T-cell epitopes. While certain T-cell clones may be able to discriminate among isoallergens or homologous allergens, more relevant clinical information might be expected from experiments looking on the induction of T-cell proliferations using T-cell lines or even primary cultures.

Based on extensive *in vitro* investigations, recombinant model allergens which share most of the relevant antigenic determinants with natural molecules can be identified.

2.3. The Basophil Histamine Release to Evaluate the Biological Activity of Recombinant Allergens

To term a recombinant IgE-binding protein, allergen, its potential to elicit effector cell activation has to be demonstrated. This can be done by skin testing, by sensitizing animals and subsequent challenge or by using basophil release assays (16). The capacity of recombinant tree and grass pollen allergens to induce specific *in vitro* histamine release

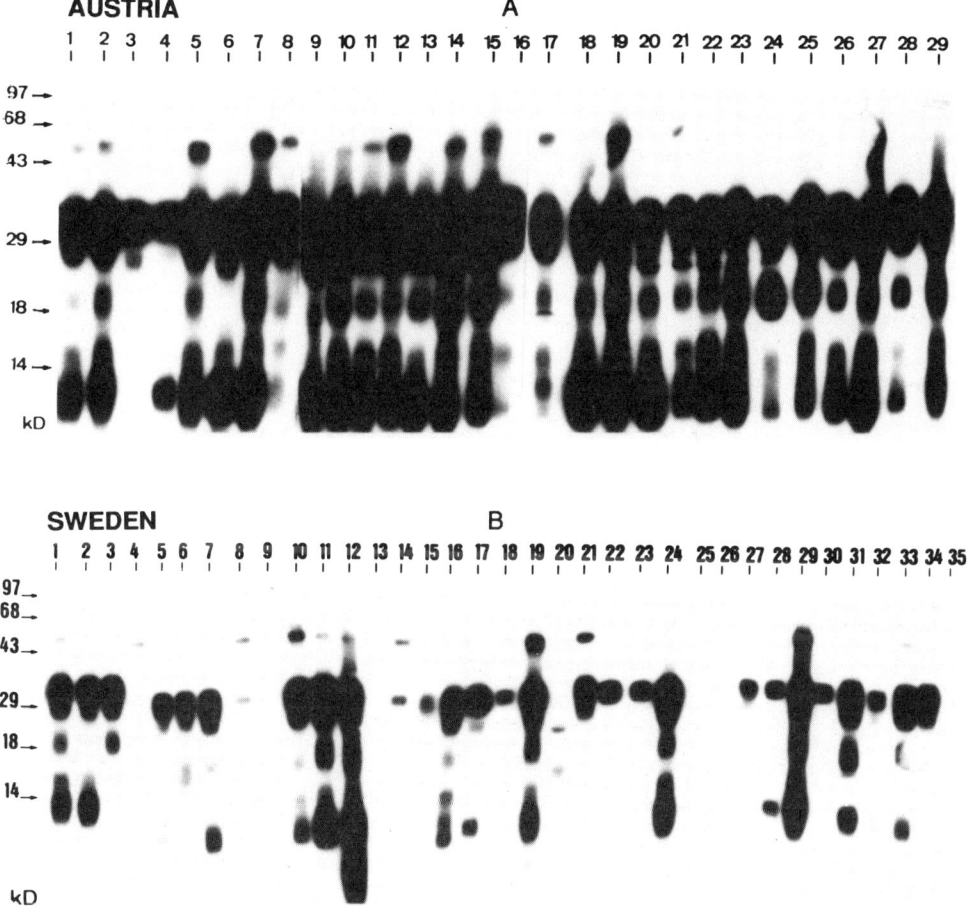

Figure 1. Sera from Austria (Fig. 1A) (n=29) and Sweden (Fig. 1B) (n=35) were tested for IgE-reactivity to nitrocellulose blotted natural timothy grass pollen allergens. Bound IgE was detected with [125] I labelled anti-human IgE antibodies (RAST, Pharmacia, Uppsala, Sweden).

from patients basophils has been well documented (17–19). No toxic release of mediators was observed up to concentrations of 100µg/ml. Recombinant tree pollen allergens (Bet v 1 (20), Bet v 2 (21)) and recombinant timothy grass pollen allergens (Phl p 1 (14), Phl p 2 (22), Phl p 5 (23)) elicited specific histamine release depending on the presence of specific serum IgE. The basophil release assay is hence considered as suitable method to evaluate recombinant allergen preparations for biological activity before *in vivo* experiments are started.

Table 1A. Austrian sera shown in Figure 1 were probed for IgE reactivity to ELISA plate coated purified recombinant timothy grass pollen allergens (rPhl p 1, rPhl p 2 and rPhl p 5) and recombinant birch profilin (rBet v 2). Bound IgE is displayed as optical density (OD) subtracted by background levels obtained with sera from non-allergic individuals. Total serum IgE levels and timothy grass pollen specific IgE as measured by CAP are displayed in kU/l

patient	total IgE (kU/l)	RAST timothy (kU/l)	ELISA rPhl p 1 OD	ELISA rPhl p 2 OD	ELISA rPhl p 5 OD	ELISA rBet v 2 OD
Austria						
1	180	50.2	0.71	0.37	0.28	0.02
2	510	>100	>2.00	0.50	1.39	1.07
3	181	26.6	1.45	0.02	0.01	0.05
4	205	74.7	1.32	0.30	0.00	0.06
5	568	>100	>2.00	0.63	1.50	0.00
6	1018	>100	>2.00	>2.00	0.08	0.01
7	>2000	>100	>2.00	>2.00	>2.00	0.02
8	413	53.1	1.17	0.02	0.24	0.01
9	508	98.5	0.67	0.37	0.33	0.28
10	1963	>100	1.94	1.06	>2.00	0.01
11	525	>100	1.21	0.50	1.71	0.01
12	611	>100	1.57	0.58	>2.00	0.00
13	370	72.1	0.96	0.25	1.16	0.01
14	1275	>100	>2.00	0.30	>2.00	0.00
15	928	>100	>2.00	0.17	>2.00	0.01
16	1380	28.5	0.34	0.01	0.10	0.00
17	238	25.1	0.26	0.12	0.25	0.02
18	>2000	>100	>2.00	>2.00	>2.00	0.01
19	1174	>100	>2.00	1.31	1.74	0.00
20	768	92.8	0.84	0.63	0.23	0.00
21	518	36.2	0.66	0.05	0.09	0.00
22	175	49.4	0.34	0.06	0.40	0.00
23	406	>100	>2.00	0.01	0.51	0.03
24	445	52.1	0.71	0.01	0.76	0.00
25	271	82.5	0.72	0.03	0.74	0.00
26	402	99.0	1.25	0.01	0.42	0.00
27	969	>100	>2.00	0.01	1.32	0.02
28	205	51.1	0.81	0.01	0.17	0.00
29	1217	>100	>2.00	0.49	1.93	0.01

Table 1B. Swedish sera shown in figure 1

patient	total IgE (kU/l)	RAST timothy (kU/l)	ELISA rPhl p 1 OD	ELISA rPhl p 2 OD	ELISA rPhl p 5 OD	ELISA rBet v 2 OD
Sweden						
1	>2000	66.6	0.69	0.22	1.39	0.00
2	88.2	12.0	0.28	0.07	0.22	0.00
3	382	12.1	0.10	0.00	0.33	0.02
4	255	1.32	0.04	0.01	0.00	0.00
5	178	16.2	0.84	0.07	0.56	0.01
6	383	4.43	0.05	0.02	0.23	0.01
7	174	11.8	0.03	0.05	0.40	0.00
8	51.3	2.94	0.08	0.02	0.02	0.00
9	1793	0.63	0.06	0.05	0.06	0.06
10	610	37.8	0.24	0.01	0.49	0.02
11	1522	95.2	1.64	0.99	1.75	0.01
12	>2000	>100	>2.00	>2.00	>2.00	>2.00
13	746	1.82	0.08	0.03	0.03	0.00
14	1163	2.78	0.03	0.02	0.06	0.00
15	1668	2.97	0.03	0.00	0.10	0.01
16	1013	20.9	0.25	0.00	0.34	0.01
17	>2000	32.7	1.13	0.08	0.00	0.01
18	301	2.40	0.12	0.00	0.01	0.00
19	393	58.9	1.01	0.30	0.48	0.13
20	315	2.23	0.03	0.00	0.11	0.01
21	239	5.97	0.23	0.02	0.04	0.01
22	1326	7.42	0.25	0.01	0.00	0.01
23	84.5	7.58	0.21	0.01	0.02	0.01
24	333	>100	>2.00	0.43	0.98	0.00
25	157	2.78	0.07	0.04	0.03	0.00
26	367	1.31	0.13	0.02	0.03	0.02
27	164	3.43	0.17	0.02	0.05	0.01
28	103	6.83	0.27	0.04	0.00	0.01
29	786	>100	1.18	0.51	0.69	0.65
30	1007	8.23	0.22	0.00	0.01	0.01
31	511	48.3	0.26	0.12	0.66	0.02
32	29.9	7.78	0.10	0.03	0.06	0.02
33	227	15.1	0.39	0.00	0.16	0.00
34	138	28.6	0.84	0.00	0.10	0.00
35	181	0.82	0.06	0.01	0.02	0.00

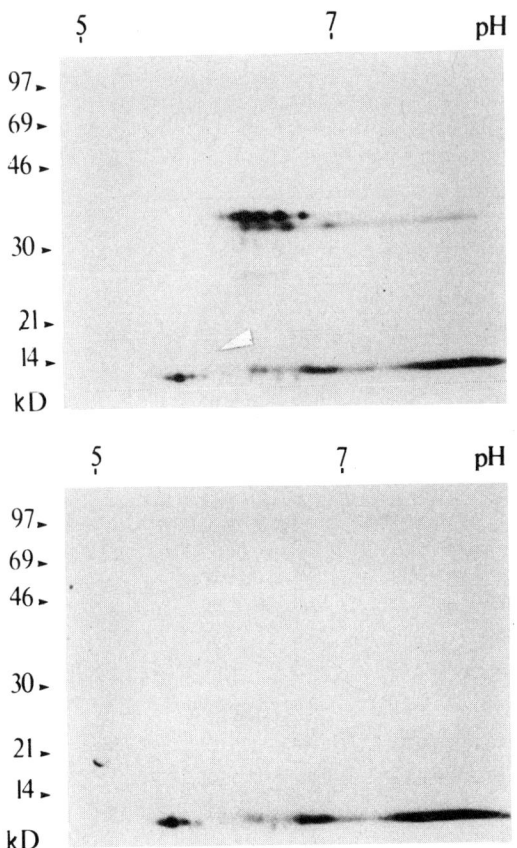

Figure 2. Serum IgE-reactivity of a grass pollen allergic individual with IgE specific for group 1 and group 2/3 allergens with two-D-separated timothy grass pollen extract. The upper blot was probed with the serum after preincubation with *Escherichia coli* proteins (negative control) while the serum used for the lower blot was preincubated with purified recombinant Phl p 1. Molecular weights are displayed on the left side of the blots and pH values are shown on top of each blot.

3. *IN VIVO* EVALUATION OF RECOMBINANT ALLERGENS

3.1. Experimental Animal Models for Type I Allergy Based on Recombinant Allergens

The induction of IgE-antibodies in animals by using adjuvants (24, 25) or by inhalation (26) represents a well established system to investigate the mechanisms underlying allergic diseases. While experimental animal models have been set up with a number of different protein antigens (e.g. ovalbumin), only a few allergens which are relevant for human allergy have been tested. Using animal models two questions have been addressed.

3. 1. 1. Does Sensitization Against a Few Recombinant Allergens Lead to the Induction of cross-Reactive IgE Antibodies and Allergic Responses to Different Allergen Sources? To establish a close to man model of Type I allergy, rhesus monkeys were injected with recombinant birch pollen allergens Bet v 1 and Bet v 2 using Al(OH)$_3$ as adjuvant (27). The skin testing in Figure 3 shows that rBet v 1 and rBet v 2 induced a battery of IgE-antibodies which crossreacted with homologous allergens present in pollen and plant derived food. Bet v 1 injected monkeys showed skin reactions with birch and hazel pollen and Bet v 2 injected monkeys reacted with birch pollen, hazel pollen, timothy grass pollen and celery.

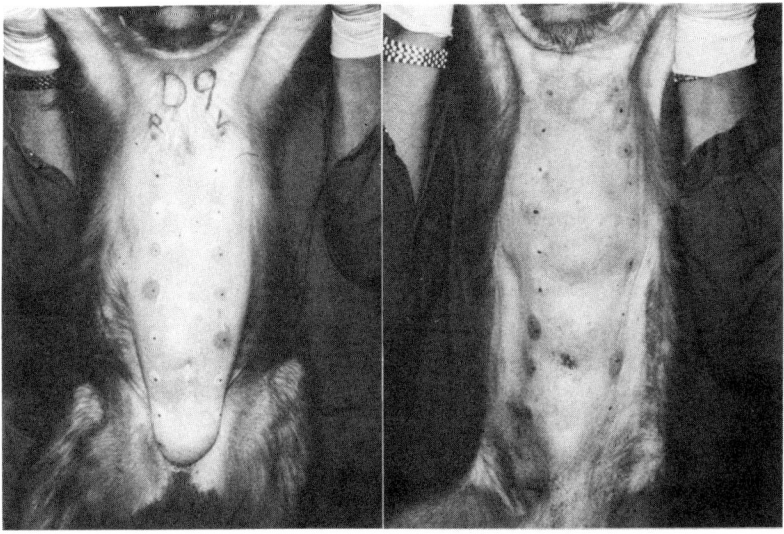

Bet v 1 monkey		Bet v 2 monkey	
hazel pollen	celery	hazel pollen	timothy pollen
celery	timothy pollen	rBet v 1	hazel pollen
birch pollen	rBet v 1	timothy pollen	celery
histamine	hazel pollen	NaCl	birch pollen
NaCl	histamine	birch pollen	rBet v 2
rBet v 2	rBet v 2	histamine	rBet v 1
timothy pollen	NaCl	celery	histamine
rBet v 1	birch pollen	rBet v 2	NaCl

Figure 3. Two rhesus monkeys which were sensitized with recombinant Bet v 1 (left monkey) or with recombinant Bet v 2 (right monkey) were tested for skin reactivity with natural allergen preparations, recombinant allergens and controls as indicated below. The extravasation of Evans Blue corresponds to the skin reactivity.

These data emphasize that due to structural similarity, sensitization against single allergens can trigger allergic crossreactivity with different allergen sources. Sensitized rhesus monkeys produced specific IgE antibodies, showed specific T-cell proliferation and basophil histamine release as well as positive bronchial reactions. IgE responses could be induced in adult male and female rhesus monkeys of different genetic background (27).

3. 1. 2. Can We Study the Immunogenicity and/or Allergenicity of Certain Recombinant Allergens in Experimental Animal Models? Quantitative determinations of specific human IgE using recombinant allergens had indicated that certain allergens (major, intermediate allergens) are not only recognized by a majority of patients but also bind a high percentage of specific IgE antibodies (28, 23, 29). Bet v 1, the major birch pollen allergen, two major timothy grass pollen allergens, Phl p 5 and Phl p 1 and dog albumin were found to induce high levels of specific IgE in patients. In contrast, rather low levels of specific IgE were directed to birch profilin, Bet v 2 and Phl p 2, a major timothy grass pollen allergen (9). Using two different animal models (mice and rhesus monkeys) we have compared the potency of Bet v 1 and Bet v 2 to induce specific IgE responses when injected with Al(OH)$_3$

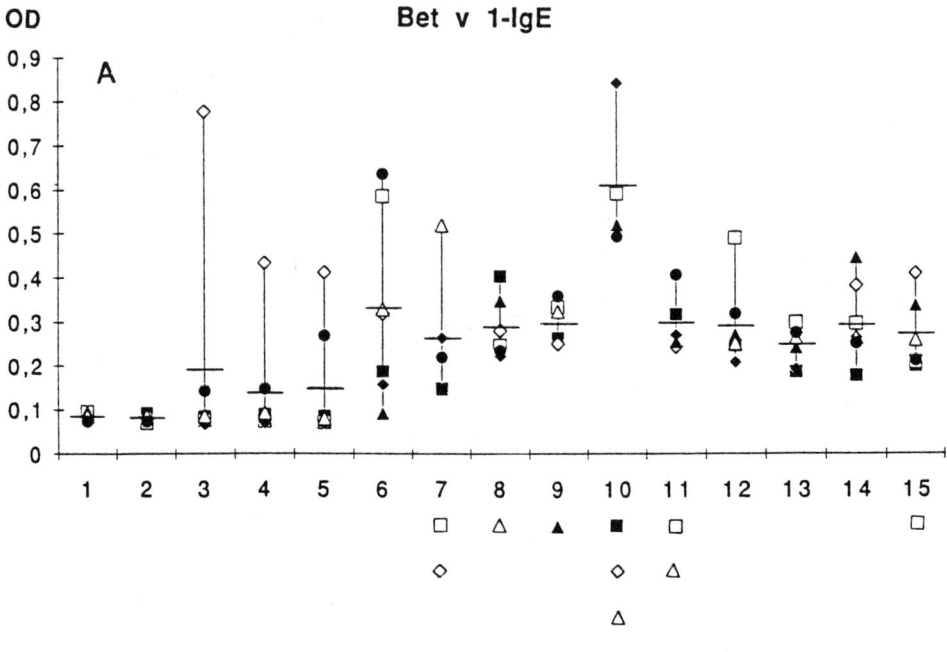

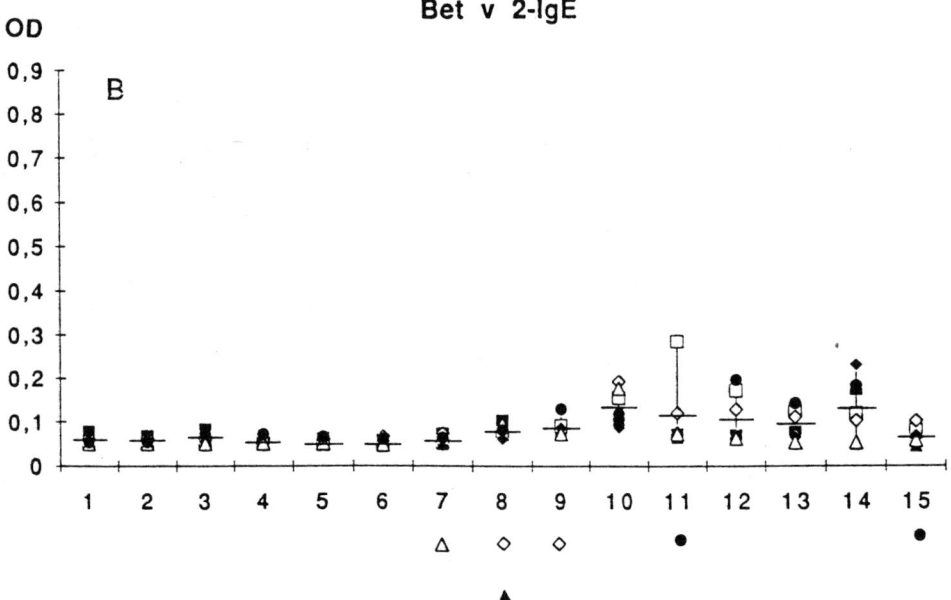

Figure 4. Development of IgE responses in mice sensitized with recombinant Bet v 1 (**A**) (1μg/injection) and Bet v 2 (**B**) (20μg/injection). Mice were immunized and bled at different time points (1: preimmune serum; 2: week 3; 3: week 5; 4: week 8; 5: week 10; 6: week 12; 7: week 16; 8: wcck 18; 9: week 25; 10: week 26; 11: week 28; 12: week 30; 13: week 35; 14: week 38; 15: week 57). 1:20 diluted sera were used to measure IgE specific for rBet v 1 and rBet v 2 by ELISA. The optical densities (OD) corresponding to the specific IgE levels are displayed for each mouse (indicated by a symbol) on the y-axis and and represent means of duplicate determinations. Mean IgE levels for the Bet v 1 and Bet v 2 groups are indicated for each time point. The symbols of those mice where specific IgE was not measured are displayed beyond the x-axis.

as adjuvant. We found that in both animal models, Bet v 1 induced at lower doses ($1\mu g$/injection) than Bet v 2 ($20\mu g$/injection) specific IgE responses and that the levels of Bet v 1 specific IgE were substantially higher than the Bet v 2 specific IgE levels (30). Figure 4 illustrates the differences of IgE responses in Bet v 1 and Bet v 2 immunized mice.

Although the use of experimental animal models for the estimation of the allergenicity of antigens is not generally accepted, particularly when adjuvants were used for induction of IgE antibodies, it was interesting to note that a major allergen, which induces high levels of specific IgE in man (Bet v 1), also induced significantly higher levels of IgE in the mouse and primate model. The lower allergenicity observed for Bet v 2 in man was observed in mice and rhesus monkeys as well. It is hence likely that experimental animal models may be useful systems to evaluate the allergenicity of allergens and perhaps to obtain informations why certain proteins are more immunogenic than others.

4. USE OF RECOMBINANT ALLERGENS FOR *IN VITRO* AND *IN VIVO* ALLERGY DIAGNOSIS

4.1. Serological Measurement of Antibody Reactivities Using Recombinant Allergens to Establish the Patients Reactivity Profile (Allergogram)-Basis for Specific Immunotherapy

Recombinant birch pollen and timothy grass pollen allergens have been made available recently in the ImmunoCAP system to allow the measurement of specific IgE at the component level. Table 2 compares traditional serological IgE measurement based on allergen extracts with the recombinant ImmunoCAP using sera from two representative patients and a non-allergic control individual.

According to traditional measurements patient #1 and #2 are positive with timothy grass pollen extract. Using recombinant timothy grass pollen allergens it is possible to dissect the IgE-reactivity profile of the patients in more detail. While patient #1 reacted exclusively with rPhl p 1, patient #2 displayed IgE reactivity against rPhl p 1 and rPhl p 5 and birch profilin, Bet v 2, which shares IgE epitopes with timothy grass profilin. According to traditional extract based measurements patient #1 would be classified as timothy grass pollen allergic and patient #2 as birch pollen and timothy grass pollen allergic. If these patients were treated by immunotherapy, patient #1 would receive timothy grass pollen extract including Phl p 2 and Phl p 5 and patient #2 birch pollen and timothy grass pollen extract containing Bet v 1 and Phl p 2 although they are not sensitized against these components. Since it cannot be excluded that patients become sensitized against such components, we believe that a component based diagnosis allowing the determination of the patients IgE-reactivity profile (allergogram) will represent a first important step towards improved specific immunotherapy. Regardless whether future forms of specific im-

Table 2. Levels of specific IgE (kU/l) directed against natural birch pollen and timothy grass pollen extract and recombinant allergens as determined by ImmunoCAP

Individual	Birch	rBet v 1	rBet v 2	Timothy	rPhl p 1	rPhl p 2	rPhl p 5
#1	<0.35	<0.35	<0.35	9.98	11.45	<0.35	<0.35
#2	3.02	<0.35	1.85	29.30	8.09	<0.35	17.76
#3	<0.35	<0.35	<0.35	<0.35	<0.35	<0.35	<0.35

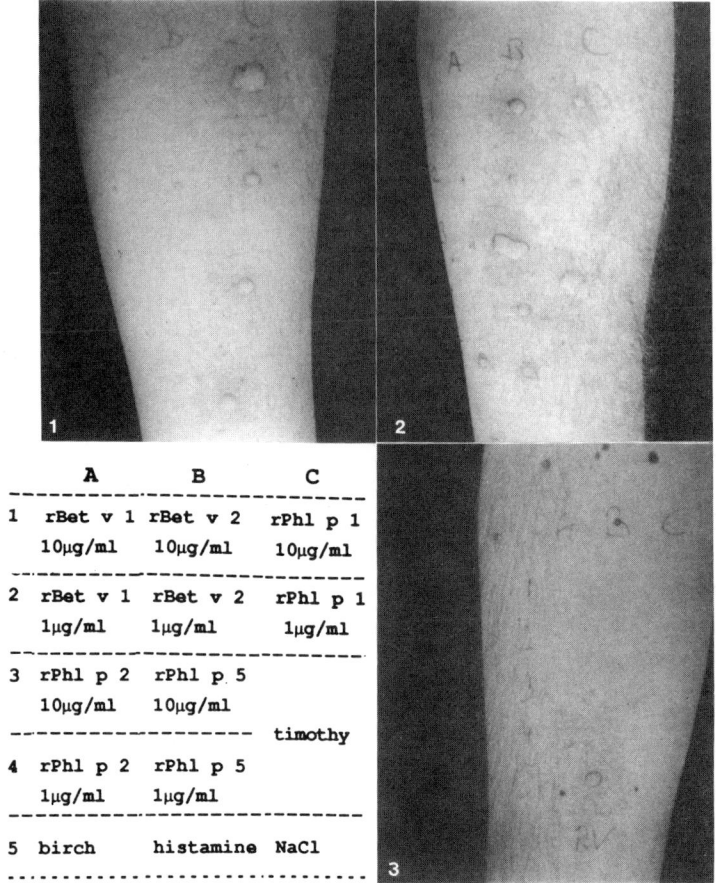

	A	B	C
1	rBet v 1 10µg/ml	rBet v 2 10µg/ml	rPhl p 1 10µg/ml
2	rBet v 1 1µg/ml	rBet v 2 1µg/ml	rPhl p 1 1µg/ml
3	rPhl p 2 10µg/ml	rPhl p 5 10µg/ml	timothy
4	rPhl p 2 1µg/ml	rPhl p 5 1µg/ml	
5	birch	histamine	NaCl

Figure 5. Biological activity of recombinant birch and timothy grass pollen allergens evaluated by skin prick testing in two allergic patients and one non-allergic individual.

munotherapy will target T-cells or comprise B-cell epitopes or make use of other allergen modifications, we believe that only those components should be selected for treatment against which the patient is sensitized.

4.2. Biological Activity of Recombinant Allergens in Man-Skin Test Diagnosis of Type I Allergy with Recombinant Allergens

After extensive *in vitro* evaluation and testing in experimental animal models, recombinant allergens may be further tested in patients. The biological activity of several recombinant allergens has been evaluated by skin testing. Recent studies with recombinant birch pollen allergens performed in 100 patients indicated that only a few recombinant allergens (Bet v 1, Bet v 2) permitted skin test diagnosis of birch pollen allergy (28, 31). As an example, Figure 5 shows the skin test results obtained in the individuals tested by serology as shown in Table 2.

The skin test results were in accordance with the serological measurements. The recombinant allergen preparations did not cause toxic effects in the non-allergic individual. It is concluded that recombinant allergens possess similar biological activity as natural extracts when used for *in vivo* testing and hence may be considered as candidates for a component based skin test diagnosis of Type I allergy.

5. ACKNOWLEDGMENTS

This study was supported in part by grant S06703 of the Austrian Science Foundation and by a grant from the "Hochschuljubiläums-stiftung" Vienna, Austria. Animal experiments shown were done with permission of the local ethics committee according to the guidelines for animal welfare. Skin testing of allergic patients with recombinant allergens was approved by the Austrian Ministry of Health and the local ethics committee.

6. REFERENCES

1. Valenta R, Kraft D. Recombinant allergens for diagnosis and therapy of allergic diseases. Curr Opin Immunol 1995;7:751–756.
2. Scheiner O, Kraft D. Basic and practical aspects of recombinant allergens. Allergy 1995;50:384–91.
3. Valenta R, Steinberger P, Duchêne M, Kraft D. Immunological and structural similarities among allergens: Prerequisite for a specific and component-based therapy of allergy. Immunol and Cell Biol 1996; in press.
4. Valenta R, Duchêne M, Vrtala S, Birkner T, Ebner C, Hirschwehr R, Breitenbach M, Rumpold H, Scheiner O, Kraft D. Recombinant allergens for immunoblot diagnosis of tree-pollen allergy. J Allergy Clin Immunol 1991;88:889–894.
5. Valenta R, Vrtala S, Ebner C, Kraft D, Scheiner O. Diagnosis of grass pollen allergy with recombinant timothy grass (*Phleum pratense*) pollen allergens. Int Arch Allergy Immunol 1992;97:287–294.
6. Bousquet J, Valenta R. *In vivo* and *in vitro* use of recombinant allergens. In: deWeck AL, (Ed.) Special report from the IUIS/WHO allergen standardization committee. ACI News 1994; 6:54–59.
7. Valenta R, Dolecek C, Laffer S, Vrtala S, Susani M, Schönheit-Kenn U, Menz G, Grönlund H, Kraft D. Diagnostic and therapeutic concepts based on recombinant allergens. In: Johansson SGO eds. Progress in Allergy and Clinical Immunology, Hogrefe&Huber Publishers 1995;3:226–233.
8. Vrtala S, Susani M, Sperr WR, Valent P, Laffer S, Dolecek C, Kraft D, Valenta R. Immunologic characterization of purified recombinant timothy grass pollen (*Phleum pratense*) allergens (Phl p 1, Phl p 2, Phl p 5). J Allergy Clin Immunol 1996;97:781–7.
9. Laffer S, Spitzauer S, Susani M, Pairleitner H, Schweiger C, Grönlund H, Menz G, Pauli G, Ishii T, Nolte H, Ebner C, Sehon AH, Kraft D, Eichler HG, Valenta R. Comparison of recombinant timothy grass pollen allergens with natural extract for diagnosis of grass pollen allergy in different populations. J Allergy Clin Immunol 1996; in press.
10. Breiteneder H, Ferreira F, Hoffmann-Sommergruber K, Ebner C, Breitenbach M, Rumpold H, Kraft D, Scheiner O. Four recombinant isoforms of Cor a 1, the major allergen of hazel pollen, show different IgE-binding properties. Eur J Biochem 1993; 212:355–62.
11. Schenk S, Hoffmann-Sommergruber K, Breiteneder H, Ferreira F, Fischer G, Scheiner O, Kraft D, Ebner C. Four recombinant isoforms of Cor a 1, the major allergen of hazel pollen pollen, show different reactivities with allergen-specific T-lymphocyte clones. Eur J Biochem 1994; 224:717–22.
12. Schenk S, Breiteneder H, Susani M, Najafian N, Laffer S, Duchêne M, Valenta R, Fischer G, Scheiner O, Ebner C. T-cell epitopes of Phl p 1, major allergen of timothy grass (Phleum pratense): Evidence for crossreacting and non-crossreacting T-cell epitopes within grass group 1 allergen. J Allergy Clin Immunol 1995;96:986–96.
13. Laffer S, Vrtala S, Duchêne M, van Ree R, Kraft D, Scheiner O, Valenta R. IgE-binding capacity of recombinant timothy grass (*Phleum pratense*) pollen allergens. J Allergy Clin Immunol 1994; 94: 88–94.
14. Laffer S, Valenta R, Vrtala S, Susani M, vanRee R, Kraft D, Scheiner O, Duchêne M. cDNA cloning of the major allergen Phl p 1 from timothy grass (*Phleum pratense*); recombinant Phl p 1 inhibits IgE binding to group I allergens from eight different grass species. J Allergy Clin Immunol 1994;94:689–698.
15. Laffer S, Duchêne M, Reimitzer I, Susani M, Mannhalter C, Kraft D, Valenta R. Common IgE-epitopes of recombinant Phl p 1, the major timothy grass pollen allergen and natural group 1 grass pollen isoallergens. Mol Immunol 1996; in press.
16. Lichtenstein LM. The mechanism of basophil histamine release induced by antigen and by the calcium ionophore A23187. J Immunol 1975; 114:1692–9.

17. Valenta R, Duchêne M, Ebner C, Valent P, Sillaber C, Deviller P, Ferreira F, Tejkl M, Edelmann H, Kraft D, Scheiner O. Profilins constitute a novel family of functional plant pan-allergens. J Exp Med 1992;175:377–385.

18. Valenta R, Sperr WR, Ferreira F, Valent P, Sillaber C, Tejkl M, Duchêne M, Ebner C, Lechner K, Kraft D, Scheiner O. Induction of specific histamine release from basophils with purified natural and recombinant birch pollen allergens. J Allergy Clin Immunol 1993; 91:88–97.

19. Ferreira F, Hoffmann-Sommergruber K, Breiteneder H, Pettenburger K, Ebner C, Sommergruber W, Steiner R, Bohle B, Sperr WR, Valent P, Kungl AJ, Breitenbach M, Kraft D, Scheiner. Purification and characterization of recombinant Bet v 1, the major birch pollen allergen. J Biol Chem 1993; 268:19574–80.

20. Breiteneder H, Pettenburger K, Bito A, Valenta R, Kraft D, Rumpold H, Scheiner O, Breitenbach M. The gene coding for the major birch pollen allergen, Bet v 1, is highly homologous to a pea diseases resistance response gene. EMBO J 1989; 8:1935–1938.

21. Valenta R, Duchêne M, Pettenburger K, Sillaber C, Valent P, Bettelheim P, Breitenbach M, Rumpold H, Kraft D, Scheiner O. Identification of profilin as a novel pollen allergen; IgE autoreactivity in sensitized individuals. Science 1991; 253:557- 560.

22. Dolecek C, Vrtala S, Laffer S, Steinberger P, Kraft D, Scheiner O, Valenta R. Molecular characterization of Phl p 2, a major timothy grass (*Phleum pratense*) pollen allergen. FEBS Lett 1993; 335:299- 304.

23. Vrtala S, Sperr WR, Reimitzer I, vanRee R, Laffer S, Müller WD, Valent P, Lechner K, Rumpold H, Kraft D, Scheiner O, Valenta R. cDNA cloning of the major allergen from timothy grass (*Phleum pratense*) pollen: characterization of the recombinant Phl p 5 allergen. J Immunol 1993;151:4773–4781.

24. Levine BB, Vaz NM. Effect of combinations of inbred strain, antigen and reagin production in the mouse. Int Arch Allergy Immunol 1970; 39:156–62.

25. Lehrer SB, Vaughan JH, Tan EM. Adjuvant activity of the histamine-sensitizing factor of Bordetella pertussis in different strains of mice. Int Arch Allergy Immunol 1975; 49:796–803.

26. Renz H, Smith HR, Henson JE, Ray BS, Irvin CG, Gelfand EW. Aerosolized antigen exposure without adjuvant causes increased IgE production and increased airway responsiveness in the mouse. J Allergy Clin Immunol 1992; 89:1127–38.

27. Ferreira F, Mayer P, Sperr WR, Valent P, Seiberler S, Ebner C, Liehl E, Scheiner O, Kraft D, Valenta R. Induction of IgE antibodies with predefined specificity in rhesus monkeys with recombinant birch pollen allergens, Bet v 1 and Bet v 2. J Allergy Clin Immunol 1996;97:95–103.

28. Menz G, Dolecek C, Schönheit-Kenn U, Ferreira F, Moser M, Schneider T, Suter M, Boltz-Nitulescu G, Ebner C, Kraft D, Valenta R. Serological and skin-test diagnosis of birch pollen allergy wth recombinant Bet v 1, the major birch pollen allergen. Clin Exp Allergy 1995;26:50–60.

29. Spitzauer S, Schweiger C, Sperr WR, Pandjaitan B, Valent P, Mühl S, Ebner C, Scheiner O, Kraft D, Rumpold H, Valenta R. Molecular characterization of dog albumin as a cross-reactive allergen. J Allergy Clin Immunol 1994; 93:614–27.

30. Vrtala S, Mayer P, Ferreira F, Susani M, Sehon AH, Kraft D, Valenta R. Induction of IgE antibodies in mice and rhesus monkeys with recombinant birch pollen allergens; different allergenicity of Bet v 1 and Bet v 2. J Allergy Clin Immunol 1996; in press.

31. Pauli G, Oster P, Deviller P, Heiss S, Bessot J, Susani M, Ferreira F, Kraft D, Valenta R. Skin testing with recombinant allergens rBet v 1 and rBet v 2. Diagnostic value for birch pollen and associated allergies. J Allergy Clin Immunol 1996; in press.

26

PRODUCTION OF A RECOMBINANT PROTEIN FROM ALTERNARIA CONTAINING THE REPORTED N-TERMINAL OF THE ALT A1 ALLERGEN

C. S. Barnes, F. Pacheco, J. Landuyt, D. Rosenthal, F. Hu, and J. Portnoy

Section of Allergy/Immunology
The Children's Mercy Hospital
Kansas City, Missouri

ABSTRACT

Allergen content of extract derived from Alternaria is somewhat variable. Allergenic molecules from Alternaria that appear as differing molecular size bands on IgE probed immunoblots may have a great deal of sequence homology and differ only in the length of the amino acid chain. One method to study this problem is to produce recombinant proteins from Alternaria. To explore these possibilities, the following experiments were performed.

A strain of Alternaria was grown on minimum salts and glucose in a fermentation container with constant stirring and aeration. Rapidly expanding mycelia were removed from the culture and mRNA was extracted. Purified mRNA was reacted with reverse transcriptase and an aliquot of first copy single strand DNA was enriched for the presence of DNA coding for an Alternaria allergen by PCR amplification. Modified DNA was then spliced into lambda gt11 phage and yielded a recombinant library with 10^5 PFU. The library was screened for the presence of allergenic proteins using IgE containing human sera from Alternaria-sensitive patients. Positive plaques were cloned.

PCR analysis of positive clones using an oligonucleotide from the reported N-terminal sequence of Alt a1 indicated an insert of 295 base pairs. Sequence analysis yielded a reading frame containing 84 amino acids and confirmed that this segment contained the code for the reported N-terminal amino acid sequence of Alt a1. A computer search for this sequence found no homologous proteins in the Entrez® sequences. Northern blotting studies on RNA purified from nine strains of Alternaria with the radiolabeled 247 BP DNA fragment indicated that this sequence was present in all strains. The 247 BP nucleotide was spliced into the Pflag® vector and clones containing insert in the proper reading frame were identified. The presence of recombinant protein in the clones was verified by

New Horizons in Allergy Immunotherapy
edited by Sehon et al. Plenum Press, New York, 1996

SDSPAGE time studies. Protein produced in time studies was shown by immunoblotting and sandwich EIA to bind human IgE from Alternaria sensitive patients.

This recombinant protein, containing amino acid sequence for Alt a1, is bound by human IgE and therefore should be useful as a model for studying allergy to the native Alternaria glycoprotein. Further research should define where this sequence occurs in the Alternaria genome and should determine the sequence of the entire protein.

INTRODUCTION

Alternaria allergens identified by SDSPAGE immunoblotting are very complex (1–5).. They may be the remnants of digestive enzymes used by the fungus to turn the environment into metabolic intermediates. They may be cell wall constituents from either spores or mycelia partially destroyed in the extraction process. They may be intracellular components lost by the mycelia into the extraction media as old mycelia die and new growth occurs. Alternaria allergens isolated thusfar exist as heavily glycosylated proteins with acidic isoelectric points(3, 4). Both the abundance of the associated carbohydrate and its variable nature have complicated characterization of native allergens To allow detailed examination of the protein components of these allergens and to determine the relative contribution of both protein and carbohydrate derived epitopes to the overall allergenicity, it is necessary to produce these proteins in a recombinant form devoid of carbohydrate moieties.

We have identified a segment of cDNA screened from a Alternaria cDNA library by IgE binding which contains the nucleotide sequence reported for the Alt a1 allergen. This nucleotide segment has been inserted into the Pflag® vector. We have identified E.coli clones which contain the insert and have used them to produce recombinant protein. The recombinant protein has been identified by specific monoclonal antibodies directed to a synthetic portion of the fusion protein. The recombinant protein has been purified chromatographically and shown to bind to IgE from pooled sera drawn from humans known to be allergic to Alternaria.

METHODS

Mycelial Preparation and RNA Extraction

A strain of *Alternaria alternata* (here designated AL 005) was obtained as described previously (6)and grown in a defined medium (7)for one week prior to harvesting. Air was bubbled through the media with constant stirring as described by Paris, et al. (8) . We have found this set of growth conditions to enhance the production of Alt aI from this strain (6). The mycelia were then separated from the culture medium by filtration through a Whatman 4 filter and the resultant dark brown mats were frozen at -70° C in 2 gram aliquots. Mycelia were frozen in liquid nitrogen and ground to a fine powder in a large mortar and pestle. Fungal ccll walls were further disrupted in a denaturing solution consisting of guanidine thiocyanate and citrate sarcosine ß-mercaptoethanol. using a Virtis 23 homogenizer. This tissue disruption procedure was repeated until all of the ground mycelia were homogenized. RNA was extracted using a Total RNA Isolation Kit (Promega Corporation, Madison, WI) according to the instructions supplied by the manufacturer. The integrity of purified RNA was determined electrophoretically on a formaldehyde denaturing 1.2 % agarose gel (FMC BioProducts Corporation, Rockland, ME).

Synthesis of First Strand DNA

Synthesis of first strand cDNA from total RNA was performed using the Riboclone® cDNA Synthesis System according to the manufacturer's instructions (Promega Corporation) (9, 10). A defined orientation strategy was planned so that an EcoR I recognition site would be on one terminus of the cDNA while an oligo $(dT)_{15}$ tail followed by a Not I recognition site would appear at the other terminal end. To amplify a fragment of the 31kD allergenic protein previously determined to be an allergen (11, 12)PCR was performed using the same Not I Primer-Adaptor as in the first strand synthesis and another primer that was derived from an N-terminal sequence determined by H Vijay and H Lowenstein (11, 13) .The 36-mer primer was synthesized by the University of Missouri-Kansas City Core Facility with the following sequence: 3' CTA GAA CCT GTG CAT CAG CGG GAC CCA CCA GTG CCC 5'. Template DNA for the PCR reaction was first strand DNA. Amplification was carried out in a MiniCycler™ thermal cycler (MJ Research) . The cycler program was 94° C for one minute, 50° C for 1 minute and 72° C for 3 minutes. The above temperature cycle was repeated 36 times. PCR products were analyzed using a 4% agarose gel (FMC BioProducts) in TAE Buffer (40 mM Tris base, 20 mM Acetic acid, 2 mM EDTA).

Preparation of cDNA for Insertion into Lambda Phage

DNA derived from the PCR products was inserted into Lambda Phage using the Riboclone® EcoR I Adaptor Ligation System (Promega Corporation) (14). Ligation and packaging of cDNA *in vitro* into the vector employed a defined orientation strategy using Lambda gt11 Sfi-Not (Promega Corporation, Madison Wisconsin). Packaging was performed with the Packagene® extract (Promega Corporation). (15, 16) . The cDNA library thus produced was amplified in host bacterial strain Y1090 and amplified library was stored short term at 4°C in the presence of chloroform or long term at -70°C. Amplified libraries were screened for successful inclusion of insert using traditional blue/clear methods and subsequently for the production of allergenic proteins with IgE containing pooled human sera from Alternaria allergic patients. Bound human IgE was detected with goat Anti-Human IgE- Alkaline Phosphatase conjugate (ε-chain specific) (Sigma) and visualized using a nitroblue tetrazolium substrate.

PCR Confirmation of Allergenic Protein and Insert Size

For production of insert DNA, we took phage containing material from individual plaques and inoculated it into rapidly growing bacterial culture. The phage was allowed to infect the bacterial culture until complete bacterial lysis was evident. Polyethylene glycol was then added to the phage containing bacterial lysate and phage particles were removed by centrifugation. Intact phage particles were digested with RNAse and then broken by chloroform treatment followed by phenol chloroform extraction and ethanol precipitation of phage DNA. DNA isolated from positive clones was subjected to PCR analysis using the non-degenerate 32-mer primer (5' CCC GTG ACC ACC CAG GGC GAC TAC GTG TCC AA 3') and oligo dT NotI. The PCR program was the same as described above. To establish the size of the Alternaria DNA insert, PCR was conducted using forward and reverse lambda gt11 sequencing primers contained in the phage sequence outside of the insert. DNA template for sequence analysis was produced either by cloning phage known to contain the 300 BP insert or by PCR amplification of the insert. Primers for sequencing included the lambda gt11 forward and reverse sequencing primers, N-terminal primer as used in PCR or a primer selected to be complementary to an area 150 base pairs into the known sequence. Sequencing primers were purchased commercially (Promega Corporation) or synthesized by the University of Missouri-Kansas City Core Facility . Sequencing was by the dideoxy method of Sanger (17) and employed either 32P autoradiography or silver staining (Promega Corporation) to visualize results.

Northern Blotting of Whole RNA

Whole RNA isolated from ten different strains of Alternaria grown in our laboratory was electrophoresed in formaldehyde denaturing 1.2% agarose and blotted by capillary mass action overnight onto nylon 66 membrane. Blotted RNA was crosslinked to the membrane by exposure to ultraviolet light . DNA for the production of radiolabeled probe was prepared by reverse transcriptase reaction of purified Alternaria RNA using a random hexamers. 247 base pair DNA for probe production was produced by PCR amplification using the 27-mer oligo (CGG AAT TCA CCA CCC AGG GCG ACT ACG) as the forward primer and the 27-mer oligo (CGG AAT TCA TCA TTC GTG CCT TTG CCG) as the reverse primer. These primers were designed from sequence information derived from the 295 BP clone. DNA purified by affinity adsorption and centrifugal elution was labeled with ^{32}P dCTP using the Decaprime® random priming method (Ambion, Dallas TX). The RNA blot was probed overnight with the radiolabeled nucleotide, washed extensively and regions of complementary nucleotide binding were visualized on a phosphorimager.

Fusion Protein Production

An oligonucleotide sequence of 247 bases including the reported sequence from the Alt aI allergen was subcloned into the Pflag® expression vector. Colonies were screened for the proper insert by restriction enzyme analysis and for expressed proteins by SDS-PAGE. Selected E. coli clones were tested using SDS-PAGE time studies to detect the presence of recombinant protein and by immunoblotting analysis using a MAB directed to the flag peptide. Recombinant protein was purified by size exclusion column chromatography on Sephadex G-25 utilizing 0.5% SDS in 0.1M TRIS buffer to maintain solubility. Purified protein was separated by SDSPAGE and blotted onto nitrocellulose(18). The blot was probed with IgE containing human sera drawn from humans known to be allergic to Alternaria, detected with horse radish peroxidase conjugated goat anti human IgE (epsilon chain specific) and visualized by a chemilluminescent method (ECL, Amersham, Arlington Heights, Illinois).

RESULTS

The library derived when the PCR amplified cDNA products were inserted into Lambda gt11 phage yielded 10^5 PFU. The recombinant plaques were screened using human IgE. IgE screening was reinforced by a second PCR determination. Positive PCR products were obtained from DNA inserts in several plaque lines. Plaques were graded for size and a clonal line containing a complete insert of 324 BP was chosen for sequence analysis and protein production.

Sequence analysis of the DNA insert using several primers (Figure 1) revealed a Alternaria cDNA sequence of 267 BP. Analysis yielded a reading frame containing 84 amino

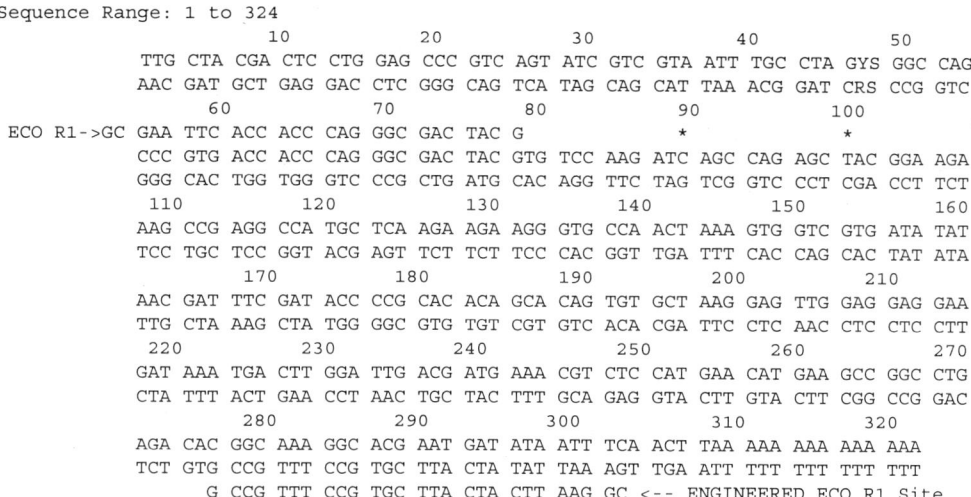

Figure 1. The complete sequence of the original cDNA insert with the positions of the PCR primers for the 247 BP DNA indicated. Bases 1–54 are part of the lambda gt11. The first base of the Alternaria cDNA is at position 55. The TGA at position 225 is a stop in E. coli.

acids and confirmed that this segment contained the code for the reported N-terminal amino acid sequence of Alt a1. The amino acid sequence, translated using the genetic code for mold mitochondria, corresponds to a peptide with a calculated molecular weight of about 9700 Daltons. A computer search for this sequence at the nucleotide level found no homologous sequence in the Entrez® sequences volume 11.

Northern blotting studies on RNA purified from 10 strains of Alternaria indicated that this sequence was present in all strains as part of a 700 BP mRNA. These experiments were performed using a radiolabeled 247 BP DNA fragment created in a separate experiment with PCR primers derived from sequence of the original insert and newly generated cDNA produced by a random priming method.

The protein produced in E. coli from the 247 BP fragment engineered into the pFlag vector is indicated in figure 2. This protein has a calculated molecular weight of 9640 and was noted by electrophoresis time studies of protein production to be approximately this size. The size was also confirmed by blotting studies using the MAB1 monoclonal specific for the Flag portion of the pFlag vector. The protein was noted to be insoluble under normal conditions but could be solubilized in solutions containing 0.5% SDS and was purified by size exclusion chromatography on sephadex G-25. Immunoblotting experiments on both whole E. coli lysate and purified fusion protein indicated that the protein bound IgE from humans known to be allergic to Alternaria.

*MKKTAIAIAVALAGFATVAQADYKDDDDKLEF***TTQGDYVSKISQSYGRKP**RPCSRRRVPTKVV VIYNDFDTPHTAQCAKELEEEDK**

Figure 2. The fusion protein produced using the Pflag vector. The Alt a1 sequence is underlined and the omp and Flag sequence intrinsic to the vector is italicized. The portion contained in the reported N-terminal of Alt a1 is in bold face. The fusion protein has a calculated MW of 9640 and a calculated pI of 7.0.

CONCLUSIONS

The cDNA identified by IgE screening from an Alternaria cDNA library was shown to contain sequence previously reported as the N-terminal amino acid sequence of Alt a1. Northern blotting studies indicated that this sequence was present in 10 strains of Alternaria as part of a 700 BP mRNA. A 247 BP portion of this sequence fused to the Pflag vector produces a recombinant protein which binds IgE from Alternaria allergic individuals.

The history of investigations into Alternaria allergy is replete with disparate results concerning the nature and molecular size of significant allergens. Possible causes of varying results include strain to strain differences, the adaptability and mutability of the fungi itself and the complexity of the allergenic proteins as to carbohydrate content and tertiary structure. This and other studies at the molecular level are providing information necessary to identify the common thread that will bind previously conflicting information into a comprehensive picture. For instance, at this point even though there may be disagreement as to the exact sequence of the complete allergen, there is overwhelming evidence that a peptide sequence identical or very similar to **PVTTQGDYVSKISQSYGRKP** is included in the Alt a1 allergen and is a significant IgE binder. The determination if this sequence exists in multiple subunits of the same protein or in more than one protein from this fungi will have to await further investigation.

REFERENCES

1. Vijay H, Burton M, Young NM. Characterization of major and hypo-allergens of Alternaria tenuis. J. Allergy Clin. Immunol 1988;81:267 (Abst).
2. Vijay HM, Huang H, Young NM, Bernstein IL. Studies On Alternaria allergens. I. Isolation of allergens from Alternaria tenuis and Alternaria solani. Int. Archs. Allergy Appl. Immunol 1979:229–239.
3. Portnoy J, Olson I, Pacheco F, Barnes C. Affinity purification of a major Alternaria allergen using a monoclonal antibody. Annals of Allergy 1990;65(2):109–14.
4. Paris S, Debeaupuis JP, Prevost MC, Casotto M, Latge JP. The 31 Kd major allergen, Alt a I1563, of Alternaria alternata. J Allergy Clin Immunol 1991;88:902–8.
5. Kroutil LA, Bush RK. Detection of Alternaria allergens by western blotting. Journal of Allergy and Clinical Immunology 1987;80:170–6.
6. Portnoy J, Pacheco F, Ballam Y, Barnes C. The effect of time and extraction buffers on residual protein and allergen content of extracts derived from four strains of Alternaria. J Allergy Clin Immunol 1993;91:130–38.
7. Schaffer N, Molomut N, Center J. Studies on allergenic extracts: I. A new method for the preparation of mold extracts using a synthetic medium. Ann Allergy 1959;17:380–4.
8. Paris S, Fitting C, Ramirez E, Latge JP, David B. Comparison of different extraction methods of Alternaria allergens. Journal of Allergy & Clinical Immunology 1990;85(5):941–8.
9. Okayama H, Berg P. High Efficiency cloning of full length cDNA. Mol Cell Biol 1982;2:161–70.
10. Gubler U, Hoffman B. A simple and very efficient method for generating cDNA libraries. Gene 1983;25:263–9.
11. Curran I, Young N, Burton M, Vijay H. Purification and characterization of a low molecular weight antigen from Alternaria alternata. J Allergy Clin Immunol 1992;89:383 (Abstract).
12. Vijay HM, Burton M, Young NM. The hypoallergen of Alternaria alternata carries a dominant epitope of the major allergen. In: Sehon AH, Kraft D, Kunkel G, eds. XIVth Cong. Eur. Acad. Allergol. Clin. Immunol. Berlin: The UCB Institute of Allergy, Brussels, 1990:14–17.
13. Matthiesen F, Olsen M, Lowenstein H. Purification and partial sequenzation of the major allergen of Alternaria alternata, Alt a 1. J of Allergy and Clin Immuno 1992;89:#386(abstr).
14. Han J, Rutter W. Lambda gt22, an improved lambda vector for directional cloning of full length cDNA. Nuc Acids Res 1987;15:6304.
15. Rosenberg S. Improved *in vitro* packaging of l DNA. *Methods Enzymol* 1987;153:95.

16. Rosenberg S, Stahl M, Kobayashi I, Stahl F. Improved in vitro packaging of E. coli phage lambda DNA: A one strain system free from endogenous phage. *Gene* 1985;38:165.
17. Sanger F, Nicklen S, Coulson A. DNA sequencing with chain terminating inhibitors. Proc. Nat. Acad. Sci. USA 1977;74:5463–7.
18. Towbin H, Staehelin T, Gordon J. Electrophoretic transfer of proteins from polyacrylamide gels to nitrocellulose sheets: procedure and some applications. Proc. Natl. Acad. Aci. U.S.A 1979;76:4350–54.

27

ISOLATION OF A CDNA CLONE ENCODING A PUTATIVE *Alternaria alternata Alt a* I SUBUNIT

M. W. De Vouge,[1] A. J. Thaker,[1] L. Zhang,[1] I. H. A. Curran,[1] G. Muradia,[1] H. Rode,[2] and H. M. Vijay[1]

[1]Life Sciences Division
Bureau of Drug Research, Drugs Directorate and
[2]Bureau of Biologics, Drugs Directorate
Health Protection Branch, Health Canada
Ottawa, Ontario, Canada

1. INTRODUCTION

Estimations of the incidence of allergies to airborne allergens range from ≈10–20% of Europeans and North Americans [1]. Examination of atopic sera has also determined that 20–30% of these individuals produce IgE to allergens from *Alternaria alternata* [2,3], implicating this mold as an important source of fungal aeroallergens. Effective immunotherapy using standardized extracts of *Alternaria* and other molds is hindered by the difficulty in developing reliable standards. High rates of somatic mutation and rapid adaptability to new environments contribute to the extreme variability of different mold isolates from similar species with respect to allergen content and composition [4–6]. Thus, the use of recombinant DNA techniques to isolate mold allergens is of potential benefit, as these proteins may be readily purified in large quantity, and in a stable form.

We have previously detected several distinct IgE-binding allergens in immunoblots of *Alternaria* extracts probed with pooled atopic sera, including strongly reactive proteins with M_rs of 14, 16, 27, 31, 32, 39, 44, 53, 78 and 93,000 [7,8]. Of these, >90% of *Alternaria*-specific atopic sera contain IgE against a major allergen isolated by several groups and termed *Alt a*-29, *Alt a* I, or *Alt a* Bd 29K [9–11]. *Alt a*-29, as characterized in our laboratory, is a disulfide-linked dimer with subunits of apparent M_rs of 14,500 and 16,000 and nearly identical N-terminal sequences [9], which are also ≈85% homologous to the N-terminal 26 residues of *Alt a* I isolated by Matthiesen *et al.* [10].

Our efforts over the past several years have been concentrated on the purification and characterization of mold allergens, including those of *A. alternata*, with the aim of facilitating the development of standardized diagnostic and immunotherapeutic extracts. Here, we have used specific IgG against purified *Alt a*-29 to isolate and characterize cDNA clones corresponding to this allergen.

New Horizons in Allergy Immunotherapy
edited by Sehon et al. Plenum Press, New York, 1996

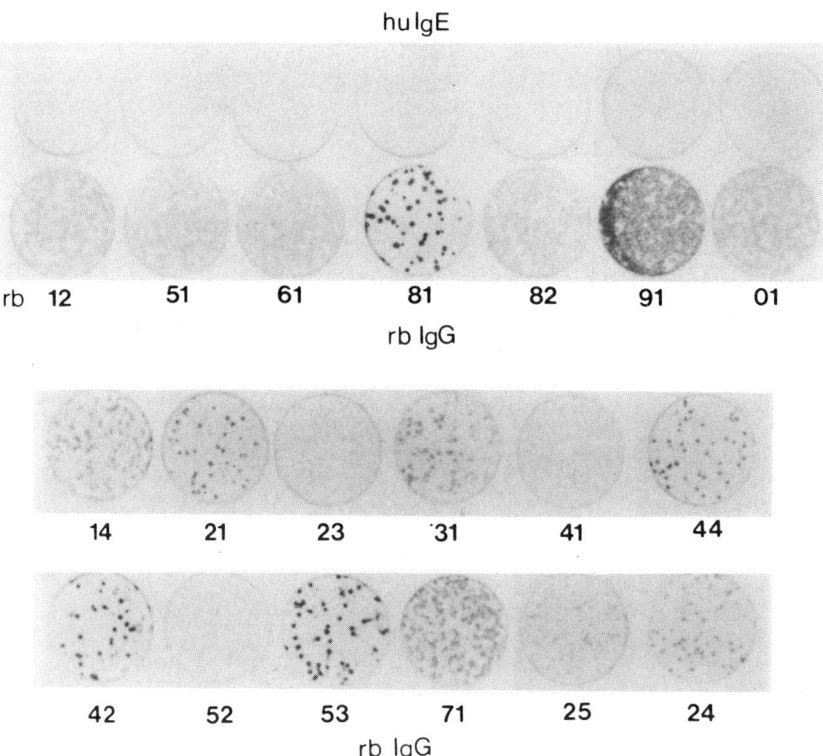

Figure 1. Immunoselection of cDNA clones reactive with rabbit anti-*Alt a*-29 IgG. Rows 1,2: Duplicate nitrocellulose membrane lifts of purified clones previously selected using rabbit anti-*Alt a*-29 IgG; membranes were immunostained using either pooled atopic IgE against *A. alternata* (hu IgE, row 1), or rabbit anti-*Alt a*-29 (rb IgG, row 2). Rows 3,4: Additional clones selected using rabbit anti-*Alt a*-29.

2. RESULTS AND DISCUSSION

2.1. Immunoselection of cDNA clones corresponding to *Alt a*-29

To immunoselect clones corresponding to *Alt a*-29, we constructed an *A. alternata*-specific cDNA library in λgt11. A total of 305,000 recombinant phage were screened using standard protocols [12], from which nineteen positive clones were obtained. The staining intensities of these positives varied considerably (Figure 1), suggesting that either sequences corresponded to more than one gene product, or similar sequences of different lengths were being selected. Surprisingly, none of the 19 positives reacted positively when immobilized plaques were immunostained with pooled human atopic IgE.

2.2. Detection of *Alt a*-29 N-Terminal Sequences in Immunopositive Clones by Southern Analysis

To determine which of the nineteen positives contained DNA sequences corresponding to the *Alt a*-29 N-terminus, PCR-amplified inserts from each were probed with an 8-

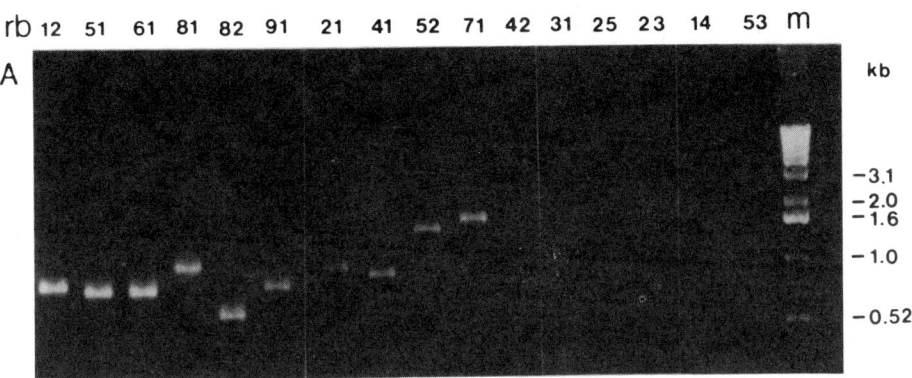

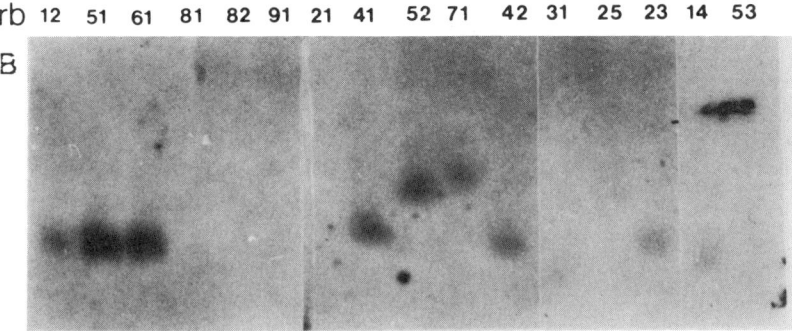

Figure 2. Agarose gel electrophoresis (A) and Southern blots (B) of representative PCR-amplified inserts from cDNA clones selected using rabbit anti-*Alt a*-29. Blots were probed with a degenerate oligonucleotide (GAAGGTGAYTACGTYGTYAAGAT) deduced from the *Alt a*-29 N-terminal peptide sequence, at 5 pmol/ml in hybridization solution (1% blocking agent, 5X SSC, 0.1% N-lauroyl sarcosine, 0.02% SDS) for 3 h at 35°C. Washes were for 2 × 5 min with (5X SSC, 0.1% SDS) at room temperature, followed by 2 × 10 min washes using (2X SSC, 0.1% SDS) also at room temperature. Positions of markers of known size are indicated in kilobase pairs (kb).

fold degenerate oligonucleotide deduced from the *Alt a*-29 N-terminal peptide sequence. After hybridizing and washing under non-stringent conditions, annealing of the probe to inserts from clones rb51 and rb61 was observed to be stronger than to inserts from any of the other clones examined (Figure 2). Additional clones that bound the probe included rb12, rb41, rb52, rb71, rb42, rb23 and rb14. The smallest clones (rb31, rb82 and rb53) may not have bound the probe because their coding sequences may not have been complete, whereas strongly immunoreactive clones rb81 and rb21 exhibited similar insert sizes (≈1 kb), but did not bind the probe, suggesting that they might possibly represent different gene products from *Alt a*-29.

2.3. Comparison of *Alt a*-29 and *Alt a* I N-Termini with Clone rb51-Derived Translated Sequence

Based on the strong hybridization observed between clone rb51 and the *Alt a*-29 N-terminal oligonucleotide, we opted to sequence clone rb51. The 660 bp rb51 cDNA clone was shown to contain an open reading frame (ORF) of 474 bp [De Vouge *et al.*, submitted]. Sequences common to the ORF were also present in eight of the other eighteen clones isolated by immunoscreening. Three clones with longer inserts contained sequences which were identified as homologous to fungal rRNAs (rb01, rb52 and rb71). One clone (rb25) appeared to contain sequences corresponding to a distinct protein which has no known homolog in gene banks. The remaining clones have not yet been investigated (of these, six did not hybridize to the degenerate oligo designed from the *Alt a*-29 N-terminal sequence). Homology searches of gene banks using the BLAST algorithm [13] failed to reveal significant sequence identity with genes encoding known proteins or allergens.

The deduced peptide sequence of the rb51 ORF encoded a peptide of 157 amino acids, with a calculated M_r of 16,960 [De Vouge *et al.*, submitted]. As shown in Figure 3, the previously determined N-terminal peptide sequences corresponded to residues 29–48 of rb51, and match the *Alt a*-29 N-terminal peptide sequence previously obtained in our laboratory at 17 of 20 positions [9]. This ORF also matches the N-terminus of *Alt a* I as determined by Matthiesen *et al.* except for two residues that were not resolved in that study [10]. In both cases, potentially variant amino acids are found at positions 30 and 40, indicating either potential differences in isoforms or polymorphic sites which mutate at high frequency between different fungal isolates. However, if additional *Alt a* I isoforms were expressed in *A. alternata*, we should have expected to immunoselect several sets of sequences differing only at these positions. Of those clones that we have isolated and sequenced, all that encode *Alt a* I appear to contain similar nucleotide sequences to rb51, suggesting that the latter hypothesis is more likely.

From the peptide sequence of rb51 ORF, analyses of hydrophobicity and predictions of protein secondary structure were carried out [De Vouge *et al.*, submitted]. The longest hydrophobic region in the rb51 ORF is within the N-terminus, from amino acids 10–23. This region also coincides with a predicted α-helical domain. As amino acids 1–28 were not previously detected in microsequenced *Alt a* I peptides, it may be speculated that the first 28 amino acids may represent a leader sequence that is cleaved from the protein during processing.

```
RB51.AA     29    SC PVTTEGDYVW KISEFYGRKP EGTY    54

NTERM1.AMI   1    AD *********V *****F**.. ....    26

NTERM2.AMI   1    AD *********V ********.. ....    26

NTERMM.AMI   1    *X *********X ********** ****    26
```

Figure 3. Comparison of previously described N-terminal peptide sequences with rb51 N-terminus. NTERM1.AMI and NTERM2.AMI represent alternative *Alt a*-29 N-terminal peptide sequences as determined by Curran *et al* [9]. NTERMM.AMI represents *Alt a* I N-terminal peptide sequences as determined by Matthiesen *et al.* [10]. Asterisks denote amino acids matching amino acids 29–54 deduced from the rb51 ORF (RB51.AA).

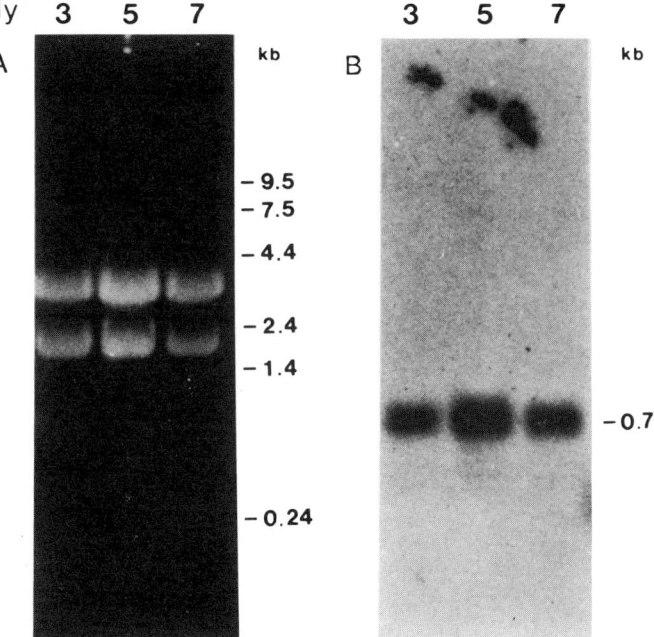

Figure 4. Northern blotting of total RNA from *A. alternata*. Total RNA was isolated by the method of Chomczynski and Sacchi [14], from cultures of *A. alternata* strain 34–016 grown in Revised Tobacco Medium for 3, 5 or 7 days. RNAs were fractionated in 1.2% formaldehyde-agarose gels (A) and transferred to nylon membrane (B). Labeled rb51 probe was hybridized to the blot overnight at 50°C. Washes were for 2 × 5 min with (2X SSC, 0.1% SDS) at room temperature and 2 × 10 min using (0.1X SSC, 0.1% SDS) at 68°C. Positions of markers of known size are indicated in kilobases (kb).

2.4. Size Analysis of rb51 Transcript by Northern Blotting of Total RNA from *A. alternata*

To determine the transcript size of rb51, total RNA was isolated from cultures of *A. alternata* strain 34–016 grown in Revised Tobacco Medium for 3, 5 or 7 days. RNAs were fractionated in 1.2% formaldehyde-agarose gels and transferred to nylon membrane. Labeled rb51 probe was hybridized to the blot overnight, and washes were carried out under stringent conditions. From the gel in panel A of Figure 4, total RNA was extracted with little or no degradation. The blot shows that rb51 hybridizes to an abundant transcript of approximately 700 bases, indicating that the clones obtained contain nearly complete cDNA sequence, and that the ORF obtained represents a complete *Alt a* I subunit.

2.5. Reactivity of Individual Human Atopic Sera against β-Galactosidase-rb42 Fusion Protein in Immunoblots

We were surprised at our inability to immunoselect *Alt a*-29 using human atopic IgE, as well as the inability of atopic IgE to immunostain immobilized phage plaques of clones selected using rabbit IgG against *Alt a*-29. Because the λgt11 vector expresses foreign sequences as the C-terminus of a β-galactosidase fusion protein, we hypothesized that the *Alt a*-29 IgE-binding epitopes were being masked by the 117 kDa β-galactosidase

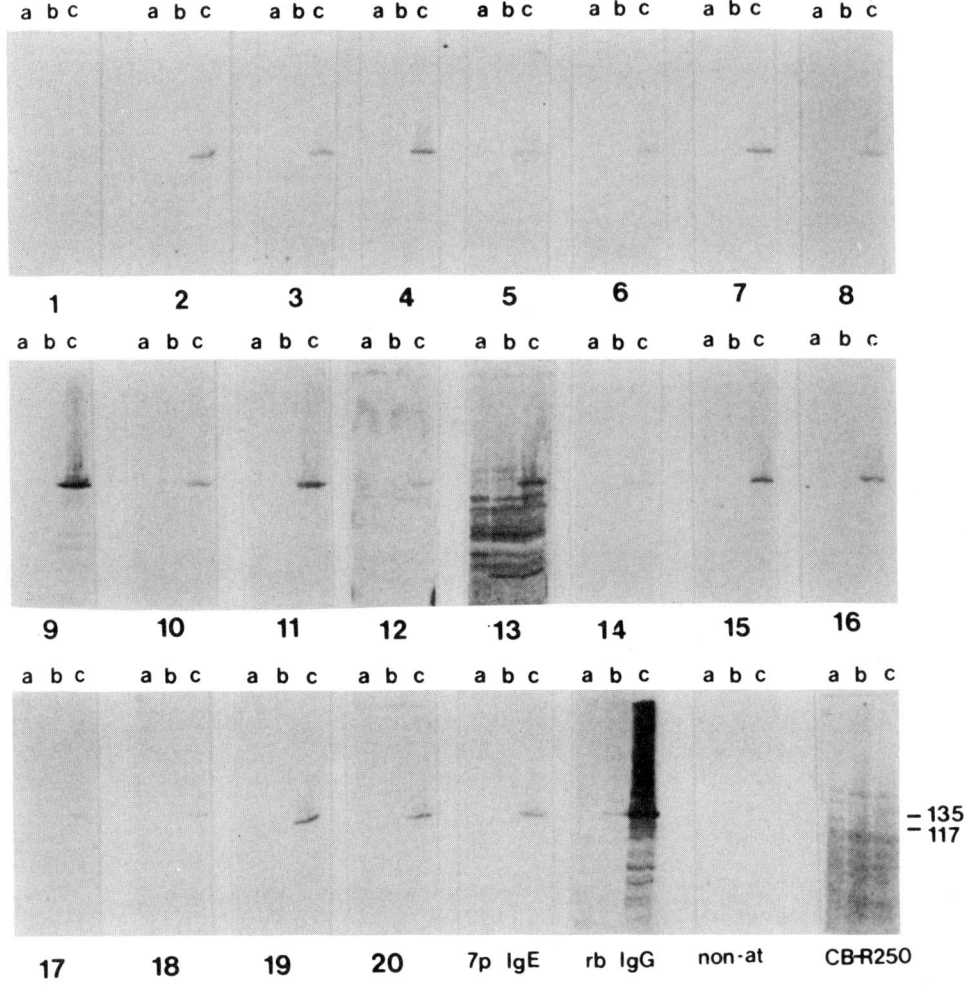

Figure 5. Reactivity of individual human atopic sera against β-galactosidase-rb42 fusion protein in immunoblots. Lanes a: lysates from lysogens of non-recombinant λgt11. Lanes b,c: uninduced and IPTG-induced lysates of clone rb42 lysogens, respectively. Blot 7p IgE was probed with pooled human atopic IgE (1:5 dilution). Blot Rb IgG was probed with rabbit anti-*Alt a*-29 diluted 1:800. Blot non-at was probed with pooled non-atopic human sera diluted 1:5. Blots 1–20 were probed with individual human atopic antisera diluted 1:5. Blot CB-R250 was stained with Coomassie blue R250. The M_rs of non-recombinant λgt11 β-galactosidase (117,000) and recombinant β-galactosidase-rb42 fusion protein (135,000) are indicated at right.

moiety of the recombinant fusion protein. Therefore, we tested individual human atopic IgE from 20 individuals allergic to *A. alternata* to assess their reactivity to the partially denatured fusion protein in immunoblots. We prepared lysogens against rb42, a clone containing an identical ORF to rb51, but which expresses the recombinant fusion protein at higher levels, since rb51 sequences bridging the β-galactosidase and *Alt a*-29 sequences contain termination codons that greatly limit expression of the recombinant fusion protein. The data in Figure 5 show that serum IgEs from 95% of these individuals reacted with the fusion protein. One antiserum (#13) exhibited too much background staining of non-recombinant β-galactosidase to be considered as positive. The β-galactosidase-rb42 fusion protein was also heavily stained with rabbit antiserum against *Alt a*-29, and was not stained using pooled non-atopic antiserum. Therefore, we have demonstrated that the isolated clone can bind IgE in human atopic sera, indicating that the expressed rb42 peptide indeed represents a bona fide *A. alternata* allergen.

3. CONCLUSIONS

In summary, we have immunoselected a 660 bp clone from an *A. alternata*-specific cDNA library constructed in λgt11. Northern analyses suggest this clone is a nearly complete transcript. The in-frame ORF within the cloned insert encodes a novel peptide of M_r 16,960. Its peptide sequence contains sequences that match the N-terminus of *Alt a*-29 at 17 of 20 positions, as well as the N-terminus of *Alt a* I at 24 of 26 positions. The N-terminal region of the peptide is highly hydrophobic, and possesses an α-helical domain and possibly signals for membrane insertion or secretion. This leader sequence may be cleaved from the mature protein. IgE from 95% of individuals atopic for *A. alternata* bind the cloned recombinant fusion protein in immunoblots, indicating that the cloned gene product is capable of acting as an allergen.

4. ACKNOWLEDGMENTS

This study was supported by the National Biotechnology Strategy [Canada].

5. REFERENCES

1. Gergen PJ, Turkeltaub PC, Kovar MG: The prevalence of allergic skin test reactivity to eight common aeroallergens in the US population: Results from the second National Health and Nutrition Examination Survey. J Allergy Clin Immunol 1987;80: 669–679.
2. Aas K, Leegard J, Aukrust L, Grimmer O: Immediate type hypersensitivity to common molds. Allergy 1980;35: 443–451.
3. Yee EG, Bahna SL: Skin testing and RAST to molds in patients with respiratory allergy. J Allergy Clin Immunol 1986;77: 200 (abstract).
4. Solvaggio JE, Burge HA, Chapman JA: Emerging concepts in mold allergy: What is the role of immunotherapy? J Allergy Clin Immunol 1993;92: 217–222.
5. Vijay HM, Huang H, Young NM, Bernstein IL: Studies on *Alternaria* allergens. IV. Comparative biochemical and immunological studies of commercial *Alternaria tenuis* batches. Int Arch Allergy Appl Immunol 1984;74: 256–261.
6. Steringer I, Aukrust L, Einarsson R: Variability of antigenicity and allergenicity in different strains of *Alternaria alternata*. Int Arch Allergy Appl Immunol 1987;84: 190–197.
7. Vijay, HM: Advanced studies on *Alternaria* mould allergens with reference to standardization; in Agashe SN (ed): Recent Trends in Aerobiology, Allergy and Immunology. New Delhi, Oxford & IBH, 1994, pp 247–277.
8. Vijay HM, Burton M, Young NM: The hypoallergen of *Alternaria alternata* carries a dominant epitope of the major allergen; in Sehon AH, Kraft D, Kunkel G (eds): Epitopes of Atopic Allergens. Proceedings of workshop, XIVth Cong Eur Acad Allergol Clin Immunol, Berlin, Sept. 1989. Brussels, UCB Institute of Allergy, 1990, pp 14–17.
9. Curran IHA, Young NM, Burton M, Vijay HM: Purification and characterization of Alt a-29 from *Alternaria alternata*. Int Arch Allergy Immunol 1993;102: 267–275.
10. Matthiesen F, Olsen M, Løwenstein H: Purification and partial sequenzation of the major allergen of *Alternaria alternata*. J Allergy Clin Immunol 1992; 89: 241 (abstract).

11. Deards MJ, Montague AE: Purification and characterization of major allergen of *Alternaria alternata*. Mol Immunol 1991;28: 409–415.
12. Huynh TV, Young RA, Davis RW: Constructing and screening cDNA libraries in λgt10 and λgt11; in Glover D (ed): DNA Cloning: A Practical Approach. Oxford, IRL Press, 1985, vol 1, pp 49–78.
13. Altschul SF, Gish W, Miller W, Myers EW, Lipman DJ: Basic local alignment search tool. J Mol Biol 1990;215: 403–410.
14. Chomczynski P, Sacchi N: Single-step method of RNA extraction by acid guanidinium thiocyanate-phenol-chloroform extraction. Anal Biochem 1987;162: 156–159.

28

PEANUT HYPERSENSITIVITY

IgE Binding Characteristics of a Recombinant *Ara h* I Protein

J. S. Stanley, R. M. Helm, G. Cockrell, A. W. Burks, and G. A. Bannon

Departments of Pediatrics and Biochemistry and Molecular Biology
University of Arkansas for Medical Sciences
Little Rock, Arkansas 72205

Peanut allergy is a significant health problem because of the potential severity of the allergic reaction, the life-long nature of the allergic hypersensitivity, and the ubiquitous use of peanut products. Milk, eggs, and peanuts are three foods which cause over 80% of food hypersensitivity reactions in children (1,2). Unlike the food hypersensitivity reactions to milk and eggs, peanut hypersensitivity reactions usually persists into adulthood and last for a lifetime (3). Despite the prevalence of peanut hypersensitivity reactions and several fatalities annually, the identification of the clinically relevant antigens is incomplete and an understanding of the immunobiology of peanut hypersensitivity is very limited (4–6).

Recombinant methodology to clone allergens provides an efficient means of producing pure polypeptides which, in their native source, form complex mixtures and are often represented in only very small amounts (7). Several inhaled allergens have been cloned, including the allergens of house dust mites (8) and pollen grains (9,10), in comparison little work has been directed toward producing recombinant food allergens. Because of the prevalence and severity of peanut hypersensitivity reactions in both children and adults, coupled with the recent identification of two peanut allergens (*Ara h* I and *Ara h* II) that are involved in this process (11,12), we set out to clone and characterize the *Ara h* I peanut allergen. Using serum IgE from peanut hypersensitive individuals, IgE reactive clones were isolated from a peanut cDNA expression library. *Ara h* I clones were then selected from this group of potential recombinant allergens by probing with a ^{32}P-labeled *Ara h I* PCR clone constructed by amplifying peanut mRNA with an *Ara h* I oligonucleotide and oligo dT (Fig. 1). After identification of a full-length *Ara h* I cDNA clone, the frequency of IgE binding by individual patients sera to the recombinant protein and purified, native *Ara h* I from whole peanut extracts was determined by immunoblot analysis. Of the 18 patients tested in this manner, 17 had IgE which recognized recombinant *Ara h* I (Table I). In general, there was good agreement between the level of IgE binding of recombinant and native *Ara h* I for each individual. For example, patients who had high levels of IgE binding to native allergen also showed high immunoreactivity with recombinant *Ara h* I

New Horizons in Allergy Immunotherapy
edited by Sehon et al. Plenum Press, New York, 1996

213

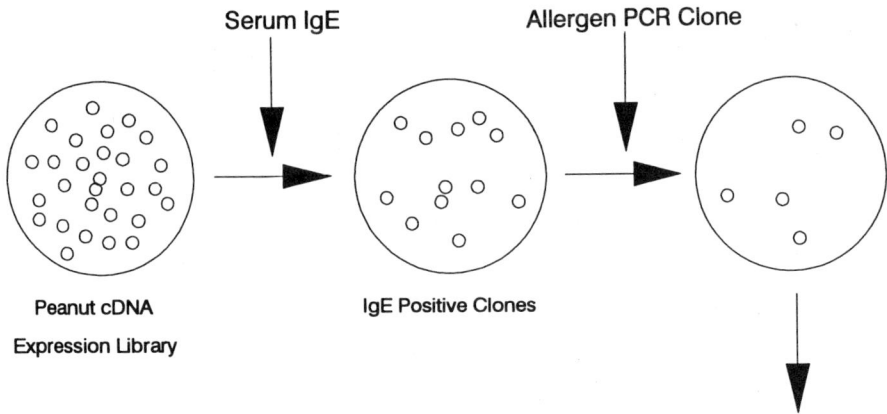

Figure 1. Strategy for isolation of *ARA h* I cDNA clones that produce IgE recognized proteins. Using Serum IgE from peanut hypersensitive individuals, IgE reactive clones were isolated from a peanut cDNA expression library as described by Burks et al. (13). *Ara h I* was then selected from this group of potential recombinant allergens by probing with a ^{32}P labeled *Ara h I* PCR clone.

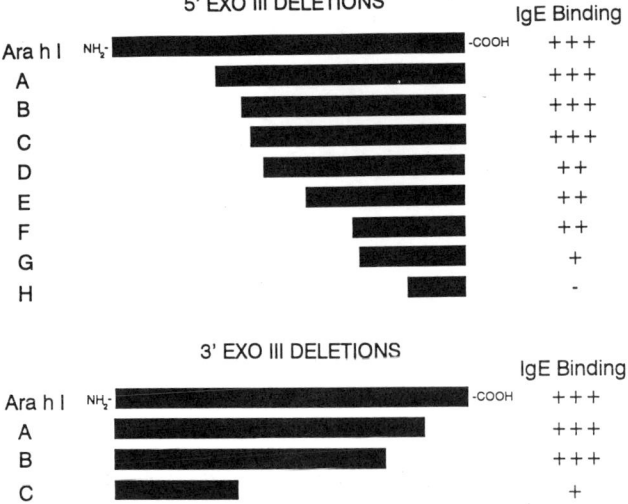

Figure 2. EXO III deletions of the intact *ARA h* I cDNA clone indicate multiple IgE binding domains. Exo III digestion from the 5' or 3' end of the full length *Ara h I* cDNA clone was used to produce shortened clones whose protein products could then be tested for IgE binding by immunoblot analysis. The pluses (+) on the right side of this figure indicate the extent of IgE binding to the protein product of each construct. All constructs bound IgE until they were reduced to the extreme carboxyl terminal (5' Exo III) or amino terminal (3' Exo III) end of the molecule. These results indicate that there are multiple IgE epitopes on the *Ara h I* allergen.

Table 1. Comparison of serum IgE binding to native and recombinant *Ara h* I protein

Patient	Native *Ara h* I	Recombinant *Ara h* I
1	+++	+++
2	+++	+++
3	+++	+++
4	+++	+++
5	+++	+++
6	++	+++
7	+++	+++
8	++	++
9	++	++
10	+	+
11	+	−
12	+	+
13	+	+
14	+	+
15	+	+
16	+	+
17	+	+
18	+	+
19	−	−

Purified *Ara h* I from whole peanut extracts or recombinant *Ara h* I protein was electrophoresed on denaturing polyacrylamide gels, blotted to nitrocellulose, and then probed with serum IgE from patients with peanut hypersensitivity (A-R) or serum IgE from an individual who is not peanut allergic (S). Patients were scored for the presence (+) or absence (−) of serum IgE to recombinant or native *Ara h* I.

protein. Patients who had low levels of IgE binding to native allergen showed low reactivity with the recombinant protein. Only one peanut sensitive individual who had serum IgE specific to native *Ara h* I had no detectable IgE which recognized the recombinant protein.

Since it appeared that the recombinant *Ara h* I protein bound IgE with the same degree/intensity as native allergen, we set out to map the major IgE binding domain(s) on the recombinant molecule. Exo III digestion from the 5' or 3' end of the full length *Ara h* I cDNA clone was used to produce shortened clones whose protein products could then be tested for IgE binding by immunoblot analysis (Fig.2). The pluses (+) on the right side of this figure indicate the extent of IgE binding to the protein product of each construct. All constructs bound IgE until they were reduced to the extreme carboxyl terminal (5' Exo III) or amino terminal (3' Exo III) end of the molecule. These results indicate that there are multiple IgE epitopes on the *Ara h* I allergen. These results are significant in that they indicate the utility of using recombinant peanut allergens for studying peanut hypersensitivity.

ACKNOWLEDGMENTS

This research was supported by the Allergy and Asthma Foundation of America.

REFERENCES

1. Sampson HA. Food hypersensitivity and atopic dermatitis: evaluation of 113 patients. J Pediatr 1985; 107:669–675.

2. Yunginger JW, Squillace DL, Jones RT, Helm RM. Fatal anaphylactic reactions induced by peanuts. Allergy Proc 1989;10:249–253.

3. Sampson HA, Mendelson L, Rosen JP. Fatal and near-fatal anaphylactic reactions to food in children and adolescents. New Engl J Med 1992; 327:380–384.

4. Metcalfe DD. Food allergens. Clin Rev Allergy 1985; 3:331–349.

5. Yunginger JW, Sweeney KG, Sturner WQ, Giannandrea LA, Teigland JD, Bray M, Benson PA, Biedrzycki L, Squillace DL, Helm RM. Fatal food-induced anaphylaxis. JAMA 1988;260:1450–1452.

6. Hoffman DR, Haddad ZH. Diagnosis of IgE mediated reactions to food antigens by radioimmunoassay. J. Allergy Clin Immunol 1974; 54:165–173.

7. Donovan GR, Baldo BA. Recombinant DNA approaches to the study of allergens and allergenic determinants. Monogr Allergy 1990; 28:52–83.

8. Thomas WR,Stewart GA, Simpson RJ, Chua KY, Plozza TM, Dilworth RJ, Nisbet A, Turner KJ. Cloning and expression of DNA coding for the major house dust mite allergen, *Der p* I in *Escherichia coli*. Int. Arch. Allergy Appl. Immunol 1988, 85:127–129.

9. Valenta R, Vrtala S, Ebner C, Kraft D, Scheiner O. Diagnosis of grass pollen allergy with recombinant timothy grass (*Phleum pratense*) pollen allergens. Int Archives Allergy Immunol 1992; 736:287.

10. Larsen JN, Stroman P, Ipsen H. PCR based cloning and sequencing of isogenes encoding the tree pollen major allergen *Car b* I from *Carpinus betulus*, Hornbeam. Mol. Immunol 1992; 29:703–711.

11. Burks AW, Williams LW, Helm RM, Connaughton C, Cockrell G, O'Brien TJ. Identification of a major peanut allergen, *Ara h* I, in patients with atopic dermatitis and positive peanut challenges. J Allergy Clin Immunol 1991; 88: 172–179.

12. Burks AW, Williams LW, Connaughton C, Cockrell G, O'Brien TJ, Helm RM. Identification and characterization of a second major peanut allergen, *Ara h* II, utilizing the sera of patients with atopic dermatitis and positive peanut challenge. J Allergy Clin Immunol 1992; 90: 962–969.

13. Burks W, Cockrell G, Stanley JS, Helm R, Bannon GA. Isolation, identification, and characterization of clones encoding antigens responsible for peanut hypersensitivity. Inter Arch Aller Immunol 1995 (In Press).

29

HUMAN T CELL CLONES AND CELL LINES SPECIFIC TO OVOMUCOID RECOGNIZE DIFFERENT DOMAINS AND CONSISTENTLY EXPRESS IL-5

P. A. Eigenmann, S. K. Huang, D. G. Ho, and H. A. Sampson

Department of Pediatrics
Division of Immunology and Allergy
School of Medicine, CMSC 1102
The Johns Hopkins Hospital
Baltimore, Maryland 21287–3923

Ovomucoid is the major egg antigen, and is composed of 3 domains (domain I: residues 1–64, domain II: residues 65–130, domain III: residues 131–186). In this study, we generated T cell lines and clones from 3 egg allergic patients (TK, PB, and XM) in order to characterize ovomucoid domain specificity and cell cytokine profile after stimulation with ovomucoid. Ovomucoid domain specificity was determined by measuring the proliferative response to each of the highly purified ovomucoid domains. Cytokine specific mRNA production was determined by reverse transcription polymerase chain reaction (RT-PCR).

The cell lines from patient TK specifically recognized domain III, whereas cell lines and clones from patient PB proliferated to domain II. The cells from patient XM were not specific to either domain. Cell lines from all 3 patients consistently expressed IL-5. In contrast, IL-4 and INF-γ mRNA production was variable in the life span of a cell line, and between different cells lines from the same individual. All clones derived from cell lines from PB and XM expressed IL-5, and one clone also expressed IL-13. However, none of the clones from patient PB expressed IL-4 or INF-γ.

The results demonstrate that ovomucoid domain specificity varies among different individuals since T cells from two different egg allergic individuals recognize different epitopes. IL-4 and INF-γ expression was highly variable, whereas all cells continually expressed IL-5. In conclusion, individual variations will have to be considered for ovomucoid specific T cell epitope mapping. Furthermore, there was no clear Th1 or Th2 cell profile expression, but all cell lines and clones expressed IL-5 mRNA.

New Horizons in Allergy Immunotherapy
edited by Sehon et al. Plenum Press, New York, 1996

217

30

ISOLATION AND CLONING OF Bet v 1-HOMOLOGOUS FOOD ALLERGENS FROM CELERIAC (Api g1) AND APPLE (Mal d1)

K. Hoffmann-Sommergruber,[1] M. Vanek-Krebitz,[1] R. Ferris,[1] G. O'Riordain,[1] M. Susani,[2] R. Hirschwehr,[1] C. Ebner,[1] H. Ahorn,[3] D. Kraft,[1] O. Scheiner[1] and H. Breiteneder[1]

[1]Inst. of General and Experimental Pathology
University of Vienna
AKH, Austria
[2]Advanced Biological Systems
Salzburg, Austria
[3]Ernst Böhringer Forschungsinstitut
Vienna, Austria

1. INTRODUCTION

Up to 70% of tree pollen allergic patients tend to display allergic reactions to a broad range of fruits and vegetables such as hazelnuts, apples, celeriac and carrots. At least part of this food intolerance is due to Bet v 1 (major birch pollen allergen) - related allergens from different plant species, as it was shown in IgE-immunoblots (1–3).

We present data on the characterization of natural Cor a 1 from hazelnuts and on the cloning and sequencing of allergens derived from celery (*Apium graveolens*) and apple (*Malus domestica*), designated Api g 1 and Mal d 1 according to the allergen nomenclature (4).

2. MATERIALS AND METHODS

2.1. Allergen-Extracts

Aqueous protein extracts from fruits, nuts and vegetables were prepared as described (2). Briefly, nuts, fruits and vegetables were washed, weighed and cut. After freeezing in liquid nitrogen, tissues were ground to fine powder and dissolved in extraction buffer (50% w/v). After centrifugation (40 000g/4°C/24h) supernatants were filtered, dialyzed, freeze dried and stored at -20°C.

New Horizons in Allergy Immunotherapy
edited by Sehon et al. Plenum Press, New York, 1996

219

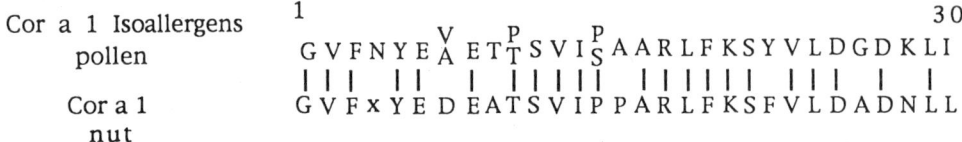

Figure 1. N-terminal Sequences from Cor a 1 allergens isolated and cloned from hazelpollen and from Cor a 1 allergen derived from hazelnuts.

2.2. Purification of Natural Food Allergens

Cor a 1 (Hazelnut). Proteins from hazelnut extracts were purified by chromatofocusing followed by C_8-RP-HPLC chromatography (5). Purified fractions of an 18kDa IgE-binding protein were subjected to SDS-PAGE and blotted to a PVDF-membrane (Millipore) and N-terminal amino acid sequence was determined by automated Edman degradation.

Api G 1 (Celery). IgE-binding proteins from celery-extract were purified by C_8-RP-HPLC. Subsequently N-terminal sequence was determined as described above.

2.3. RNA-Extraction (Celery, Apple)

RNA from apple and celery was extracted according to Chomczynski *et al.* (6). Messenger RNA was isolated by binding to biotinylated oligo(dT)-paramagnetic particles (Promega) according to the manufacturers' instructions followed by poly(A)$^+$ priming (7). Subsequent PCR using degenerated primers according to the known N-terminal sequence from Api g 1 (celery) and Mal d 1 (apple, 8) was performed.

2.4. Cloning and Sequencing of Api g 1 and Mal d 1

PCR-products were cloned into the *Eco R I* -restriction site of the plasmid pCR II of the TA cloning system (Invitrogen, San Diego, CA). Cloned inserts of identical length of 643bp (Api g 1) and 736 (Mal d 1) respectively, were sequenced according to Sanger et al.

2.5. Expression and Purification of Recombinant Food Allergens

Api g 1 encoding cDNA was subcloned into the expression plasmid pMW 175 under control of the lac UV5-promoter (9). Expression of recombinant allergen was induced by adding IPTG (1mM final concentration) to the culture medium for 4 hours. Finally, *E. coli* cells were harvested by centrifugation and disrupted by repeated freeze - thawing steps. Rec Api g 1 was purified to homogeneity by anion-exchange chromatography and hydrophobic-interaction chromatography on phenyl sepharose (10). Purified recombinant protein was quantitated by using the molar extinction coefficient (11).

2.6. SDS-Page and Immunoblotting

Total extracts and purified proteins were separated by 12% SDS-PAGE, Coomassie-stained or blotted to nitrocellulose membrane. IgE-binding proteins were detected by incu-

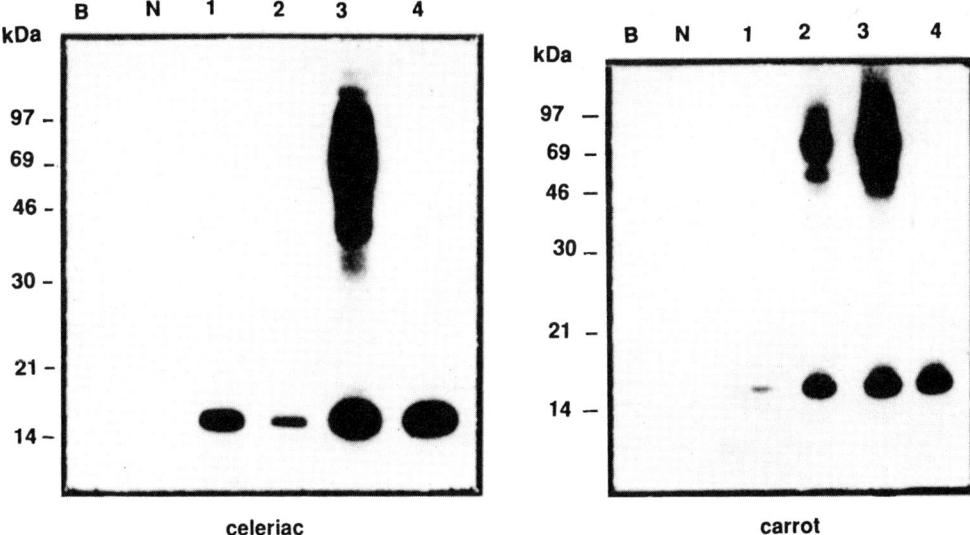

Figure 2. Immunoblots from food allergic patients: Protein extracts from cleriac (a) and carrot (b) were separated by SDS-PAGE, blotted onto nitrocellulose and tested with the same set of allergic patients sera (1–4). IgE-binding was detected by radiolabelled ^{125}I anti-human IgE as described above. (N-normal human serum, B-buffer control).

bating the blots with either individual allergic patients' sera or serum pools (serum pool from 8 allergic patients with established food allergy and serum pool from 8 patients with allergy to birch pollen) followed by radiolabelled anti-human IgE antibodies (Pharmacia). For rabbit anti-Bet v 1-IgG ,^{125}I-donkey anti-rabbit IgG was used (Pharmacia).

For inhibition experiments, a serum pool of patients with established allergy to celery (n=8), was preincubated with rBet v 1 (major birch pollen allergen; 10µg/ml). Subsequently, immunoblots were continued as mentioned above.

3. RESULTS

3.1. Immunoblots

Sera from patients with established allergy to birch pollen and with known hypersensitivity to a variety of fruits and vegetables were tested in immunoblots. They displayed IgE-binding to a range of allergens (18 - 80 kDa) present in protein extracts from carrots as well as from celery (Fig. 2).

N-Terminal Sequences from Food Allergens. **Cor a 1(hazelnut):** N-terminal sequencing of the purified 18kDa IgE-binding protein from hazelnut revealed a 73% identity to the already known Cor a 1 allergens isolated from pollen (12; Fig. 1).

Api g 1: 20 N-terminal amino acids from purified natural Api g 1 were determined by automated Edman degradation and degenerated primers constructed (Fig. 4).

Sequence Analysis of Recombinant Food Allergens. **Api g1:** Sequencing of 8 identical clones of 643bp length and a predicted molecular mass of 16,3kDa revealed 42% identity (65% similarity) to Bet v 1 (Fig. 4)

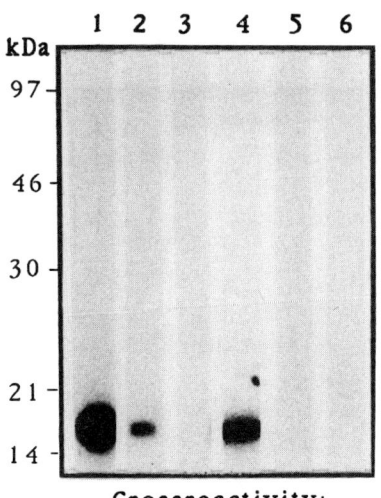

Crossreactivity:
Bet v 1 : Api g 1

Figure 3. Crossreactivity: Bet v 1 : Api g 1. Purified recombinant Api g 1 was run on SDS-PAGE, blotted onto nitrocellulose sheets and tested with serum pool from celery allergic patients (lane 1), a serum pool of birch pollen allergic patients (lane 2), celery allergic serum pool after preincubation with rec Bet v 1 (lane 3), and polyclonal rabbit anti-Bet v 1 IgG (lane 4). Detection of bound antibodies was performed as described above. (Controls: normal human serum - lane 5, buffer control lane 6).

Mal d 1: Clones isolated by PCR coding for the Bet v 1-homologue from apples revealed sequences of 736bp length with a predicted molecular mass of 17,5kDa and 60% identity (76% similarity) to Bet v 1 (Fig. 4).

Expression and Purification of recApi g 1. Api g 1 was subcloned into expression plasmid pMW 175 under control of the lac UV5-promoter, yielding 100mg purified protein per liter culture medium. Highly purified rApi g 1 was tested in immunoblots using serum pools of birch pollen allergic patients and patients with additional allergy to celery and polyclonal rabbit-anti-Bet v 1 IgG (Fig. 3 lane 1,2,4). IgE-antibodies derived from sera from either patients with established food allergy and allergy to birch pollen respectively, recognized Api g 1, yet with different intensity. Furthermore, IgE-binding of celery-allergic patients was 100% inhibited, when preincubating the serum pool with purified recombinant Bet v 1 (Fig. 3, lane 3). Polyclonal anti- Bet v 1 raised in rabbit did also recognize rApi g 1 (Fig 3, lane 5).

```
                        Bet v 1: Mal d 1: Api g 1

         1                                                                      80
Bet v 1  MGVFNYETETTSVIPAARLFKAFILDGDNLFPKVAPQAISSVENIEGNGGPGTIKKISFPEGFPFKYVKDRVDEVDHTNF

Mal d 1  ---YTF-N-F--E--PS------V--A---T--I---- KQA-IL------------T-G--SQYG---H-I-SI-EASY

Api g 1  ---QTHVL-L--SVS-EKI-QG-VI-V-TVL--A--G-YK---I.K-D-----L-I-TL-D-G-ITTMTL-I-G-NKEAL


         81                                                                     160
Bet v 1  KYNYSVIEGGPIGDTLEKISNEIKIVATPDGCSILKISNKYHTKGDHEVKAEQVKASKEMGETLLRAVESYLLAHSDAYN

                                                   P                      A        D
Mal d 1  S-S-TL---DALT--I----YET-L--CGS-ST-KS--H.---?---NI-I-E-H--VG--K-HG-FKLI----KE-P----

Api g 1  TFD----D-DILLGFI-S-ENHVVL-P-A--GS-C-TTAIF-----AV-PE-NI-YAN-QNTA-FK-L-A--I-N
```

Figure 4. Amino acid sequence comparison of Bet v 1, Mal d 1 and Api g 1. Sequence identities to Bet v 1 are marked by bars. N-terminal sequence of Api g 1 determined by Edman degradation is underlined; 3 different amino acid residues present in Mal d 1-isoforms are included.

4. DISCUSSION

The phenomenon of crossreactivities of pollen allergens and allergenic proteins derived from various food stuff is already well-observed and some are summed up as the "mugwort-celery-birch syndrome" (Lit. L. Bauer, see this volume) or the "apple-birch syndrome" (1). This crossreactivity is based on homologous IgE-binding proteins present in various tissues and species as it has been shown in IgE-immunoblotting and inhibition assays (2,3) as well as N-terminal amino acid sequencing.

Using recently cloned new Bet v 1-homologous allergens from celery (*Apium graveolens*) and apple (*Malus domestica*), crossreactivity is shown in IgE immunoblots and sequence comparison. Since 50% of allergic patients sera tested, displayed IgE-binding to Api g 1 and Mal d 1 respectively, we consider these proteins major allergens (data not shown).

Inhibition assays revealed the immunological potency of Bet v 1 - covering a broad range of possible B-cell epitopes, thus leading to a 100% inhibition of binding to rApi g 1 bound to nitrocellulose membranes, whereas preincubation with Api g 1 only succeeds in partial blocking of IgE-binding to recBet v 1 (data not shown).

This crossreactivity could not yet be demonstrated on the T-cell level, since linear T-cell epitopes known from Bet v 1 (13) are too diverse from Api g 1 coding sequence (data not shown).

Presenting sequences coding for major allergens from celery and apple, Api g 1 and Mal d 1, the spectrum of available, well defined recombinant allergens is enlarged and ready to be used for precise diagnosis for food hypersensitivity. Furthermore, we think that these purified and well defined recombinant proteins are superior to raw protein extracts containing hindering components like carbohydrates, phenolic compounds etc.

At the moment, we are unable to distinguish by positive immunoblotting to food allergens, whether patients with established birch pollen allergy have already developed food hypersensitivity or will in near future develop allergic reactions to certain vegetables and/or fruits. Nevertheless, the fact that allergenic proteins related to tree pollen allergens are present in numerous fruits and vegetables may point at their clinical relevance.

Further investigations have to be made, to decide whether a single molecule - Bet v 1 - will be sufficient to diagnose tree pollen allergy as well as related food hypersensitivity, or if the whole panel of related food allergens will be necessary.

ACKNOWLEDGMENTS

This work was supported by grant S6002-BIO from the FWF (Austria).

5. REFERENCES

1. Ebner, C., Birkner, T., Valenta, R., Rumpold, H., Breitenbach, M., Scheiner, O., Kraft, D. (1991) *J Allergy Clin Immunol* 88:588–594.
2. Hirschwehr, R., Valenta, R., Ebner, C., Ferreira, F., Sperr, W., Valent, P., Rohac, M., Rumpold, H., Scheiner, O., Kraft, D. (1992) *J Allergy Clin Immunol* 90:927–936.
3. Ebner, C., Hirschwehr, R., Bauer, L., Breiteneder, H., Valenta, R., Ebner, H., Kraft, D., Scheiner, O. (1995) *J Allergy Clin Immunol* (in press).
4. WHO/IUIS (1994) Allergen nomenclature *ACI News* 6, 38–44.

5. Ferreira, F., Hoffmann-Sommerguber, K., Breiteneder, H., Pettenburger, K., Ebner, C., Sommergruber, W., Steiner, R., Bohle, B., Sperr, W., Valent, P., Kungl, A., Breitenbach, M., Kraft, D., Scheiner, O. (1993) *J Biol Chem* 268:19574–19580.
6. Chomczynski P., Sacchi, N. (1987) *Anal Biochem* 162:156–159.
7. Sambrook, J., Fritsch, E.F., Maniatis, T. (1989) Molecular cloning: a laboratory manual 2nd edn, Cold Spring Harbor Laboratory, Cold Spring Harbor, N.Y.
8. Vieths, S., Schoening, B., Peterson, A. (1994) *Int Arch Allergy Immunol* 104:399–404.
9. Studier, F., Rosenberg, A., Dunn J., Dubendorff, J. *Methods in Enzymology* 185: 60 - 89.
10. Susani, M., Hoffmann-Sommergruber, K., Ferreira, F., Jertschin, P., Ahorn, H., Breiteneder, H., Kraft, D., Scheiner, O. (1995) *FEBS Letters*, submitted.
11. Gill, S.C., von Hippel, P.H., (1989) *Anal Biochem* 182:319–326.
12. Breiteneder, H., Ferreira, F., Hoffmann-Sommergruber, K., Ebner, C., Breitenbach, M., Rumpold, H., Kraft, D., Scheiner, O. (1993) *Eur J Biochem* 212:355–362,
13. Ebner, C., Szepfalusi, Z., Ferreira, F., Jilek, A., Valenta, R., Parronchi, P., Maggi, E., Romagnani, S., Scheiner, O., Kraft, D. (1993) *J Immunol* 150:1047–1054.

31

IGE AND MONOCLONAL ANTIBODY REACTIVITIES TO THE MAJOR SHRIMP ALLERGEN Pen a 1 (TROPOMYOSIN) AND VERTEBRATE TROPOMYOSINS

Gerald Reese, Deborah Tracey, Carolyn B. Daul, and Samuel B. Lehrer

Tulane University Medical Center
Department of Medicine
Section of Clinical Immunology and Allergy
1700 Perdido Street, New Orleans, Louisiana, 70112

1. ABSTRACT

Pen a 1, the major shrimp allergen from brown shrimp *Penaeus aztecus* has been identified as the muscle protein tropomyosin. To identify Pen a 1 IgE binding sites, the reactivities of Pen a 1-specific monoclonal antibodies (mAbs) and shrimp-allergic subjects' IgE to shrimp and homologous mammalian tropomyosins were analyzed. Pen a 1, purified by preparative SDS-PAGE and commercially obtained porcine, bovine and rabbit tropomyosin were cleaved by CNBr or digested by endoproteinases Lys-C, Glu-C, trypsin, Arg-C and chymotrypsin. Reactivities of Pen a 1-specific mAbs and IgE to the resulting peptides were analyzed by dot blot and immunoblotting. The dot blot analysis showed that mAbs and IgE antibodies did not react with any of the mammalian tropomyosins. The immunoblot analysis showed that all Pen a 1 digests bound IgE or mAbs. However, not all peptides in each digest possessed an IgE binding site. IgE binding intensity and frequency varied by subject and peptide digest. IgE and mAb reactivity patterns were similar but no mAb reproduced the IgE binding patterns indicating that subjects' IgE bound some epitopes that were not recognized by the Pen a 1-specific mAbs. These studies suggest that IgE-binding epitopes are restricted to certain parts of the Pen a 1 molecule, Pen a 1 may have several similar epitopes, and that Pen a 1 epitopes do not appear to be located in the highly homologous parts of the tropomyosin molecule.

2. INTRODUCTION

At least 13 IgE-binding bands had been identified in the extract of brown shrimp (*Penaeus aztecus*). Eighty-two percent of subjects' sera bound to a 36 kD protein, desig-

New Horizons in Allergy Immunotherapy
edited by Sehon et al. Plenum Press, New York, 1996

225

nated as Pen a 1, the only major allergen in shrimp [1]. Pen a 1-like bands were also detected in other crustacea such as crawfish (*Procambarus clarkii*), crab (*Callinectes sapidus*) and lobster (*Panulirus argus*) suggesting a common crustacea allergen [2, 3]. Pen a 1 was identified as the muscle protein tropomyosin by sequencing a 21 amino acid residue peptide obtained by endoproteinase digestion and HPLC purification [1, 4]. This amino acid sequence showed a 60 to 87% sequence homology with tropomyosins ranging from human to fruitfly tropomyosin [4, 5]. The aim of this study was the immunoblot analysis of IgE and Pen a 1-specific mAb reactivities to Pen a 1, homologous vertebrate tropomyosins and their fragments. For these purposes the major shrimp allergen Pen a 1 was purified by preparative SDS-PAGE and purified Pen a 1, chicken, rabbit, beef and porcine tropomyosin were cleaved with CNBr and endoproteinases. The resulting peptide-containing digests were analyzed by immunoblot and dot blot of digests with patients' IgE and Pen a 1-specific mAbs.

3. MATERIAL AND METHODS

3.1. Subjects' Sera

Sera were collected from atopic shrimp-sensitive individuals, with histories of respiratory, dermatologic, or gastrointestinal symptoms occurring within one hour of shrimp ingestion. All individuals were skin test positive (wheal ≥3 mm) to shrimp and demonstrated elevated levels of IgE antibodies (RAST binding ≥3%) to shrimp extract.

3.2. Purification of Pen a 1

Pen a 1 was purified by preparative SDS-PAGE (Model 491 PrepCell, Biorad). Shrimp extract [6] was separated on the 28 mm ID column using Laemmli's discontinuous SDS-PAGE buffer system [7]. A 15 mm-high stacking gel (5%T, 1.5%C) was poured on top of the 60 mm-high separation gel (10%T, 1.5%C). The fractions were analyzed by SDS-PAGE and immunoblotting using a serum pool of shrimp-allergic subjects and Pen a 1-specific (mAbs). Fractions that contained pure Pen a 1 were pooled, dialyzed and lyophilized.

3.3. Production of Monoclonal Antibodies (mAbs)

BALB/c mice were immunized twice at days 1 and 7 with 5 µg of purified Pen a 1. After five weeks, spleen cells were fused with P3X63Ag8.U1 myeloma cells (ATCC CRL 1597) using PEG fusion technique [8, 9]. Cells were screened for antibody-producing hybridomas by ELISA, checked for specificity by immunoblotting and cloned by limiting dilution.

3.4. Peptide Production

100 µg purified Pen a 1 or tropomyosin from beef, pork, rabbit and chicken (Sigma) were incubated overnight in the dark at room temperature in 10% CNBr in 70% formic acid [10]. CNBr products were lyophilized. For endoproteinase digestion, 100 µg tropomyosin were denatured in 50 µl denaturation buffer (50 mM Tris/HCl pH 8.0, 6 M urea, 5 mM DTT) followed by 1:8 dilution in protease buffer (Lys-C: 25 mM Tris/HCl pH

7.7, 1 mM EDTA, Glu-C I: 50 mM NH_4CH_3COO/CH_3COOH pH 4.0; Glu-C II: 50 mM Na_2HPO_4/NaH_2PO_4 pH 7.8; trypsin: 50 mM Tris/HCl pH 7.6, 1 mM $CaCl_2$; alkaline protease: 50 mM Tris/HCl pH 9.0, 5 mM $CaCl_2$; Arg-C: 50 mM Tris/HCl pH 7.5, 1 mM $CaCl_2$, 2 mM DTT; chymotrypsin: 50 mM Na_2HPO_4/NaH_2PO_4 pH 7.0). One μg of enzyme was added and Pen a 1 was digested overnight at 37°C.

3.5. Peptide SDS-PAGE and Immunoblotting

The buffer system of Schägger and von Jagow [11] with slight modifications was used. A 10 mm-high stacking gel (5%T, 2.5%C) was poured on top of the 60 mm-high separation gel (17.5%T, 2.5%C). The cleavage products were diluted in sample buffer and boiled for 5 min. The separated peptides were electrophoretically transferred [12] onto CNBr-activated nitrocellulose membranes [13]. The individual IgE and mAb reactivities were detected using alkaline phosphatase-labeled, monoclonal anti-human-IgE (Southern Biotechnology Associates) and goat anti-mouse-IgG+IgM (Jackson Immunoresearch Laboratories) in combination with the chemiluminescence substrate CSPD (Tropix).

3.6. Dot Test

1 μl of tropomyosins (1 μg/μl) and their digests (1 μg/μl) were applied onto CNBr-activated nitrocellulose membrane. After air-drying and blocking with TBS-Tween, the dot blots were incubated in diluted patients' serum pool (1:100) and mAbs (1:2), respectively. The IgE and mAb reactivities were detected as described above.

4. RESULTS

4.1. Shrimp Tropomyosin Pen a 1

All cleavage procedures, with the exception of alkaline protease digestion, resulted in IgE-binding peptides. Not all Pen a 1 fragments bound IgE or mAbs. Seven/8 shrimp-allergic subjects reacted with Pen a 1 peptides. The IgE binding intensity and frequency varied by subject and peptide digest. For example, Arg-C fragments bound IgE of 6 subjects whereas trypsin fragments were detected by only 3 subjects' IgE; individual subjects reacted up to 7/8 Pen a 1 digests (Table 1). Depending on the digest, the IgE-binding peptides had a molecular weight as high as 20 kD and as low as 4 kD. Six/9 of the Pen a 1-specific mAbs reacted with Pen a 1 peptides and all 6 to IgE-binding peptides. Six/8 cleavage procedures (CNBr, Lys-C, Glu-C I, Glu-C II, trypsin, Arg-C) produced both IgE and mAb binding peptides whereas the digestion with chymotrypsin produced only IgE binding peptides. IgE and mAb reactivities showed similar but not identical binding patterns (Figure 1). An 8 kD CNBr peptide was detected by both mAb 8 and IgE whereas a 14 kD peptide was only detected by mAb 8. The mAbs 1 to 4 showed their strongest reactivities to an 18 kD Lys-C fragment whereas the most intense IgE binding occurred to 10 to 18 kD fragments.

4.2. Beef, Pork, Rabbit and Chicken Tropomyosin

Pen a 1-specific mAbs and Pen a 1-specific IgE of shrimp-allergic subjects did not bind to any of the vertebrate tropomyosins both by dot blot and immunoblot analysis (Figure 2).

Table 1. Intensity of individual IgE and mAb reactivities (– to ++++) to Pen a 1 digests. mAb reactivities representing mAb binding with IgE-binding Pen a 1 peptides are shaded

	Reactivities of																
	Subjects (IgE)								Monoclonal Antibodies								
digest	1	2	3	4	5	6	7	8	1	2	3	4	5	6	7	8	9
CNBr	++++	–	–	++	++	++	–	++	–	–	–	–	–	–	–	++	–
Lys-C	++++	–	–	++++	++++	++	++	–	+++	+++	+++	+++	+++	–	–	+++	–
Glu-C I	++++	–	–	+++	++	+	–	–	–	++	++	++	–	–	–	–	–
Glu-C II	++++	–	–	+++	++	–	–	–	–	++	++	++	–	–	–	–	–
trypsin	+++	–	++	–	+	–	–	–	–	+	+	+	–	–	–	–	–
alkaline protease	–	–	–	–	–	–	–	–	–	–	–	–	–	–	–	–	–
Arg-C	++++	–	++	++	++++	++++	+++	–	–	+++	+++	+++	+++	–	–	+++	–
chymotrypsin	++++	–	+++	+++	+	–	–	–	–	–	–	–	–	–	–	–	–

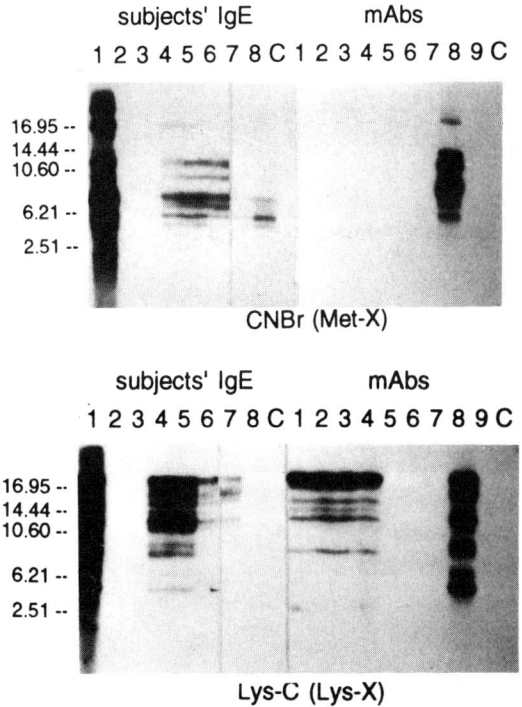

Figure 1. Comparison of IgE and mAb reactivities to CNBr and Lys-C cleavage-derived Pen a 1 fragments.

5. DISCUSSION

Immunologically active, IgE-binding Pen a 1, purified by preparative SDS-PAGE, was cleaved by CNBr and endoproteinases Lys-C, Glu-C, trypsin, alkaline protease, Arg-C and chymotrypsin. With the exception of alkaline protease digestion, all cleavage procedures resulted in IgE-binding peptides. Not all peptides generated bound IgE. indicating that IgE-binding epitopes are restricted to certain parts of Pen a 1. cleavage by CNBr, Lys-C, trypsin, Glu-C and Arg-C resulted in mAb-binding peptides. In contrast to IgE reactivities, chymotrypsin fragments were not detected by any mAb. Since the same mAb reacted

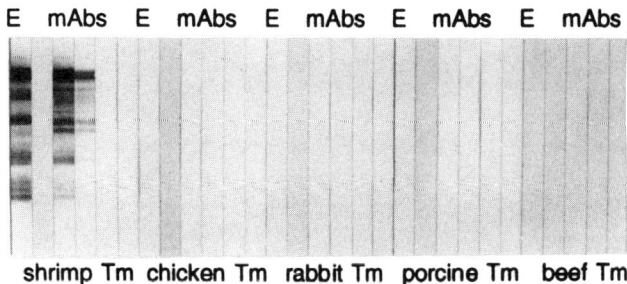

Figure 2. IgE and mAb reactivities to Lys-C peptides of shrimp (Pen a 1), chicken, rabbit, porcine and beef tropomyosins (Tm's).

to different peptides from the same digest, Pen a 1 may have several similar epitopes. The comparison of IgE and mAb reactivities demonstrated similar but not identical binding, indicating that these Pen a 1-specific mAbs and subjects' IgE bound to different epitopes. Pen a 1-specific mAbs and IgE did not bind highly homologous vertebrate tropomyosins from chicken, rabbit, beef and pork indicating that IgE and mAb binding epitopes may be restricted to the variable parts of Pen a 1. Further sequence analysis and epitope mapping of Pen a 1 and other tropomyosins will advance our understanding of the molecular basis and pathogenesis of shrimp allergy in particular and food allergy in general.

6. ACKNOWLEDGMENT

This study was supported by a grant from the National Fisheries Institute (NFI).

7. REFERENCES

1. Daul CB, Slattery M, Reese G, Lehrer SB: Identification of the major brown shrimp (*Penaeus aztecus*) as the muscle protein tropomyosin. Int Arch Allergy Clin Immunol 1994;105:49–55.
2. Daul CB, Slattery M, Morgan JE, Lehrer SB: Identification of a common major crustacea allergen. J Allergy Clin Immunol 1992;89:194.
3. Halmepuro L, Salvaggio JE, Lehrer SB: Crawfish and lobster allergens: Identification and structural similarities with other crustacea. Int Arch Allergy Appl Immunol 1987;84:165–72.
4. Daul CB, Slattery M, Morgan JE, Lehrer SB: Common crustacea allergens: identification of B cell epitopes with shrimp-specific monoclonal antibodies; in Kraft D, Sehon A (eds): Molecular Biology and Immunology of Allergens. Boca Raton, CRC Press, 1993, pp 291–294.
5. Daul CB, Slattery M, Lehrer SB: Shared antigenic/allergenic epitopes between shrimp Pen a I and fruit fly extract. J Allergy Clin Immunol 1993;91:341.
6. Daul CB, Morgan JE, Waring NP, McCants ML, Hughes J, Lehrer SB: Immunologic evaluation of shrimp-allergic individuals. J Allergy Clin Immunol 1987;80:716–721.
7. Laemmli UK: Cleavage of structural proteins during the assembly of the head of bacteriophage T4. Nature 1970;227:680–685.
8. Goding JW: Antibody production by hybridomas. J Immunol Methods 1980;39:285–308.
9. Kehler G: The technique of hybridoma production; in Lefkovits I, Pernis B (eds): Immunological Methods, Academic Press, New York, 1981, vol 2, pp 285–298.
10. Gross E: The cyanogen bromide reaction. Methods Enzymol 1967;11:238–255.
11. Schägger H, von Jagow G: Tricine-sodium dodecyl-polyacrylamide gel electrophoresis for the separation of proteins in the range from 1 to 100 kDa. Anal Biochem 1987;166:368–379.
12. Kyhse-Andersen J: Electroblotting of multiple gels: a simple apparatus without buffer tank for rapid transfer of proteins from polyacrylamide to nitrocellulose. J Biochem Biophys Methods 1984;10:203–209.
13. Demeulemester C, Peltre G, Laurent M, Pankeleux D, David B: Cyanogen bromide-activated nitrocellulose membranes: A new tool for immunoprint techniques. Electrophoresis 1987;8:71–73.

32

IMMUNOMODULATION WITH T CELL REACTIVE PEPTIDES

Barbara P. Wallner and Mohammad Luqman

ImmuLogic Pharmaceutical Corporation
610 Lincoln Street
Waltham, Massachusetts 02154

1. INTRODUCTION

The tremendous advances made in the identification and characterization of major environmental allergens over the last decade have made it possible to design therapies which are targeted to specific points in the allergic cascade. Proposed therapies include those which modulate either the activity or the production of cytokines, the binding of IgE to FcεRI on effector cells or the production of IgE antibodies. Considerable attention also has been given to treatments which directly modulate allergen-specific T cell responses[1-3]. This concept has been realized in the therapeutic treatment of allergies with soluble allergenic extracts. Immunotherapy in this form has proven to be efficacious[4-6] and in some studies, clinical benefits have been correlated directly with downregulation of allergen specific T cell responses, such as T cell proliferation and cytokine production[7-11].

Immunotherapy with soluble allergenic extracts, although successful, carries the risk of severe IgE mediated side effects due to interactions of the full length allergens with their specific IgE antibodies following administration[4-6]. A logical therapeutic approach therefore is to take advantage of the observation that certain regions (epitopes) within an antigen (or allergen) are sufficient to elicit immune responses to that antigen. When immunodominant T cell epitopes are administered under non-immunogenic conditions, unresponsiveness of the immune system to subsequent immunogenic challenges with that antigen is observed[12-14]. In most cases, immunodominant T cell epitopes are distinct from sequences that interact with antibodies and in the case of allergens can therefore be dissected away from IgE antibody binding regions. Peptides then can be administered at high concentrations over a short period of time leading to downregulation of allergy associated immune functions without eliciting IgE mediated side effects. In this paper, the determination of clinical peptide candidates, their effect on primary immune responses in murine models, as well as their effect on allergic symptoms in a clinical trial setting will be discussed.

New Horizons in Allergy Immunotherapy
edited by Sehon et al. Plenum Press, New York, 1996

231

2. IMMUNOLOGICAL BASIS FOR IMMUNOTHERAPY

The modulation of T cell responses observed during immunotherapy is analogous to effects seen in a number of experimental models, where administration of antigens under tolerizing conditions causes downregulation of antigen specific T cell responses to subsequent immunogenic challenges with the respective antigen[14,15]. In these studies, T cell unresponsiveness was demonstrated by the inability of T cells to proliferate or to produce cytokines in response to antigenic stimuli. The involvement of T cell derived cytokines in the initiation and maintenance of the allergic state has been well established. Allergic effector cells such as mast cells, eosinophil and basophils require cytokines for their growth, differentiation, as well as for their priming and activation to degranulate in response to allergen.[16–19]. Thus the success of immunotherapy with soluble allergenic extracts may at least in part be due to the inhibition of secretion of T cell derived cytokines that drive the allergic state. The improvement of clinical symptoms during immunotherapy prior to any significant changes in IgE levels, implies that an earlier stage of the allergic cascade must be affected by the treatment.

For a positive immune response to occur, the initial signal transmitted to T cells via the TCR must be accompanied by other activating costimulatory events[15]. These events range from interactions between cell surface receptor/ligand pairs on T cells and APCs such as CD28 and B7[20], the secretion of lymphocyte specific cytokines and growth factors, to the release of inflammatory mediators by a number of effector cells.(for review, see Mueller and Jenkins[21]). The type of costimulatory events and the sequence in which they occur define the quantitative and qualitative T cell responses to an antigen. In the absence of activating cofactors T cells become unresponsive to subsequent challenges with the antigen possibly due to their inability to produce cytokines required for proliferation and subsequent events of the immune response. It has been shown that T cell anergy caused by blocking certain costimulatory signals during antigen presentation can be overcome by the addition of cytokines such as IL-2, IL-4 or IL-7[22,23].

Another variable to be considered is the route of administration. Although, by itself, the route of administration does not influence the therapeutic outcome, the mechanisms by which that outcome is affected is dependent on the route and dose of administration. Orally, subcutaneously, intravenously or intranasally administered peptides all exert similar effects on immune responses or disease modulation[24–26]. The mechanism by which this is accomplished however is dependent on a number of different factors. For example, repeated subcutaneous or intravenous injections of peptides lead to suppression of cytokine production from antigen specific T cells. This occurs either through induction of T cell anergy, or at very high peptide concentrations, through apoptosis of peptide specific T cells[14,27], (M. Luqman manuscript in preparation). Modulation of immune responses by peptides via the mucosal system can occur through anergy when administered intranasally or orally at high peptide concentrations[24,25]. Oral administration of full length antigens can induce anergy at high dose and works by eliciting production of suppressor factors at repeated low doses[28–30]. The importance of antigen presentation by thymic dendritic cells in the induction of peripheral T cell tolerance has recently been shown by Weiner and coworkers[31]. Although our understanding is still incomplete with regard to the relationship between the route of administration and the precise mechanism of induction of T cell unresponsiveness, it has become apparent that the micro-environment in which antigen presentation occurs dictates the functional consequences of T cell responses.

3. DEFINING PEPTIDE PRODUCT CANDIDATES

In defining peptides to be included in a therapeutic product, aspects of T cell activation must be considered. (1) The major histocompatibility complex (MHC) haplotypes within the human population are diverse and different MHC alleles exhibit different peptide specificities. (2) Most allergens contain more than one T cell reactive epitope, some of which are clearly dominant in terms of stimulation of T cell proliferation or cytokine production *in vitro*.

To account for the diversity of MHC haplotypes, a large panel of allergic patients must be tested in order to define a peptide candidate. An immunogenic peptide containing T cell reactive epitopes of an antigen is recognized by its specific T cell receptor (TCR) when presented in the context of class II major histocompatibility complex (MHC) on the surface of an antigen presenting cell (APC). This recognition is highly specific for the TCR and dependent on the amino acid sequence of the peptide as well as on its physical interactions with residues of the peptide binding groove of particular MHC class II molecules[32]. Despite this high level of specificity, some peptides will bind to different MHC alleles[33]. In fact, it is advantageous to find peptides that are promiscuous in their binding to MHC, in order to derive a therapeutic that will benefit a broad spectrum of patients[34]. We have found for example, that two peptides identified to contain immunodominant epitopes for the cat allergen *Fel d 1* (discussed below) are recognized by 80–90% of patients tested (Garman, R.D., manuscript in preparation). Although, these peptides are 27 amino acids long and probably contain more than one T cell reactive epitope, promiscuity of interaction between these peptides and different HLA alleles almost certainly contributes to the high frequency of recognition.

The immunogenicity of a peptide is not only dictated by its ability to be presented by the HLA molecule, but also by the magnitude of the T cell response. Thus the objective is to define peptides which elicit strong T cell responses. The peptides that contain dominant T cell epitopes of an allergen are selected based on their ability to stimulate T cell reactivity in *in vitro* assays in the majority of allergic patients tested. Typically, T cell epitopes which elicit strong T cell responses *in vitro* are also potent tolerogens of primary immune responses in *in vivo* animal models[14,35]. The relative magnitude of T cell responses to synthetic overlapping peptides spanning the entire region of the allergen is determined using allergen specific T cell lines or clones established from atopic patient peripheral blood lymphocytes. In this way, T cell reactive epitopes have been determined for a number of allergens including grass pollen[36], cat pelt[14], house dust mite[37], birch pollen[38], and bee venom PLA$_2$[39]. Our approach in defining T cell epitope containing peptides has been to establish allergen specific T cell lines rather than T cell clones, because this assures that the total potential TCR repertoire for antigenic epitopes within the allergen is retained. In addition, T cell lines, but not clones, allow a direct comparison of T cell reactivity within an entire set of overlapping peptides in individual patients and within a patient population (Garman, R. et al, manuscript submitted).

The relative importance of T cell responses to individual peptides are assessed by taking into account both the magnitude of T cell responses to each peptide and the frequency of response within the patient population tested. In this way, T cell reactive epitope maps can be established which allow the identification of peptides containing dominant epitopes. Figure 1 shows the T cell epitope map of *Fel d 1*, clearly distinguishing two regions at the N-terminus of the chain I of *Fel d 1* from minor regions in the rest of the allergen. For the definition of clinical peptide candidates, immunodominant regions are remapped for the location of T cell reactive epitopes by using a different set of over-

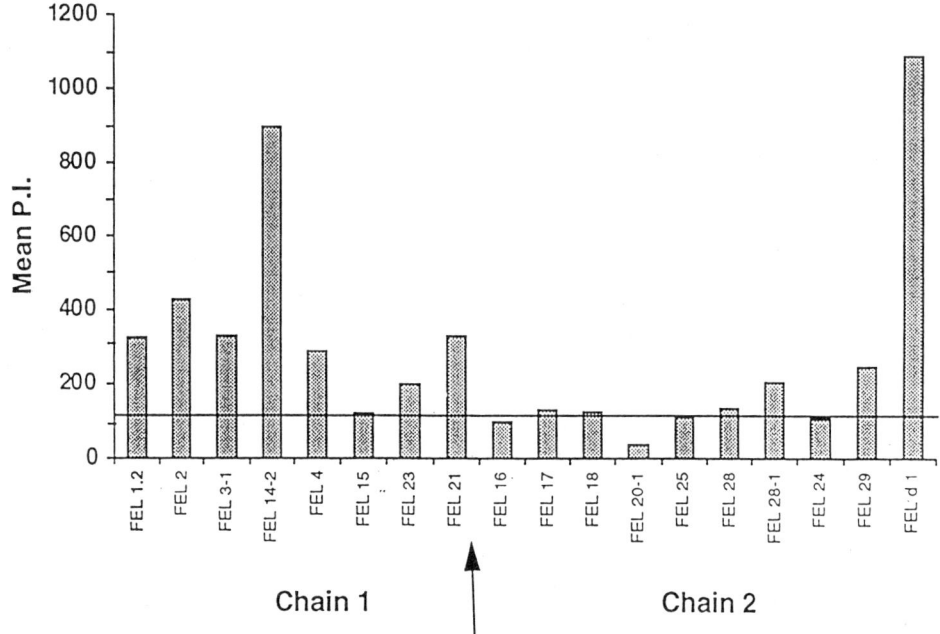

Figure 1. T cell epitope map of *Fel d* 1. Peripheral blood lymphocytes from cat allergic individuals (n=43) were cultured with full length *Fel d* 1 to establish *Fel d* 1 specific T cell lines. Aliquots of these lines were tested with an overlapping set of *Fel d* 1 specific peptides for their ability to stimulate T cell proliferation. The magnitude of the T cell response for each peptide (expressed as fold stimulation over the background) multiplied by the percent frequency of peptide response in the patient population gives a value (positivity index) which allows the evaluation of the relative T cell relativity of each peptide within the total peptide set. Numbers on the X axis indicate peptides; the Y axis represents the mean positivity index (P.I.).

lapping peptides of various lengths covering these regions. In this way, the shortest peptide sequence still retaining the T cell reactive epitopes originally identified can be determined[40]. Using this approach, two peptides, IPC-1 and IPC-2, specific for the N-terminal sequence of *Fel d* 1 have been identified and developed as product candidates. Since it is essential that peptides developed as therapeutic candidates, lack IgE antibody binding epitopes, both IPC-1 and IPC-2 have been tested rigorously in *in vitro* histamine release assays using blood basophils from cat allergic individuals as well as in ELISA based IgE binding assays for their IgE binding reactivity (Garman, R. et al, manuscript submitted). These two peptide candidates have been tested in clinical trials for their effectiveness to downregulate allergic symptoms and the results from one study will be discussed below. Applying similar strategies described above, we have defined clinical peptide candidates specific for other allergens including ragweed pollen *Amb a* I, house dust mite *Der p* I and *Der p* II; grass pollen *Lol p* I and *Lol p* V, as well as for Japanese cedar pollen *Cry j* I (B. Wallner, unpublished results).

4. PRECLINICAL STUDIES FOR PEPTIDE BASED IMMUNOTHERAPY

The ability of soluble antigens or antigenic peptides to induce peripheral T and B cell unresponsiveness has been demonstrated in a number of different experimental model systems[14,15,23]. Peptides containing immunodominant T cell epitopes for antigens such as the major allergen in cat pelt extract, *Fel d* 1[14] the house dust mite allergen, *Der p* I[24,25], and type II collagen[41] have been used successfully in murine and rat models to induce T cell unresponsiveness to subsequent immunogenic challenge with the peptide or the full length protein from which they were derived. Typically, unresponsiveness has been assessed by measuring the ability of isolated T cells to proliferate or secrete cytokines in response to antigen or by the absence of antigen specific antibody synthesis *in vivo*.

Briner and co-workers[14] established that the two peptides derived from chain I *Fel d* 1, IPC-1 and IPC-2, when administered subcutaneously in PBS, substantially diminish T cell responses to subsequent immunogenic challenges with peptides or with full-length chain I *Fel d* 1. T cells from treated mice showed a decreased ability to synthesize cytokines of both the TH_1 and TH_2 phenotype, namely IL-2, IL-4, IL-3 and IFN-γ[14]. In the present study, we were able to extend these findings to show that peptide treatment also resulted in reduced synthesis of IL-5 and IL-10 and in the reduction of eosinophil infiltration into airways. In this set of experiments, $B6CBAF_1$ mice were treated with peptides IPC-1 and IPC-2 subcutaneously in PBS five and ten days before challenge with chain 1 *Fel d* 1 in adjuvant (CFA or alum). Fourteen days after administration of *Fel d* 1 in adjuvant, mice were challenged intratraehaly with chain 1 *Fel d* 1 and bronchial lavages were collected for eosinophil count. Control mice received only PBS injection without peptides. As shown in Figure 2, the number of eosinophil infiltrating airways in mice treated with peptides was only 30% of the number observed in control mice.

Lymphocytes from mice treated with IPC-1 and IPC-2 as described above, when challenged with antigen *in vitro* secreted substantially lower amounts of IL-2, IL-5, IL-10, and IL-4 than control mice (Figure 3). These cytokines, in addition to other TH_2 type cytokines such as IL-6, GMCSF and IL-13 contribute substantially to allergic responses[17,18]. IL-4 and IL-10 inhibit TH_1 type inflammatory responses[42] while they promote mast cell differentiation and growth[43]. IL-5 induces eosinophil growth and differentiation and functions as a chemotactic factor for eosinophils[19,44]. IL-5, IL-4, and GMCSF prime and activate basophils and mast cells to degranulate in response to crosslinking agents[16]. Incubation of human basophils with IL-3, IL-5, or GMCSF *in vitro* primes and activates these cells so that the concentration of allergen required for histamine release is dramatically reduced (M. Kasaian, personal communication). Together, these results indicate that quantitative as well as qualitative changes in cytokine production after peptide treatment can modulate allergic effector cell function and immune responses in addition to regulating IgE antibody production. The murine model described above also illustrates that peripheral T cell unresponsiveness to full length antigen after peptide treatment affects physiological responses to the antigen.

Peptide therapy also has been shown to be effective in inhibiting disease progression in a series of rodent models for autoimmune diseases. Administration of peptides immunoreactive with autoantigen specific T cells in PBS or IFA abrogate disease onset or reverses ongoing disease in models such as collagen-induced RA[41],IDDM[45] and EAE (a model for human MS). For example, specific peptides of myelin basic protein (MBP), prevent, or reverse MBP induced EAE, and reduce incidence of disease relapse when administered under tolerogenic conditions[35,46].

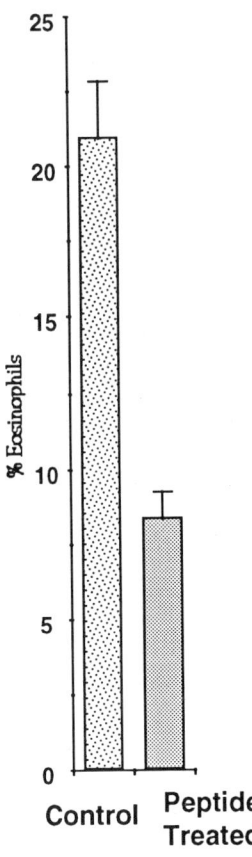

Figure 2. Control and peptide-injected mice were challenged intratrachealy with chain 1 *Fel d* 1 in PBS. 48 h after the challenge, bronchial lavage was collected and cells were spun down onto slides using a cytocentrifuge. Slides were stained with Wright's stain and put under oil immersion for cell count. Results are expressed as percentage of total cells.

5. CLINICAL STUDY RESULTS ON THE EFFECTIVENESS OF PEPTIDE TREATMENT FOR ALLERGIES

The effect of cat allergen *Fel d* 1 derived peptides, IPC-1 and IPC-2 were examined for their clinical efficacy in a double blinded, placebo controlled clinical trial. Peptides were administered subcutaneously once per week for four weeks at 3 different doses (7.5 µg, 75 µg and 750 µg) and their effect evaluated before and after peptide treatment by comparing allergic symptoms during exposure to cats in a room where cats were housed continuously and *Fel d* 1 levels monitored. Patients treated with the 75 µg and 750 µg doses showed statistically significant decreases in nose and lung symptoms 6 weeks after treatment. A trend analysis showed a dose related improvement in total allergic symptom scores with 86.4% of the patients improving about 50% or more in the high dose groups, compared to 62.5 % of patients in the placebo group improving about 20%[47] (Norman, P. et al, manuscript in preparation). As had been observed previously in immunotherapy studies with soluble extracts[4], allergen specific serum IgE antibody levels had not decreased at the time when clinical benefits could be observed. However since the treatment extended only over a period of 4 weeks, a decrease of allergen specific IgE antibody production had not been expected. No measurements of T cell derived cytokine production were performed in this study and the mechanism by which peptide therapy affected allergic symptoms must still be determined. By analogy to animal models, one can speculate

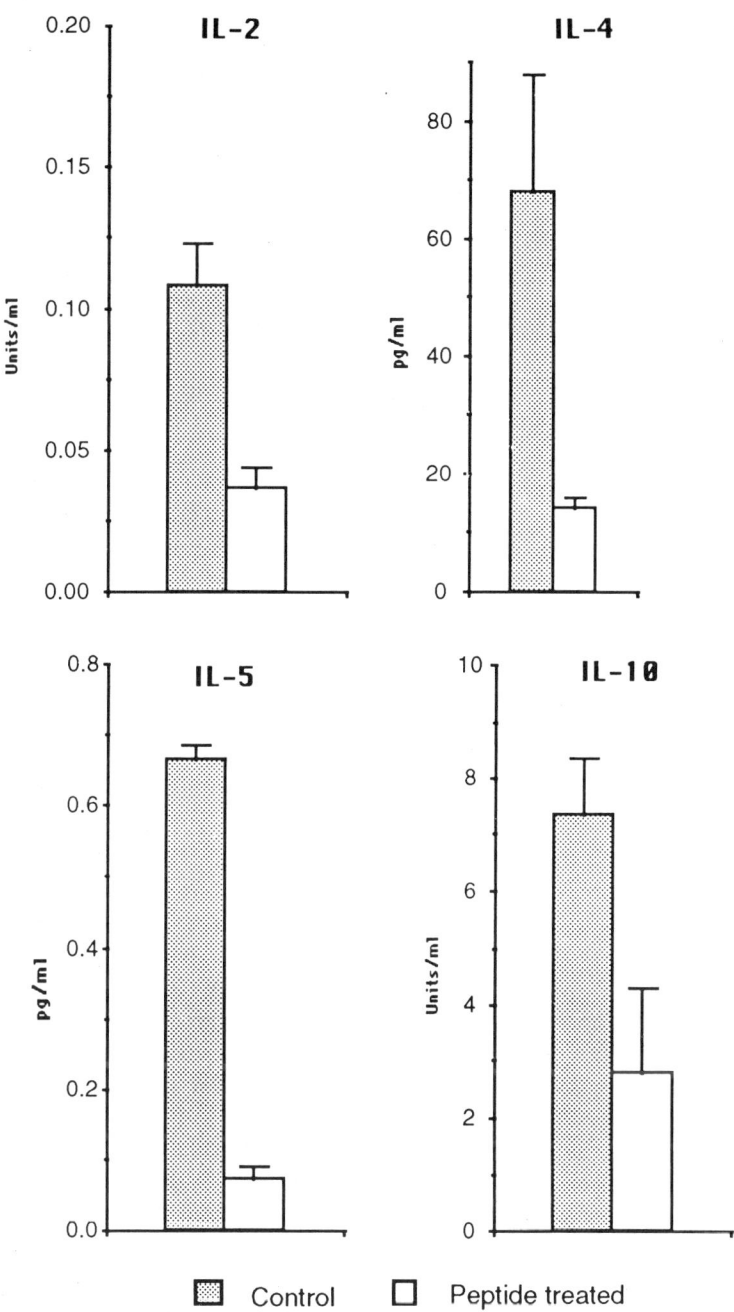

Figure 3. CD4+ enriched T cells from spleens of control and peptide injected mice were stimulated *in vitro* with 150 μg of chain 1 *Fel d* 1 in the presence of irradiated splenocytes as APC. Supernatants were removed at 24h for IL-2, 48h for IL-4, and at day 5 for IL-5 and IL-10 detection. IL-2 and IL-4 levels in the culture S/N were determined by indicator cell lines CTLL and CT4.5 respectively according to published procedures (Briner, et al). IL-4 and IL-5 amounts were determined using ELISA kits according to vendor's recommendation (Endogen Inc., Boston, MA).

that the immediate improvement of clinical symptoms observed may be a consequence of a decrease in the production of specific cytokines involved in the maintenance of the allergic state.

The mechanism by which peptide therapy modulates allergic immune responses both, in murine models as well as in human studies has to be further studied. Well controlled assays performed during future clinical trials will help to elucidate the mechanism of peptide therapy in allergic patients.

REFERENCES

1. Gefter, M. L. 1992. A new generation of antigens for immunotherapy. In *Current therapy in allergy, immunology, and rheumatology*. L.M. Lichtenstein and A. Fauci, eds. C. V. Mosby, St. Louis, MO, p. 376.
2. O'Hehir, R. E., R. D. Garman, J. L. Greenstein, and J. R. Lamb. 1991. The specificity and regulation of T cell responsiveness to allergens. *Annu. Rev. Immunol. 9*:67.
3. Schad, V. C., R. D. Garman, and J. L. Greenstein. 1991. The potential use of T cell epitopes to alter the immune response. *Seminars in Immunology 3*:217.
4. Creticos, P. S. 1992. Immonologic changes associated with immunotherapy. In *Immunology and allergy clinics of North America: immunotherapy of IgE-mediated disorders*. P.A. Greenberger, ed. W. B. Saunders, Philadelpha, PA, p. 13.
5. McHugh, S. M., B. Lavelle, D. M. Kemeny, S. Patel, and P. W. Ewan. 1990. A placebo-controlled trial of immunotherapy with two extracts of Dermatophagoides pteronyssinus in allergic rhinitis, comparing clinical outcome with changes in antigen-specific IgE, IgG, and IgG subclasses. *J. Allergy Clin. Immunol. 86(4)*:521.
6. Lichtenstein, L. M., K. Ishizaka, and P. S. et al Norman. 1973. IgE antibody measurements in ragweed hay fever: Relationship to clinical severity and the results of immunotherapy. *J. Clin. Invest. 52*:472.
7. Greenstein, J. L., J. P. Morgenstern, and J. et al LaRaia. 1992. Ragweed immunotherapy decreases T cell reactivity to recombinant *Amb a* I.1. *J. Allergy Clin. Immunol. 89*:322.(Abstract)
8. Secrist, H., C. J. Chelen, Y. Wen, J. D. Marshall, and D. T. Umetsu. 1993. Allergen immunotherapy decreases interleukin-4 production in CD4+ T cells from allergic individuals. *J. Exp. Med. 178*:2123.
9. Varney, V. A., Q. A. Hamid, M. Gaga, S. Ying, M. Jacobson, A. J. Frew, A. B. Kay, and S. R. Durham. 1993. Influence of grass pollen immunotherapy on cellular infiltration and cytokine mRNA expression during allergen-induced late-phase cutaneous responses. *J. Clin. Invest. 92*:644.
10. Jutel, M., W. J. Pichler, D. Kkrbic, A. Urwyler, C. Dahinden, and U. R. Muller. 1995. Bee venom immunotherapy results in decrease of IL-4 and IL-5 and increase of IFNγ secretion in specific allergen-stimulated T cell cultures. *J. Imm. 154*:4187.
11. Tokushima, M., M. L. Sanz, M. D. de las Marinas, and A. Oehling. 1990. Lymphocyte response to IgE regulatory factors in allergic patients during the course of immunotherapy. *Allergol. Immunopathol. (Madr.) 18*–2:69.
12. Lamb, J. R., B. J. Skidmore, N. Green, J. M. Chiller, and M. Feldmann. 1983. Induction of tolerance in influenza virus immune T lymphocyte clones with synthetic peptides of influenza haemagglutinin. *J. Exp. Med. 157*:1434.
13. Schwartz, R. H. 1990. A cell culture model for T lymphocyte clonal anergy. *Science 248*:1349.
14. Briner, T. J., M-C. Kuo, K. M. Keating, B. L. Rogers, and J. L. Greenstein. 1993. Peripheral T cell tolerance induced in naive and primed mice by subcutaneous injection of peptides from the major cat allergen. *Proc. Natl. Acad. Sci. 90*:7608.
15. Mueller, D. L., M. K. Jenkins, and R. H. Schwartz. 1989. Clonal expansion versus functional clonal inactivation: a costimulatory signalling pathway determines the outcome of T cell antigen receptor occupancy. *Annu. Rev. Immunol. 7*:445.
16. Schleimer, R. P., C. P. Derse, B. Friedman, S. Gillis, M. Plaut, L. M. Lichtenstein, and D. W. Jr. MacGlashan. 1989. Regulation of human basophil mediator release by cytokines. I. Interaction with antiinflammatory steroids. *J. Immunol. 143*:1310.
17. Kay, A. B., S. Ying, V. Varney, M. Gaga, S. R. Durham, R. Moqbel, A. J. Wardlaw, and Q. Hamid. 1991. Messenger RNA expressing of the cytokine gene cluster, interleukin-3 (IL-3), IL-4, IL-5 and granulocyte/macrophage colony-stimulating factor in allergen-induced late phase reactions in atopic subjects. *J. Exp. Med. 173*:775.

18. Robinson, D., Q. Hamid, A. Bentley, S. Ying, A. B. Kay, and S. R. Durham. 1993. Activation of CD4+ T cells, increased Th2-type cytokine in RNA expression and eosinophil recruitment in bronchoavellar lavage after inhalation challenge in patients with atopic asthma. *J. Allergy Clin. Immunol. 92*:313.

19. Ohnishi, T., H. Kita, D. Weiler, S. Sur, J. G. Sedgwick, W. J. Calhoun, W. W. Busse, S. S. Abrams, and G. J. Gileich. 1993. IL-5 is the predominant eosinophil-active cytokine in the antigen-induced pulmonary late phase reaction. *Am. Rev. Respir. Dis. 147*:901.

20. Krummel, M. F. and J. P. Allison. 1995. CD28 and CTLA-4 have opposing effects on the response of T cells to stimulation. *J. Exp. Med. 182*:459.

21. Mueller, D. L. and M. K. Jenkins. 1995. Molecular mechanisms underlying functional T-cell unresponsiveness. *Current Opinion in Immunology 7*:375.

22. Boussiotis, V. A., D. L. Barber, T. Nakarai, G. J. Freeman, J. G. Gribben, G. M. Bernstein, A. D. D'Andrea, J. Ritz, and L. M. Nadler. 1994. Prevention of T cell anergy by signaling through the γ_c chain of the IL-2 receptor. *Science 266*:1039.

23. DeSilva, D. R., K. B. Urdahl, and M. K. Jenkins. 1991. Clonal anergy is induced *in vitro* by T cell receptor occupancy in the absence of proliferation. *J. Immunol. 147*:3261.

24. Hoyne, G. F., M. G. Callow, M-C. Kuo, and W. R. Thomas. 1994. Inhibition of T-cell responses by feeding peptides containing major and cryptic epitopes: Studies with the Der p I allergen. *Immunology 83*:190.

25. Hoyne, G. F., R. E. O'Hehir, D. C. Wraith, W. R. Thomas, and J. R. Lamb . 1993. Inhibition of T cell and antibody responses to house dust mite allergen by inhalation of the dominant T cell epitope in naive and sensitized mice. *J. Exp. Med. 178*:1783.

26. Metzler, B. and D. C. Wraith. 1993. Inhibition of experimental autoimmune encephalomyelitis by inhalation but not oral administration of the encephalitogenic peptide: influence of MHC binding affinity. *Int. Immunology 5*:1159.

27. Critchfield, J. M., M. K. Racke, J. C. Zuniga-Pflücker, B. Cannella, C. S. Raine, J. Goverman, and M. J. Lenardo. 1994. T cell deletion in high antigen dose therapy of autoimmune encephalomyelitis. *Science 263*:1139.

28. Miller, A., O. Lider, and H. L. Weiner. 1991. Antigen-driven bystander suppression after oral administration of antigens. *J. Exp. Med. 174*:791.

29. Miller, A., O. Lider, A. B. Roberts, M. B. Sporn, and H. L. Weiner. 1992. Suppressor T cells generated by oral tolerization to myelin basic protein suppress both *in vitro* and *in vivo* immune responses by the release of transforming growth factor b after antigen-specific triggering. *Proc. Natl. Acad. Sci. USA 89*:421.

30. Friedman, A. and H. L. Weiner. 1994. Induction of anergy or active suppression following oral tolerance is determined by antigen dosage. *Proc. Natl. Acad. Sci. USA 91*:6688.

31. Khoury, S. J., L. Gallon, W. Chen, K. Betres, M. E. Russell, W. W. Hancock, C. B. Carpenter, M. H. Sayegh, and H. L. Weiner. 1995. Mechanisms of acquired thymic tolerance in experimental autoimmune encephalomyelitis: thymic dendritic-enriched cells induce specific peripheral T cell unresponsiveness in vivo. *J. Exp. Med. 182*:357.

32. O'Sullivan, D., T. Arrhenius, J. Sidney, M. F. delGuercio, M. Albertson, M. Wall, C. Oseroff, S. Southwood, S. M. Colon, F. C. Gaeta, and A. Sette. 1991. On the interaction of promiscuous anti-genic peptides with different DR alleles. Identification of common structural motifs. *J. Immunol. 147*:2663.

33. Hammer, J., P. Valsasnini, and K. et al Tolba. 1993. Promiscuous and allele-specific anchors in HLA-DR binding peptides. *Cell 74*:197.

34. Marshall, K., A. Liu, J. Canales, B. Perahia, B. Jorgensen, R. Gantzos, B. Aguilar, B. Devaux, and J. Rothbard. 1994. Role of the polymorphic residues in HLA-DR molecules in allele-specific binding of peptide ligands. *J. Immunol. 152*:4946.

35. Samson, M. F. and D. E. Smilek. 1995. Reversal of acute experimental autoimmune encephalomyelitis and prevention of relapses by treatment with a myelin basic protein peptide analogue modified to form long-lived peptide-MHC complexes. *J. Imm. 155*:2737.

36. Bungy Poor Fard, F. A., Y. Latchman, S. Rodda, M. Geysen, I. Roitt, and J. Brostoff. 1993. T cell epitopes of the major fraction of ryegrass *Lolium perenne* (*Lol p* I) defined using overlapping peptides *in vitro* and *in vivo*. I. Isoallergen clone 1A. *Clin. Exp. Immunol. 94*:111.

37. Higgins, J. A., S. Keswani, and E. R. et al Jarman. 1991. T cell determinants in the group II allergen of *D. pteronyssinus. Allergy 47*:14.

38. Ebner, C., S. Schenk, Z. Szepfalusi, K. Hoffman, F. Ferreira, M. Wilheim, O. Scheiner, and D. Kraft. 1993. Multiple T cell specificities for Bet v I, the major birch pollen allergen, within single individuals. Studies using specific T cell clones and overlapping peptides. *Eur. J. Immunol. 23*:1523.

39. Kuo, M., A. Lussier, A. Brauer, J. F. Bond, and J. L. Greenstein. 1989. Epitope mapping of T cell recognition of pholpholipase A$_2$. *J. Allergy Clin. Immunol. 83*:251.(Abstract)

40. Wallner, B. P. and M. L. Gefter. 1994. Immunotherpy with T-cell-reactive peptides derived from allergens. *Allergy 49*:302.

41. Ku, G., M. Kronenberg, and D. J. et al Peacock. 1993. Prevention of experimental autoimmune arthritis with a peptide fragment of type II collagen. *Eur. J. Immunol. 23*:591.

42. Powrie, F., S. Menon, and R. L. Coffman. 1993. Interleukin-4 and interleukin-10 synergize to inhibit cell mediated immunity in vivo. *Eur. J. Immunol. 23*:3043.

43. Thompson-Snipes, L., V. Dhar, M. W. Bond, T. R. Mosmann, K. W. Moore, and D. Rennick. 1991. Interleukin-10: a novel stimulatory factor for mast cells and their progenitors. *J. Exp. Med. 173*:507.

44. Seminario, M-C. and G. J. Gilrich. 1994. The role of eosinophils in the pathogenesis of asthma. *Current Opinion in Immunology 6*:860.

45. Aichele, P., D. Kyburz, P. S. Ohashi, B. Odermatt, R. M. Zinkernagel, H. Hengartner, and H. Pircher. 1994. Peptide-induced T-cell tolerance to prevent autoimmune diabetes in transgenic mouse model. *Proc. Natl. Acad. Sci. USA 91*:944.

46. Gaur, A., B. Wiers, A. Liu, J. Rothbard, and C. G. Fathman. 1992. Amelioration of autoimmune encephalomyelitis by myelin basic protein synthetic peptide-induced anergy. *Science 258*:1491.

47. Norman, P. S., J. L. Ohman, A. A. Long, P. S. Creticos, M. L. Gefter, Z. Shaked, R. A. Wood, P. A. Eggleston, L. M. Lichtenstein, N. H. Jones, and C. F. Nicodemus. 1995. Follow on study of the first clinical trial with T cell defined peptides from cat allergen *Fel d* I. *J. All. Clin. Imm. 95–1*:259.(Abstract)

33

MOLECULAR CLONING AND IMMUNOLOGICAL CHARACTERIZATION OF THE GROUP 7 ALLERGENS OF HOUSE DUST MITES

H. D. Shen,[1] K. Y. Chua,[2] K. H. Hsieh,[3] and W. R. Thomas[4]

[1]Department of Medical Research
Veterans General Hospital-Taipei
[2]Institute of Immunology and
[3]Department of Pediatrics
National Taiwan University
College of Medicine
Taipei, Taiwan, Republic of China
[4]Institute for Child Health Research
Perth, Australia

The group 7 allergens of house dust mites (both Der p 7 and Der f 7) have been characterized by cDNA cloning. The cDNA clone HD6 of Der p 7 isolated by using human IgE contained DNA encoding a 215 residue protein. The cDNA encoding Der f 7 was amplified using the polymerase chain reaction and cloned into *E. coli*. It encoded a 213 residue protein containing a predicted 17 amino acid leader sequence, no cysteines and a single N-glycosylation site similar to Der p 7. An amino acid sequence identity of 86% of Der f 7 to that of Der p 7 was found. No homologues of both sequences to those of proteins in the data banks were found.

Both Der p 7 and Der f 7 have been expressed as fusion proteins with the glutathione S-transferase (GST). The allergenicity of both fusion proteins was studied by comparing their IgE-binding to that of the Der p 2-GST fusion protein. The results showed that 88% and 46% of the 41 asthmatic sera tested were IgE-positive for Der p 2 and Der p 7, respectively. All of the 19 Der p 7-positive sera showed IgE reactivity to Der p 2. However, 10 (53%) of the 19 samples showed anti-Der p 7 IgE count indices higher than the indices to Der p 2. Seventeen (41%) sera showed IgE-binding to both Der p 7 and Der f 7. Der f 7-specific IgE antibodies were detected in 19 of the 41 (46%) asthmatic sera tested with the degree of binding usually about 30% of that to Der p 7 consistent with the exposure of the patients to *D. pteronyssinus*.

MoAbs against the group 7 allergens were obtained by immunization of BALB/c mice with recombinant Der p 7 and Der f 7, respectively. Results from 2D-immunoblot

New Horizons in Allergy Immunotherapy
edited by Sehon et al. Plenum Press, New York, 1996

analysis showed that components in extracts of *D. pteronyssinus* and *D. farinae* with MWs of about 31, 30 and 26 kDs and pI values from about 5.7 - 6.0 reacted with MoAbs produced. This reduce to 2 bands with MWs of 27 and 26 kDs after treatment with N-glycosidase F suggesting that the 31 and 30 kD reactivities may be different glycosylation products of Der p 7 with a MW of about 27 kD. MoAbs generated may also be used further in the purification and quantitation of the group 7 allergens of house dust mites.

It has therefore been shown that the newly described group 7 allergens of *D. pteronyssinus* and *D. farinae* are of interest because (i) they often elicit IgE antibodies responses as large as those to the major allergen Der p 2 and (ii) because they appear in mite extracts with multiple molecular weights.

REFERENCES

Shen HD, Chua KY, Lin KL, Hsieh KH, Thomas WR. Molecular cloning of a house dust mite allergen with common antibody binding specificities with multiple components in mite extracts. Clin Exp Allergy 23:934–40, 1993.

Shen HD, Chua KY, Lin WL, Hsieh KH, Thomas WR. Characterization of the house dust mite allergen Der p 7 by monoclonal antibodies. Clin Exp Allergy 1995, in press.

Shen HD, Chua KY, Lin WL, Hsieh KH, Thomas WR. Molecular cloning and immunological characterization of the house dust mite allergen Der f 7. Clin Exp Allergy 1995, in press.

Shen HD, Chua KY, Lin WL, Chen HL, Hsieh KH, Thomas WR. IgE and monoclonal antibody binding by the mite allergen Der p 7. Clin Exp Allergy, submitted.

This work was supported by the National Science Council and Veterans General Hospital-Taipei of the Republic of China and the Australian National Health and Medical Research Council, Australia.

34

EPITOPE STRUCTURE OF RECOMBINANT ISOALLERGENS OF Bet v 1

Jørgen Nedergaard Larsen, Susanne Hauschildt Sparholt,
and Henrik Ipsen

ALK-Abelló Research
Bøge Allé 10–12
DK-2970 Hørsholm, Denmark

1. INTRODUCTION

The presence of isoallergens has been demonstrated in all pollen allergens so far studied. A definition of isoallergens may be cited from the publication of the allergen nomenclature (1): "Similar molecules are designated as isoallergens when they share the following common biochemical properties: a. similar molecular size; b. identical biological function, if known, e.g. enzymatic action; and c. > 67% identity of amino acid sequences." Thus, isoallergens differ in aminoacid sequence and show extensive immunochemical cross-reactivity.

Isoallergenic variation may be studied from different angles. When analysed by 2-D electrophoresis and immunoblotting using a rabbit antiserum raised by immunization with purified Bet v 1, a birch pollen extract may be shown to display approx. 25 spots representing isoallergenic variants of Bet v 1. Other approaches based on genetic methodology such as sequencing of multiple clones or the analysis of genomic DNA by Southern blotting concurrently establishes isoallergenic variation as a feature inherent in pollen allergens.

It is to be expected from current models of protein structure, that even single aminoacid substitutions are likely to have a significant effect on the topography of the protein antigen. Thus, even single aminoacid substitutions are likely to affect the affinities of particular antibodies, as well as they may affect the affinities, with which T-cell epitopes bind to HLA-D molecules, or the affinities of the interactions between the T-cell epitope/HLA-D complexes and T-cell receptors.

We have taken an interest into the study of epitope structures of isoallergens since we would like to address the significance of possible differences in epitope structure between isoallergens for the prospect of using for specific immunotherapy single isoallergens in the form of recombinant allergens or synthetic peptides.

New Horizons in Allergy Immunotherapy
edited by Sehon et al. Plenum Press, New York, 1996

2. MATERIALS AND METHODS

2.1 Materials

Pollen extract and rabbit antibodies raised against purified Bet v 1 were prepared as described (2). Monoclonal antibodies (mAbs) were raised in BALB/c mice against purified Bet v 1 or Car b 1.

2.2 Methods

Methods that are not described in detail below were performed according to standard procedures.

2.2.1. Recombinant Allergens. RNA was purified from *Betula verrucosa* pollen (Allergon) using a procedure based on phenol extraction followed by LiCl precipitation (3). Oligo(dT)-cellulose (Boehringer Mannheim) affinity chromatography was performed batch-wise in tubes. Double stranded cDNA synthesis was performed using a commercially available kit (Amersham). The gene encoding Bet v 1 was subsequently specifically amplified in a polymerase chain reaction (PCR), as described (4). The PCR products were cloned into the non-fusion expression plasmids pKK223–3 using *Eco*RI and *Hin*dIII or pKK233–3 using *Nco*I and *Hin*dIII, all restriction sites encoded by the PCR primers. The clones identified by three digit numbers in this communication were expressed in these vectors and recombinant allergens were purified by affinity chromatography using Hi-Trap (Pharmacia) columns coupled with Bet v 1 specific mAb. After elution at pH 2.8 the recombinant allergens were extensively dialysed against phosphate buffered saline. The clones identified by four digit numbers in this communication were subcloned by PCR into the protein fusion vector pMAL-c (New England Biolabs), expressed, and fusion protein was subsequently purified by amylose column affinity chromatography. Recombinant allergen with autentic aminoterminal was released by cleavage using factor X_a, followed by purification by gel filtration (5). All recombinant allergens were more than 95 % pure as judged by digital scanning of silver stained SDS polyacrylamide gels.

2.2.2. Quantitative Chemilumenescence Immuno Inhibition Assay. DynaTech Micro-Lite 2 ELISA trays were coated with 0.1 ml 20mg/ml murine monoclonal antibodies produced in serum free media. After overnight incubation the wells were blocked, washed and incubated for 1 hour with 0.1 ml antigen solution. Antigen solution was a mixture of a dilution series of recombinant Bet v 1 isoallergen and a constant amount of biotinylated highly purified nBet v 1. After washing the wells were incubated for 15 min. with acridiniumester labelled avidin. Wells were finally washed and counted in an ELISA luminometer. Inhibition percentage was calculated as 100*(1-(cpmx - cpm100%)/(cpm0% - cpm100%)) based on average of duplicate experiments.

2.2.3. T-Cell Cloning and Stimulation Assay. Bet v 1 reactive T-cell clones were isolated from a donor clinically allergic to birch pollen. The clones were generated from freshly isolated peripheral blood mononuclear cells and from a long term Bet v 1 reactive T-cell line using standard limiting dilution techniques in the presence of irradiated autologous Eppstein-Barr virus transformed B-cells, 10^3 /well, and irradiated allogeneic PBMCs, 10^4 /well, as antigen presenting cells, 0.5 µg/ml of PHA (Sigma), 10% Lymphocult T (Biotest Folex), and 10 µg/ml of Bet v 1. Growing clones were split when necessary and restimulated every 12 days.

Antigen-specific proliferation was assessed by stimulation of the T-cells, 10^4 /well, by serial dilutions of antigen using irradiated autologous EBV-transformed B-cells as APCs. The cells were cultured for 4 days, the last 12–18 h in the presence of tritiated methylthymidine, 0.5 µCi/well. Finally, the cultures were harvested and specific incorporation expressed as mean cpm of triplicate cultures.

3. RESULTS AND DISCUSSION

3.1. Recombinant Isoallergens of Bet V 1

Gene cloning using PCR amplification is a rather efficient way of obtaining massive amounts of clones in a single experiment, which may be used when some sequence of the gene of interest is available. In this study we have analysed the epitope structure of 6 rBet v 1 isoallergens. Analyses comprise, apart from nucleotide sequencing, quantitative measurement of antibody binding using a small panel of murine monoclonal antibodies and reactivity with T-cells illustrated by 2 clones in standard stimulation assays. The deduced aminoacid sequences of the 6 isoallergens are shown in fig. 1. The sequences are very similar displaying from 1 to 5 aminoacid substitutions. The sequence designated Bet v 1 is identical to the Bet v 1 sequence originally published by H. Breiteneder et al. (6) and to clone #224 and #2230 in this study. Clones designated by a three digit number were expressed as non-fusion proteins in expression vector pKK223 and the recombinant allergens were purified by affinity chromatography using a monoclonal anti Bet v 1 antibody. Clones designated by a four digit number were expressed in pMAL-c as fusion proteins with 'maltose binding protein' as fusion partner, and the fusion proteins were purified by affinity chromatography using an amylose column. Purified fusion proteins were subsequently cleaved by incubation with factor X_a protease, and the recombinant allergen with autentic aminoterminal sequence was then purified by gel filtration (5).

The 6 purified recombinant isoallergens of Bet v 1 were adjusted to equal concentrations based on quantitative measurents by rocket immunoelectrophoresis.

```
          1        10        20        30        40        50        60        70        80
Bet v 1  GVFNYETETTSVIPAARLFKAFILDGDNLFPKVAPQAISSVENIEGNGGPGTIKKISFPEGFPFKYVKDRVDEVDHTNFK
   167   --------------------------------------------------------------------------------
   226   ---------------------G-------------------------------------------G--------------
   280   --------------------------------------------------------------------------------
  2226   ------   ---------------------------------------------------------G-L------------
  2227   -------------------------------------------------------------------L-------------

               90       100       110       120       130       140       150       159
Bet v 1  YNYSVIEGGPIGDTLEKISNEIKIVATPDGGSILKISNKYIITKGDHEVKAEQVKASKEMGETLLRAVESYLLAHSDAYN
   167   ----------V-------------------CV----------N-------------------------------------
   226   --------M--------------------------------------------N-----------------------   -
   280   -----------------------------------------------------R--------------------------
  2226   ----------------------------CV----------N---------------------------------------
  2227   --------------------------------------------------------------------------------
```

Underlined sequence represent synthtic peptides reactive with T-cell clones described in this study.
- denotes aminoacid identities.

Figure 1. Deduced aminoacid sequences of recombinant Bet v 1 isoallergens.

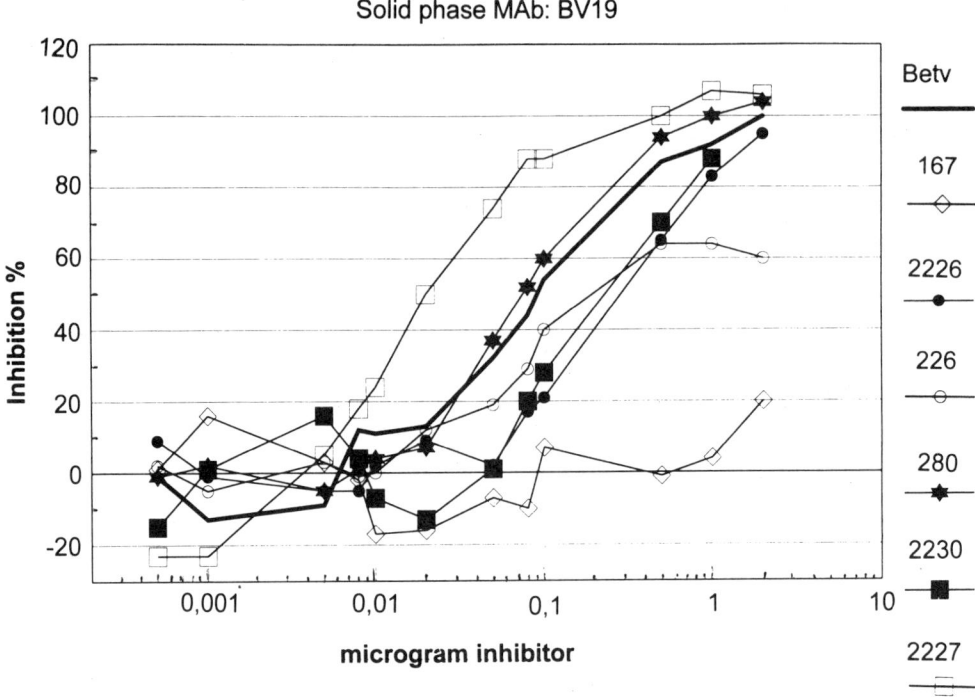

Figure 2. Chemilumenescence immuno inhibition assay.

3.2. Chemiluminescence Immuno Inhibition Assays

Fig. 2 shows an example of data from the chemiluminescence immuno inhibition as-says, and fig. 3 is a summary of data from all experiments. 3 recombinant isoallergens, i.e. al-lergens expressed from clones #280, #2227 and #2230, inhibited the binding of labelled Bet v 1 to the solid phase coated with monoclonal antibody 100% for all 5 antibodies tested. The se-quences of these clones are very similar differing in only one aminoacid. This result is in agreement with earlier results obtained by analysis of clone #224(4), which is identical in se-quence to clone #2230. The 3 other recombinant isoallergens inhibited the binding of Bet v 1 less than 100% for one or more of the monoclonal antibodies tested. The gene product of clone #226 inhibited the binding of Bet v 1 to MAb BV19 only 60%, whereas the gene prod-uct of clone #2226 did not at all inhibit the binding of Bet v 1 to MAb CB11. CB11 was raised by immunization with purified Car b 1, the major allergen of the related tree *Carpinus betu-lus*, hornbeam, and is cross-reactive with Bet v 1 from pollen. One isoallergen, the gene prod-uct of clone #167, did not inhibit the binding of Bet v 1 to any of the monoclonal antibodies BV18, BV19 or CB11, in concentrations up to 20 μg/ml, a concentration which inhibited the binding of Bet v 1 to MAbs BV09 and BV10 100%. The sequences of these three clones dif-fer from the Bet v 1 sequence originally published in 4 or 5 aminoacids.

We conclude from these data that the epitope structure of recombinant isoallergens of Bet v 1 differ. These results fit nicely with a model, in which aminoacid substitutions induce local pertubations in the surface topography, causing differences in the affinity of the binding of particular antibodies. We have not yet conducted similar experiments using

Inhibition %	BV09	BV10	BV18	BV19	CB11
nBet v 1	100	100	100	100	100
buffer	0	0	0	0	0
#280 #2227 #2230	=	=	=	=	=
#226	=	=	=	<	=
#2226	=	=	* =	=	<<
#167	=	=	<<	<<	<<

For clarity reasons operators indicate inhibition capacity relative to nBet v 1.

Figure 3. (Table) Summary of inhibition assays.

IgE, since the polyclonal nature of IgE is likely to blur the picture, however, we do consider the experiments using murine monoclonal antibodies as a model system for human IgE reactivity.

3.3 T-Cell Stimulation Assays

Four of the six purified recombinant isoallergens were probed in standard T-cell stimulation assays using two CD4$^+$ T-cell clones. One clone, JNP08, has been found to react with a synthetic peptide covering position 126–140, whereas clone JNL26 react with a synthetic peptide covering position 19–33, see fig. 4. Whereas clone JNP08 is stimulated by all four recombinant isoallergens, clone JNL26 is stimulated by all four but the gene product of clone #226. Examination of the deduced aminoacid sequences reveal, that both clone #226 and clone #280 contain aminoacid substitutions within the region 126–140, which are apparently insignificant for the ability to stimulate T-cell clone JNP08. However, only clone #226 contain an aminoacid substitution within the region 19–33. This substitution is an Asp→Gly where a negative charge is replaced by a neutral aminoacid. Apparently this substitution abrogates the ability of this recombinant isoallergen to stimulate T-cell clone JNL26.

On the basis of these results we conclude that also with respect to T-cell epitopes, the epitope structure of recombinant isoallergens of Bet v 1 differ. These results are in agreement with current models of epitope structure of T-cell epitopes, in which two or three aminoacid residues are critical for the binding of the T-cell epitope to the HLA-D molecule for antigen presentation, and a few other aminoacid residues are critical for the

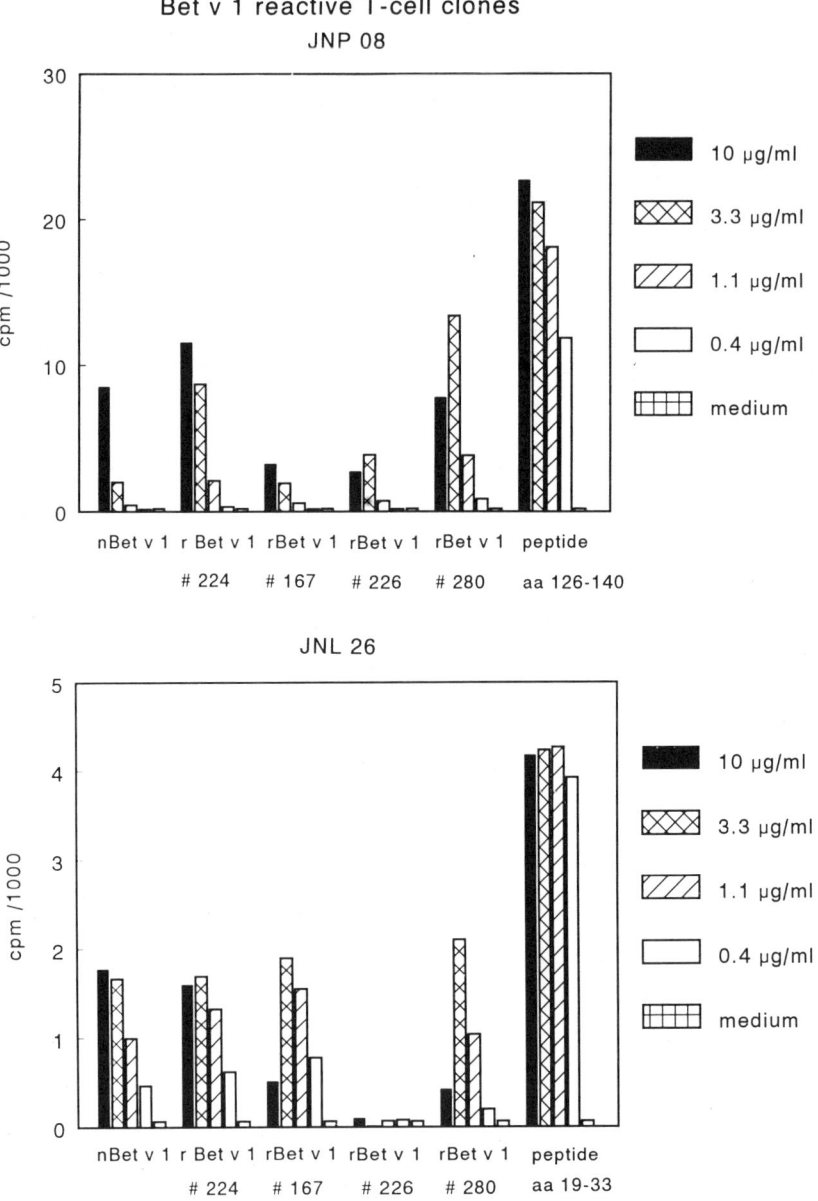

Figure 4. Isoallergen specific T-cell reactivity.

specific recognition by the T-cell receptor, whereas other aminoacids may be substituted without significant effect.

3.4 Prospect for Using Recombinant Allergens for Immunotherapy

The observation that isoallergens show differences in epitope structure both with respect to B- and T-cell epitopes seem to add a tremendous complexity to the problem of finding agents for specific immunotherapy, which are more readily standardized than the extracts in current use. However, our results, as well as those of other groups, point to the fact, that some recombinant isoallergens are more generally reactive than others. For Bet v 1 the isoallergen originally described (6), identical in sequence with the product of clone #224 and #2230 of this study, is reactive with all antibodies as well as T-cells so far tested. Furthermore, we have shown in inhibition assays using serum IgE from allergic patients, that this isoallergen is as effective in inhibition as is the purified allergen from natural sources. It seems therefore likely that by careful selection among isoallergens, it may be possible to obtain a panel of broadly reactive recombinant isoallergens as candidates for the replacement of the extracts used for specific immunotherapy today. Ignoring the problem of lack of minor allergens, it remains to be determined whether recombinant allergens will be as efficient in immunotherapy as the natural mixture of isoallergens present in the extracts. In our opinion the answer to this question is dependent on the mechanism of immunotherapy, which is only partly known. If, on the one hand, immunotherapy works by down regulating the existing immune response leading to IgE synthesis, the target of the treatment most likely is all specificities directed towards all isoallergens, demanding the presence of all possible epitopes in the agent used. If, however, on the other hand, immunotherapy works by starting a new immune response based on IgG and/or IgA production, the use of recombinant allergens may be feasible after all, since once started the immune response will by natural mechanisms develop specificities directed towards all isoallergens that share epitopes with the molecule used for therapy. If this model is indeed correct it follows that B-cell epitopes are indispensable for a successful outcome.

4. REFERENCES

1. King TP, Hoffmann D, Løwenstein H, Marsh DG, Platts-Mills TAE, Thomas W: Allergen Nomenclature. ACI News 1994; 6: 38–44.
2. Ipsen H, Hansen OC: The NH_2-terminal amino acid sequence of the immunochemically partial identical major allergens of Alder (*Alnus glutinosa*) *Aln g* I, Birch (*Betula verrucosa*) *Bet v* I, Hornbeam (*Carpinus betulus*) *Car b* I, and Oak (*Quercus alba*) *Que a* I pollens. Mol Immunol 1991; 28: 1279–1288.
3. Larsen JN, Strøman P, Ipsen H: PCR based cloning and sequencing of genes encoding the tree pollen major allergen *Car b* I from *Carpinus betulus* (hornbeam). Mol Immunol 1992; 29: 703–711.
4. Larsen JN, Casals AB, From NB, Strøman P, Ipsen H: Characterization of recombinant *Bet v* I, the major pollen allergen of *Betula verrucosa* (White Birch), produced by fed-batch fermentation. Int Arch Allergy Immunol 1993; 102: 249–258.
5. Spangfort et al. This issue.
6. Breiteneder H, Pettenburger K, Bito A, Valenta R, Kraft D, Rumpold H, Scheiner O, Breitenbach M: The gene coding for the major birch pollen allergen *Bet v* I, is highly homologous to a pea disease resistance response gene. EMBO J 1989; 8: 1935–1938.

35

CHARACTERISATION OF RECOMBINANT ISOFORMS OF BIRCH POLLEN ALLERGEN Bet v 1

M. D. Spangfort,[1] H. Ipsen,[1] S. H. Sparholt,[1] S. Aasmul-Olsen,[1] P. Osmark,[2] F. M. Poulsen,[2] M. Larsen,[3] E. Mørtz,[3] P. Roepstorff,[3] and J. N. Larsen[1]

[1]ALK Laboratories
Hørsholm, Denmark
[2]Carlsberg Research Laboratories
Copenhagen, Denmark
[3]Odense University
Odense, Denmark

1. ABSTRACT

Three isoforms of the major birch pollen allergen, Bet v, 1 from *Betula verrucosa* have been expressed as recombinant proteins in *E. coli* and purified. The immunochemical properties of recombinant isoforms (rBet v 1) differed on immunoblots when compared using Mabs and birch pollen allergic patients serum IgE. 2-D gel analysis showed that recombinant isoforms with different epitope structure can focus under the same protein spot after electrophoresis. The structure of conformational epitopes can be distorted by amino acid substitutions even when T-cell epitopes are not affected as judged by T-cell proliferation studies.

2. INTRODUCTION

The major birch pollen allergen Bet v 1 is a protein with an apparent molecular weight of 17 kDa. About 20 different isoforms of Bet v 1 can be identified in birch pollen extract by 2-D immunoblotting using monospecific antibodies [1,2]. Using Mabs or sera from individual birch pollen allergic patients, differences in individual reactivity towards different isoforms suggest differences in epitope structure [1]. These observations are in agreement with a model in which differences in amino acid sequence induces differences in epitope structure. However, a detailed characterisation of the epitope structure and molecular properties of Bet v 1 is lacking due to difficulties of isolating individual Bet v 1 isoforms from pollen extract. In this work, we have addressed this problem by producing

New Horizons in Allergy Immunotherapy
edited by Sehon et al. Plenum Press, New York, 1996

251

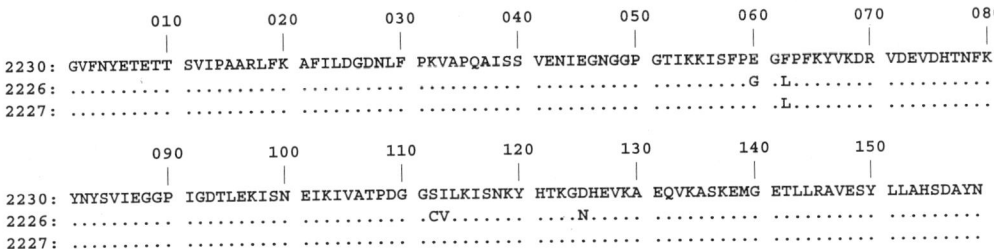

Figure 1. Isoforms of Bet v 1 expressed as recombinant proteins in *E. coli.*

purified Bet v 1 isoforms as recombinant proteins in order to compare their immuno-chemical and molecular properties.

3. MATERIAL AND METHODS

RNA was purified from *Betula verrucosa* pollen and genes encoding Bet v 1 were specifically amplified by PCR as in [3]. The products were subcloned into the maltose-binding protein fusion vector pMAL-c and expressed in *E. coli*. Affinity purified fusion protein was enzymatically clevaged into its two protein constituents by incubation with Factor Xa, followed by gel filtration to isolate rBet v 1.

4. RESULTS AND DISCUSSION

The primary amino acid sequences of the rBet v 1 isoforms 2230, 2227 and 2226 as deduced from their respective genes are shown in Fig. 1. The purified isoforms were characterised by SDS-PAGE, analytical gelfiltration, mass spectrometry, N-terminal sequencing and NMR spectroscopy.

4.1. Immunological Characterisation

Fig. 2 show that isoform 2227 is recognised by all Mabs tested, whereas isoform 2230 does not bind Mab BV12. Isoform 2227 and 2230 differ by a hydrophobic amino acid substitution, Phe to Leu, which apparently abolish BV12 binding. The reactivity of isoform 2226 on immunoblots was generally weaker compared to other isoforms. It did however, react readily with a polyclonal rabbit anti-Bet v 1 antibody. Recombinant iso-forms were also tested on immunoblots against a pool of birch pollen allergic patients se-rum IgE. Isoforms 2227 and 2230 strongly bound patients IgE, whereas no IgE-binding to 2226 could be detected. This demonstrates that relatively small changes in the amino acid composition can have large effects on the structure of conformational epitopes. The anti-genic activity of recombinant Bet v 1 isoforms was further characterised by their ability to induce T-cell proliferation in a longterm Bet v 1 reactive T-cell line (not shown). All three isoforms elicited a strong proliferation response in rates comparable to naturally occurring Bet v 1.

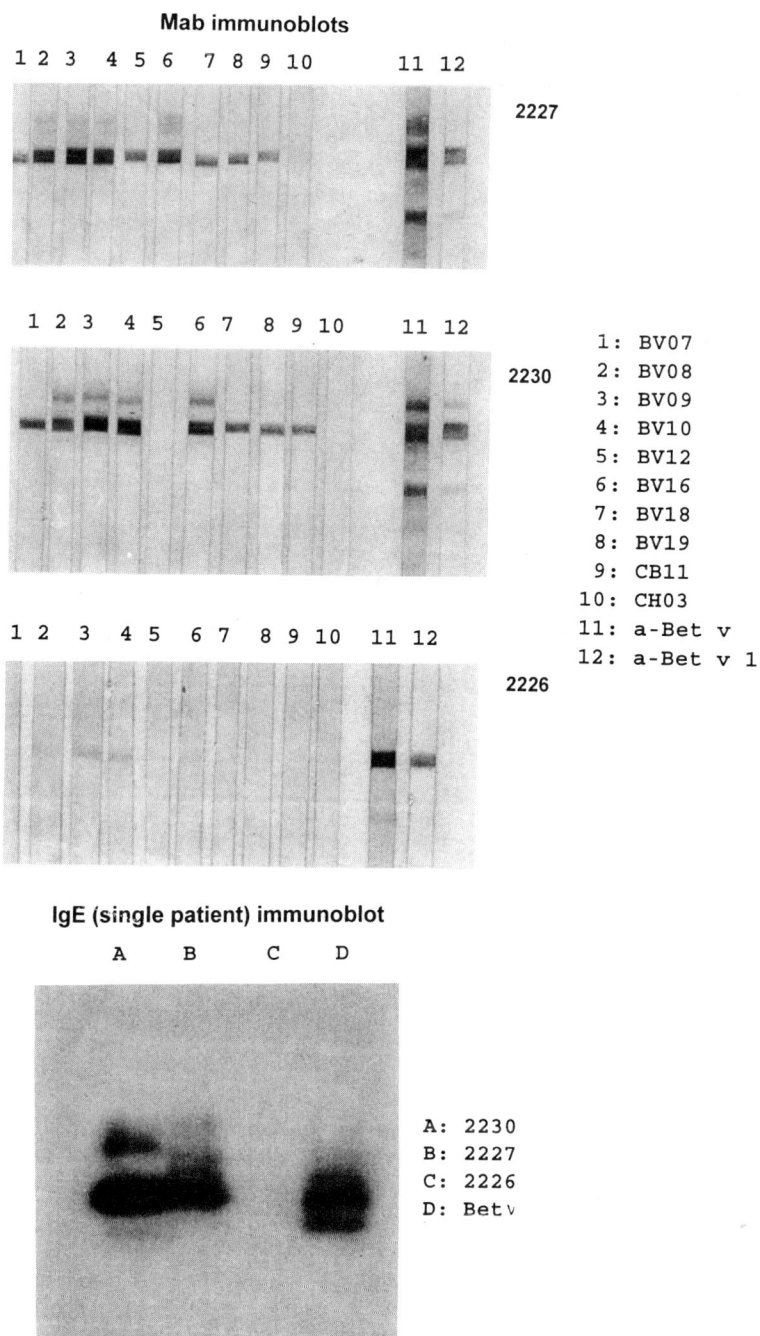

Figure 2. Immunoblotting of purified recombinant Bet v 1 against a panel of Mabs (left) and against birch pollen allergic patients serum IgE (right).

4.2. 2-D Gel Electrophoresis of Bet v 1 Isoforms and Birch Extract

When analysed by 2-D electrophoresis (not shown), isoforms 2230 and 2227 gave identical 2-D profiles which demonstrates that different isoforms can be located under the same protein spot on a 2-D gel. Since isoform 2227 but not 2230 reacts with Mab BV12, it also demonstrates that isoforms with different epitope structure can be present under the same 2-D gel protein spot. Thus, the resolution power of the 2-D gel system is limited as it cannot account for the full spectrum of immunochemical and sequence heterogeneity of Bet v 1. Apart from a major protein spot, all isoforms gave rise to up to three additional minor spots which probably represents artefacts generated by the 2-D gel system.

In summary, although these data suggests that even single amino acid substitutions apparently affects epitope structure, the reported immunochemical characterisation is limited to immunoblots only. In theory, the lack of reactivity against Mabs and/or serum IgE could be accounted for by incorrect re-folding of the protein after SDSPAGE. Further characterisation using fluid-phase inhibition assays are in progress.

5. REFERENCES

1. Løwenstein, H., Sparholt, S.H., Klysner, S.S., Ipsen, H., and J.N. Larsen (1995), Int. Arch. Allergy Immunol. (*in press*).
2. Jarolim, A., Rumpold, H., Endler, T., Ebner, H., Breitenbach, M., Scheiner, O. and D. Kraft (1989) Allergy 44: 385–395.
3. Larsen, J.N., Casals, A.B., From, N. B., Strøman, P. and H. Ipsen. (1993), Int. Arch. Allergy Immunol. 102:249–258.

36

*LOL p*II ALLERGEN

Production and Characterization of the Recombinant Protein and Human Antibody Fragments

Alessandro Sidoli,[1] Claudia De Lalla,[1] Elena Tamborini,[1] Anna Brandazza,[1] and Paolo Arosio[2]

[1]Dibit
Department of Biology and Technology
San Raffaele Scientific Institute
Via Olgettina, 58. 20132 Milano, Italy
[2]Department of Biomedical Technologies
University of Brescia
Spedali Civili, Brescia

INTRODUCTION

Grass pollen allergens are a major cause of allergy affecting about 75% of allergic patients (1). The perennial rye grass *Lolium perenne* is the most important species that produces allergenic pollen world-wide, due to its large use for forage and turf. Earlier studies showed that this pollen contains at least 17 allergens ranging in size from 12 to 89 kDa (2). They have been grouped on the basis of molecular size and electrophoretic mobility, and it has been recognised that most of these proteins exist in multiple isoforms which may differ in allergenicity. Recent work to isolate, clone and sequence cDNAs for the various allergens has somehow simplified the analysis of these proteins and it is expected to produce new concepts for diagnosis and therapy of grass pollen allergies (3). It has been recognised that *Lol p*I and *Lol p*V are the major IgE binding allergens, they have similar size (27–35 Kda) and no significant amino acid sequence homology (4–7). They both exist in multiple forms (6,7), the origin and allergenicity of which have not been clarified. *Lol p*I is localised in the cytoplasm and it is exported on the surface of the pollen (8), while *Lol p*V is addressed to amyloplasts (9), a localisation that seems to facilitate the diffusion of the allergen in the air and to trigger attacks of asthma (10).

*Lol p*II is another important class of isoallergens (11). It is composed of a group of acidic proteins of about 11 kDa with various isoforms. It has the same molecular weight as *Lol p*III class, these being basic proteins, which cross react with *Lol p*II as determined by means of human, goat and rabbit antibodies (12). The only sequenced representatives of

New Horizons in Allergy Immunotherapy
edited by Sehon et al. Plenum Press, New York, 1996

255

the two groups: *Lol p*IIA and *Lol p*IIIB showed an identical size of 97 residues and 59% amino acid sequence identity (13,14). *Lol p*I, II and III appear to be cross reactive at the T cell level (15), and a T cell epitope has been mapped in a region of *Lol p*I which has some homology with the sequences of *Lol p*II and III (9,16).

RESULTS AND DISCUSSION

*Lol p*II is recognised as an important allergen to which 45% of subjects allergic to grass pollen are sensitive (11). It is present in various isoforms, one of which, *Lol p*IIA has been purified and the amino acid sequence determined by direct sequencing (13). This allowed us to design oligonucletide primers to clone a cDNA encoding for *Lol p*II by PCR amplification from pollen mRNA (17). The amino acid sequence we have determined is fully consistent with the one reported by Ansari et al. (13) except for the residue Arg77 to Trp. The cDNA, encoding for a protein truncated at 4 and 5 residues at the N- and C-termini, respectively, was subcloned in an expression vector in fusion with the C-terminus of human ferritin, thus obtaining large amounts of a chimeric protein which retained the high stability and quaternary structure of the ferritin (a 24-mer protein) and which exposed on the surface the allergenic peptide. This approach demonstrated that the *Lol p*II we cloned binds IgEs of allergic subjects and it induces positive reactions in skin prick tests in sensitive subjects. It was concluded that it has allergenic properties similar to the natural *Lol p*II (17).

In order to obtain the mature form of the allergen, the coding region of the complete sequence of *Lol p*II was subcloned in the pET12c vector in fusion with the *omp*T leader peptide for secretion into *E. coli* periplasm (18). This construct encodes for the complete 97 amino acid sequence of *Lol p*II with and N-terminal extension of 10 unrelated residues. *E. coli* transformed with the recombinant plasmid expressed intracellularly *Lol p*II protein with uncleaved *omp*T peptide, and in the periplasmic space the mature form. Conditions were found to induce the accumulation of a high proportion of the protein in the periplasmic space. This, joined to the high solubility of the protein in water, facilitated the purification of the recombinant protein (Table 1) allowing us to obtain 10 mg of homogenous protein from 1 litre of cell culture, a yield that may be improved, if needed.

Biochemical Properties

The protein is soluble in water and in high ionic strength, it resists to pH values in the range 2–9, and to temperatures above 80°C. The high solubility, the intrinsic fluorescence emission spectra (excitation at 295 nm) with maxima at 344 nm, which shift to 355 nm after denaturation in 6 M Guanidine HCl, and the far UV CD spectra, with minima at 198 and 212 nm, strongly suggest that the protein has a folded conformation, probably like the natural protein. Preliminary NMR studies indicate that the protein has a significant proportion of β-sheet structure, likely without helical segments. The protein elutes in a single peak of about 14 Kdal from Superdex 75 columns, and shows a single band of pI 5.8 on polyacrylamide gel isoelectric focusing. These properties are similar to the ones described for the natural *Lol p*II: a soluble and small monomeric globular protein (13).

Immunological Properties

The IgEs of some subjects allergic to *Lolium perenne* specifically recognised the recombinant *Lol p*II in blotting and in ELISA assays. Binding was inhibited by preincuba-

Table 1. Production of recombinant *Lol p*II

Purification step	Total proteins[a] (mg)	r*Lol p*II (mg)	Purity (%)
E. coli growth[b]	5 g cells	-	-
Periplasmic extraction	100	40	40
Dialysis in water	50	35	70
Preparative electrophoresis	10	10	100

[a] From 1 litre of bacterial culture
[b] Conditions: growth at 25°C followed by induction with 1 mM IPTG for 3 hr

tion of the sera with pollen extracts, and, more important, the binding of IgEs to the natural *Lol p*II in western blotting was completely inhibited by preincubation of the sera with recombinant *Lol p*II (18). In a limited number of samples we observed that all positive *Lol p*II sera recognised the natural *Lol p*II as well as the recombinant one. Preparations of recombinant *Lol p*II induced strong allergic response in skin prick tests on two allergic subjects, and not in non-allergic controls. They also induced histamine release from basophils of allergic subjects. Recombinant *Lol p*II elicited antisera in rabbits that cross react with the natural *Lol p*II present in the extracts of *L. perenne* pollen. Cross reactivity was observed between natural and recombinant *Lol p*II, and not with other proteins of the pollen extract, including *Lol p*I. Data of the immunological characterisations are summarised in table 2, showing that natural and recombinant forms are apparently analogous.

Recombinant Anti-*Lol p*II Human Fabs

The display of antibody fragments on philamentous phages has provided a powerful tool to make antibodies of predefined binding specificity. The fragments are fused to the minor coat protein pIII, and then phages can be easily selected by panning techniques. In order to isolate high affinity human antibodies for *Lol p*II we used a recently developed combinatorial library (19). This library was generated from a highly diverse repertoires of heavy and light chains entirely *in vitro* from a bank of human germ line V gene segments. Recombination of the repertoires in bacteria produced a large synthetic repertoire (about 6.5×10^{10}) of Fab fragments displayed on philamentous phages. After 5 cycles of biopanning on a solid phase r*Lol p*II we isolated 17 specific phages binders, as determined by ELISA tests. By subsequent cloning, the antibody sequences were then expressed as soluble Fab fragments in the periplasms of transformed bacteria. Four of these Fabs were pu-

Table 2. Immunological properties of *Lol p*II

Assay	Rec *Lol p*II	Natural *Lol p*II
IgE binding[a]	+	+
IgG binding[b]	+	+
rFab binding[c]	+	+
Skin prick test[d]	+	+
Histamine release[d]		

[a] Evaluated by blotting and ELISA assays with sera of allergic subjects.
[b] Rabbit IgG, evaluated by blotting experiments.
[c] Blotting experiments with 4 different clones of recombinant human Fabs.
[d] Experiments with natural proteins were performed with total soluble extracts form *L. perenne* pollen.

rified by immobilised metal affinity chromatography (IMAC) (20) taking advantage of a His-tag fused to the H-chain of the antibody. This simple procedure yielded homogenous preparations of the Fabs, about 1–2 mg per litre of culture. The antibodies bound recombinant as well as natural *Lol p*II in Western blotting experiments. In ELISA they showed specific binding to recombinant *Lol p*II which could be displaced by preincubation with an excess of *L. Perenne* pollen extract .

The kinetics parameters of association and dissociation of the recombinant Fab (clone 1) to r*Lol p*II were analysed by BIAcore surface plasmon resonance technique. The recombinant allergen was immobilised on the dextran matrix, and various concentrations of the Fab were injected in the instrument for the reaction with the immobilised protein. Real time monitoring of the reactions of binding and unbinding allowed to calculate a k_{on} of 1×10^6 M^{-1}, sec^{-1}, and a k_{off} of 2×10^{-3} sec^{-1}. The Fab showed an affinity constant (Ka) of 5×10^8 M^{-1}, a value that can be considered high for a monovalent antibody fragment.

Epitope Mapping

Three types of antibodies to *Lol p*II were available to us, they are produced by different cell types and are selected by different means: human IgEs, rabbit IgGs, and human Fab fragments, which are produced by *E. coli* and selected *in vitro*. Preliminary analyses indicated a partial competition between IgEs and rFabs which could be attributed to epitope sharing or to steric interference. The different affinities of the various antibodies complicated the identification of its binding sites by competition experiments. In order to identify the *Lol p*II sequences preferentially recognised by the three types of antibodies we synthesised overlapping peptides of 20–25 residues covering the whole *Lol p*II sequence. Peptide binding to antibodies was analysed either directly in ELISA and Dot/Blot tests, or in competition experiments in which we monitored the inhibition of the antigen-antibody binding in the ELISA tests as caused by various concentrations of the peptides. The results, summarised in table 3, indicate that human IgEs and rFabs bind to the same peptides, mostly localized in the central region of the molecule, suggesting that they may have common epitopes. In contrast rabbit IgGs bound preferentially peptides of the the C-terminal region of the molecule.

Table3. Epitope mapping by synthetic peptides

Antibodies	Peptides (residue numbers)						
	A (1-23)	B (15-39)	C (27-50)	D (39-64)	E (52-75)	F (64-88)	G (75-97)
IgE[b]	-	-	+	+++	-	+	-
IgG[c]	-	-	-	-	-	-	++++
rFabs[d]	-	-	++	+++++	-	+	-

[a] Results of ELISA tests with solid-phase r*Lol p*II and enzyme-labelled secondary antibodies. Various concentrations of the peptides were added to the wells together with the antibodies and the relative binding judged by the inhibition of the response. The semi-quantative results are shown.
[b] Polyclonal IgEs from a single allergic subject.
[c] Polyclonal rabbit IgGs.
[d] Analysis of three different monoclonal recombinant Fabs.

CONCLUSIONS

We have obtained two types of recombinant proteins that may be useful as a model for the study of rye grass allergies: the allergen *Lol p*II and specific human Fab fragments. The allergen appears to be remarkably similar for biochemical and immunological properties to the natural one, can be easily obtained in large amounts, and now work is in progress to evaluate the clinical significance of the determination of IgE specific for it. The human Fab antibodies show high affinity, which can be increased by the construction of bivalent molecules. These reagents may be useful not only for diagnosis of allergies, but also to approach new passive therapeutic treatments based on the evidence that they share some epitopes with IgE antibodies. Future mutational studies will be addressed to evaluate the possibility to alter/eliminate the IgE binding sequences of *Lol p*II, to provide novel concepts for desensitisation therapies.

ACKNOWLEDGMENTS

We are grateful to Dr. G. Musco for NMR studies.

REFERENCES

1. Wutrich B.(1989) Epidemiology of the allergic diseases: are they really on the increase? Int. Arch. Allergy Appl. Immunol. 90, 3–10.
2. Ford D. and Baldo B.A. (1986) A re-examination of rye-grass (*Lolium perenne*) pollen allergens. Int. Arch. Allergy Appl. Immunol. 81, 193–203.
3. Baldo B.A. and Donovan G.R. (1988) The structural basis of allergenicity: recombinant DNA-based strategies for the study of allergens. Allergy 43, 81–97.
4. Marsh D.G., Milner, F.H. and Johnson P. (1966) The allergenic activity and stability of purified allergens from the pollen of common rye grass (*Lolium perenne*). Int. Arch. Allergy 29, 521–535.
5. Kahn C.R. and Marsh D.G. (1986) Monoclonal antibodies to the major *Lolium perenne* (rye grass) pollen allergen *Lol p*I (Rye I) Mol. Immunol. 23, 1281–1288
6. Ong E.K., Griffith I.J., Knox B.R. and Singh M.B. (1993) Cloning of a cDNA encoding a group-V (group IX) allergen isoform from rye-grass pollen that demonstrates specific antigenic immunoreactivity. Gene 134, 235–240.
7. Perez. M., Ishioka G.Y., Walker L.E. and Chesnut, R.W. (1990) cDNA cloning and immunological characterization of the rye grass allergen *Lol p* I J. Biol. Chem. 265, 16210–16215.
8. Staff I., Taylor P.E., Smith P., Singh M.B., Knox R.B. (1990) Cellular localization of water soluble, allergenic proteins in rye-grass (*Lolium perenne*) pollen using monoclonal and specific IgE antibodies with immunogold probes. Histochem. J. 22, 276–290.
9. Singh M.B., Hough T., Theerakulpisut P., Avjioglu A., Davies S., Smith P.M., Taylor P., Simpson R.J., Ward L.D., McCluskey J., Puy R. and Knox B.R. (1991) Isolation of a cDNA encoding a newly identified major allergenic protein of rye-grass pollen: intracellular targeting to the amyloplast. Proc. Natl. Acad. Sci. USA 88, 1384–1388.
10. Knox R.B. (1993) Grass pollen, thunderstorms and asthma. Clin. Exper. Allergy 23, 354–359.
11. Freidhoff L.R., Kautzky E.E., Grant J.H., Meyers D.A. and Marsh D.G. (1986) A study of the human immune response to *Lolium perenne* (Rye) pollen and its components, *Lol p* I and *Lol p* II (Rye I and Rye II). J. Allergy Clin. Immunol. 78, 1190–1201.
12. Ansari A.A., Kihara T.K. and Marsh D,G. (1987) Immunochemical studies of *Lolium perenne* (rye grass) pollen allergens, *Lol p* I, II and III. J. Immunol. 139, 4034–4041.
13. Ansari A.A., Shenbagamurthi P. and Marsh D.G. (1989) Complete amino acid sequence of a *Lolium perenne* (perennial rye grass) pollen allergen, *Lol p* II. J. Biol. Chem. 264, 11181–11185.
14. Ansari A.A., Shenbagamurthi P. and Marsh D.G. (1989) Complete primary structure of a *Lolium perenne* (perennial rye grass) pollen allergen, *Lol p* III: comparison with known *Lol p* I and II sequences. Biochem. 28, 8665–8670

15. Baskar S., Parronchi P., Mohapatra S., Romagnani S. and Ansari A.A. (1992) Human T cell responses to purified pollen allergens of the grass, *Lolium perenne*. J. Immunol. 148, 2378–2383

16. Bungy Poor Fard G.A., Latchman Y., Rodda S., Geysen M., Roitt I. and Brostoff J. (1993) T cell epitopes of the major fraction of rye grass *Lolium perenne* (*Lol p* I) defined using overlapping peptides in vitro and in vivo. Isoallergen clone 1A. Clin. Exp. Immunol. 94, 111–116.

17. Sidoli A., Tamborini E., Giuntini I., Levi S., Volonte' G., Paini C., De Lalla C., Siccardi A.G., Baralle F.E., Galliani S. and Arosio P. (1993) Cloning, expression and immunological characterization of recombinant *Lolium perenne* allergen *Lol p* II. J. Biol. Chem.. 268, 21819–21825.

18. Tamborini E., Brandazza A., De Lalla C., Musco G., Siccardi A., Arosio P. and Sidoli A. (1995) Recombinant allergen *Lol p* II: expression, purification and characterization. Mol. Immunol., in press.

19. Griffiths AD, Williams SC, Hartley O, et al, (1994) Isolation of high affinity human antibodies directly from large synthetic repertoires. EMBO J. 13, 3245–3260.

20. Crowe J, Dobeli H, Gentz R, Hochuli E., Stuber D. and Henco K.(1994) 6XHis-Ni-NTA chromatography as a superior technique in recombinant protein expression/purification. Methods Mol. Biol. 31, 371–387.

37

CHARACTERIZATION OF GROUP 1 ALLERGENS FROM ELEVEN GRASS SPECIES

S. Aasmul-Olsen,[1] P. A. Würtzen,[1] M. Lombardero,[2] H. Løwenstein,[1] and H. Ipsen[1]

[1]ALK-ABELLÓ Group
Bøge Allé 10–12, 2970 Hørsholm, Denmark
[2]ALK-ABELLÓ Group
Miguel Fleta, 19 - 28037 Madrid, Spain

1. INTRODUCTION

Grass pollens are one of the most important allergen sources throughout the world[1]. The grasses constitutes a large and diverse group of plants counting over 10,000 individual species. Despite the taxonomical diversity, a number of common features, with respect to allergenenecity[2], is apparent.

The pollens of all grass species investigated so far contain the allergen groups 1, 2 and 3, whereas group 5 allergens do not seem to be present in the subtropical species (e.g. *Cynodon dactylon*, *Paspalum notatum* etc.).

The group 1, 2 and 3 allergens exhibit a high degree of intra-group similarity, both with respect to physico-chemical parameters[3,4], aminoacid sequence identity (85–93%)[5–8] and immuno-chemical reactivity/cross-reactivity[9–14]. Additionally, groups 1 and 2/3 exhibit inter-group amino acid identity (approx. 60%)[15–20].

The group 5 allergens from various grass species, though physicochemically and immunochemically similar, exhibit a higher degree of amino acid sequence diversity (72–90% identity)[21–24]. Further, all grass pollen allergen groups seem to exist in multiple isoforms distributed throughout the pH range 4 to approximately 9[25–27]. The charge microheterogeneity observed, most probably originates from a few substitutions of charged amino acids.

2. MATERIALS AND METHODS

2.1. Pollen Extracts

Pollens from eleven grass species *Dactylis glomerata* (Dac g), *Festuca pratensis* (Fes p), *Lolium perenne* (Lol p), *Poa pratense* (Poa p), *Avena elatior* (Ave e), *Holcus la-*

New Horizons in Allergy Immunotherapy
edited by Sehon et al. Plenum Press. New York. 1996

261

natus (Hol l), *Phleum pratense* (Phl p), *Secale cereale* (Sec c), *Cynodon dactylon* (Cyn d), *Paspalum notatum* (Pas n) and *Sorghum halepense* (Sor h) were obtained from Allergon, Sweden. Crude extracts of the pollens were prepared in 0.125 M NH_4HCO_3 pH 8.3 (1:10 w/v), dialysed against water and lyophilized.

2.2. Antibodies

Serum samples were obtained from 13 grass pollen allergic patients (positive clinical history, positive SPT (grass) and RAST (Phl p)). Murine monoclonal antibodies were raised towards either Cyn d 1 or Lol p 1.

2.3. 1 and 2D SDS-Page

SDS-PAGE (16%T, 2%C) was performed with reduced (DTT) protein samples (0.5–30 µg) and the gels were either silverstained or electroblotted to nitrocellulose membranes. The first dimension IEF gels (Immobilon, 3–10.5, Pharmacia) for the 2D-SDS-PAGE were run for 22950 Vh and either silver stained or transferred to the top of SDS-PAGE gels after incubation in sample buffer containing SDS and mercaptoethanol. The nitrocellulose membranes were developed with monoclonal antibodies (diluted 1:1000 v/v) or patient sera (diluted 1:40 v/v).

2.4. Purification of Grass Pollen Allergens

Group 1 and 2/3 allergens from eleven grass species were purified by a combination of hydrophobic interaction chromatography on Phenyl Sepharose and size exclusion chromatography. 50 mg of crude pollen extract dissolved in 1.0 M $(NH_4)_2SO_4$, 0.05 M NaAcetate pH 5.0 were applied on a Phenyl Sepharose column (10 ml) equilibrated in the same buffer. The proteins were eluted from the column according to the following proce-

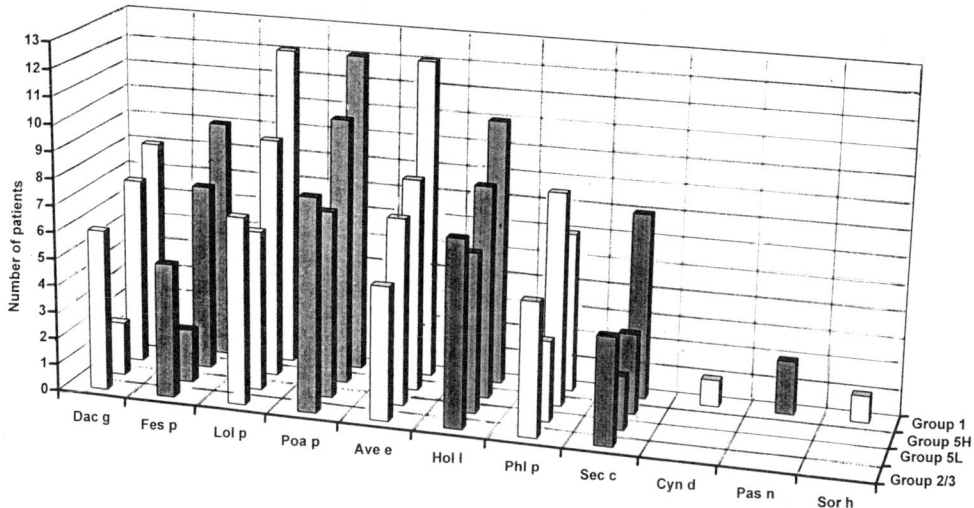

Figure 1. Summary of the SDS-PAGE immunoblot reactivity towards individual allergens from eleven grass species of IgE from thirteen patients.

dure: Fraction 1: two column volumed (2 x V_T, 20 ml) in 1.0 M $(NH_4)_2SO_4$, 0.05 M NaAcetate pH 5.0; Fraction 2: 2 x V_T 0.05 M NaAcetate pH 5.0; Fraction 3: 2 x V_T PBS pH 7.4; Fraction 4: 2 x V_T 0.05 M Na_2HCO_3 pH 10.0 and Fraction 5: 2 x V_T 50% (v/v) ethylen-glycol in 0.05 M Na_2HCO_3 pH 10.0. Fraction 1 contained primarily group 1 and 2/3 allergens, fraction 4 and 5 contained group 5 allergens. Fraction 1 was further processed on a S75 Superdex column yielding isolated group 1 and group 2/3.

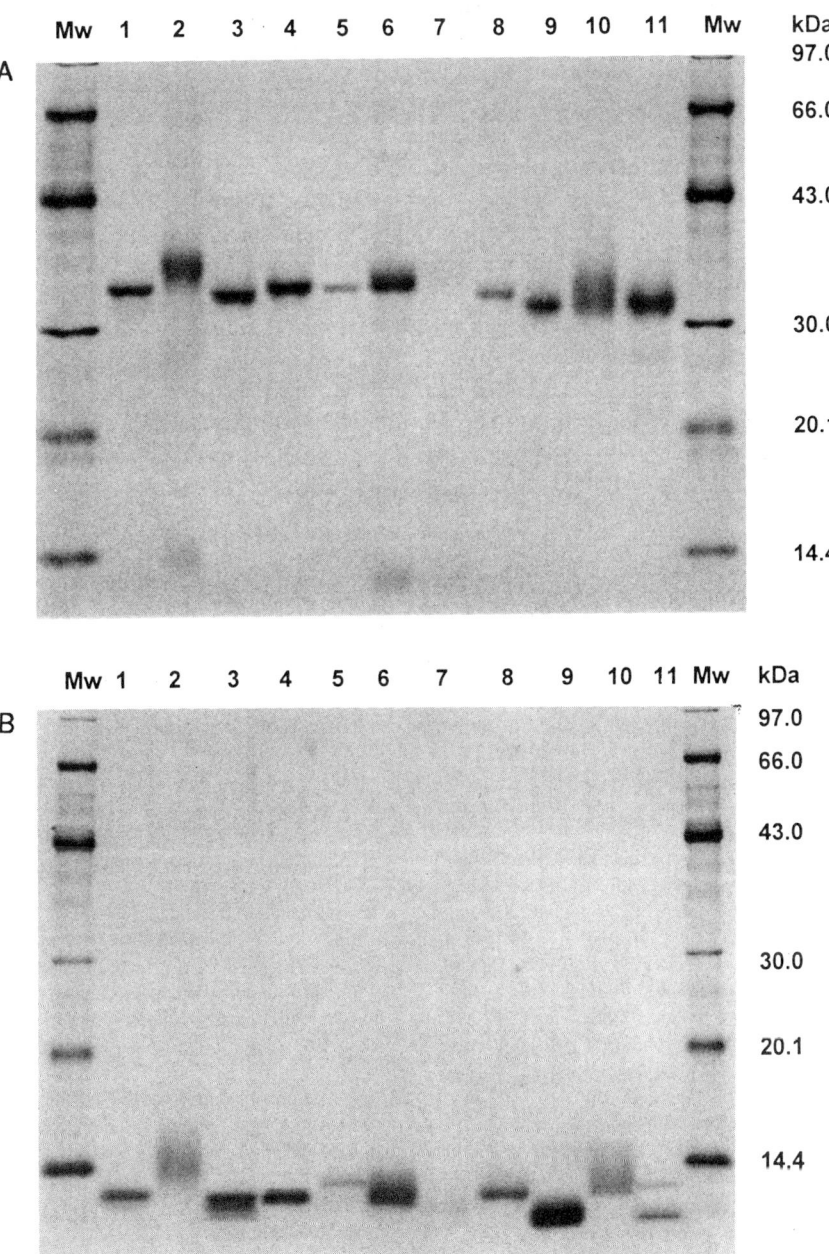

Figure 2. Silver stained SDS-PAGE of isolated group 1 (A) and group 2/3 (B) allergens from eleven grass species. 1-Dac g, 2-Fes p, 3-Lol p, 4-Poa p, 5-Ave e, 6-Hol l, 7-Phl p, 8-Sec c, 9-Pas n, 10-Sor h and 11-Cyn d.

3. RESULTS AND DISCUSSION

IgE immunoblot analysis of the reaction of 13 individual sera with eleven grass species indicates that group 1 seem to be the most important allergen, followed by group 5 and 2/3 (Fig. 1).

Patient IgE cross-react extensively with the various allergens from the different grass species although few of the sera reacted with the major allergens of subtropical grass species. The majority of the patients reacted with the major allergens of Lol p, Poa p and Ave e, whereas fewer reacted with the other grasses tested indicating a difference in the epitope pattern of the individual major allergens from the various grass species. Immunoblots performed with seven group 1 specific monoclonal antibodies (not shown) confirm the apparent differences in epitope pattern observed with IgE immunoblots.

The group 1 and 2/3 allergens from the eleven grass species were purified by a combination of hydrophobic interaction chromatography and size exclusion chromatography and the purified allergens were characterized by 1D-SDS-PAGE (Fig. 2) and 2D-SDS-PAGE (silver stain and immunoblots).

The group 1 allergens from the various grass species exhibit a high degree of heterogeneity with respect to pI (not shown). Some of the group 1 allergens seem to consist of isoforms covering both the acidic and alkaline pH range whereas others only seem to produce isoforms in the acidic pH range. Further, 2D-immunoblotting with monoclonal antibodies clearly indicates that various isoforms contain different subsets of antibody binding epitopes.

4. REFERENCES

1. Wuthrich, B. Epidemiology of the allergic diseases. Are they really on the increase? Int Arch Allergy Appl Immunol 90, 3–10, 1989.
2. Martin, BG., Mansfield, LE., Nelson, HS. Cross-allergenecity among the grasses. Ann Allergy 54, 54–99, 1985.
3. Suphioglu, C., Singh, MB., Knox, RB. Peptide mapping analysis of group 1 allergens of grass pollens. Int Arch Allergy Immunol 102, 144–151, 1993.
4. Cottam, G.P.; Moran, D.M.; Standring, R. Physicochemical and immunochemical characterization of allergenic proteins from rye-grass (Lolium perenne) pollen prepared by a rapid and efficient purification method. Biochem J 234, 305–310, 1986.
5. Perez M., Ishioka G.Y., Walker L.E., Chesnut R.W. cDNA cloning and immunological characterization of the rye grass allergen Lol p I. J Biol Chem 265, 16210–16215, 1990.
6. Griffith I.J., Smith P.M., Pollock J., Theerakulpisut P., Avjioglu A., Davies S., Hough T., Singh M.B., Simpson R.J. Ward L.D., Knox R.B. Cloning and sequencing of Lol pI, the major allergenic protein of ryegrass pollen. FEBS Lett. 279, 210–215, 1991.
7. Laffer, S., Valenta, R., Vrtala, S., Susani, M., van Ree, R., Kraft, D., Scheiner, O., Duchene, M., Complementary DNA cloning of the major allergen Phl p 1 from thimothy grass (Phleum pratense), recombinant Phl p 1 inhibits IgE binding to group 1 allergens from eight different grass species. J Allergy Clin Immunol 94, 689–698, 1994.
8. Petersen, A., Scramm, G., Bufe, A., Schlaak, M., Becker, WM. Structral investigations of the major allergen Phl p 1 on the complementary DNA and protein level. J Allergy Clin Immunol 95, 987–994, 1995.
9. Esch, RE., Klapper, DG. Identification and localization of allergenic determinants on grass group 1 allergens using monoclonal antibodies. J Immunol 142, 179–184, 1989.
10. Singh, MB., Knox, RB. Grass pollen allergens. Antigenic relationships detected using monoclonal antibodies and dot blotting immunoassay. Int Arch Allergy Appl Immunol 78, 300–304, 1985.
11. Matthiesen, F., Løwenstein, H. Group V allergens in grass pollens II. An investigation of group V allergens in pollens from ten grasses. Clin Exp Allergy 21, 309–320, 1991.
12. Matthiesen, F., Schumacher, MB., Løwenstein, H. Characterization of the major allergen of Cynodon dactylon (bermuda grass) pollen, Cyn d 1. J Allergy Clin Immunol 88, 763–774, 1991.

13. Esch, RE., Klapper, DG. Isolation and characterization of a major cross-reactive grass group 1 allergenic determinant Mol Immunol 26, 557–561, 1989.

14. van Ree, R., van Leeuwen, WA., Vandenberg, M., Weller, HH., Aalberse, RC. IgE and IgG cross-reactivity among Lol p 1 and Lol p 2/3 - Identification of the C-termini of Lol p 1, 2 and 3 as cross-reactive structures. Allergy 49, 254–261, 1994.

15. Sidoli, A., Tamborini, E., Giuntini, I., Levi, S., Volonte, G., Paini, C., De Lalla, C., Siccardi, AG., Baralle, FE., Galliani, S. and Arosio, P. Cloning, expression and immunological characterization of recombinant Lolium perenne allergen Lol p II. J Biol Chem 268, 21819–21825, 1993.

16. Ansari, AA., Shenbagamurthi, P., Marsh, DG. Complete amino acid sequence of a Lolium perenne (Perennial Rye Grass) pollen allergen, Lolp II. J Biol Chem 264, 11181–11185, 1989.

17. Dolecek, C., Vrtala, S., Laffer, S., Steinberger, P., Kraft, D., Scheiner, O.,Valenta, R. Molecular characterization of PHL P II a major timothy grass (Phleum pratense) pollen allergen FEBS Lett. 335, 299–304, 1993.

18. Roberts, AM., Van Ree, R., Cardy, SM., Bevan, LJ. and Walker, MR. Recombinant pollen allergens from Dactylis glomerata: preliminary evidence that human IgE cross-reactivity between Dac g II and Lol p I/II is increased following grass pollen immunotherapy Immunology 76, 389–396, 1992.

19. Ansari, AA., Shenbagamurthi, P., Marsh, DG. Complete primary structure of a Lolium perenne (perennial rye grass) pollen allergen, Lol P III: Comparison with known Lol P I and II sequences. Biochemistry 28, 8665–8670, 1989.

20. Roberts, AM., Bevan, LJ., Flora, PS., Jepson, I., Walker, WR. Nucleotide sequence of cDNA encoding the group-II allergen of Cocksfoot Orchard grass (Dactylis glomerata), Dac g II. Allergy 48, 615–623, 1993.

21. Ong, EK., Griffith, IJ., Singh, MB. Cloning of a cDNA encoding a group V (group IX) allergen isoform from Rye grass pollen that demonstrates antigenic immunoreactivity. Gene 134, 235–240, 1993.

22. Vrtala, S., Sperr, WR., Reimitzer, I., van Ree, R., Laffer, S., Müller, WD., Valent, P., Lechner, K., Rumpold, H., Kraft, D. cDNA cloning of a major allergen from Thimothy grass (Phleum pratense) pollen - Characterization of the recombinant Phl p V allergen. J Immunol 151, 4773–4781, 1993.

23. Silvanovich, A., Astwood, J., Zhang, L., Olsen, E., Kisil, F., Sehon, A., Mohapatra, S., Hill, R. Nucleotide sequence analysis of three cDNAs coding for Poa p IX isoallergens of Kentucky bluegrass pollen J Biol Chem 266, 1204–1210, 1991.

24. Bufe, A., Becker, WM., Schramm, G., Petersen, A., Mamat, U., Schlaak, M. Major Allergen Phl p Va (Timothy Grass) Bears at Least Two Different IgE Reactive Epitopes J Allergy Clin Immunol 94, 173–181, 1994.

25. Petersen, A., Schramm, G., Becher, WM., Schlaak, M. Comparison of 4 grass pollen species concerning their allergens of group V by 2D immunoblotting and microsequencing. Biol Chem Hoppe-Seyler 374, 855–861, 1993.

26. Petersen, A., Becher, WM., Schlaak, M. Examination of microheterogeneity in grass pollen allergens. Electrophoresis 13, 736–739, 1992.

27. Petersen, A., Becher, WM., Schlaak, M. Epitope analysis of isoforms of the major allergen Phl p V by fingerprinting and microsequencing. Clin Exp Allergy 24, 250–256, 1994.

38

A MAJOR ALLERGEN INVOLVED IN IgE MEDIATED COCKROACH HYPERSENSITIVITY IS A 90 kD PROTEIN WITH MULTIPLE IgE BINDING DOMAINS

Ricki M. Helm,[1] Gael Cockrell,[1] J. Steve Stanley,[1] Richard Brenner,[2]
A. Wesley Burks,[1] and Gary A. Bannon[1]

[1]Arkansas Children's Hospital Research Institute
University of Arkansas for Medical Sciences
Little Rock, Arkansas
[2]USDA/MVERL
Gainesville, Florida[2]

The role of the cockroach as an etiologic agent of respiratory allergic disorders is well documented (1–3). Positive skin test reactivity to whole body cockroach extracts is second only to the house dust mite of the indoor allergens; however, the identification of clinically relevant antigens and an understanding of the immunobiology of cockroach-induced asthmatic reactions is just beginning (4). The prevalence of asthma induced by cockroach exposure has been coupled with the identification of major cockroach allergens ranging in molecular weight from 6,000 to 100,000 daltons (5–10). In earlier experiments, we documented the in vitro translation of RNA from German cockroaches for the presence of IgE-binding proteins (11). In this report, we describe the isolation of a cDNA clone from a cDNA library derived from the German cockroach (*Blattella germanica*) encoding a major allergen, Bla g 90 kD.

A cDNA expression library was constructed (Lambda ZAP XR., La Jolla, CA) using German cockroach poly A+ RNA and oligo dT primers. The library was screened using IgE antibody from a cockroach-sensitive patient with documented asthma and skin test reactivity to whole body cockroach extracts (12). Bound IgE was detected with radiolabeled anti-IgE (Sanofi Diagnostics, Chaska, MN). Positive IgE-binding plaques were purified to homogeneity, and re-screened with non-cockroach sensitive serum to control for non-specific, IgE binding.

IgE immunoblot SDS-PAGE analysis of expressed recombinant allergens were performed according to standard procedures (13,14). Clones producing IgE-binding proteins ranged from 50 to 90 kD. Clone 4G, expressing a 90 kD allergen, was selected for further study. The recombinant protein expressed from clone 4G in E. coli XL Blue cells showed

New Horizons in Allergy Immunotherapy
edited by Sehon et al. Plenum Press, New York, 1996

267

strong IgE binding in sera from 17 of 22 (77%) individuals with cockroach-sensitivity. The recombinant protein failed to bind IgE in serum pools from either mite or Alternaria-sensitive individuals identifying this to be a major specific German cockroach allergen.

Preliminary DNA sequencing revealed several important pieces of information. Direct DNA sequence analysis of clone 4G revealed repeated portions throughout the gene. A gamma ^{32}P-labeled oligonucleotide from this repeat region was used to probe restriction enzyme digestion of clone 4G. The probe hybridized to more than one of the digested insert bands indicating repeated sequences. Southern blot analysis, using purified random primer labeled ($-^{32}$P—dCTP), 4 kb insert of clone 4G as a hybridization probe, demonstrated a high degree of sequence identity among 10 different IgE-binding cDNA clones. In addition, dideoxy thymidine DNA sequencing reactions of the same 10 cDNA clones using the M13 forward primer identified identical patterns.

The exact extent to which these clones, as well as the repeat sequences within these clones, occur in genes isolated from our cDNA library and their contribution as IgE binding epitopes remains to be determined. The recombinant cockroach allergens we have identified will allow further application of this technology to improve our understanding of the mechanisms and management of this major indoor aeroallergen.

REFERENCES

1. Bernton HS, McMahon TF, Brown H. Cockroach asthma. Br J Dis Chest 1972; 66:61.
2. Hulett AC, Dockhorn RJ. House dust mite (D. farinae) and cockroach allergy in a midwestern population. Ann Allergy 1979; 42:160.
3. Kang B, Vellody D, Homburger H, Yunginger JW. Cockroach cause of allergic asthma. Its specificity and immunologic profile. J Allergy Clin Immunol 1979, 63:80–86.
4. Chapman MD. Cockroach allergens: a common cause of asthma in North American cities. Insights in Allergy 1993; Vol 8, no.6.
5. Helm RM, Squillace DL, Jones RT, Brenner RJ. Shared allergenic activity in Asian (*Blattella asahinai*), German (*Blattella germanica*), American (*Periplaneta americana*), and Oriental (*Blatta orientalis*) cockroach species. Int Arch Allergy Appl Immunol 1990; 92:154–61.
6. Schou C. Lind P, Fernandez-Caldas E, Lockey RF, Lowenstein H. Identification and purification of an important cross-reactive allergen from American (*Periplaneta americana*) and German (*Blattella germanica*) cockroach. J Allergy Clin Immunol 1990; 86:935–46.
7. Wu CH, Lan JL. Cockroach hypersensitivity: isolation and partial characterization of major allergens. J Allergy Clin Immunol 1988; 82:727–35.
8. Pollart SM, Mullins DE, Vailes LD. Identification, quantification and purification of cockroach allergens using monoclonal antibodies. J Allergy Clin Immunol 1991; 87:511–521.
9. Stankus RP, O'Neill CE. Antigenic/allergenic characterization of American and German cockroach extracts. J Allergy Clin Immunol 1988; 81:563–70.
10. Helm RM, Burks AW, Williams LW, Brenner RJ. Isolation of the 36 kD German cockroach allergen using Fast Protein Liquid Chromatography. Int Arch Allergy Immunol 1994; 103:59–66.
11. Helm RM, Cockrell G, Sharkey P, Brenner R, Burks AW. In Vitro translation of RNA from the German cockroach *Blattella germanica*. Mol Immunol 1993; 30:1685–88.
12. Scheiner O, Bohle B, Breitenbach M, Breitenbach H, Duchene M, Ebner C, Ferreira F, Hirschwehr R, Hoffman-Sommergruber K, Pettenberg K, Rumpold H, Steiner R, Tejkl M, Valenta R, Kraft D. RAs: Production and possible clinical implications. In: Advances in Allergology and Clinical Immunology. Goddard P, Bousquet J, Michel FB, eds. The Parthenon Publishing Group. Carnforth, Park Ridge, UK, USA, 115.
13. Laemmli UK. Cleavage of structural proteins during the assembly of the head of bacteriophage T4. Nature 1970; 227:680–85.
14. Towbin H, Staehelin T, Gordon J. Electrophoretic transfer of proteins from polyacrylamide gels to nitrocellulose sheets: procedures and some applications. Proc Natl Acad Sci 1979; 76:4350–54.

39

MOLECULAR CHARACTERIZATION OF *Hor v* 9

Conservation of a T-Cell Epitope Among Group IX Pollen Allergens and Human VCAM and CD2

James D. Astwood[1] and Robert D. Hill[2]

[1]Monsanto Company
700 Chesterfield Parkway North
St. Louis, Missouri, 63021
[2]Department of Plant Science
University of Manitoba
Winnipeg, Manitoba, Canada, R3T 2N2

1. ABSTRACT

We have cloned, sequenced and expressed a recombinant group IX pollen allergen from barley (*Hordeum vulgare*). *Hor v* 9 is a polypeptide of 313 amino acids. The *Hor v* 9 cDNA clone was engineered into the *E. coli* protein expression vector pMAL and expressed as a fusion of maltose binding protein and truncated *Hor v* 9. Polyclonal antibodies to the fusion protein were raised in mice. Cross-reactive proteins, RNA and DNA homologues were found in many agricultural species including wheat, rye, triticale, oats, maize, sunflower and flax. The presence of group IX-like proteins in a variety of agricultural crops may represent a previously uncharacterized aeroallergenic occupational hazard. Sequence comparisons of the barley allergen, *Hor v* 9, with *Poa p* 9 and other cloned group IX pollen allergens revealed putative structural domains common to all. These include a signal peptide, two conserved immunoglobulin-like motifs, a 150 amino acid highly conserved carboxyterminal domain and a carboxyterminal transmembrane helix. This structural arrangement is also found in cell adhesion molecules. The highly conserved T-cell epitope previously characterized and mapped in group IX allergens (and present in *Hor v* 9) was found in several human cell adhesion molecule sequences (VCAM, NCAM and CD2). This T-cell epitope corresponded to the most highly conserved amino acid residues common to all group IX homologues sequenced to date. CD2 and VCAM are known to play a role in allergic inflammation: VCAM is involved in the recruitment of lymphocytes to sites of inflammation, and cross-linking CD2 leads to T-cell activation. We anticipate that the similar structural arrangement of group IX allergens and human cell adhesion molecules, as well as the presence of a T-cell epitope common to group IX pol-

New Horizons in Allergy Immunotherapy
edited by Sehon et al. Plenum Press, New York, 1996

len allergens and cell adhesion molecules, will have important consequences in the natural history of the atopic immune response.

2. INTRODUCTION

Homologues of Kentucky bluegrass (*Poa pratensis*) group IX pollen allergens (1) have been identified and cloned in other grass species such as Ryegrass (*Lolium perenne*)(2) and Timothy (*Phleum pratense*)(3). We have shown previously by western, northern and Southern analysis that group IX allergens are present in many agricultural crop species, especially cultivated barley (*Hordeum vulgare*), which we designate *Hor v* 9(4). Epitopes have been mapped for the group IX allergens in Kentucky bluegrass (5) and Timothy (3). We describe the cloning and expression in *E. coli* of a *Hor v* 9 cDNA, clone 9742 from the agricultural crop barley. Clone 9742 encodes a protein highly homologous to the *Poa p* 9 isoallergens. Clone 974, comprising approximately the carboxyterminal two-thirds of clone 9742, was sub-cloned into the *E. coli* expression vector, pMAL, from which affinity purified MBP::974 fusion protein was obtained. Antibodies to this fusion protein were used to screen other agricultural crops for the presence of group IX proteins. Finally, we investigate whether the extensive amino acid sequence homology among group IX sequences of several grass species could be exploited to describe important structural domains of group IX allergens.

3. RESULTS

3.1. Cloning and Sequence of *Hor v* 9

A barley pollen cDNA library, prepared in lambda-zap II (Stratagene), was screened by standard techniques (6) with the Kentucky bluegrass *Poa p* 9 allergen clone c7.2, a fragment of *Poa p* 9 clone KBG41 (7). Twenty-five positively hybridizing plaques were identified, of which seven were sequenced (please see Table 1). Clones 94, 95, 96, and 97 were found to be unique. Clone 97 appeared to be a partial-length clone and had the greatest sequence similarity to KBG41. Clone 97 was used to re-screen the library to obtain two additional partial cDNAs (clones 971 and 974) and the full-length clone 9742. Clone 9742 contained an open reading frame encoding 313 amino acids, included a possible signal peptide (8) to yield a mature polypeptide of 286 amino acids. The mature polypeptide contains a potential glycosylation site (9). Clone 9742 also included a polyadenylation signal and poly(A) tail.

3.2. Subcloning of 974 into the *E. coli* Protein Expression Vector pMAL

Barely pollen clone 974 was sub-cloned (6) into the *E.coli* protein expression vector, pMAL (New England Biolabs). A fusion of maltose binding protein (MBP) and clone 974 produced a 65 kDa protein. The MBP::974 fusion protein was purified from *E. coli* extracts using a bound maltose affinity column. Purified MBP::974 fusion protein was used to immunize mice, and produce anti-MBP::974 serum by standard protocols (10)(please see Figure 1). Anti-MBP::974 antibody identified a single 30 kDa band in barley pollen extracts, designated *Hor v* 9.

Table 1. Barley pollen cDNAs identified by *Poa p* 9 allergen clone c7.2

| Clone No. | Insert (nt) | mRNA (nt) | Similarity[1] of barley pollen cDNAs to clone 9742 (%) | |
			Nucleotide	Amino Acid
9742	1339	1450		
974	894	1450	100 (445-1339)	100
971	841	1450	100 (348-1189)	100
97	625	1450	100 (694-1314)	100
96	350	1200	Not similar	
95	574	1900	82 (765-1339)	93
94	601	1600	Not similar	

[1] The region of similarity to clone 9742 is indicated in brackets.

3.3. Survey of Agricultural Species for *Hor v* 9 Homologues

Proteins and mRNA were extracted from pollen of species listed in the Table 2 below. Western blots (shown in Figure 2) of pollen proteins were performed with anti-974 antibody and revealed cross-reactive proteins in all species tested except canola (*Brassica napus*). Total RNA was also extracted from the pollen of these species, and northern blots probed with ^{32}P labelled clone 9742 revealed cross-hybridizing transcripts in cultivated Rye (*Secale cereale*), wheat (*Triticum aestivum*) and Kentucky bluegrass. Southern blots of genomic DNA from species listed in Table 2 probed with ^{32}P labelled clone 9742 revealed cross-hybridizing genes in cultivated Rye, wheat and maize (*Zea mays*). Results of

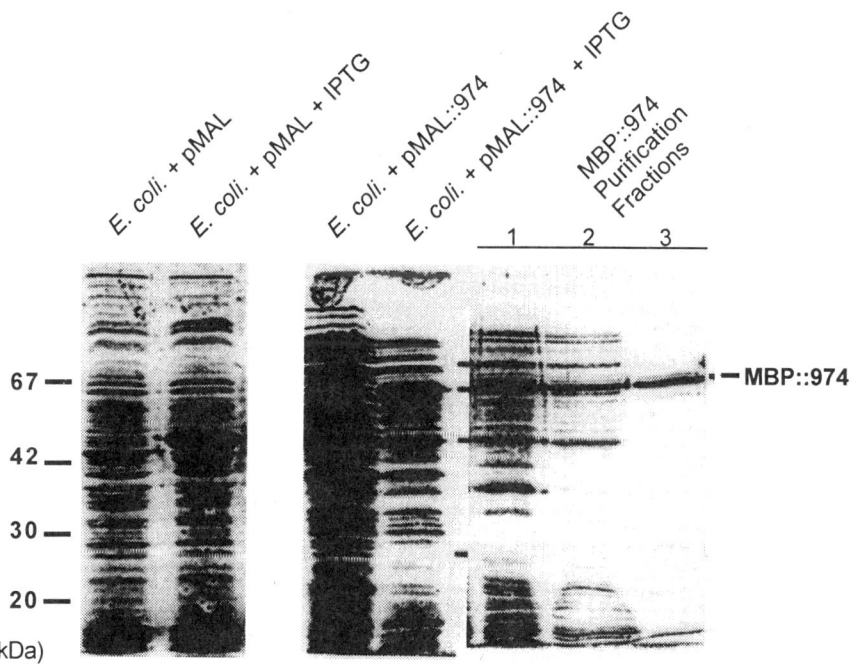

Figure 1. Purification of clone 974 protein as a Maltose binding fusion protein expressed by pMAL plasmid in *E. coli*.

Table 2. Hor v 9 Homologues in agricultural species

Species	Pollen Proteins (kDa)	Pollen mRNAs (kb)	Genomic DNA *Eco* R I (kbp)
Hordeum vulgare	(28), 30, (57)	1.4	10.5
Poa pratensis	30	1.4	n.t.
Secale cereale	28	1.4	10
Triticum aestivum	33	1.4	10
Triticale	28, 30	-	-
Avena sativa	33	-	-
Zea mays	57	-	11
Helianthus annus	28	n.t.	n.t.
Linum usitassimum	57	-	n.t
Brassica napus	-	-	-

Notes to table: - = none detected, n.t.= not tested, ( ) = faint band.

western, northern and Southern blots (Table 2) together show that group 9 homologues exist in a variety if agricultural species. In addition, homologues can be detected by nucleic acid cross-hybridization in especially *gramineae* species.

3.4. Conservation of Antibody Binding Epitopes in 7 Pollen Allergens Including *Hor v* 9

The extensive cross-reactivity and cross-hybridization observed in barley, Kentucky bluegrass, Rye, wheat and maize suggested that immunologically important epitopes may be conserved among these species, and group IX homologues generally. An amino acid sequence alignment of representative group IX homologues *Poa p* 9, *Hor v* 9 and *Lol p* 1b (11) using the computer program FASTA (12), indicated exceptionally high amino acid sequence similarity (please see Figure 3). To determine whether antibody binding epitopes

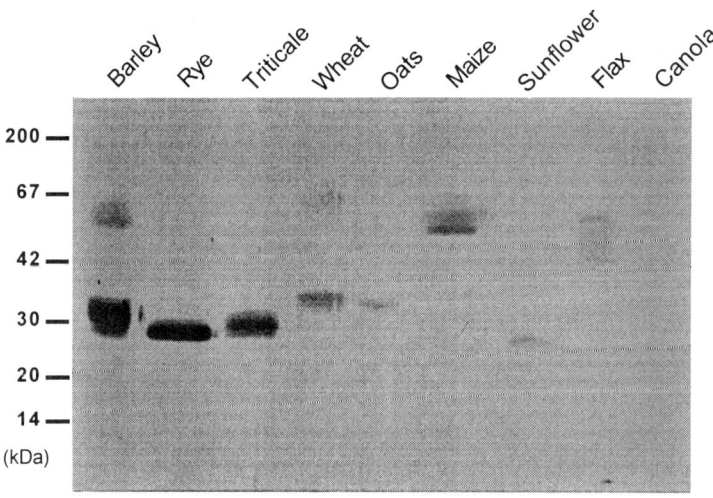

Figure 2. Western blot of pollen proteins in agricultural crop species which cross-react with anti-MBP::974 (*Hor v* 9) antibody.

```
Horv 9  mansgrehsavprrrnlvalv-prhgcYAEFSLYVCVGNINAPFPVFNRT     49
KBG41   ..----v.qytvalfla....agpaas..ADVG.GAPATLAT.ATPAAPA     46
LolpIb  ..----vqkytvalflrrgprggpgrs..ADAG.TPAAAATPATPAAIPA     46

Horv 9  TFIANAGIE-AELEPHFLLLLFTFSSSSSFFTLLKTMIHFTDRSDNKNKA     98
KBG41   AGYTP.APAG.APKATTDEQKLIEKINAG.KAAVAAAAGVPAVDKY.TFV     96
LolpIb  GGWREGDDRR..AAGGRQR.ASRQPWPPLPTPLRRTSSRSSRPPSPSPPR     96

Horv 9  MMRGREFRKATFAEVLKGAAGQIAGQSSSMAKLSSSLELSYKLAYDKAQG    148
KBG41   ATF.TASN.....A.STEPK.AA.AS.NAV--.T.K.DAA.....KS.E.    144
LolpIb  AS------------------SPTSAAKAPG.IPK.DTA.CV..-..AE    125

Horv 9  ATPEAKYDAYVATLTESLRVISGTLEVHSVKPAAEEVKG--VPAGELKAI    196
KBG41   ..............S.A..I.A......A....G....A--I.....QV.    192
LolpIb  .H.RGQVRRLRHCPHR.....A.A....A....T...PAAKI.T...QIV    175

Horv 9  DQVDAAFRTAATAADAAPANDKFTVFESLQQGPSRKPRGGAYESYKFIPA    246
KBG41   .K.....KV.....N...........AAFNDAIKAST....Q.......    242
LolpIb  .KI....KI.....N...T.........AFNKALNECT...NRPTSSS.P    225

Horv 9  LEAAVKQAYAATVAAAPEVKFTVFQTALSKAINAMTQAGKVAKPAAAATA    296
KBG41   .......S......T..A..Y...E...K...T..S..Q.A......V..    292
LolpIb  SRPRSSRPTPPPSP......YA..EA..T...T.....Q.AG......AT    275

Horv 9  TATVAAGAAATAGNYKV                                    313
KBG41   ...G.V...TG.VGAATGAATAAAGGYKTGAATPTAGNYKV            333
LolpIb  A.ATV.T.....AA.LPPPLLVVQSLISLLIYY                    308
```

Figure 3. Amino acid sequence alignment of *Hor v 9*, *Poa p 9*, and *Lol p* Ib; (.) indicate identical amino acids, (-) inicate gaps.

mapped for *Poa p* 9 are present in all group IX proteins, alignments of *Hor v 9*, *Poa p* 9 (KBG31, KBG41 and KBG60), *Phl p* 5 (3), *Phl p* 5a, and *Lol p* Ib (11) were made (4). Table 3 shows that the epitopes are found in all of these species, and that they are highly conserved, having few amino acid substitutions (4).

3.5. Sequence Motif Predictions Based on Homologous Grass Pollen Allergens

An amino acid sequence similarity plot (13) of the group IX pollen allergens listed above showed that all shared epitopes (5) in Table 3 also correspond to the most highly conserved segments of these proteins (please see Figure 4). In addition, the group IX pollen allergen sequences were imported into the Antherpro (14) suite of protein structure prediction computer programs. Antherpro predicted a transmembrane sequence in the carboxyterminal region of all seven group IX proteins. Finally, it can be seen that the carboxyterminal domain (relative amino acid position 200 to 400) of the seven allergens is more highly conserved than the amino terminal domain (Figure 4).

Searches of the GenBank, EMBL, PIR and SwissProt sequence databases using FASTA (12) revealed small similarities between group IX epitopes and several cell adhesion proteins (VCAM, NCAM and CD2). Based on the domain structure predicted by the

Table 3. Conservation of epitopes in seven grass pollen allergens

Epitope Number	*Poa p* 9 (KBG60) Amino Acid Sequence	Consensus Amino Acid Sequence
2	SYGAPATPAA	(G̲/S)YG(X̲)PATPAA
4	PAAGYTPAAP	PAAGYTPAAP
21-22	YKLAY	YKLAY
25	KYDDYVALTS	KYD̲A̲YVATLS
31	EVKATPAGEL	EVKA(I̲/V̲)PAGEL
33-34	VDAAF	VDAAF
38	FTVFEAAFND	FTVFEAAFND
41	TGGAYQSYKF	TGGAY(Q/E̲)SYKF
42	QSYKFIPALE	(Q/E̲)SYKFIPALE
44	AAVKQSYAAT	AAVKQ(S/A̲)YAAT
55	AATGAATAAA	AATGAATAA(T̲/A)

a) Variable residues are indicated in parentheses (i.e. G/S = glycine or serine), and "X" indicates "any amino acid". Substitutions in the concensus relative to KBG60 are double underlined.

similarity plot in Figure 4, the presence of a putative transmembrane span in all seven grass pollen homologues, the presence of a putative signal peptide, and the presence of conserved epitopes, we have developed a generalized domain structure for this group of pollen allergens. We note that this generalized structure is reminiscent of the generalized structure of cell adhesion molecules such as VCAM, NCAM and CD2 (15); and this structure is depicted in Figure 5.

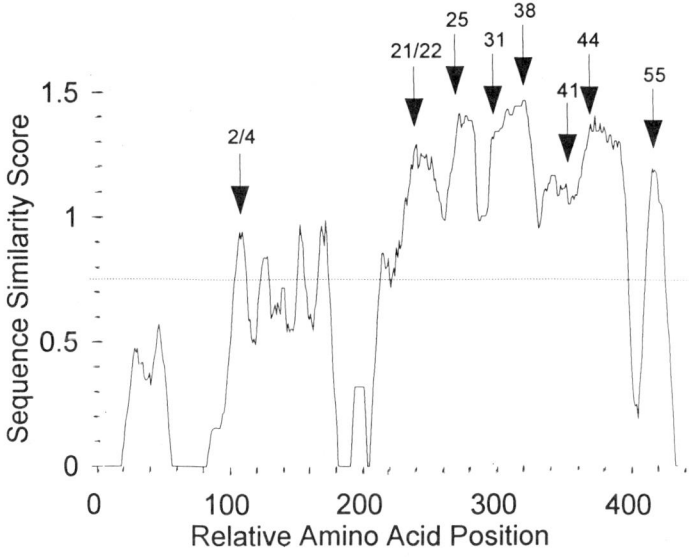

Figure 4. Similarity plot of group IX pollen allergen homologues (4). Similarity scores were calculated to indicate conservation of amino acid residues relative to a consensus sequence of seven group IX homologues. *Poa p* 9 epitopes are indicated by number (as in Table 3).

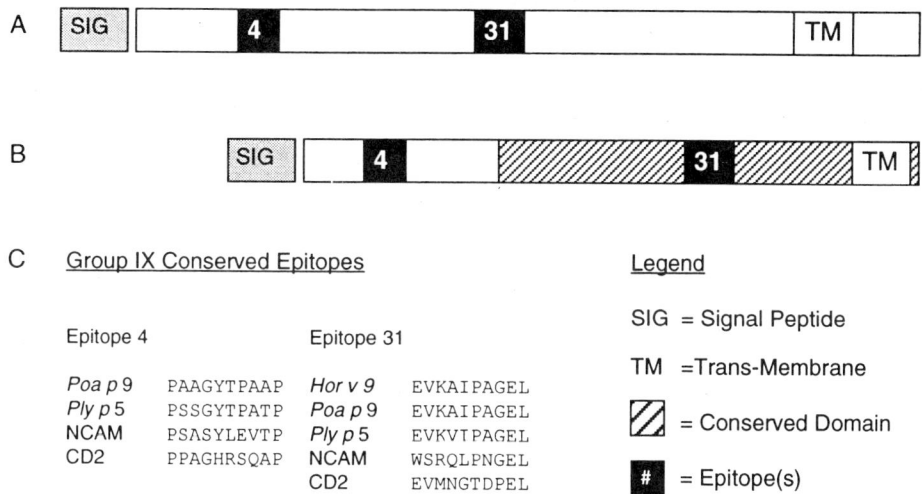

Figure 5. Generalized domain structure of cell adhesion molecules (A) and group IX pollen allergens (B). Epitopes (C) as in Table 3.

4. DISCUSSION

Western, and northern and Southern blotting experiments showed that cognates for barley *Hor v 9* exist in a variety of species, including the important cereal crops wheat, rye, Triticale, maize, and oats (*Avena sativa*). The apparent ubiquity in *Gramineae* of group IX allergens implies that allergen cognates have an important role in the biology of pollen. The *Hor v 9* amino acid sequence predicted by clone 9742 contains several structural motifs which suggest a role in the extracellular matrix. *Hor v 9* contains a signal peptide and an asparagine sequon for glycosylation, which imply protein secretion. Sequence comparisons of *Hor v 9* to the related isoallergens *Poa p 9*, *Phl p 5* and *Lol p* 1b indicated that the region of greatest similarity occurs in the carboxyl terminal region. Thus, the amino terminal domain corresponding to $Ala_{(1)}$ to $Ser_{(107)}$ in *Hor v* IX can be described as highly variable. The role of the variable domain is not obvious, except that it probably confers unique properties to each group IX isoform. For example, it has recently been shown that *Phl p 5* has RNAse activity (Bufe *et al.*, this volume). This activity could be unique to the Timothy pollen allergens and could be conferred by the aminoterminal domain.

Group IX pollen allergens have domain structure similar to the immunoglobulin motif superfamily of cell adhesion molecules (such as VCAM, NCAM and CD2) involved in cell surface recognition (15). In addition, two epitopes common to all group IX homologues may be present in these cell adhesion molecules. NCAM is a neural cell adhesion molecule which has been implicated in the regulation of axonal growth (16). VCAM is a vascular cell adhesion molecule involved in the recruitment of lymphocytes and monocytes to sites of inflammation (16). CD2 is expressed predominantly on thymocytes and T-lymphocytes and is a T-cell receptor for antigen presentation (17). A common domain structure and the possibility of common epitopes between pollen allergens and cell adhesion molecules suggests a potential for interaction at the cellular level, an interaction that could be important to the atopic immune response. The Ig-like motifs may trigger a similar auto-immune mechanism which has been proposed for profilin (18). Now that recombinant pollen allergens are being exploited as diagnostic and therapeutic agents (this volume) in the treatment of atopic allergies, we suggest that therapeutic polypeptides be engineered so as to avoid the inclusion of possible human Ig sequences like those similar to epitope 4 and epitope 31 identified in the group IX pollen allergens, especially since epitope 31 is a highly conserved human T-cell epitope (19).

5. ACKNOWLEDGMENTS

We thank the National Science and Engineering Research Council of Canada, the Canadian Wheat Board, and Monsanto Company. We also thank Sharon M. Gubbels for critically reviewing this manuscript.

6. REFERENCES

1. Silvanovich, A., Astwood, J., Zhang, L., Olsen, E., Kisil, F., Sehon, A., Mohapatra S. and Hill, R. (1991) Nucleotide sequence analysis of three cDNAs coding for *Poa p* IX isoallergens of kentucky bluegrass pollen. *J. Biol. Chem.* **266**, 1204–1210.
2. Ong, E.K., Griffith, I.J., Knox, R.B. and Singh, M.B. (1993) Cloning of a cDNA encoding a group-V (group IX) allergen isoform from rye-grass pollen that demonstrates specific immunoreactivity. *Gene* **134**, 235–240.
3. Vrtala, S., Sperr, W.R., Reimitzer, I., van Ree, R., Laffer, S., Muller, W-D., Valent, P., Lechner, K., Rumpold, H., Kraft, D., Scheiner, O., and Valenta, R. (1993) cDNA cloning of a major allergen from Timothy grass (*Phleum pratense*) pollen, characterization of the recombinant *Phl p* V allergen. *J. Immunol.* **151**, 4773–4781.
4. Astwood, J.D., Mohapatra, S.S., Ni, H. and Hill, R.D. (1994) Pollen allergen homologues in barley and other crop species. *Clin. Exp. Allergy* **25**, 66–72.
5. Zhang, L., Olsen, E., Kisil, F.T., Hill, R.D., Sehon, A.H., and Mohapatra, S.S (1992) Mapping of antibody binding epitopes of a recombinant *Poa p* IX allergen. *Mol. Immunol.* **29**, 1383–1389.
6. Sambrook, J., Fritsch, E.F., and Maniatis, T. (1989) *Molecular cloning: a laboratory manual, second edition.* Cold Spring Harbour: Cold Spring Harbour Laboratory Press.
7. Mohapatra, S.S., Hill, R., Astwood, J., Ekramoddoullah, A.K.M., Olsen, E., Silvanovich, A., Hatton, T., Kisil, F.T. and Sehon, A.H. (1990) Isolation and characterization of a cDNA clone encoding an IgE-binding protein from kentucky bluegrass (Poa pratensis) pollen. Int. Arch. Allergy Appl. Immunol. 91, 362–368.
8. von Heijne, G. (1985) Signal sequences, the limits of variation. *J. Mol. Biol* **184**, 99–105.
9. Hunt, L.T. and Dayhoff, M.O. (1970) The occurrence in proteins of the tripeptides Asn-X-Ser and Asn-X-Thr and of bound carbohydrate. *Biochem. Biophys. Res. Commun.* **39**, 757–765.
10. Harlow, E and Lane, P. (1988) *Antibodies, A Laboratory Manual.* Cold Spring Harbour: Cold Spring Harbour Laboratory Press.
11. Singh, M.B., Hough, T., Theerakulpisut,P., Avjioglu, A., Davies, S., Smith, P.M., Taylor, P., Simpson, R.J., Ward, L.D., McCluskey, J., Puy, R. and Knox, R.B. (1991) Isolation of cDNA encoding a newly identified major allergenic protein of rye-grass pollen: intracellular targeting to the amyloplast. *Proc. Natl. Acad. Sci.* USA **88**, 1384–1388.
12. Pearson, W.R. and Lipman, D.J. (1988) Improved tools for biological sequence comparison. *Proc. Natl. Acad. Sci.* USA **85**, 2444–2448.
13. Deveraux, J., Haeberli, P., and Smithies, O. (1984) A comprehensive set of sequence analysis programs for the VAX. *Nuc. Acids Res.* **12**, 387–395.
14. Georjon, C., Deleage, G. and Roux, B. (1991) ANTHEPRO: an interactive graphic software for analyzing protein structures from sequences. *J. Mol. Graph.* **9**, 188–190.
15. Williams, A.F. and Barclay, A.N. (1988) The immunoglobulin superfamily - domains for cell surface recognition. *Ann. Rev. Immunol.* **6**, 381–405.

16. Obrink, B. (1993) Cell adhesion and the cell-cell contact proteins. In *Guidebook to the extracellular matrix and adhesion proteins.* (Kreis, T and Vale, R., eds). Oxford: Oxford University Press, pp. 109–114.

17. Canonica, G.W., Ciprandi, G., Buscaglia, S., Pesce, G. and Bagnasco, M. (1994) Adhesion molecules of allergic inflammation: recent insights into their functional roles. *Allergy* **49**, 135–141.

18. Valenta, R., Duchene, M., Pettenburger, K., Sillaber, C, Valent P., Breitenbach, M., Rumpold, H., Kraft, D. and Scheiner, O. (1991) Identification of profilin as a novel pollen allergen; IgE autoreactivity in sensitized individuals. *Science* **253**, 557–560.

19. Mohapatra, S.S., Mohapatra, S., Yang, M., Ansari, A.A., Parronchi, P., Maggi, E., and Romagnani, S. (1994) Molecular basis of cross-reactivity among allergen-specific human T cells: T-cell receptor $V\alpha$ gene usage and epitope structure. *Immunology* **81**, 15–20.

40

CYTOKINE AND DRUG MODULATION OF TNFα IN MAST CELLS

Tong-Jun Lin, Antonio Enciso, Elyse Y. Bissonnette, Agnes Szczepek, and
A. Dean Befus

Pulmonary Research Group
Department of Medicine
University of Alberta
Edmonton Alberta, Canada, T6G 2S2

1. INTRODUCTION

Mast cells (MC) are critical effector cells in allergic reactions, but also have the potential to regulate immune responses through the cytokines they produce (Table 1). These MC-derived multifunctional mediators (first mediator pool) recruit and activate other effector cells such as neutrophils, eosinophils and monocytes/macrophages, as well as MC themselves to produce a broader spectrum of mediators in large amounts (second mediator pool) to amplify the response (Figure 1). Because of the limitation of space, this brief review focuses on the production and regulation of the first mediator pool in MC.

2. MAST CELLS AS A SOURCE OF MULTIPLE CYTOKINES

Of the growing number of cytokines identified from MC (Table 1), tumor necrosis factor α (TNFα) is the best described. Human dermal[1,2] and mucosal MC (MMC),[3,4] human mast cell line (HMC-1),[5,6] freshly isolated mouse[7,8] or rat[9] peritoneal MC (PMC), mouse MC lines[10] and rat basophilic leukemia (RBL) cells[11,12] synthesize and release TNFα. Interestingly, MC constitutively synthesize and release a substantial amount of TNFα without obvious stimulation, a marked distinction from that of macrophages, T cells and B cells which contain little or no preformed TNFα bioactivity without stimulation. For example, unstimulated mouse PMC contain approximately twice as much TNFα bioactivity as LPS-stimulated mouse peritoneal macrophages.[8] Our experiments[9] also showed that freshly isolated rat PMC and intestinal mucosal MC (IMMC) constitutively synthesize and release a substantial amount of TNFα. Although the biological significance of constitutive release of TNFα from MC is unclear, MC-generated TNFα is a major mediator in neutrophil recruitment and infiltration.[13] MC also release TNFα in response to stimuli such as antigen/anti-IgE,[8] substance P[10], calcium ionophores[14] and PMA.[8]

New Horizons in Allergy Immunotherapy
edited by Sehon et al. Plenum Press, New York, 1996

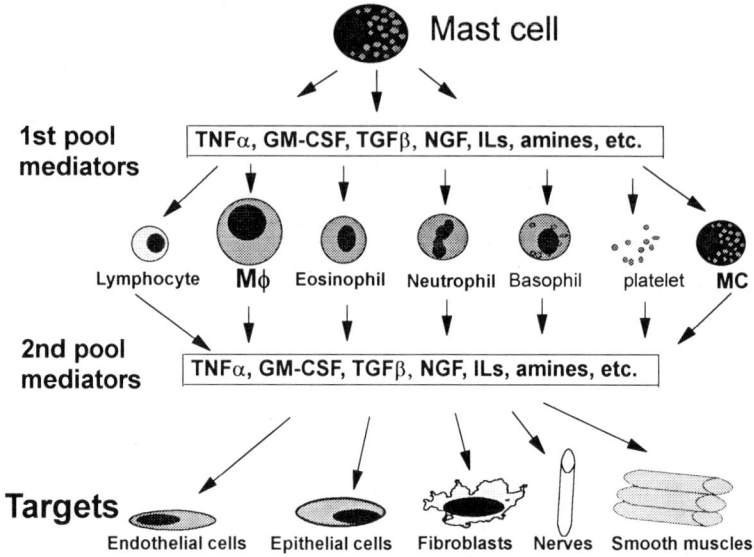

Figure 1. Mast cell mediators in allergy and inflammation.

Granulocyte macrophage colony-stimulating factor (GM-CSF) not only plays a role in the functional activity of MC,[15] but is also produced by MC.[16] Both mRNA and protein for GM-CSF are produced by several MC lines.[16,17] Another important cytokine produced by a mouse MC line,[18] dog mastocytoma cells[19] and freshly isolated rat PMC (EY Bissonnette and AD Befus, submitted) is transforming growth factor-β (TGFβ). TGFβ production seems not to be an artifact of cell culture, since antibody specific for TGFβ markedly diminished MC-dependent collagen gene expression of fibroblasts in MC-reconstituted W/Wv mice *in vivo*.[20] Treatment of isolated rat PMC with anti-TGFβ1 antibodies enhanced TNFα-dependent cytotoxicity, suggesting an autocrine role for MC-derived TGFβ1 (EY Bissonnette and AD Befus, submitted). MC have recently been recognized as a source of nerve growth factor (NGF), a mediator with profound effects on mast cell survival, gene expression and mediator secretion.[21–23] Some murine MC lines express mRNAs for four members of β-chemokines (macrophage inflammatory proteins (MIP) 1α and 1β, T-cell-activation antigen 3 (TCA3), and JE).[24,25] I-309 and monocyte chemotactic protein 1 (MCP-1) are human homologues of murine TCA3 and JE respectively. The human MC line, HMC-1, expresses multiple chemokine mRNAs for β-chemokines (I-309, MCP-1, MIP-1α, MIP-1β and RANTES) and α-chemokine (IL-8), and chemokine proteins for I-309 and MCP-1.[26] β-Chemokines including MIP-1α, MCP-1 and RANTES are potent stimulators of MC migration and mediator release.[27–29] Rat PMC and some MC lines produce leukemia inhibitory factor (LIF) mRNA or protein, a pluripotent cytokine important in the regulation of immune and inflammatory responses.[30] However, there is limited information on the effects of LIF, IL-6 and IL-11, members of a subfamily of cytokines with similar predicted structures and functional redundancy in their actions, on MC function.

MC lines or *in vivo*-derived MC express mRNAs or proteins for almost all the interleukins known (IL-1,2,3,4,5,6,8,10,12,13) as shown in Table 1. Human tissue MC or *in vivo*-derived rodent MC which express multiple phenotypic differences from *in vitro*-de-

Table 1. Cytokines produced by different population of mast cells

	human mast cells		rodent mast cells	
	normal mast cells	Cell line	Freshly isolated	Cell lines
TNFα	p[a] (1-5)	m[b], p (5,6)	m, p (7-9,14)	m, p (10-12)
GM-CSF				m, p (16,17)
TGFβ			m, p (20)	m, p[c] (18)
NGF			m, p (21)	
IFNγ				m (24,28)
β-chemokines[d]		m,p (28)		m (24,25)
LIF			m (30)	m, p (30)
IL-1	p (5)	m, p (5,6)		m, p (24)
IL-2				m (32)
IL-3		m, p (5,33)	p (32)	m, p (32)
IL-4	p (4)	m (33)		m, p (24,32,34)
IL-5	p (4)			m (24,32)
IL-6	p (4,5)	p (5)	p (14)	m, p (24,32)
IL-8	p (5,35)	m, p (33,35)	p (36)	
IL-10		m (37)		m (38)
IL-12				m (34)
IL-13		m (37,39)		m, p (39)

[a]p: evidence for protein, [b]m: evidence for mRNA, [c]Dog mastocytoma cells also produce TGFβ₁ (J. Clin. Invest. 1992; 90:35-41). [d]For individual chemokines: see text. Numbers in parentheses are references.

rived MC lines, synthesize and secrete several cytokines (Table 1). However, it should be recognized that in current literature, some cytokines (GM-CSF, IFNs, β-chemokines, IL-2, 10, 12 and 13) have only been found in MC lines, not in *in vivo* derived MC. Moreover, only cytokine mRNAs instead of proteins for IFNγ, most β-chemokines, IL-2, IL-10 and IL-12 were found. Given the significant MC heterogeneity, including substantial differences in mediator contents and sensitivity to cytokines and pharmacological agents, it is not surprising that the amounts and types of cytokines produced by various populations of

MC are variable. Indeed, the spectrum of MC cytokines, the kinetics of cytokine release, and sensitivity to specific stimuli vary significantly among various MC populations.[5,6,24]

Furthermore, several interesting issues are worthy of mention. Firstly, MC-generated mediators (Table 1) include both Th1 (IFNγ, IL-2, 12) and Th2 (IL-4, 5, 6, 10, 13) type cytokines which show reciprocal regulation on T and B lymphocyte functions. However, it is unclear to what extent this reciprocal Th1 and Th2 -type cytokine interaction affects MC function. Secondly, there is no information on IL-9 producing capability of MC, although IL-9 shows significant effects on MC development and function.[31] Thirdly, given that MC respond to most of the cytokines listed in Table 1, MC likely express receptors for these cytokines. However most of these MC-cytokine receptors are not characterized. Finally, the regulation of MC cytokine production is poorly understood. Given the complexity of possible effects of MC-derived cytokines and the space limitation, we will restrict the subsequent discussion to MC-derived TNFα because of its significant role in allergy and inflammation and its constitutive production by resting MC.

3. MODULATION OF TNFα IN MAST CELLS

3.1. Cytokine Inhibition of MC TNFα Production

IFN-α/β and -γ, TGFβ and IL-10 inhibit TNFα production by MC. Although IFNs enhance the cytotoxic activity of natural killer (NK) cells and monocytes/macrophages, IFN-α/β and IFN-γ do not stimulate the cytotoxic activity of rat PMC, but inhibit TNFα-dependent cytotoxicity in concentration and time dependent manners.[9] Preincubation of MC for 2 h with 100 and 200 U/ml of IFN-γ and IFN-α/β, respectively, inhibited PMC cytotoxicity against WEHI-164 target cells. Lower concentrations of IFN-γ (12.5 U/ml) and IFN-α/β (25 U/ml) inhibited cytotoxicity of PMC after 8 h preincubation. Our experiments also demonstrated that both IFN-α/β and IFN-γ inhibited TNFα-dependent cytotoxicity of IMMC. Furthermore, treatment of rat MC lines (HRMC and RCMC) with IFN-α/β and IFN-γ inhibited TNFα-dependent cytotoxicity and downregulated mRNA levels of TNFα in dose and time dependent manners.

In contrast to IFN, IL-10 shows similar inhibitory effects on TNFα-dependent cytotoxicity in both MC and monocytes/macrophages. We have demonstrated that spontaneous and antigen(Ag)-induced TNFα production by rat PMC are inhibited by IL-10 in a dose-dependent manner (20 to 200 U/ml) (TJ Lin and AD Befus, unpublished data). Concurrent incubation of PMC with IL-10 for 3, 6, 12 and 24 h significantly inhibited Ag-stimulated and spontaneous TNFα production. At 200 U/ml, IL-10 inhibited more than 90% of spontaneous and Ag-induced TNFα production by rat PMC, unlike IFN-α/β and -γ and TGFβ which at optimal concentrations only inhibit TNFα-dependent cytotoxicity in rat PMC by 30–50%. Thus, IL-10 is the potent inhibitor of MC TNFα production.

Recently, we demonstrated that TGF-β1 suppresses TNFα and histamine secretion from rat PMC (EY Bissonnette and AD Befus, submitted). *In vitro* treatment of rat PMC with TGF-β1 (10–9 and 10–10 M) inhibited TNFα-dependent cytotoxicity (29% and 27%, respectively). At least 2 h pretreatment with TGF-β1 was required to inhibit MC TNFα-dependent cytotoxicity. This inhibitory effect of TGF-β1 was abrogated by antibody to TGF-β1. Furthermore, the treatment of purified PMC with anti-TGF-β1 antibody alone significantly increased the release of TNFα, suggesting that TGF-β1 may regulates MC TNFα production in an autocrine manner.

It is interesting that stem cell factor (SCF) and IL-4, both have major positive effects on MC development and function, but appear to have little effect on MC TNFα production. Our experiments and others[40] have established that SCF is an important microenvironmental factor which regulates release of MC histamine and arachidonic acid metabolites, and MC development. However, treatment of rat PMC with SCF at the doses of 2 to 500 ng/ml for 3, 6, 12, 24 h did not affect the spontaneous and Ag-induced TNFα production (TJ Lin, EY Bissonnette and AD Befus, submitted). Similarly, IL-4 which showed significant promotion on MC growth and mediator release,[40] has no effects on TNFα mRNA expression in both resting and ionomycin-activated HMC-1 cells.[6,33] Thus, the regulation of TNFα in MC is distinct from that of other mediators such as histamine and arachidonic acid metabolites.

3.2. Drug Inhibition of MC TNFα Production

The anti-allergic drugs and prostanoids which exhibit inhibitory effects on MC TNFα production include sulfasalazine, sodium cromoglycate (SCG), nedocromil sodium (NED), adrenergic β2 receptor agonists (salbutamol, salmeterol and isoproterenol), cyclosporine A (CsA), FK506, corticosteroids (dexamethasone, DEX) and prostaglandins (PG E1, E2 and misoprostol).

We have established that sulfasalazine inhibits MC TNFα-dependent cytotoxicity in a concentration dependent manner (more than 95% inhibition at high dose) (EY Bissonnette, A Enciso and AD Befus, submitted). One metabolite of sulfasalazine, sulfapyridine, but not the other metabolite, 5-aminosalicylic acid (5-ASA), also inhibits MC cytotoxicity, but is less potent than sulfasalazine. Both pretreatment of rat PMC with sulfasalazine and addition of sulfasalazine to PMC, 0.5 to 12 h after the cytotoxic assay (16 h) has started, significantly inhibited MC cytotoxic activity. Furthermore, significant inhibition by sulfasalazine of TNFα-dependent cytotoxicity of fixed MC in the absence of released TNFα suggests a direct interaction between sulfasalazine and MC membrane-bound TNFα. Moreover, northern blot analysis showed that TNFα mRNA of PMC was significantly reduced by sulfasalazine (77%). Taken together, these observations suggest that sulfasalazine inhibits MC TNFα-dependent cytotoxicity by multiple mechanisms: competitive inhibition of soluble and membrane TNFα, and depression of TNFα mRNA level and release of TNFα.

The cromone family comprises SCG and the more recently developed NED. Our laboratory found that both SCG and NED significantly inhibited TNFα-dependent cytotoxicity of rat MC (27% and 37%, respectively). Furthermore, treatment of MC with NED significantly reduced TNFα mRNA (71%). Thus, the inhibition of TNFα production by MC may be one of the therapeutic mechanisms of SCG and NED in the treatment of allergic disorders.

The anti-inflammatory effect of β2-adrenergic agonists on TNFα activity of human MC was established in our laboratory.[41] Human skin MC were used in TNFα-dependent cytotoxicity and histamine release assays. Significant inhibition ($p < 0.05$) of TNFα activity was observed at 10 nM of all β2-agonists tested (salbutamol, salmeterol and isoproterenol). Almost complete inhibition was observed with 100 nM of salbutamol (93.8 ± 3.9%, n=5). The IC50 were 14.9, 31.2 and 20.2 nM for salbutamol, salmeterol and isoproterenol respectively. Thus, the inhibition of human MC TNFα activity and histamine release may be important in the actions of β2-agonists in asthma.

CsA, FK506 and DEX are potent immunosuppressive agents and have significant inhibitory effects on TNFα production in mouse MC lines.[42,43] It was suggested that these immunosuppressive agents can have at least three actions that interfere with the pathogenesis of IgE and MC-dependent inflammatory reactions: suppression of the IgE-dependent increase in TNFα mRNA by MC, inhibition of the IgE-dependent production of TNFα protein by MC, and diminution of the responsiveness of target cells to TNFα.[42]

Prostaglandins, such as PGE1, PGE2, and misoprostol but not PGD2 significantly inhibit TNFα release from rat freshly isolated PMC and IMMC in picomolar to nanomolar concentrations.[44,45] These effects may contribute to the protective and anti-inflammatory effects of prostaglandins in the gastrointestinal tract and elsewhere.

4. CONCLUSION

One of the consequences of MC activation is the initiation of MC-leukocyte cascade (Figure 1) in which MC-derived cytokines (Table 1) contribute to the recruitment and activation of secondary effector cells, which in turn provide additional mediators important to the progression of the response. The recognition that MC-derived cytokines may be responsible for many of the biologically and clinically important consequences of MC activation may have therapeutic implications. Management of MC-initiated pathogenesis may include downregulation of the MC-derived first mediator pool (such as inhibition of MC-TNFα production by IL-10, IFNs and drugs), suppression of other effector cell-derived secondary mediator pool and diminution of the responsiveness of target cells to mediators (such as inhibition by CsA and corticosteroids).

REFERENCES

1. Walsh LJ, Trinchieri G, Waldorf HA, Whitaker D and Murphy GF. *Proc. Natl. Acad. Sci. USA.* 1991; 88:4220.
2. Benyon RC, Bissonnette EY, and Befus AD. *J. Immunol.* 1991; 147:2253.
3. Bradding P, Feather IH, Bardin PG, Heusser CH, Holgate ST and Howarth PH. *J. Immunol.* 1993; 151:3853.
4. Bradding P, Roberts JA, Britten KM, Montefort S, Djukanovic R, Mueller R, Heusser CH, Howarth PH and Holgate ST. *Am. J. Respir. Cell Mol. Biol.* 1994; 10:471.
5. Grabbe J, Welker P, Moller A, Dippel E, Ashman LK and Czarnetzki BM. *J. Invest. Dermatol.* 1994; 103:504.
6. Sillaber C, Bevec D, Butterfield JH, Heppner C, Valenta R, Scheiner O, Kraft D, Lechner K, Bettelheim P and Valent P. *Exp. Hematol.* 1993; 21:1271.
7. Young JD, Liu CC, Butler G, Cohn ZA and Galli SJ. *Proc. Natl. Acad. Sci. USA.* 1987; 84:9175.
8. Gordon JR and Galli SJ. *Nature* 1990; 346:274.
9. Bissonnette EY and Befus AD. *J. Immunol.* 1990; 145:3385.
10. Ansel JC, Brown JR, Payan DG and Brown MA. *J. Immunol.* 1993; 150:4478.
11. Richards AL, Okuno T, Takagaki Y and Djeu JY. *J. Immunol.* 1988; 141:3061.
12. Baumgartner R, Yamada K, Deramo VA and Beaven MA. *J. Immunol.* 1994; 153:2609.
13. Zhang Y, Ramos BF and Jakschik B. *Science* 1992; 258:1957.
14. Leal-Berumen I, Conlon P and Marshall JS. *J. Immunol.* 1994; 152:5468.
15. Meade R, Neddermann KM, Greenfield RS, Braslawsky G and Bursuker I. *J. Leuk. Biol.* 1993; 54:523.
16. Chung SW, Wong PMC, Shen-Ong G, Ruscetti S, Ishizaka T and Eaves CJ. *Blood* 1986; 68:1074.
17. Nishikomori R, Kawai M, Jung EY, Tai G, Miyajima A, Arai N, Mayumi M and Heike T. *J. Immunol.* 1995; 154:694.
18. Hu ZQ, Yamazaki T, Cai Z, Yoshida T and Shimamura T. *Immunology* 1994; 82:482.
19. Pennington DW, Lopez AR, Thomas PS, Peck C and Gold WM. *J. Clin. Invest.* 1992; 90:35.
20. Gordon JR and Galli SJ. *J. Exp. Med.* 1994; 180:2027.
21. Leon A, A. Buriani A, Dal Toso R, Fabris M, Romanello S, Aloe L and Lev-Montalcini R. *Proc. Natl. Acad. Sci. USA.* 1994; 91:3739.
22. Horigome K, Bullock ED and Johnson EM Jr. *J. Biol. Chem.* 1994; 269:2695.

23. Horigome K, Pryor JC, Bullock ED and Johnson EM Jr. *J. Biol. Chem.* 1993; 268:14881.

24. Burd PR, Rogers HW, Gordon JR, Martin CA, Jayaraman S, Wilson SD, Dvorak AM, Galli SJ and Dorf ME. *J. Exp. Med.* 1989; 170:245.

25. Oh CK and Metcalfe DD. *J. Immunol.* 1994; 153:325.

26. Selvan RS, Butterfield JH and Krangel MS. *J. Biol. Chem.* 1994; 269:13893.

27. Alam R, Kumar D, Anderson-Walters D and Forsythe PA. *J. Immunol.* 1994; 152:1298.

28. Taub D, Dastych J, Inamura N, Upton J, Kelvin D, Metcalfe D and Oppenheim J. *J. Immunol.* 1995; 154:2393.

29. Mattoli S, Ackerman V, Vittori E and Marini M. *Biochem. Biophy. Res. Commun.* 1995; 209:316.

30. Marshall JS, Gauldie J, Nielsen L and Bienenstock J. *Eur. J. Immunol.* 1993; 23:2116.

31. Renauld JC, Kermouni A, Vink A, Louahed J and Van Snick J. *J. Leuk. Biol.* 1995; 57:353.

32. Plaut M, Pierce JH, Watson CJ, Hanley-Hyde J, Nordan RP and Paul WE. *Nature* 1989; 339:64.

33. Buckley MG, Williams CMM, Thompson J, Pryor P, Ray K, Butterfield JH and Coleman JW. *Immunology* 1995; 84:410.

34. Smith TJ, Ducharme LA and Weis JH. *Eur. J. Immunol.* 1994; 24:822.

35. Moller A, Lippert U, Lessmann D, Kolde G, Hamann K, Welker P, Schadendorf D, Rosenbach T, Luger T and B.M. Czarnetzki BM. *J. Immunol.* 1993; 151:3261.

36. Zhang Y, Ramos BF, Jakschik B, Baganoff MP, Deppeler CL, Meyer DM, Widomski DL, Fretland DL and Bolanowski MA. *Inflammation* 1995; 19:119.

37. Szczepek A and Befus AD. *Clin. Immunol. Immunopathol.* 1995;76:S115(Abstr).

38. Moore KW, Vieira P, Fiorentino DF, Troustine ML, Khan TA and Mosmann TR. *Science* 1990; 248:1230.

39. Burd PR, Thompson WC, Max EE and Mills FC. *J. Exp. Med.* 1995; 181:1373.

40. Coleman JW, Holliday MR, Kimber I, Zsebo KM and Galli SJ. *J. Immunol.* 1993;150:556.

41. Bissonnette EY and Befus AD. *Am. J. Respir. Crit. Care Med.* 1994; 149:A805(Abstr).

42. Wershil BK, Furuta GT, Lavigne JA, Choudhury AR, Wang ZS and Galli SJ. *J. Immunol.* 1995; 154:1391.

43. Fruman DA, Bierer BE, Benes JE, Burakoff SJ, Austen KF and Katz HR. *J. Immunol.* 1995; 154:1846.

44. Hogaboam CM, Bissonnette EY, Chin BC, Befus AD and Wallace JL. *Gastroenterology.* 1993; 104:122.

45. Leal-Berumen I, O'Byrne P, Gupta A, Richards CD and Marshall JS. *J. Immunol.* 1995; 154:4759.

41

SYNTHESIS AND STORAGE OF REGULATORY CYTOKINES IN HUMAN EOSINOPHILS

Redwan Moqbel[*]

Department of Allergy and Clinical Immunology
National Heart and Lung Institute
University of London
London, United Kingdom

1. INTRODUCTION

Eosinophils are prominent cells in allergic inflammation, asthma, and immune reactions against parasitic helminths.[1,2] The association between eosinophils and asthma has been extensively documented. Large numbers of eosinophils and their granule products have been observed in the airways of patients with asthma,[2] and an inverse correlation between the degree of bronchial hyperreactivity and peripheral blood eosinophilia was shown in subjects in whom a late-phase response developed after antigen challenge.[3] With use of fiberoptic bronchoscopy it was possible to correlate the number of activated eosinophils with the degree of bronchial hyperresponsiveness.[4] However, despite this close association, the evidence of a cause and effect relationship between eosinophil products and tissue damage remains unproven.

The accumulation of eosinophils into the site of the inflammatory focus in allergic-type responses is believed to be regulated by a complex series of events that involves T cells and cytokines[1,5,6] Cytokines, particularly interleukin-3 (IL-3), IL-5, and granulocyte-macrophage colony-stimulating factor (GM-CSF), influence eosinophil growth, maturation, and differentiation. IL-5 is of particular interest because it is unique in that it promotes terminal differentiation of precursors committed to the eosinophil lineage[7] Eosinophil survival is also prolonged as a result of incubation with IL-3, IL-5 and GM-CSF[8-10]. In addition to the latter three cytokines, interferon-γ (IFNγ) and tumour necrosis factor-α prime eosinophils and activate them for a number of effector functions[11,12].

Eosinophils, originally considered as "end cells" incapable of synthesizing novel proteins, have now been shown to synthesize and release a number of regulatory cytoki-

---

[*] Address for Correspondence: Department of Medicine, Pulmonary Research Group, 574 Heritage Medical Research Centre, University of Alberta, Edmonton, Alberta, Canada, T6G 2S2. Tel: (1) (403) 492–7168; Fax: (1) (403) 492–5329; E-mail: rmoqbel@asthma.med.ualberta.ca.

New Horizons in Allergy Immunotherapy
edited by Sehon et al. Plenum Press, New York, 1996

287

nes. Here, I review recent advances in the field of eosinophil cytokine synthesis, storage and release in association with allergic inflammation and asthma.

2. INTERLEUKINS

2.1. Interleukin-1

Murine eosinophils were shown to express mRNA for IL-1α, using *in situ* hybridization[13], and IL-1α protein was detected in supernatants following stimulation. The ability of human eosinophils to synthesize IL-1α was examined by Weller *et al.*[14] in cells obtained from a hypereosinophilic patient. Eosinophils contained transcripts for IL-1α mRNA both before and after stimulation with phorbol esters. The expression of IL-1α protein was also detectable by immunocytochemistry. IL-1α release was shown to be associated with the induction of cytokine-induced HLA-DR expression suggesting that eosinophils may act as antigen presenting cells.

2.2. Interleukin-2 (IL-2)

We recently showed that an average of 10% of freshly isolated, unstimulated blood eosinophils showed cytoplasmic staining for IL-2[15]. Using a cell fractionation method, the majority of IL-2 was shown to be stored in eosinophil granules and co-eluted with granule markers; minor peaks were detected in the cytosolic and membrane fractions. Immunogold-labelled intact eosinophils revealed IL-2 immunoreactivity in association with eosinophil crystalline granule cores[15]. Bossé *et al.*[16] also demonstrated the presence of mRNA signals for IL-2 in human eosinophils following elegant in-cell RT-PCR followed by *in situ* hybridization.

2.3. Interleukin-3 (IL-3)

Ionomycin-treated eosinophils produced IL-3 at concentrations equivalent to 50% of the capacity of mononuclear cells[17]. Thus, IL-3 may be an additional autocrine factor that can be produced and utilised by the eosinophil following stimulation. Of interest two immunosuppressants, FK-506 and rapamycin, inhibited calcium ionophore A23187-induced production of IL-3 and GM-CSF from eosinophils[18]. Also rapamycin, unlike FK-506, suppressed IL-5-induced prolongation of eosinophil survival. Such immmonosuppressive agents may have an important modulating role in eosinophil-associated allergic reactions.

2.4. Interleukin-4 (IL-4)

Initial studies using double *in situ* hybridization and immunocytochemical (ICC) staining of bronchial biopsies and BAL cells from atopic asthmatic subjects indicated that very few EG2+ cells co-expressed IL-4 mRNA[19]. However, by RT-PCR, we detected IL-4 mRNA in highly purified blood eosinophils obtained from atopic asthmatics[20]. About 30% of these cells were IL-4-immunoreactive. Like IL-2, eosinophil-derived IL-4 was found stored in association with their cationic granules as assessed by cell fractionation and cell lysis (repeated freeze-thawing revealed an average of 75 pg/ml of IL-4 per 10^6 cells). Eosinophils incubated with serum-coated Sephadex beads released physiological concentrations of IL-4 into the supernatants, thus confirming that these cells synthesize and secrete this important pro-inflammatory cytokine. These observations suggest that eosinophil, through IL-4, may play an important regulatory role in the development and maintenance of the allergic inflammatory response.

2.5. Interleukin-5 (IL-5)

Eosinophils infiltrating mucosa of active coeliac patients express mRNA for IL-5[21]. By *in situ* hybridization, IL-5 mRNA was identified in peripheral blood eosinophils from the hypereosinophilic syndrome. IL-5 mRNA expression in eosinophils was also demonstrated, *in vivo*, in bronchoalveolar lavage cells obtained from asthmatic subjects[22,] and patients with eosinophilic cystitis[23] and eosinophilic heart disease[21]. IL-5 was released following stimulation IgA-, IgE- or IgG-immune complexes but was co-localised to eosinophilic granules by immunogold staining[23], suggesting that this cytokine is also stored intracellularly in association with eosinophil granules. By simultaneous *in situ* hybridization and immunocytochemistry on nasal biopsy tissue from atopic rhinitic subjects following allergen exposure it was possible to co-localize IL-5 mRNA to MBP$^+$ eosinophils[19]. However, only 5.4% of the total leucocyte population were IL-5 mRNA$^+$/MBP$^+$ as compared with 83.2% IL-5 mRNA$^+$/CD3$^+$ and 18% IL-5 mRNA$^+$/tryptase$^+$.

2.6. Interleukin-6 (IL-6)

We studied the expression of IL-6 mRNA in normal density eosinophils[24], and showed that approximately 20% of unstimulated eosinophils were IL-6 mRNA$^+$. This percentage was elevated (55%) following stimulation with IFN-γ. Transcription of IL-6 mRNA was confirmed by Northern blot analysis. Translation of the product was detected by immunocytochemistry in which staining was also "granular", and IL-6 release from cultured eosinophils before and after stimulation was measured[24]. As with a number of eosinophil-derived cytokines, we showed that eosinophil IL-6 was stored in association with the crystalloid granules[25]. The capacity of blood eosinophils obtained from both normal and hypereosinophilic donors to synthesize IL-6 and its constitutive expression have been confirmed using reverse transcription polymerase chain reaction (RT-PR) and *in situ* hybridization[26]. In this study, neutrophil granulocytes from healthy individuals were also shown to express variable levels of IL-6 although this was rapidly down-regulated following culture of cells, *in vitro*. The precise significance and biological role of eosinophil-derived IL-6 is yet to be determined. IL-6 plays an important role in the regulation of the immune response by modulating T and B lymphocyte functions as well as priming granulocytes and endothelial cells.

2.7. Interleukin-8 (IL-8)

Highly purified eosinophils cultured *in vitro* with calcium ionophore released IL-8 into the supernatant[27], release was inhibited by the immunosuppressant agent cyclosporin A and by cycloheximide. IL-8 mRNA was demonstrated by PCR amplification following stimulation and IL-8 immunoreactivity was detected by immunocytochemical staining with granular appearance suggesting that this cytokine may also reside in the cell in a stored form[27]. While IL-8 appears to be a very abundant eosinophil cytokine its precise role in allergic inflammation remains unknown.

3. GROWTH FACTORS AND COLONY STIMULATING FACTORS

3.1. Transforming Growth Factor-α and β (TGFα & TGFβ)

TGFα was detected in tissue eosinophils found in abundance in close proximity to the site of oral squamous carcinoma[28]. The latter type of tumour is known to be associated with increases in the level of tissue eosinophils. TGFα mRNA the protein were co-localized to eosinophils. The observation was confirmed in peripheral blood eosinophils from hyper-eosinophilic syndrome patients. It is now known that eosinophils, both *in vivo* and *in vitro*, have a constitutive expression of mRNA for TGFα. This observation was confirmed in eosinophil-associated wound healing in the rabbit skin tissues[29]. Epithelial wound healing coincided with TGFα expression in the Syrian hamster cheek pouch mucosa. Normal hamster bone marrow eosinophils were also shown to express TGFα mRNA and the protein[30].

TGFβ1 mRNA was identified in eosinophils from patients with blood eosinophilia[31], and was localized in nasal tissue from a patient with allergic rhinitis but not in normal nasal mucosa[32]. By a combination of *in situ* hybridization and specific eosinophil staining, approximately 50% of the eosinophils which accumulated in the polyp tissue were TGFβ1 mRNA+. Immunoreactivity for TGFβ1 in eosinophils was confirmed using immunocytochemical staining. TGFβ1 has also been localized to eosinophils in nodular sclerosis-associated Hodgkin's disease[33], and immunoreactivity was detected mainly at the margins of sites of new collagen synthesis in the vicinity of areas rich with Hodgkin/Reed/Sternberg (H/RS) cells. Probing for TGFβ1 revealed that the major sites for TGFβ1 mRNA expression were confined to eosinophils, but not H/RS cells. TGFβ1 plays an important role in tissue repair by promoting fibroblast growth and activation and can exert its effects on extracellular matrix by stimulation of collagen synthesis. Thus, eosinophils, through the production of this cytokine, may contribute towards structural abnormalities, observed in inflammatory conditions and asthma, such as stromal fibrosis and basement membrane thickening.

3.2. GranuLocyte-Macrophage Colony-Stimulating Factor (GM-CSF)

Using *in situ* hybridization, we showed that normal density human eosinophils transcribe and translate mRNA for GM-CSF after stimulation with either IFN-γ or the calcium ionophore A23187[34]. GM-CSF mRNA was co-localized to the stimulated eosinophil using a combination of *in situ* hybridization and histochemistry (Carbol chromotrope 2R), or immunocytochemistry (EG2)[34]. A concurrent study demonstrated the release of eosinophil-derived GM-CSF following stimulation of cells with ionomycin[17], and presented elegant evidence for an autocrine effect of eosinophil-derived GM-CSF on prolongation of eosinophil survival. Ionomycin-induced, GM-CSF-dependent, enhancement of eosinophil survival was blocked by cyclosporin A, which suggests that the beneficial effect of the latter in chronic corticosteroid-dependent asthma[35] may be related to the direct effect of the drug on eosinophil cytokine synthesis. We have recently shown by cell fractionation and immunogold-labelling that GM-CSF is stored in association with crystalloid granules of eosinophils obtained from asthmatic subjects[36]. Following ultra-centrifugation of post-nuclear supernatant of eosinophil subcellular components on a 0–40% Nycodenz gradient in sucrose buffer, GM-CSF co-eluted with granule proteins and enzymes (i.e. major basic protein, eosinophil cationic protein, eosinophil peroxidase, aryl sulphatase and β-hexosaminidase), but not in fractions associated with CD9 activity (a marker for eosinophil plasma membrane). The presence of granule-stored GM-CSF in eosinophils from asthmatics has important implications in terms of their activation eithre by autocrine, paracrine or juxtacrine signalling mechanisms.

GM-CSF mRNA and immunoreactivity have also been detected in eosinophils, *in vivo*, in association with nasal polyposis[37]. By *in situ* hybridization and counterstaining with chromotrope 2R, approximately 30% of eosinophils infiltrating the polyp tissue expressed mRNA for GM-CSF. The presence of GM-CSF mRNA expression was confirmed in human bronchoalveolar lavage (BAL) eosinophils obtained from asthmatic subjects after endobronchial allergen challenge[22].

3.3. Tumour Necrosis Factor-α

By *in situ* hybridization, 44%-100% of blood eosinophils obtained from normal subjects or patients with hypereosinophilia were positive for TNFα mRNA[38] and the stored protein was detected by immunocytochemical staining. The spontaneous release of eosinophil TNFα from atopic individuals, *in vitro*, was inhibitable by cycloheximide pretreatment. Infiltrating eosinophils in necrotizing enterocolitis were also shown to express TNFα mRNA, suggesting a role for these cells in the pathogenesis of intestinal necrosis[39]. TNFα immunogold positive signals were co-localized to the matrix compartment of the specific secondary granules of eosinophils obtained from patients with the idiopathic hypereosinophilic syndrome[40].

4. CHEMOKINES

4.1. RANTES

Highly-purified human blood eosinophils were shown to express mRNA for RANTES, a C-C chemokine with potent eosinophil chemotactic and activating properties, as detected by RT-PCR[41]. This was confirmed by *in situ* hybridization where 7–10% of peripheral blood eosinophils expressed RANTES mRNA in the absence of stimulus. This increased to 25% following incubation with IFNγ, but not ionomycin, *in vitro*. These cells also showed specific immunoreactivity with an anti-RANTES mAb. By ELISA, human blood eosinophils were shown to contain a median of 7300 pg of RANTES per 10^6 cells. Following stimulation of these cells with serum-coated particles, *in vitro*, 24% of this total was secreted into culture supernatants in physiologically-relevant quantities. The eosinophil-derived RANTES was shown to be bioactive (in eosinophil chemotactic assays) and its activity was inhibited by an anti-RANTES antibody. The capacity of human eosinophils to synthesize and translate mRNA for RANTES in association with allergic inflammation, *in vivo*, was also demonstrated in allergen-induced late-phase cutaneous reactions in atopic volunteers[41].

4.2. Macrophage Inflammatory Protein-1α

A high percentage of blood eosinophils (39%-91%) obtained from hypereosinophilic patients showed positive mRNA expression for the chemokine MIP-1α[38]. In contrast, eosinophils obtained from normal donors exhibited weak or undetectable expression. *In vivo*, the majority of eosinophils infiltrating nasal polyp tissue had strong expression for MIP-1α mRNA; the expression was also confirmed by Northern blot analysis.

5. CONCLUSIONS

Thus, eosinophils synthesize, store and release a wide array of cytokines as well as basic granule-derived proteins and lipid mediators. This functional versatility has a number of implications on the potential role of the eosinophil in allergic tissue reactions. Eosinophils might act to amplify the allergic response which, in asthma for example, would enhance tissue damage, but in helminth infections could promote adaptive immunity. On the other hand, eosinophil cytokine production may be a redundant process in the spectrum of immune and inflammatory systems. Conversely, as stated eosinophils may be involved in tissue repair and remodelling by, for example, promoting collagen synthesis through release of TFGα and β. It is not known whether eosinophil-derived cytokines act synergistically with other eosinophil mediators, i.e. basic proteins, LTC_4 and PAF. Eosinophils have also been shown to express MHC (Class II) molecules, elaborate IL-1α and act as antigen-presenting cells. Eosinophils might function as specialised APCs in certain situations such as helminthic infections. Although the control and regulation of eosinophilia associated with asthma and allergic disease are not yet fully understood, it is likely to be dependent on IL-3, IL-5 and GM-CSF release from T cells, mast cells and eosinophils themselves. The recent advances in eosinophil-derived cytokines suggest that the capacity of this cell to participate in effector functions during allergic type reactions may be greater than hitherto assumed.

The relative contribution of eosinophil-derived cytokines to the development and maintenance of inflammatory reactions associated with allergic reactions, asthma and allied disorders remains to be determined. Although the amounts of cytokines generated by these cells appear less than that produced by T lymphocytes, the synthesis of these cytokines and their storage and potential autocrine and paracrine usage may have particular pathophysiological relevance.

6. ACKNOWLEDGMENTS

The author wishes to acknowledge the invaluable help of his colleagues, Professor AB Kay, Drs Sun Ying, SR Durham, CJ Corrigan, F Levi-Schaffer, L Taborda-Barata, Q Hamid, TM Newman as well as J Barkans, P Kimmitt, Qiu Meng and J North, at the National Heart & Lung Institute, London, UK. The experiments described here were supported by grants from the Medical Research Council and the Wellcome Trust, UK.

7. REFERENCES

1. Kay AB, Moqbel R, Durham SR, MacDonald AJ, Walsh GM, Shaw RJ, Cromwell O, Mackay JA. Leucocyte activation initiated by IgE- dependent mechanisms in relation to helminthic parasitic disease and clinical models of asthma. *Int Arch Allergy Clin Immunol* !985; 77:69–72.
2. Wardlaw AJ, Moqbel B. The eosinophil in allergic and helminth related inflammatory responses. In: Moqbel R, ed. Allergy and immunity to helminths. London: Taylor & Francis, 1992: 54–86.
3. Durham SR, Kay AB. Eosinophils, bronchial hyperreactivity and late-phase asthmatic reactions. *Clin Allergy* 1985; 15:411–8.
4. Azzawi M, Bradley B, Jeffery PK *et al.* Identification of activated T lymphocytes and eosinophils in bronchial biopsies in stable atopic asthma. *Am Rev Respir Dis* 1990; 142: 1407–13.
5. Corrigan CJ, Kay AB. T cells and eosinophils in the pathogenesis of asthma. *Immunol Today* 1992; 13–501–7.
6. Kay AB. Asthma and inflammation. *J Allergy Clin Immunol* 1991; 87: 893–910.

7. Clutterbuck EJ, Hirst EMA, Sanderson CJ. Human interleukin 5 (IL-5) regulates the production of eosino-phils in human bone marrow cultures: comparison and interaction with IL-1, IL-3, IL-6 and GM-CSF. *Blood* 1988; 73: 1504–11.

8. Rothenburg ME, Owen WF, Silberstein DS, Soberman RJ, Austen KF, Stevens RL. Eosinophils co-cultured with endothelial cells have increased survival and functional properties. *Science* 1987; 237: 645–7.

9. Owen WF, Rothenburg ME, Silberstein DS, *et al.* Regulation of human eosinophil viability, density and function by granulocyte/macrophage colony-stimulating factor in the presence of 3T3 fibroblasts. *J Exp Med* 1987; 166: 129–41.

10. Rothenburg ME, Owen WF, Silberstein DS, *et al.* Human eosinophils have prolonged survival, enhanced functional properties and become hypodense when exposed to human interleukin 3. *J Clin Invest* 1988; 81: 1986–92.

11. Valerius T, Repp R, Kalden JR, Platzer E. Effects of interferon on human eosinophils in comparison with other cytokines. *J Immunol* 1990; 145:2950–8.

12. Silberstein DS, David JR. The regulation of human eosinophil function by cytokines. *Immunol Today* 1987; 8:380–5.

13. Del Pozo V, De Andres B, Martin E, *et al.* Murine eosinophils and IL-1: alpha IL-1 mRNA detection by *in situ* hybridization. Production and release IL-1 from peritoneal eosinophils. *J Immunol* 1990; 144:3117–22.

14. Weller PF, Rand TH, Barrett T, Elovic A, Wong DTW, Finberg RW. Accessory cell function of human eosi-nophils: HLA-DR-dependent. MHC-restriction antigen presentation and interleukin-1α formation. *J Immunol* 1993; 150:2554–62.

15. Levi-Schaffer F, Barkans J, Newman TM, Sun Ying, Wakelin M, Hohenstein R, Barak V, Lacy P, Kay AB, Moqbel R. Identification of interleukin-2 in human peripheral blood eosinophils. *Immunology* (in press).

16. Bossé M, Audett M, Ferland C, Pelletier G, Chu HW, Dakhama A, Lavigne S, Boulet L-P, Laviolette M. Human eosinophils transcribe and translate mRNA for interleukin-2. *Immunology* (in press).

17. Kita H, Ohnishi T, Okubo Y, Weiler D, Abrams JS, Gleich GJ. GM-CSF and Interleukin-3 release from hu-man peripheral blood eosinophils and neutrophils. *J Exp Med* 1991; 174: 743–8.

18. Hom JT, Estridge T. FK-506 and rapamycin modulate the functional activities of human peripheral blood eosinophils. *Clin Immunol Immunopathol* 1993; 68:293- 300.

19. Sun Ying, Durham SR, Barkans J, Masuyama K, Jacobson M, Rak S, Lowhagen O, Moqbel R, Kay AB, Hamid Q. T cells are the principal source of interleukin-5 mRNA in allergen-induced allergic rhinitis. *Am J Respir Cell Mol Biol* 1993; 9:356–60.

20. Moqbel R, Sun Ying, Barkans J, Newman TM, Kimmitt P, Wakelin M, Taborda- Barata L, Qiu Meng, Cor-rigan CJ, Durham SR, Kay AB. Identification of mRNA for interleukin-4 in human eosinophils with gran-ule localization and release of the translated product. 1995; *J Immunol.* (in press).

21. Desreumaux PA, Janin A, Colombel JF, *et al.* Interleukin-5 mRNA expression by eosinophils in the intesti-nal mucosa of patients with coeliac disease. *J Exp Med* 1992; 175:293–6.

22. Broide H, Paine M, Firestein G. Eosinophils express interleukin-5 and granulocyte macrophage-colony-stimulating factor mRNA at sites of allergic inflammation. *J Clin Invest* 1992; 90:1414–24.

23. Dubucquoi SP, Desreumaux P, Janin A, *et al.* Interleukin 5 synthesis by eosinophils: association with gran-ules and immunoglobulin-dependent secretion. *J Exp Med* 1994; 179:703–8.

24. Hamid Q, Barkans J, Abrams JS, Qiu Meng, Sun Ying, Kay AB, Moqbel R. Human eosinophils synthesize and secrete interleukin-6, in vitro. *Blood* 1992:; 80:1496–501.

25. Moqbel R, Lacy P, Levi-Schaffer F, Mannan M, North J, Gomperts B, Kay AB. Interleukin-6 as a granule-associate dpre-formed mediator in peripheral blood eosinophils (PBE) from asthmatic subjects. *Am J Respir Crit Care Med* 1994; 149: A836.

26. Melani C, Mattia GF, Silvani A, *et al.* Interleukin-6 expression in human neutrophil and eosinophil periph-eral blood granulocytes. *Blood* 1993; 81:2744–9.

27. Braun Rk, Franchini M, Erard F, *et al.* Human peripheral blood eosinophils produce and release inter-leukin-8 on stimulation with calcium ionophore. *Eur J Immunol* 1993; 23:956–60.

28. Wong DTW, Weller PF, Galli SJ, *et al.* Human eosinophils express transforming growth factor α. *J Exp Med* 1990; 172: 673–81.

29. Todd R, Donoff BR, Chiang I, *et al.* The eosinophil as a source of transforming growth factor alpha in healing cutaneous wounds. *Am J Pathol* 1991; 138:1307–13.

30. Wong DT, Donoff RB, Yang J, *et al.* Sequential expression of transforming growth factors α and β-1 by eosinophils during cutaneous wound healing in the hamster. *Am J Pathol* 1993; 143: 130–2.

31. Wong DTW, Elovic A, Matossian K, *et al.* Eosinophils from patients with blood eosinophilia express trans-forming factor β_1. *Blood* 1991; 78:2702–42.

32. Ohno I, Lea RG, Flanders KC, *et al.* Eosinophils in chronically inflamed human upper airway tissues ex-press transforming growth factor-β1 gene. (TGF-β_1). *J Clin Invest* 1992; 89:1662–8.

33. Kadin M, Butmarc J, Elovic A, Wong D. Eosinophils are the major source of transforming growth factor-β1 in nodular sclerosing Hodgkin's disease. *Am J Pathol* 1993; 142:11–6.

34. Moqbel R, Hamid Q, Ying S, Barkans J, Hartnell A, Tsicopoulos A, Wardlaw AJ, Kay Ab. Expression of mRNA and immunoreactivity for the granulocyte/macrophage-colony stimulating factor (GM-CSF) in activated human eosinophils. *J Exp Med* 1991; 174; 749–52.

35. Alexander AG, Barnes NC, Kay Ab. Trial of cyclosporin A in corticosteroid-dependent chronic severe asthma. *Lancet* 1992; 339:324–8.

36. Levi-Schaffer F, Lacy P, Severs NJ, Newman TM, North J, Gmperts B, Kay AB, Moqbel R. Association of granulocyte/macrophage colony-stimulating factor with the crystalloid granule of human eosinophils. *Blood* 1995; 85:2579–2586.

37. Ohno I, Lea R, Finotto S, *et al.* Granulocyte/macrophage colony-stimulating factor (GM-CSF) gene expression by eosinophils in nasal polyposis. *Am J Respir Cell Mol Biol* 1991;505–10.

38. Costa JJ, Matossian K, Resnick MB, *et al.* Human eosinophils can express the cytokines tumor necrosis factor-α and macrophage inflammatory protein-1α. *J Clin Invest* 1993; 91:2673–84.

39. Tan X, Hsueh W, Gonzalez-Crussi F. Cellular localization of tumor necrosis factor (TNF)-α transcripts in normal bowel and in necrotizing enterocolitis; TNF gene expression by Paneth cells, intestinal eosinophils, and macrophages. *Am J Pathol* 1993; 142: 1858–65.

40. Beil WJ, Weller PF, Tzizik Dm, Galli Sj, Dvorak AM. Ultrastructural immunogold localization of tumor necrosis factor-α to the matrix compartment of eosinophils secondary granules in patients with idiopathic hypereosinophilic syndrome. *J Histochem Cytochem* 1993; 41:1611–5.

41. Sun Ying, Qiu Meng, Taborda-Barata, Corrigan CJ, Barkans J, Assoufi B, Moqbel R, Durham SR, Kay AB. Human eosinophils express mRNA encoding RANTES and store and relrease physiologically-active RANTES protein. Submitted for publication.

42

ALLERGEN DOSE DEPENDENT CYTOKINE PRODUCTION REGULATES SPECIFIC IgE AND IgG ANTIBODY PRODUCTION

Kurt Blaser[*]

Swiss Institute of Allergy and Asthma Research (SIAF)
Davos, Switzerland

1. ABSTRACT

The elicitation of a specific immune response against allergens depends on the recognition of antigenic determinants (epitopes) by specific T and B lymphocytes. In order to determine the relevant epitopes for human T and B cells and their features in the regulation and production of specific IgE and/or IgG antibodies, we have investigated the immune response to bee venom phospholipase A2 (PLA) in allergic and non-allergic subjects. This enzyme represents the major allergen in bee sting allergy. It consists of 134 amino acid residues with a carbohydrate side chain at position 13 and is available as recombinant protein. We have developped PLA-specific T-cell clones from bee sting allergic and non-allergic human subjects. Using a panel of dodecapeptides overlapping in 10 residues and a large set of 18 - 25 mer overlapping peptides, we detected three epitopes that were recognized by peripheral blood T-cells and T-cell clones. A fourth determinant involved the carbohydrate moiety on Asn[13] of PLA. Whereas the CHO-depending epitope seems to be mostly active in allergics, the other three epitopes are equally recognized by peripheral blood mononuclear cells (PBMC) of both allergic and non-allergic individuals. In T-cell clones, the ratio of IL-4/IFNγ cytokines and the quality of the activating signal depend on the strength of the binding of the MHC-II/Ag/TcR complex between APC and T-cells. The number of antigen-specific APC-T-cell contact sites can be varied *in vitro* by changing the dose of antigen added to the cell culture. While isotype switch for both IgE and IgG4 requires IL-4, this cytokine suppresses antigen-specific IgG4 production by already switched B-cells. Therefore, IL-4 and IFNγ display counterregulatory effects on the production of IgE being responsible for atopic states and IgG4 antibodies which are signs of a normal immune response to allergen and act as protective

* Correspondence: K. Blaser, PhD, Swiss Institute of Allergy and Asthma Research (SIAF), CH-7270 Davos Platz, Switzerland, Tel. 41–81–43 70 83, FAX 41–81–43 16 07.

New Horizons in Allergy Immunotherapy
edited by Sehon et al. Plenum Press. New York. 1996

295

antibodies. The combination of this counter-regulation of IgE and IgG4 antibodies with the fundamental law of mass action for chemical equilibrium reactions revealed that the antigen concentration governs to a great part the ratio of IL-4/IFNγ secretion and therefore the formation of IgE and IgG and allergy or protection, together with the equilibrium constant K, which represents immunological individuality and a measure of Ag presentation.

2. INTRODUCTION

Antibody responses to allergens represent appropriate models to elucidate the regulatory mechanisms of different antibody classes or isotypes. Excessive IgE antibody production against allergens generally leads to immediate type allergic reactions, whereas specific IgG production, in particular the formation of IgG4 antibodies, reflects normal, protective immunity to the same agent.

Specific antibodies to allergens are elicited after differentation and clonal expansion of B-lymphocytes. These steps are under the control of specific T-lymphocytes and depend on soluble factors that are released upon T-cell activation (1). The qualitative and quantitative composition of the cytokines, in particular Interleukin-4 (IL-4) and gamma-Interferon (IFNγ), regulates the isotype formation in B-cells (2). Since the pattern of generated cytokines is associated with the antigenic peptide structure bound to the MHC haplotype and recognized by the specific T-cell receptor (TcR) (3), a better knowledge of the single components involved in the ternary MHC/peptide/TcR complex is crucial to understand the development of IgE antibody-mediated allergic diseases and their therapy in comparison to the IgG related immunity.

The major allergen in bee sting allergy is represented by the bee venom phospholipase A2 (PLA) (4). Recently it was demonstrated that 99% of bee venom allergic patients react against commercial preparations of PLA and 96% against recombinant PLA produced in E.coli (5). Other allergens, such as hyaluronidase and melittin are of minor importance. Therefore, the immune response to PLA represents an ideally defined model to study the regulation of an antigen-specific human IgE and IgG4 antibody response in allergic and non-allergic individuals. PLA is a glycoprotein of 14 to 16 kDa consisting of 134 amino acid residues with a carbohydrate side chain at position Asn^{13} (6). Its three-dimensional crystal structure and biochemical function are well defined (7). At initial response to bee sting generally low affinity IgG1 anti-PLA antibodies are elicited (8), but after repeated exposure most subjects elicit high affinity IgG4 antibodies to PLA. In contrast, some individuals generate high levels of PLA-specific IgE antibodies and develop bee sting allergy (4). However, their allergic or non-allergic state is not merely defined by the content of specific IgE antibodies, but rather by the ratio of allergen-specific IgE and IgG4 antibodies as Fig. 1 demonstrates. The average PLA-specific IgE/IgG4 ratio in bee venom in allergic patients is about 100 times higher than in healthy subjects. It is known that IgE antibody formation by B-cells requires T-cell contact and IL-4 for isotype switch (9), but also the isotype switch to IgG4 depends on IL-4 (10). The basic mechanisms leading to a preferential IgE or IgG4 production as observed in the different groups of individulals remains to be identified.

Our work was aimed to define cytokine patterns and epitope specificity of T-cells derived from allergic and non-allergic subjects and their correlation with IgE and IgG isotype expression in B-cells.

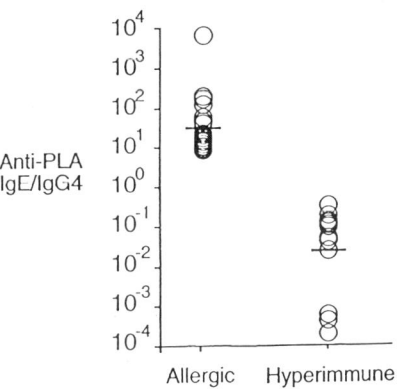

Figure 1. The allergic or non-allergic state in bee venom sensitized individuals is characterized by the ratio of anti-PLA IgE and IgG4 antibody ratios in serum.

3. ALLERGIC AND NON-ALLERGIC INDIVIDUALS RECOGNIZE THE SAME EPITOPES FOR T-CELLS IN PLA

The differences in cytokine secretion between T-cells derived from IgE producing allergic and IgG4 producing non-allergic subjects were mostly quantitative. Therefore, the molecular features of individual allergen recognition may be of more importance. By screening the epitope specificity of PLA-specific T-cell clones with overlapping PLA-derived dodeca- and octadeca-peptides, three immunodominant sites in the PLA molecule could be mapped (11). These T-cell epitopes are represented by the peptides PLA$^{40-63}$, PLA$^{74-92}$ and PLA$^{107-131}$ as demonstrated in Fig. 2.

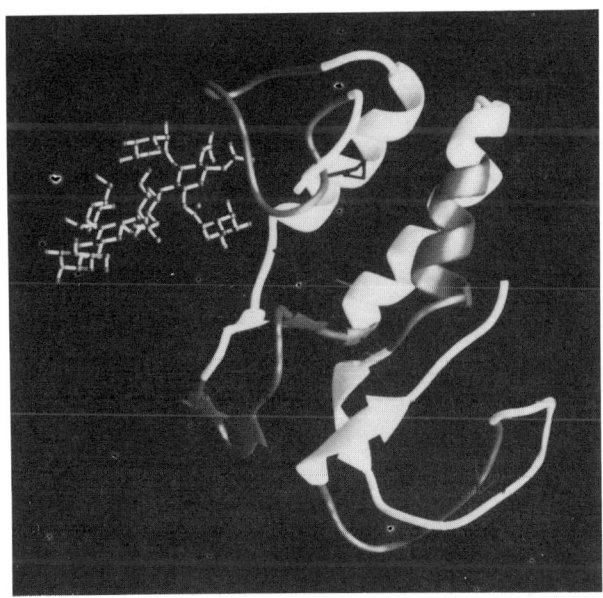

Figure 2. T-cell epitopes in bee venom PLA as found by overlapping synthetic peptides in specific T-cell clones and in PBMC of allergic and non-allergic subjects sensitized to bee sting. One epitope includes the oligosaccharide at position Asn^{13} (provided by Dr. C. Broger, Hoffmann-La Roche Ltd. Basel Switzerland).

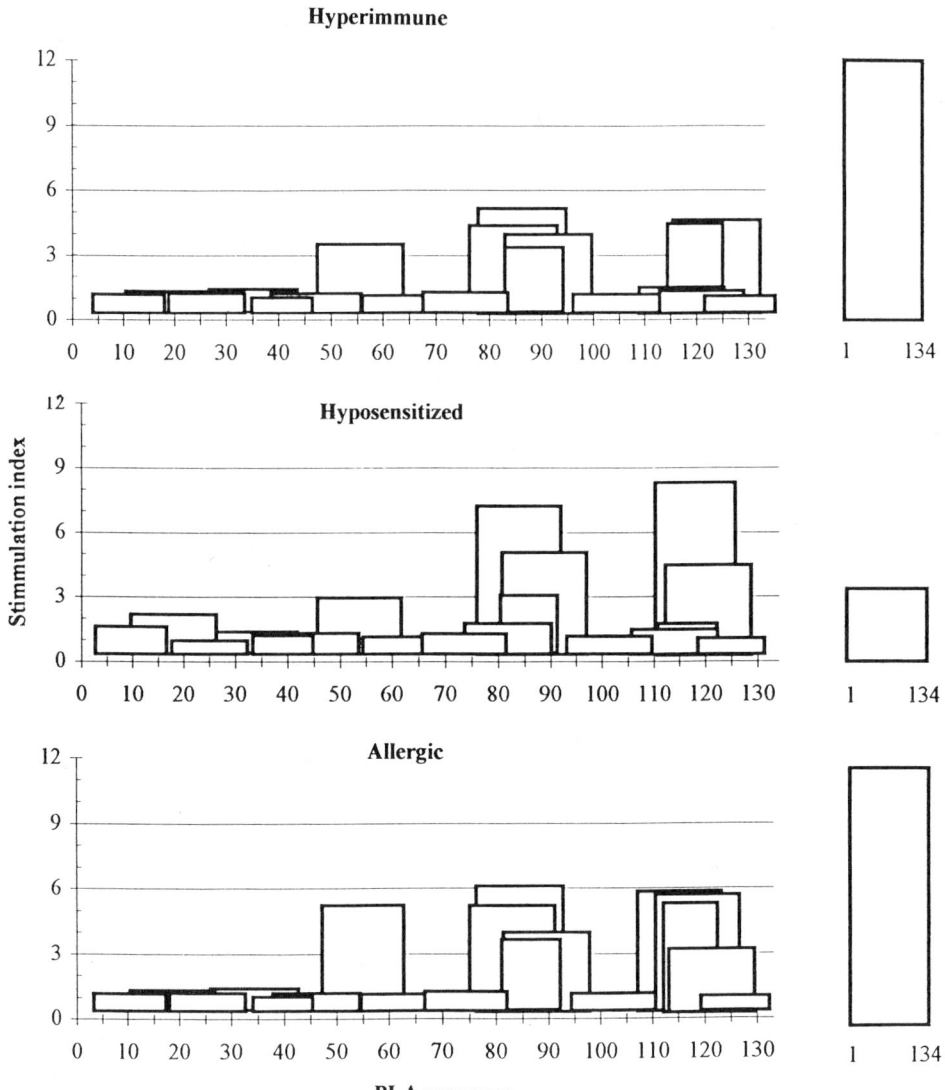

Figure 3. T-cell proliferation of unfractioned PBMC from bee sting-sensitized donors. PBMC from allergic (n = 20), hyposensitized (n = 8), and hyperimmune (n = 12) subjects were stimulated with PLA and PLA-derived peptides. Each bar represents the geometrical mean of the Stimulation Index (SI) induced by optimal Ag concentrations.

Primary *in vitro* proliferation of unfractioned PBMC isolated from allergic or from hyposensitized or hyperimmune individuals to the three PLA-derived peptides was restricted to the same immunogenic sites as found in T-cell clones and no other of the overlapping PLA peptides was active in any sensitized subject (Fig. 3). Same patterns of epitope reactivity were detected among these groups of individuals, although proliferative responses were generally higher in allergic than in non-allergic donors (Fig. 3). Thus, three linear epitopes are involved in T-cell recognition of PLA, independent of the individuals IgE or IgG levels or whether they were allergic or not. Among the bee venom allergic patients >90% responded to the peptide corresponding to $PLA^{107-131}$, 70% recognized PLA^{74-92} and 34% of patients responded to PLA^{40-63}. Moreover, 70% recognized both epitopes PLA^{74-92} and $PLA^{107-131}$. The same recognition pattern was observed in hyperimmune, non-allergic subjects, whereas T-cell proliferation in response to the same peptides PLA^{74-92} and $PLA^{107-131}$ were significantly less in successfully hyposensitized patients. Only one out of 40 tested donors, a hyposensitized patient, did not respond significantly in the primary *in vitro* response to at least one of the 19 overlapping octadeca-peptides spanning the entire PLA molecule. These peptides do not bind IgE antibodies and do not elicit skin reactions in allergic patients.

4. PLA EXPRESSES A CARBOHYDRATE DEPENDENT T-CELL EPITOPE

Some of our T-cell clones generated from allergic subjects could not be mapped to any of the linear peptide sequences in PLA, although they expressed clear reactivity to this allergen. Using native PLA in comparison to non-glycosylated native and recombinant PLA as well as a number of different analogues to glycosylated and non-glycosylated PLA, we were able to demonstrate a glycosylation-dependent T-cell epitope being recognized by several T-cell clones of different allergic individuals (12). The recognition of this epitope was HLA-DR restricted. The isolated carbohydrate moiety alone did not trigger T-cell growth and the PLA response was abrogated after selective and stepwise enzymatic deglycosylation of the native PLA (12). So far, such carbohydrate-dependent T-cell epitopes have been found in experimental animal models. Whether they play a special role in IgE induction and allergy remains to be established.

5. THE IL-4/IFNγ CYTOKINE PHENOTYPE OF PLA-SPECIFIC T-CELL CLONES DEPENDS ON THE DOSE OF ALLERGEN

A panel of $CD4^+$ T-cell clones specific to PLA was established from PBMC of human subjects allergic, hyposensitized or immune to bee sting (13). Depending on the T-cell clone maximal stimulation required 1 to 100 µg/ml of PLA (13). Following high dose antigen stimulation, all clones produced IL-4, IFNγ and granuloyte-macrophage colony-stimulating factor (GM-CSF) beside other cytokines (13). However, both absolute and relative amounts of secreted cytokines depended on the antigen concentration in the culture containing antigen presenting cells (APC) together with a defined T-cell clone. Either autologous B-cells or PBMC were used as APC (13, 14). Moreover, the PLA-specific T-cell clones could be classified according to the increasing or decreasing ratio of IL-4/IFNγ production in response to increasing allergen doses (14). Certain clones, mostly derived from allergic or hyposensitized individuals, required higher threshold amounts of allergen for IFNγ induction and expressed increasing IL-4/IFNγ ratios following stimulation with increasing concentrations of PLA (13, 14) (Fig. 4). Accordingly, the generation of different IL-4/IFNγ ratios depends on the amount of the allergen added to the culture (15). As observed in a typical ThO clone producing at optimal stimulatory conditions both IL-4 and IFNγ in comparable amounts, stimulation of IL-4 required less allergen and IFNγ re-

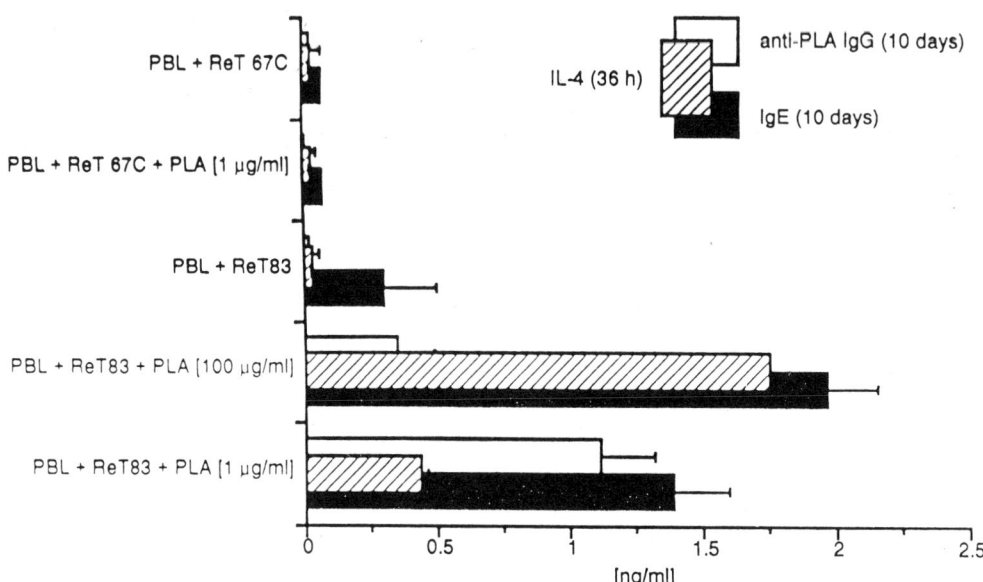

Figure 4. Different ratios of IL-4/IFNγ and IgE/IgG4 depend on the antigen concentration. Whereas IL-4 is required for the induction of both IgE and IgG4, it suppresses the IgG4 production in already switched B-cells. ReT83 is a PLA specific Th2 and ReT67C a PLA non-specific T-cell clone, which were added to a culture of autologous PBMC (15).

quired up to 10 times higher treshold amounts for its induction than IL-4. At low antigen dose the T-cell clone showed a clear Th2 cytokine pattern. Increasing allergen concentrations however, favored the IFNγ production, whereas IL-4 decreased at high allergen contents in the culture.

6. ALLERGEN-DOSE DEPENDENT IgE AND IgG PRODUCTION TO PLA

The production of IgG4 antibodies by already switched mature B-cells depends on the presence of IFNγ (15). This was demonstrated in two different *in vitro* systems which were used to study the role of cytokines in the development of allergen-specific IgE and IgG antibodies (15). In one system, PBMC of PLA sensitized subjects were stimulated with pockeweed mitogen (PWM). In this case, a typical Th1 cytokine pattern was induced, showing high IFNγ and little IL-4 production (15). The addition of IL-4 and/or blocking anti-IFNγ antibody decreased, respectively abrogated the specific IgG4 response, whereas the IgE formation increased (15). The other system consisted of B-cells or PBMC supplemented with defined T-cell clones specifically responding to PLA. In this latter case, the secreted cytokine pattern depended on the properties of the specific T-cell clone used in the experiment and the amount of allergen added to the culture. Increases in IL-4 correlated positively with IgE production and negatively with IgG4.

The counter-regulatory effects of IL-4 and IFNγ on already switched mature B-cells may reflect the physiological situation during allergen immunotherapy in which high allergen doses are repeatedly injected over a longer period of time. These results clearly demonstrate, that the modulation of a T-cell cytokine pattern by the dose of the antigen or allergen may be a driving force for differential IgE and IgG antibody formation resulting in either allergy or immunoprotection.

7. CONCLUSIONS

Antigen stimulation of PLA-specific T-cell clones, which were generated from human subjects demonstrating different stages of allergy or immunity to bee sting, induced differential cytokine profiles at certain antigen concentrations *in vitro*. However, at high allergen doses most T-cell clones from both allergic and non-allergic subjects showed cytokine patterns related to the Th0 phenotype including both IL-4 and IFNγ production at high amounts. Differences among the two groups were observed in the ratio of IL-4 and IFNγ produced by the T-cells. Depending on the dose of antigen, allergics displayed a lower capacity of IFNγ production, especially at low antigen-doses. In contrast IFNγ production was favored at high allergen doses. Therefore, the dose of allergen is a major driving force in the generation of cytokine patterns either demonstrating high (Th2) or low (Th1) IL-4/IFNγ ratios. This is particulary interesting, since IL-4 enhances IgE production and suppresses specific IgG4 antibody formation, once the B-cells have undergone isotype-switch. T-cell epitope mapping of PLA-specific T-cell clones demonstrated three linear main immunogenic sites in the PLA molecule, which were recognized by unfractioned PBMC from all groups of donors, independent whether the individuals were allergic to PLA or not. In general however, higher proliferative responses were found in patients with IgE mediated allergy to bee sting. Accordingly, T-cell recognition of PLA is directed against the same three immunogenic determinants independently whether a subject is atopic or not. This is against the existence of special allergenic epitopes and suggests that other factors beside the T-cell epitope-specificity may be more relevant for the induction of IgE antibodies. A fourth epitope however, seems to be preferentially recognized by T-cells of allergics. It includes the carbohydrate moiety at amino acid residue 13. However, the immunological consequences related to the recognition of this glycan-containing structure has to be further investigated.

Recently we have suggested that one of the cytokine regulating elements might be related to a particular HLA-class II expression of the bee stung individuals (11, 14, 15). Following antigen internalization, immunogenic peptides generated in the endosomal compartment of APC bind to HLA-class II molecules to be further exported to the cell surface of the APC and presented to PLA-specific T-cells. If the affinity of this HLA-II/peptide complex is low, then only few contact sites between T-cells and APC will be displayed. A low density of these complexes will generate a weak activation, but it might still be sufficient to trigger the T-cell and the induction of IL-4. This might be the case in allergic individuals of which the T cells secrete high amounts of IL-4 but low IFNγ and therefore favor the formation of IgE. HLA-class II molecules expressing high affinity to the immunogenic peptides will display a higher density of HLA-II/peptide complexes on the surface of APC and will induce stronger T-cell activation, generating sufficient amounts of IFNγ to suppress IgE and to enhance IgG4 antibody production. Following the chemical law of mass action for equilibrium reactions the number of complexes between MHC-II, the peptide and the TcR can be increased by higher peptide concentrations (Fig.

3). Since in activated cells the number of surface expressed MHC-II and TcR molecules may be constant, the only relevant factor which can be varied by external means in the equilibrium reaction remains the concentration of the antigen/allergen (Fig. 4). This may already find its application in immunotherapy, were repeated injections of high allergen doses over a longer period of time are administrated. Moreover, this mathematical expression relates the immunological and genetical individuality of antigen recognition to the chemical equilibrium constant K or to the standard free-energy change G° of the individual MHC-II/peptide/TcR complex reaction according to the Gibb's law of thermodynamics. This constant K may therefore also represent a measure for antigen presentation. Accordingly, the change in free-energy of the MHC-II/peptide/TcR formation is decisive for the generation of particular cytokine patterns by T-cells, which finally lead to either disease or a healthy immune state. Although further investigations are required to validate this model, such mechanisms may explain the existence and the change in allergen-specific IgE/IgG4 ratios observed in allergic patients after prolonged bee venom immunization in immunotherapeutical treatments. Moreover, since immunogenic epitopes are also potent tolerogens (16), immunization of allergic patients with allergen derived peptides could be used to induce T-cell unresponsiveness to bee sting without risk of anaplylactic reactions.

8. ACKNOWLEDGMENTS

We thank Dr. C. Broger, Hoffmann-La Roche Ltd. Basel for protein modeling. This work was supported by the Swiss National Science Foundation grants Nr. 31.26357.84 and 31.39177.93.

Chemical Mass Action Law

HLA-D	+	AG	HLA-D/AG	1
HLA-D/AG	+	TcR	HLA-D/AG/TcR	2

HLA-D	+	AG	+	TcR	HLA-D/AG/TcR	3

$$\frac{[\text{HLA-D/AG/TcR}]}{[\text{HLA-D}]\,[\text{AG}]\,[\text{TcR}]} = K$$

$[\text{HLA-D}] = \text{const.} = 1$, $[\text{TcR}] = \text{const.} = 1$, $[\ ]$: concentration, K : constant

$$[\text{HLA-D/AG/TcR}] \quad = \quad K\ [\text{AG}]$$

Figure 5. The thermodynamic laws of chemical equilibrium reactions can be applied to the activation process of antigen-specific T-cells. The formation of MHC-II/peptide/TcR complexes between APC and T-cell leads to T-cell activation, proliferation and cytokine production. The only componend in the system that can be changed, is the concentration of antigen or T-cell epitope [peptide]. The equilibrium constant K of the reaction reflects the immunological individuality and represents a measure for antigen presentation. According to the Gibb's law of thermodynamics, the equilibrium constant K includes the change of free-energy $^{-}G^{\circ}$ of the reaction. Therefore, the induction of either a Th2 cytokine pattern and development of an allergic state or of a ThO pattern and normal immunity, may depend only on the $^{-}G^{\circ}$ of the antigen-specific interaction between APC and T-cells and the antigen concentration.

9. REFERENCES

1. Zubler, R.H., Werner-Favre, C., Wen, L., Sekita, K.I. & Straub, C. *Immunol. Rev.* **99**, 281–299 (1987).
2. Finkelmann, F.D., Holmes, J., Katona, I.M., Urban, J.F., Beckmann, M.P., Park, L.S., Schooley, K.A., Coffman, R.L., Mosmann, T.R. & Paul, W.E. *Annu. Rev. Immunol.* **8**, 303–333 (1990).
3. Soloway, P., Fish, S., Passmore, H., Gefter, M., Coffee, R. & Manser, T. *J. Exp. Med.* **174**, 847–858 (1991).
4. Müller, U., Dudler, T., Schneider, T., Crameri, R., Fischer, H., Skrbic, D., Maibach, R., Blaser, K. & Suter, M. *J. Allergy Clin. Immunol.* in press.
5. Müller, U., Dudler, T., Schneider, T., Crameri, R., Fischer, H., Blaser, K. &Suter, M. *Allergo J.* **2**, 60–61 (1993).
6. Kuchler, K., Gmachl, M., Sippl, M.J. & Kreil, G. *Eur. J. Biochem.* **184**, 249–254 (1989).
7. Scott, D.L., Otwinowski, Z., Gelb, M.H. & Sigler, P.B. *Science* **250**, 1563–1566 (1990).
8. Aalberse, R.C, van der Gaag, R. & van Leeuwen, J. *J. Immunol.* **130**, 722–726 (1983).
9. Heusser, C.H., Brinkmann, V., Delespesse, G., Kilchherr, E., Blaser, K. & Le Gros, G. *Allergy Clin. Immunol. News* **3**, 47–56 (1991).
10. Nüsslin, H.G. & Spiegelberg, H.L. *J. Clin. Lab. Ana.* **4**, 414–419 (1990).
11. Carballido, J.M., Carballido-Perrig, N., Kägi, M.K., Meloen, R.H., Wüthrich, B., Heusser, C.H. & Blaser, K. *J. Immunol.* **91**, 3582 (1993).
12. Dudler, T., Altmann, F., Carballido, J.M. & Blaser, K. *Eur. J. Immunol.* **25**, 538–542 (1995).
13. Carballido, J.M., Carballido-Perrig, N., Terres, G., Heusser, C.H., & Blaser, K. *Eur. J. Immunol.* **22**, 1357–1363 (1992).
14. Carballido, J.M., Carballido-Perrig, N., Heusser, C.H. & Blaser, K. *Int. Arch. Allergy Immunol.* **99**, 366–373 (1992).
15. Carballido, J.M., Carballido-Perrig, N., Oberli-Schrämmli, A., Heusser, C.H. & Blaser, K. *J. Allergy Clin. Immunol.* **4**, 758–767 (1994).
16. Gammon, G. & Sercarz, E. *Nature* **342**, 183–185 (1989).

43

THE ROLE OF ACCESSORY CELL PRODUCTS IN THE REGULATION OF T CELL CYTOKINE PRODUCTION

M. L. Kapsenberg,[1] C. M. U. Hilkens,[1] T. C. T. M. van der Pouw Kraan,[2] E. A. Wierenga,[1] and A. Snijders[1]

[1]Department of Cell Biology and Histology
Academic Medical Center
Meibergdreef 15, 1105 AZ Amsterdam, The Netherlands
[2]Department of Clinical and Experimental Immunology
Central Laboratory Blood Transfusion Service
Plesmanlaan 125, 1066 CX Amsterdam, The Netherlands

1. TH1 AND TH2 CYTOKINE-MEDIATED IMMUNE RESPONSES

The balance between specific cellular and humoral immune responses is determined largely by cytokines secreted by CD4$^+$ T lymphocytes after activation upon recognition of antigen presented by antigen-presenting accessory cells (AC). Subsets of CD4$^+$ T cells secreting high levels of the Th1 cytokine IFN-γ and low levels of Th2 cytokines favor cellular immunity characterized by delayed type hypersensitivity, which is particularly efficient for the clearing of certain intracellular parasites. Secretion of low levels of IFN-γ and high levels of the Th2 cytokines IL-4 and IL-5 favors humoral immunity, characterized by immediate type hypersensitivity mediated by antigen-specific IgE (via IL-4) and late phase hypersensitivity, mediated by eosinophilia (via IL-5) and these responses are considered to be efficient for the clearing of certain helmith species. CD4$^+$ T cells secreting balanced levels of Th1 and Th2 cytokines, although less efficient in clearing intracellular parasites and the helminth types, induce mixed cellular and humoral (without IgE) responses that are often sufficient for the many other immune activities.

2. REGULATION OF THE PRODUCTION OF TH1 AND TH2 CYTOKINES BY ACCESSORY CELL-DERIVED FACTORS

In vivo mouse model studies and in vitro experiments with human cells imply that the balance between Th1 and Th2 cytokines is determined by various physiological fac-

New Horizons in Allergy Immunotherapy
edited by Sehon et al. Plenum Press, New York, 1996

305

tors. Because T cells are optimally susceptible to such factors when they are activated, factors produced by antigen-presenting AC are of great importance. In this respect, the finding that IL-12 induces the outgrowth of Th1 cells, due to selective induction and stimulation of IFN-γ levels of Th cells, is most relevant[1,2]. PGE$_2$, another compound released by AC, selectively inhibits the secretion of the Th1 cytokine IFN-γ[3,4,5]. Recently, we obtained evidence that AC regulate IFN-γ levels of Th cells through the opposite effects of IL-12 and PGE$_2$ in a model using LPS-stimulated monocytes and CD3 mAb-activated human Th cells (Hilkens et al., submitted for publication). These opposite effects of IL-12 and PGE$_2$ are exerted via independent mechanisms. The IFN-γ level in Th cells, therefore, is determined by the net levels of IL-12 and PGE$_2$. Various parameters influence the levels of IL-12 and PGE$_2$ including the type of stimulus, the type of AC and the different kinetics of IL-12 and PGE$_2$ synthesis. Because IL-12 is secreted earlier than PGE$_2$, simultaneous stimulation of monocytes and T cells results in the stimulation of the IFN-γ level due to early IL-12 release, whereas 24 h prestimulation of monocytes results in a suppressed IFN-γ level due to overexpression of PGE$_2$.

To date, the requirements for the induction and regulation of IL-12 and PGE$_2$ production are poorly studied. Here we will discuss some recent findings from our and other laboratories, focussing on the induction and regulation of the IL-12 production.

3. INDUCTION OF IL-12 PRODUCTION

Bioactive IL-12 is a 70 kD heterodimer composed of a 35 and a 40 kD subunit[6]. The 35 kD subunit is only secreted as part of bioactive p70 IL-12, whereas the 40 kD subunit may be secreted as a biologically inactive homodimer, which has no bioactivity[7]. IL-12 is secreted by many AC types, incuding B cells, dendritic cells[8] and macrophage subsets and epithelial cells[9] and these cells have in common that they show constitutive or inducible expression of MHC class II molecules and therefore, may act as antigen-presenting cells. Although some cell types show a constitutive expression of one of the IL-12 subunits, the production of bioactive IL-12 must be induced by stimulation. For instance, monocytes only express p35 or p40 mRNA after activation with bacteria or bacterial compounds, such Staphylococcus aureus Cowan strain I and LPS.

Recently, sensitive ELISA techniques became available for the detection of p40 and p70 IL-12 production. Analysis of the secretion products of LPS-stimulated monocytes in whole blood showed that the production of the p40 subunit is optimal at 1 - 1000 ng/ml LPS, whereas the p70 production gradually rises in this concentration range, suggesting that the synthsis of the p35 and p40 subunits are induced by different mechanisms and that p70 production is determined by the production of the p35 subunit (Snijders et al., manuscript submitted for publication). Due to the uncorrelated production profiles, the excess of p40 over p70 production varies from about 500 (at 1 ng/ml LPS) to 150 (at 1000 pg/ml LPS)-fold.

4. REGULATION OF IL-12 PRODUCTION BY CYTOKINES

It was previously shown that the production of IL-12 is highly regulated by different cytokines[10,11,12]. We found that the mechanisms of regulation are rather complex [Snijders et al., submitted for publication]. The production of bioactive p70 and p40 are both stimulated by IFN-γ and suppressed by IL-10 and IL-4, although the dose response curves were markedly different. The effects of IFN-γ and IL-10 on p40 production were weaker, resulting in an even larger excess of p40 over p70 production. At high doses (> 100 U/ml), IL-4 strongly inhibits p70 and p40 production, but at lower doses the effects on p70 production were only marginal, showing a slight donor-dependent stimulation or suppression of p70 secretion, in conditions in which p40 secretion was suppressed in all donors. Notably, at all IL-4 doses p40 production still exceeded p70 production more than 10-fold. Prostaglandin (PG) E_2 suppresses the secretion of p70 and p40 IL-12 equally well, thereby not changing the high ratio between p40 and p70 production [van der Pouw Kraan et al., submitted for publication]. Strong effects on IL-12 secretion were accompanied by effects on p35 and p40 mRNA levels, as analysed by RT-PCR, indicating that the induction and regulation of bioactive IL-12 production is predominantly determined by regulation of p35 mRNA levels (Snijders et al. manuscript submitted for publication).

These observations have interesting implications. The different characteristics of regulation of p70 and p40 IL-12 production by IFN-γ, IL-10 and IL-4 highly suggests that, like for the induction of the production, the mechanisms of regulation of production of the p35 and p40 subunits by these cytokines, are different. Furthermore, the finding that p40 production exceeded p70 production in all conditions of regulation, implies that the inhibitory and stimulatory effects on bioactive p70 IL-12 are determined by the regulation of the production of the p35 subunit.

5. INTERREGULATION BETWEEN AC-DERIVED FACTORS

IL-12 and its inhibitors IL-10 and PGE_2 are simultaneously secreted by human monocytes. IL-12 production, therefore, may be subject to suppression by endogenous IL-10 and PGE_2 levels. Indeed, we found that IL-12 production by LPS-stimulated monocytes is considerably enhanced by blocking endogenous IL-10 production with neutralizing antibody and enhanced to a lesser extent by blockers of PGE_2 production. These findings may have implications for the mechanisms of stimulation of IL-12 production by IFN-γ and low doses of IL-4. Since both cytokines inhibit the production of IL-10, stimulation of IL-12 production by IFN-γ and IL-4 may, at least partially, follow indirectly from inhibition of endogenous IL-10 production.

6. THE NETWORK OF TYPE 1 AND TYPE 2 FACTORS AND IMPLICATIONS FOR ATOPIC ALLERGY

Many studies collectively imply the existence a tight network of the Th1 response-associated factors IL-12 and IFN-γ (type 1 factors), which bias to delayed type hypersensitivity, and the Th2 response-associated factors PGE_2 and IL-4 (type 2 factors), which bias to humoral responses eventually with immediate type hypersensitivity. A first feature of the network is that there is some degree of cooperation within the type 1 and type 2 pathways. The pathway to delayed hypersensitivity is strengthened by the mutual stimulations of IL-12 and IFN-γ production. Also the pathway to immediate hypersensitivity is strengthened by the fact that PGE_2 strongly stimulates the IL-4-induced switch to IgE in B cells[13]. A most remarkable second feature of the network is the high degree of mutual suppressive effects between the type 1 and type 2 factors. IL-4 suppresses IL-12 production and PGE_2 suppresses IL-12 as well as IFN-γ production. Earlier findings were that IFN-γ suppresses IL-4 secretion and that IL-12 selectively suppresses the IL-4-induced IgE switch[14].

Immediate hypersensitivity reactions followed by late phase responses, as observed in atopic patients, probably follow from an aberrant balance between type 1 and type 2 factors. Various studies, including our own, have reported on a shift to high IL-4 (and IL-5) and low IFN-γ production in allergen-specific Th cells from atopic individuals. Furthermore, purified monocytes from severe atopic dermatitis patients show an elevated production of PGE_2[15] (Snijders et al,. unpublished results). Data on the level of IL-12 production by monocytes from atopics are not available, up to now. However, it may be expected from the interactions of the cytokines of the network that in the course of the allergen response, IL-12 secretion in AC will be hampered due to the lower levels of feedback stimulation by Th cell-derived IFN-γ and by the feedback inhibition by enhanced levels of IL-4 and PGE_2.

The network of interactions implies that the study of the role of factors in the etiology of atopic allergic immune reactions requires the analysis of the production of such factors in experiments excluding the direct interference by their regulators. Most studies published on this issue to date have been performed in mixed cell populations and do not fully meet this requirement.

REFERENCES

1. Hsieh C-S., S.E. Macatonia, C.S. Tripp, S.F. Wolf, A. O'Garra and K.M. Murphy. 1993. Development of Th1 CD4[+] T cells through IL-12 in Lysteria-induced macrophages. Science 260:547.
2. Manetti R., P. Parronchi, M.G. Giudzi, M-P. Piccini, E. Maggi, G. Trinchieri and S. Romagnani. 1993. Natural killer stimulatory factor (interleukin-12) induces T helper type 1 (Th1)-specific immune responses and inhibits the development of IL-4-producing cells. J. Exp. Med. 177:1199.
3. Betz M, and B. Fox. 1991. PGE_2 inhibits production of Th1 cytokines but not Th2 cytokines. J. Immunol. 146:108.
4. Snijdewint F.G.M., P. Kalinski, E.A. Wierenga, J.D. Bos and M.L. Kapsenberg. 1993. Prostaglandin E_2 differentially modulates cytokine secretion profiles of human helper T lymphocytes. J. Immunol. 150:5321.
5. Hilkens C.M.U., H. Vermeulen, R.J.J. van Neerven, F.G.M. Snijdewint, E.A. Wierenga and M.L. Kapsenberg. 1995. Differential modulation of T helper type 1 (Th1) and Th2 cytokine secretion by PGE_2 critically depends on IL-2. Eur. J. Immunol. 25:59.
6. Trinchieri G. 1993. Interleukin-12 and its role in the generation of Th1 cells Immunol. Today 14:335.
7. Ling P., M. Gately, U. Gubler, A.S. Stren, P. Lin, K. Hollfelder, C. Su, Y-C. E. Pan and J. Hakimi. 1995. Human IL-12 p40 homodimer binds to the IL-12 Receptor but does not mediate biological activity. J. Immunol. 154:116.
8. Macatonia S.E., N.A. Hosken, M. Litton, P. Vieira, C-I. Hsieh, J.A. Culpepper, M. Wysocka, G. Trichieri, K.M. Murphy and A. O'Garra. 1995. Dendritic cells produce IL-12 and direct the development of Th1 cells from naive CD4[+] T cells. J. Immunol. 154:5071.
9. Müller G., J. Saloga, T. Germann, I. Bellinghausen, M. Mohamadzahdeh, J. Knop and A. Enk. 1994. Identification and induction of human keratinocyte-derived IL-12. J. Clin. Invest. 94:1799.
10. Kubin M., J.M. Chow and G. Trinchieri. 1994. Differential regulation of IL-12, TNFα and IL-1β production in human myeloid leukemia cell lines and peripheral blood cells. Blood 83:1847.
11. D.Andrea A., M. Aste-Amezaga, N.M. Valiante, X. Ma, M. Kubin and G. Trinchieri. 1993. IL-10 inhibits human lymphocyte interferon-γ production by suppressing natural killer cell stimulatory factor/IL-12 synthesis in accessory cells. J. Exp. Med. 178:1041.
12. van der Pouw Kraan T.C.T.M., L.C.M. Boeije, R.J.T. Smeenk, J. Wijdenes and L.A. Aarden. 1995. PGE_2 is a potent inhibitor of human interleukin-12 production. J. Exp. Med. 181:775.
13. Roper R.L., D.H. Conrad, D. Brown, G. Warner and R.P Phipps. 1990. PGE_2 promotes IL-4-induced IgE and IgG1 synthesis. J. Immunol. 145:2644.
14. Morris C., K.B. Madden, J.J. Adamovicz, W.C. Gause, B.R. Hubbard, M.C. Gately and F.D. Finkelman. 1994. Effects of IL-12 om in vivo cytokine gene expression and Ig isotype selection. J. Immunol. 152:1047.
15. Jacob T., B.N. Huspith, Y.W. Latchman, R. Rycroft and J. Brostoff. 1990. Depressed lymphocyte transformation and the role of prostaglandins in atopic dermatitis. Clin Exp. Immunol. 79:380.

44

IN VIVO DIRECTION OF CD4 T CELLS TO TH1 AND TH2–LIKE PATTERNS OF CYTOKINE SYNTHESIS

Kent T. HayGlass,[1] Mingdong Wang,[1] Randall S. Gieni,[1*] Cynthia Ellison,[2] and John Gartner[2]

[1]Department of Immunology
[2]Department of Pathology
University of Manitoba
Winnipeg, Canada. R3E 0W3

1. SUMMARY

Factors that influence the initial development, and continued maintenance, of Th1 or Th2-like responses in vivo play a pivotal role in determining immune effector mechanisms and clinical outcome. Here, we review recent developments in this area with particular emphasis on (i) the ability of chemically modified exogenous antigens to preferentially activate Th1-dominated responses in vivo and (ii) the role played by NK cells in initial commitment of naive exogenous antigen-specific T cells to Th1 or Th2-like cytokine synthesis. We find that NK cell depletion of naive mice prior to immunization with OVA (which induces balanced Th0 like responses), or a high Mr polymer (that preferentially elicits OVA-specific Th1-dominated responses), fails to influence the development of cytokine or specific antibody responses. The results argue that NK cells do not play an essential role in shaping induction of immune responses to exogenous antigens, the most common class of inhalant allergen.

2. INTRODUCTION

Cytokine production by T lymphocytes, or accessory cells involved in their triggering, is pivotal in determining the intensity, *and type,* of immune response that develops upon antigen exposure. With CD4 T cells controlling the activation of B cells, macrophages and CD8 cells, the activation of naive CD4 cells by antigen is arguably the most

---

* Present address: Department of Pediatrics, Stanford University, Stanford, California.

New Horizons in Allergy Immunotherapy
edited by Sehon et al. Plenum Press, New York, 1996

important event in the generation of adaptive immunity (1). Although many experimental tools can be used experimentally to activate CD4 T cells, physiologic activation results from cognate interaction between mature peripheral T cells and MHC Class II$^+$ APC. Initial CD4 T cell action results primarily in synthesis of IL-2. The T cell is then highly sensitive to other signals which further shape its ultimate response. Of these, cytokine mediated signals are of pivotal importance (reviews, 2–4).

A decade ago, studies with murine, later human, CD4 T cell clones identified two major populations with distinct patterns of cytokine synthesis and function, designated Th1 and Th2. These prototypes are now recognized as polar extremes in the spectrum of T cell activation. Subsequent research has expanded the number of T cell subsets involved; identified important sub-classes of cytokine gene expression (5–7), differences between Th1/Th2 clones in mouse vs. humans (i.e., in IL-10 expression, 4,8) and distinct similarities with patterns of CD8 T cell activation (9–11). However, the key point is that the association of Th1/Th2-*like* cytokine synthesis patterns with activation and maintenance of distinct effector mechanisms *in vivo* and subsequent clinical outcome (exacerbation or self-limiting disease, protection or hypersensitivity, etc.) is widely demonstrable in human and animal responses. This correlation between induction of specific patterns of cytokine synthesis in vivo and the resulting clinical consequences applies to antigens ranging from simple, highly purified peptides to complex replicating parasites (4,9,12–15). We argue that the question of whether single T cells *in vivo* conform explicitly to the Th1/Th2 paradigm defined in clones (an issue yet to be resolved due to the technical demands) is a moot point. Recognition of the existence of Th1 or Th2-*like responses at the T cell population level,* and recent progress in development of strategies allowing preferential activation (or inhibition) of specific patterns of cytokine synthesis *in vivo* (16–21) promises substantial changes in our understanding of the mechanisms of, and therapeutic approaches to, hypersensitivity, transplantation, immunization, resistance to parasitic infections, autoimmunity, and a variety of immunologic disorders.

Immediate hypersensitivity is the most widespread immunological disorder in humans. Allergies represent the most prevalent (and rapidly increasing) chronic health problem among individuals ≥ 15 years of age (22). We utilize a murine model of human immediate hypersensitivity to ovalbumin (OVA), a common allergen in humans that also elicits strong IgE responses in mice. We previously developed a novel approach for chemically modifying OVA to yield a high Mr polymer termed OA-POL. Its salient characteristic is its ability to selectively activate a specific (protective) pattern of CD4 cytokine synthesis within the OVA-specific repertoire. Thus, OA-POL exposure (ip in saline, without adjuvants) leads to decreased Th2-like activity, indicated by substantially reduced IL-4 and IL-10 production, and increased Th1-like activation, as indicated by markedly enhanced IFNγ levels relative to the cytokine response induced following administration of unmodified OVA (18,23–25). These changes in cytokine synthesis are responsible for 95–99% inhibition of primary and secondary anti-OVA IgE, and 250–1000 fold increases in IgG$_{2a}$ responses in OA-POL treated mice (16). Most importantly, these effects do not reflect transient phenomena best observed in acute (~2 week) experiments, but reflect stable changes in OVA-specific T cell memory responses, persisting for over 18 months in the absence of additional treatment despite multiple OVA (alum) booster immunizations (26). In contrast, unmodified OVA, or OVA polymerized by previous approaches (27), given under the same conditions (i.e., analogous to those used in human allergen immunotherapy), elicits a Th0 (or balanced Th1/Th2-like) response that very effectively stimulates enhanced IgG1 synthesis *in vivo* (as does clinical immunotherapy) but fails to alter cytokine (IL-4/10,IFNγ) or other antibody (IgE or IgG$_{2a}$) responses.

3. RESULTS AND DISCUSSION

Recently, we have utilized limiting dilution analysis (LDA) to more precisely characterize changes in the CD4 response to OVA (25). Specifically, we determined the precursor frequencies of OVA-specific CD4 T cells activated by native and modified OVA, and the relative frequencies of IFNγ IL-4 and IL-10 producing cells stimulated by the two forms of antigen. Highly enriched CD4 cells from OVA or OA-POL treated mice (administered ip in the absence of adjuvants, see references 18,25 for detailed methods) were analyzed. Examination of the frequency of clonogenic CD4 T cells in OA-POL vs. OVA treated mice, expressed here as the ratio of their frequencies for purposes of comparison (OA-POL:OVA), indicates that the two forms of antigen are essentially equivalent in their capacity to stimulate T cell activation (Figure 1, OA-POL: OVA ratio of OVA-specific proliferation: 0.97 ± 0.22, n=3 independent experiments).

However, a substantial difference is evident in the nature of the allergen-driven cytokine response elicited by the two forms of antigen. The frequency of IFNγ producing CD4 T cells is some ten fold higher in OA-POL treated mice (OA-POL: OVA ratio = 10.2 ± 2.1; n=3). In contrast, IL-10 producing CD4 T cells are some 5 fold less frequent in mice administered OVA. (OA-POL: OVA ratio = 0.18 ± 0.06). Indeed, the net effect of the differences in the frequency of CD4 cells responding to OVA-specific stimulation by IFNγ and/or IL-10 synthesis is a reversal from a situation where IL-10 producers outnumber IFNγ producers by 4:1 (upon OVA administration) to one where IFNγ producers outnumber IL-10 producers 11:1 (upon OA-POL administration, 25). This net 47 fold change reflects a substantial quantitative, but more importantly, *qualitative shift* in the dominant response stimulated by native and chemically modified antigen.

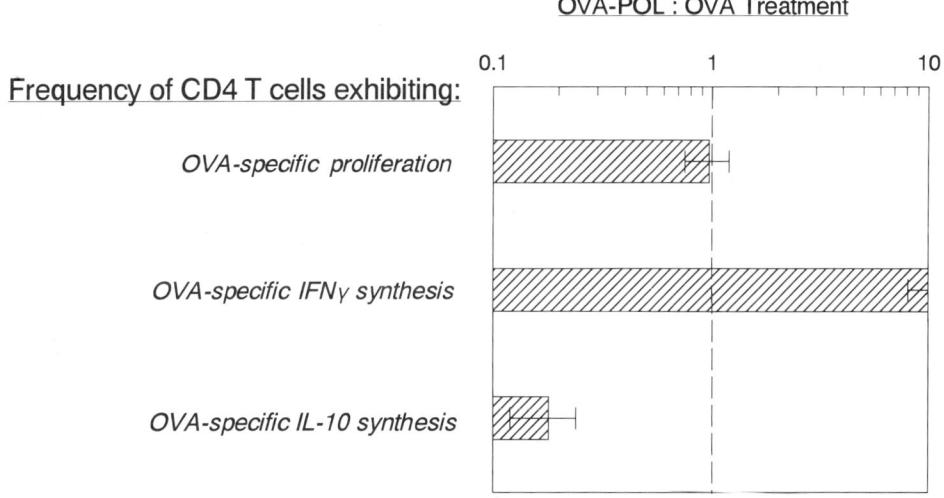

Figure 1. Minimal estimates of the *precursor frequency* of OVA-specific CD4 T cells in OVA (in saline) and OA-POL (in saline)-treated C57Bl/6 mice were determined by limiting dilution analysis (25). Independent analysis was made of the frequency of clonogenic (proliferation), IFNγ and IL-10 producing, antigen-specific CD4 T cells. The data are expressed here as the *ratio* (± S.E.M.) of the frequencies obtained in order to facilitate comparison between the two forms of antigen. Data presented are derived from a minimum of three independent experiments for each parameter.

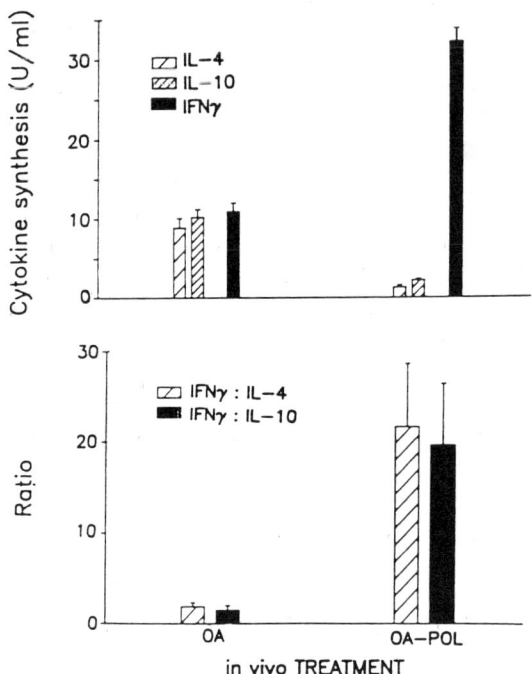

Figure 2. Bulk culture analysis of the *intensity* of OVA-specific cytokine responses stimulated by OVA vs. OA-POL administration in vivo. These data, previously presented in detail in reference 18, reflect mean values (± S.E.M.) from a minimum of four independent experiments. Copyright permission of The Rockefeller University Press.

The ability of OA-POL to preferentially select for dominance of Th1-like cytokine synthesis patterns *in vivo* among OVA-specific CD4 T cells is similarly seen in analyses of the *intensity* of cytokine production in bulk culture (Figure 2). As such it stands in marked contrast to the balanced pattern of cytokine synthesis elicited by most exogenous antigens, including unmodified OVA. We reasoned that these two forms of the same antigen provide a useful tool with which to examine the impact of different influences on initial T cell activation. They allow examination of activation of naive (for that antigen) normal T cells *in vivo* responding to typical exogenous antigens under physiologic conditions.

Much evidence supports a pivotal role for the cytokines present in the environment of the naive T cell during initial cognate antigen-dependent activation. Thus, IL-4 appears to be the key cytokine in steering newly activated CD4 T cells towards IL-4 production while IL-12 and IFNγ play a similar role in promoting Th1-like activation. Much attention has focussed on the initial sources and stimuli that drive production of these cytokines. One intriguing hypothesis (5,28) suggests a role for the natural immune response in selecting for Th1 vs. Th2-like cytokine dominance. T and NK cells are the only known sources of IFNγ. Stimulation of NK, unlike T cells, leads to very rapid, intense IFNγ production even when these cells are in a resting, non-preactivated state (29). Thus NK cells, perhaps secondary to APC derived IL12 production, have been suggested as important sources of IFNγ that act to prevent potentially hazardous Th2-like cytokine production from dominating following exposure to most antigens. Indeed, several investigators have obtained compelling indirect evidence of a role for NK cells in shaping the initial induction (d.1–3 post immunization or infection) of Th1-like responses *in vivo*. The strongest evidence comes from bacterial (30), protozoal (31,32) or viral infection.

Table 1. Impact of *in vivo* administration of anti-NK1.1 mAb PK136 on *in vivo* development of OVA-specific responses

In vivo Treatment		IFNγ	IL-4	IL-10	IgE
d-2,±1	d.0	(U/ml)	(U/ml)	(U/ml)	(d.10 Titer)
—	OVA (alum)	31.0±2.8	16.3±4.0	26.1±3.9	860
anti-NK1.1	OVA (alum)	28.2±3.6	15.9±3.3	20.8±5.5	1140

C57Bl/6 mice were treated ip with anti-NK 1.1 (PK136) ascites, normal mouse IgG (not shown) or saline on d.-2 and +1. All mice were OVA (alum) immunized on d.0 and sacrificed at d.5 for bulk culture (18) or were bled at d.10 for determination of serum OVA-specific IgE levels (23). Data reflect mean cytokine production and geometric mean serum IgE PCA titers.

Our interest was in evaluating the role of NK cells in soluble antigen driven responses, the class of antigens of primary relevance in immediate hypersensitivity. We hypothesized that *in vivo* NK cell depletion prior to immunization would lead to a less Th1-like, more Th2-like, cytokine and antibody response. Specifically, we reasoned that if NK cells play an essential role in shaping the developing OVA-specific response, their depletion immediately prior to antigen exposure should markedly influence (i) antigen driven cytokine synthesis in short term culture and (ii) the balance of OVA-specific IgE vs. IgG2a synthesis *in vivo*.

We first examined the OVA-specific cytokine and antibody response obtained in anti-ASGM1 treated BALB/c and control normal rabbit Ig treated mice. This treatment is highly effective in depleting NK cell function in normal mice and, in poly I:C treated mice that exhibit enhanced NK cell activity (32,33,39). However, NK cell depletion *in vivo* immediately prior to OVA immunization did not lead to detectable decreases in IFNγ responses, nor increases in IL-4/IL10 in antigen stimulated bulk culture (39).

These data were obtained using antigen stimulated spleen cells in short term bulk culture (method: reference 18). One might argue that NK cell activity would be localized elsewhere (ie. at the injection site), obscuring any difference in antigen-stimulated cytokine production by spleen or lymph node cells removed for culture. We therefore examined the whole animal effector response since we have previously demonstrated for this system (18,23), as numerous other groups have for other antigens, that there is a tight association between the nature of the cytokine response and the *in vivo* effector mechanisms that result. We therefore examined OVA-specific serum IgE responses (which could be anticipated to *increase* in the absence of NK-dependent Th1 activation) and IgG2a (which we could anticipate to *decrease*). However, neither primary or secondary IgE, IgG1 nor IgG2a responses differed between control and anti-ASGM1 treated mice (data not shown, 39).

Well aware that ASGM1 is expressed on activated T cells as well as NK cells, we also employed an *in vivo* NK cell depletion model initially developed by Koo and colleagues (34). Anti-NK1.1 treated C57Bl/6 mice were found to exhibit no detectable NK cell function, even in groups administered poly I:C 18h prior to sacrifice, confirming the effectiveness of this widely used approach for in vivo depletion. Comparison of OVA-specific IgE production (intensity and kinetics) in NK-depleted mice revealed no differences relative to those obtained in untreated control or normal mouse IgG treated mice. Similarly, IgG1 and IgG2a responses were unaffected. Direct analysis of cytokine (IL-4, IL-10 and IFNγ) synthesis also failed to indicate any difference between NK-depleted and control mice (Table 1 and reference 39).

Native OVA was selected for initial examination because it is a "typical" exogenous antigen, not yielding a strongly polarized Th1 or Th2-like response *in vivo*. We recently determined the impact of NK cell depletion on responses induced by high Mr OA-POL polymers— taking advantage of the capacity of this exogenous antigen to induces Th1-polarized cytokine and effector (antibody) responses in vivo. In data obtained to date (n= 3 independent experiments) NK cell depletion had no detectable impact on the ability of this antigen to preferentially elicit Th1-like responses in vivo.

4. CONCLUSIONS

The studies above describe further characterization of one of a number of antigens that elicit a polarized pattern of cytokine gene expression, and consequently dictate effector responses *in vivo* (reviews 5,13,35–37). What distinguishes this approach is that it is one of the few strategies by which one can actively **select** the response to be generated rather than obtain the default response stimulated by "inherently" Th1 or Th2-like stimuli. Indeed, it demonstrates that responses to Ags believed inherently Th1 or Th2-like can be readily manipulated.

There is persuasive evidence that NK cells, by virtue of their ability to promptly produce IFNγ following non-cognate activation, are pivotal in the development of protective, Th1-like, responses to several infectious agents (5, 30–32). A previous report (38), largely based on immunocytochemical analysis, suggested that this may also be the case for exogenous antigens such as ovalbumin. However, the data presented above, based on analysis of cytokine and antibody production in OVA-immunized normal and NK deficient mice, strongly suggests that the role of NK cells in influencing initial activation of the exogenous antigen specific CD4 T cell response is minimal.

5. ACKNOWLEDGMENTS

We thank W. Stefura for expert technical support and K. Risk for excellent secretarial assistance. This work was supported by grants from the MRC of Canada to KH and JG. KH holds an MRC Scientist salary award.

6. REFERENCES

1. Janeway, C.A., Jr. and Bottomly, K. 1994. Signals and signs for lymphocyte responses. *Cell* 76:275.
2. Seder, R.A. and Paul, W.E. 1994. Acquisition of lymphokine-producing phenotype by CD4+ T cells. *Annu. Rev. Immunol.* 12:635.
3. O'Garra, A. and Murphy, K. 1994. Role of cytokines in determining T-lymphocyte function. *Curr. Opin. Immunol.* 6:458.
4. Romagnani, S. 1994. Lymphokine production by human T cells in disease states. *Ann. Rev. Immunol.* 12:227.
5. Paul, W.E. and Seder, R.A. 1994. Lymphocyte responses and cytokines. *Cell* 76:241.
6. Kelso, A., and Gough, N.M. 1988. Coexpression of granulocyte-macrophage colony-stimulating factor, gamma interferon, and interleukins 3 and 4 is random in murine alloreactive T-lymphocyte clones. *Proc. Natl. Acad. Sci. USA* 85:9189.
7. Street, N.E., Schumacher, J.H., Fong, T.A.T. *et al.* 1990. Heterogeneity of mouse helper T cells. Evidence from bulk cultures and limiting dilution cloning for precursors of Th1 and Th2 cells. *J. Immunol.* 144:1629.
8. Moore, K. W., O'Garra, A., de Waal Malefyt, R., Vieira, P., and Mosmann, T. R. 1993. Interleukin-10. *Ann. Rev. Immunology.* 11:165.
9. Salgame, P., Abrams, J.S., Clayberger, C., *et al.* 1991. Differing lymphokine profiles of functional subsets of human CD4 and CD8 T cell clones. *Science* 254:279.

10. Croft, M., Carter, L., Swain, S.L. and Dutton, R.W. 1994. Generation of polarized antigen-specific CD8 effector populations: Reciprocal action of interleukin (IL)-4 and IL-12 in promoting Type 2 versus Type 1 cytokine profiles. *J. Exp. Med.* 180:1715.

11. Kemeny, D.M., Noble, A., Holmes, B.J. and Diaz-Sanchez, D. 1994. Immune regulation: a new role for the CD8⁺ T cell. *Immunol. Today* 15:107.

12. King, C. L., and Nutman, T. B. 1992. Biological role of helper T cell subsets in helminth infections. *Chem. Immunol. 54:136.*

13. Sher, A., Gazzinelli, R. T., Oswald, I. P., Clerici, M., Kullberg, M., Pearce, E. J., Berzofsky, J. A., Mosmann, T. R., James, S. L., Morse, H. C. III, and Shearer, G. M. 1992. Role of T cell derived cytokines in the downregulation of immune responses in parasitic and retroviral infection. *Immunol. Rev. 127:183.*

14. Modlin, R. L., and Nutman, T. B. 1993. Type 2 cytokines and negative immune regulation in human infections. *Curr. Op. Immunol. 5:511.*

15. Marrack, P. and Kappler, J. 1994. Subversion of the immune system by pathogens. *Cell* 76:323.

16. HayGlass, K.T. and Stefura. W. 1991. Antigen-specific modulation of murine IgE and IgG$_{2a}$ responses with glutaraldehyde-polymerized allergen is independent of MHC haplotype and Igh allotype. *Immunology* 73:24.

17. Bretscher, P.A., Wei, G., Menon, J.N., *et al.* 1992. Establishment of stable, cell-mediated immunity that makes "susceptible" mice resistant to *Leishmania major. Science* 257:539.

18. Yang, X., Gieni, R., Mosmann, T.R. and HayGlass, K.T. 1993. Chemically modified antigen preferentially elicits induction of Th1-like cytokine synthesis patterns *in vivo. J. Exp. Med.* 178:349.

19. Salk, J., Bretscher, P.A., Salk, P.L. *et al.* 1993. A strategy for prophylactic vaccination against HIV. *Science* 260:1270.

20. Afonso, L.C., Scharton, T.M., Vieira, L.Q. *et al.* 1994. The adjuvant effect of interleukin-12 in a vaccine against *Leishmania major. Science* 263:235.

21. Trinchieri, G. and Scott, P. 1994. The role of interleukin 12 in the immune response, disease and therapy. *Immunol. Today* 15:460.

22. "Chronic Health Problems" in 1991. *Health Status of Canadians: Report of the 1991 General Social Survey.* Statistics Canada, 1994, p. 175.

23. HayGlass, K.T. and Stefura, W.P. 1991. Anti-IFNγ treatment blocks the ability of glutaraldehyde polymerized allergens to inhibit specific IgE responses. *J. Exp. Med.* 173:279.

24. Gieni, R.S., Yang, X. and HayGlass, K.T. 1993. Allergen-specific modulation of cytokine synthesis patterns and IgE resonses *in vivo* with chemically modified allergen. *J. Immunol.* 150:302.

25. Gieni, R., Yang, X., Kelso, A. and HayGlass, K.T. Limiting dilution analysis reveals reciprocal regulation of IFNγ and IL-10 CD4 T cell frequencies following exposure to chemically modified allergen. (Submitted, 1995).

26. HayGlass, K.T., Gieni, R. and Stefura, W. 1991. Long-lived reciprocal regulation of antigen-specific IgE and IgG$_{2a}$ responses in mice treated with glutaraldehyde-polymerized ovalbumin. *Immunology* 73:407.

27. Patterson, R., Suszko, I.M. and McIntire, F.C. 1973. Polymerized ragweed antigen E. I. Preparation and immunologic studies. *J. Immunol.* 110:1402.

28. Romagnani, S. 1992. Induction of T$_H$1 and T$_H$2 responses: a key role for the 'natural' immune response? *Immunol. Today* 13:379.

29. Trinchieri, G. 1992. Natural killer (NK) cells. In: Encyclopedia of Immunology. Eds: I.M. Roitt and P.J. Delves, London, p. 1136.

30. Teixeira, H.C. and Kaufmann, S.H.E. 1994. Role of NK1.1⁺ cells in experimental listeriosis. NK1⁺ cells are early IFN-γ producers but impair resistance to *Listeria monocytogenes* infection. *J. Immunol.* 152:1873.

31. Scharton, T. M., and Scott, P. 1993. Natural killer cells are a source of interferon γ that drives differentiation of CD4⁺ T cell subsets and induces early resistance to *Leishmania major* in mice. *J. Exp. Med. 178:567.*

32. Denkers, E.Y., Gazzinelli, R.T., Martin, D. and Sher, A. 1993. Emergence of NK1.1⁺ cells as effectors of IFN-γ dependent immunity to *Toxoplasma gondii* in MHC class I-deficient mice. *J. Exp. Med.* 178:1465.

33. Tiberghien, P., Longo, D.L., Wine, J.W. *et al.* 1990. Anti-asialo GM1 antiserum treatment of lethally irradiated recipients before bone marrow transplantation: evidence that recipient natural killer depletion enhances survival, engraftment, and hematopoietic recovery. *Blood* 76:1419.

34. Koo, G.C., Dumont, F.J., Tutt, M. *et al.* 1986. The NK-1.1(-) mouse: A model to study differentiation of murine NK cells. *J. Immunol.* 137:3742.

35. Modlin, R.L. and Nutman, T.B. 1993. Type 2 cytokines and negative immune regulation in human infections. *Curr. Op. Immunol.* 5:511.

36. Locksley, R.M. 1994. Th2 cells: Help for helminths. *J. Exp. Med.* 179:1405.

37. Marrack, P. and Kappler, J. 1994. Subversion of the immune system by pathogens. *Cell* 76:323.

38. Bogen, S.T., Fogelman, Ilana and Abbas, A.K. 1993. Analysis of IL-2, IL-4, and IFN-γ-producing cells *in situ* during immune responses to protein antigens. *J. Immunol.* 150:4197.

39. Wang, M.D., Ellison, C., Rempel, J.D., Gartner, J., and HayGlass, K.T. 1995. The role of NK cells in initial CD4 T cell activation by Th0-like and Th1-like exogenous antigen. (manuscript submitted).

45

CONTROVERSIAL ISSUES AND POSSIBLE ANSWERS ON THE ANTIGEN-SPECIFIC REGULATION OF THE IgE ANTIBODY RESPONSE

Kimishige Ishizaka,[1] Tatsumi Nakano,[1] Yasuyuki Ishii,[1] Yun-Cai Liu,[1] Toshifumi Mikayama,[2] and Akio Mori[1]

[1]La Jolla Institute for Allergy and Immunology
La Jolla, California 92037
[2]Pharmaceutical Laboratory
Kirin Brewery Co.
Maebashi, Japan

1. INTRODUCTION

In the past 10 years, the major approaches for the regulation of the IgE antibody response by many investigators have been focused to isotype-specific suppression of the IgE synthesis. However, another approach to be considered is to suppress the antibody response to the allergens to which the allergic patients are sensitive. In this presentation, we would like to discuss the possibility to regulate the antibody response in antigen-specific manner, and scientific evidence for the presence of such a mechanism.

About 25 years ago, Dick Gershon described antigen-specific suppressor T (Ts) cells, which regulate the antibody response in antigen-specific manner. Subsequently, Tada and his co-workers found that extracts of antigen-specific Ts cells contained a unique factor that had affinity for the nominal antigen and suppressed the antibody response to the homologous antigen. Many investigators reproduced these findings in various antigen systems, and Ts and TsF became popular research subjects for the next 10 years. After the T cell receptors on helper and cytotoxic T cells were identified, however, many controversial issues were raised on Ts cells and TsF, and the majority of cellular immunologists became suspicious about the presence of Ts cells. Thus, research on Ts and TsF became an unpopular subject in immunology in spite of several thousand previous publications on this subject. Nevertheless, antigen-specific regulation of the antibody response is a kind of dream for immunologists. If this can be achieved, one may expect that the principles may be applied to control autoimmune diseases and allergic diseases without affecting the abilities for protection against infectious agents.

New Horizons in Allergy Immunotherapy
edited by Sehon et al. Plenum Press, New York, 1996

Fortunately, or unfortunately, we found that a product of antigen-specific Ts cell hybridomas could regulate the *in vivo* IgE antibody response to homologous antigen (1). At that time, we were studying the mechanism for isotype-specific regulation of the IgE antibody response, and found a unique cytokine, glycosylation inhibiting factor (GIF) which is involved in the selective formation of IgE suppressive factors (2). Since the major cell source of GIF appeared to be antigen-specific Ts cells, Dr. Paula Jardieu, who was working with us at that time, tried to establish ovalbumin (OVA)-specific Ts cell hybridomas and tested for the formation of GIF. Many hybridomas constitutively secreted GIF which failed to bind OVA. Upon antigenic stimulation with antigen-pulsed syngeneic macrophages, however some of the hybriodmas, such as 231F1 cells, produced GIF that had affinity for OVA. Thus, she purified OVA-binding GIF from culture supernatants of the antigen-stimulated Ts hybridoma cells using OVA-coupled Sepharose, and the partially purified factor was tested for the ability to regulate the *in vivo* antibody responses of syngeneic mice. We realized that the OVA-binding GIF suppressed the *in vivo* antibody response to DNP-OVA, but failed to suppress the anti-DNP antibody response to DNP-KLH (1). Our major interests were the mechanisms through which the antigen-specific GIF or TsF could regulate the antibody response. However, we realized that no immunologist would accept such a finding, until we can resolve various controversial issues on Ts cells and TsF, and biochemically characterize the antigen-specific GIF. Therefore, we spent several years to identify the factors.

2. UNIQUENESS OF ANTIGEN-SPECIFIC Ts CELLS AND BIOACTIVE GIF

First of all, many immunologists were suspicious about the presence of T cell receptors (TCR) on Ts hybridomas (3). However, a representative OVA-specific Ts hybridoma, 231F1 cells express both TCRβ chain and CD3, as determined by immunofluorescence (4). Indeed, many Ts hybridomas (5,6) and Ts clones (7) established by several groups of investigators express CD3 and TCRαβ. Then, what is unique for the Ts cells? We speculated that the production of GIF may be unique for Ts cells. Indeed, our experiments in collaboration with Martin Dorf showed that several hapten-specific TsF produced by Ts hybridomas bound to anti-GIF antibodies. The acid eluate from anti-GIF immunosorbent had both GIF bioactivity and TsF activity (8). These findings suggest that GIF may be a subunit or component of TsF. Thus, we isolated nonspecific GIF from the culture supernatant of 231F1 cells (9), and obtained a cDNA clone encoding the GIF peptide (10). Expecting homology between murine GIF and human GIF, we have also isolated human GIF cDNA using the mouse GIF cDNA as a probe. Nucleotide sequence of the cDNA clones indicate that mouse GIF cDNA and human GIF cDNA encode a 13 kDa peptide of 115 amino acids, and human GIF has 90% homology with mouse GIF at the amino acid level. Rabbit polyclonal antibodies against *E.coli*-derived recombinant 13 kDa peptide bound hybridoma-derived bioactive GIF, indicating that the cDNA actually encode GIF (10). However, we obtained several unexpected findings. First of all, the nucleotide sequence of human GIF cDNA was identical to that of human MIF cDNA described by Weiser and David (11), except for a single base. One may predict that amino acid sequence of human GIF is different from human MIF by one amino acid. Nevertheless, neither the recombinant GIF formed in *E.coli* nor that formed by Ts hybridoma, or that obtained by transfection of GIF cDNA in mammalian cells had MIF activity at the level of 1 μg/ml. Another unexpected finding was that not only Ts cells but also various cell line cells contained

Table 1. GIF bioactivity of purified 13 kDa peptide from murine and human cell line cells

Species	Cell source of GIF[a]	GIF activity in culture supernatant	13 kDa peptide for bioactivity[b]*
Murine	231F1	+	5
	CKB-Ts3	+	15
	12H5	-	>100[c]
	A20.3	-	>250[c]
	AtT-20	-	>500[c]
Human	AC5	+	10
	31E9	+	10
	BUC	-	1000

[a] 231F1 and CKB-Ts3 cells are suppressor T cell hybridomas. AC5 and 31E9 cells are GIF-producing human T cell hybridomas.

[b] The 13 kDa peptide was affinity purified by using anti-GIF-Affigel 10. The purity and concentration of the peptide was determined by SDS/PAGE. Numbers in the column show the minimum peptide concentration required for detection of GIF bioactivity.

[c] Production of 13 kDa peptide was limited. The GIF bioactivity was not detectable at the concentration tested.

* ng/ml

mRNA that hybridized with GIF cDNA in Northern blot analysis. Indeed, culture supernatant of the cell line cells contained a 13 kDa peptide, which bound anti-GIF in Western blot (12). However, only the culture supernatants of Ts hybridomas had GIF bioactivity. Thus, we isolated the 13 kDa peptide using anti-GIF-coupled Affigel, and tested for GIF bioactivity of the peptide. As shown in Table 1, the 13 kDa peptide from both murine and human Ts hybridomas had high GIF bioactivity, whereas the peptide from non-suppressor cells did not. However, nucleotide sequence of the cDNA encoding the 13 kDa peptide from the five murine cell line cells in Table 1 was exactly the same as that described for murine GIF cDNA (10). These findings suggested to us the possibility that bioactive GIF and inactive GIF peptides have identical amino acid sequences, and that the bioactivity of the GIF peptide is generated by post-translational modification.

We tested the hypothesis by using stable transfectants of human GIF cDNA in BMT10 monkey kidney cells. One of the stable transfectants was established by transfection of hGIF cDNA in a mammalian expression vector pEFneo. Although the GIF peptide does not contain a signal peptide sequence, the stable transfectant (BTH cells) secreted a substantial quantity of the GIF peptide (Table 2). However, the peptide did not have GIF bioactivity. Thus, we made a device for the secretion of the GIF peptide through the constitutive secretory pathway. For this purpose, we expressed a chimeric cDNA encoding a fusion protein consisting of N-terminal pro-region of calcitonin precursor and human GIF, so that the fusion protein will be translocated into endoplasmic reticulum. Based on the deduced amino acid sequence of the fusion protein, one may expect that the protein will be cleaved by a furin-like endoproteinase at Golgi for the secretion of mature GIF peptide (13). Indeed, transfection of the chimeric cDNA in BMT10 cells resulted in the secretion of the 13 kDa peptide. As shown in Table 2, the recombinant 13 kDa peptide secreted by the transfectant of the chimeric cDNA was as active as the Ts hybridoma-derived GIF. In contrast, even 1 μg/ml of the recombinant GIF peptide obtained by the transfection of GIF cDNA (BTH cells) failed to show GIF bioactivity. It is well known that a peptide is modified in endoplasmic reticulum and Golgi. These results, therefore, indicate that a certain post-translational modification of the peptide in endoplasmic reticulum was responsible

Table 2. Bioactivity of the 13 kDa peptide was formed by stable transfectants

		GIF in supernatant		GIF in cytosol	
Source	cDNA Transfected	Yield[a] μg	Activity[b] ng/ml	Yield[a] μg	Activity[b] ng/ml
BTH	hGIF	3.5	>1000	25.0	>1200
BCTH	pro-CT-hGIF	2.1	15	4.5	>500
2FH2	hGIF	6.0	10	80.0	1000
231F1	none	0.3	5	5.0	1000

a)13 kDa peptide was affinity-purified from culture supernatant or cytosol. Yield represents micrograms of the peptide obtained from 100 ml of culture supernatant or cytosol of the cells recovered from the culture.
b)Concentration of the 13 kDa peptide required for the detection of GIF bioactivity.

for the generation of biologic activity. However, if one transfects the human GIF cDNA into mouse Ts hybridoma, 231F1 cells, the recombinant human 13 kDa peptide secreted by the stable transfectant (2FH2 cells) was bioactive (Table 2). It should be noted that the same plasmid was used to establish BTH and 2FH2 clones, but only the product of 2FH2 cells was bioactive. The results indicate that murine Ts cells can modify the recombinant human peptide to biologically active human GIF. However, we realized that cell lysates of the 231F1 cells and 2FH2 cells contained a large quantity of the 13 kDa peptide which reacts with anti-GIF. Fractionation of post-nuclear fractions showed that essentially all of the intra-cellular GIF peptide is present in the cytosol. Furthermore, bioactivity of the cytosolic GIF peptide in the 2FH2 cells was 100 fold less than that recovered from culture supernatant of the same cells. It appears that Ts cells convert a portion of inactive GIF peptide in cytosol to bioactive GIF during the process of secretion (12).

When we initiated molecular cloning of GIF, we expected that production of the GIF peptide is unique for Ts cells. However, uniqueness of Ts was not the ability of synthesizing the peptide, but the existence of the machinery for a certain post-translational modification which is required for the generation of bioactivity of the peptide. We do not know what this machinery is, nor the nature of the post-translational modification. Neither N-glycosylation nor phosphorylation appears to be involved. At present, the best explanation for the conversion of inactive GIF to bioactive GIF is conformational transition of the peptide (12).

3. EPITOPE SPECIFICITY OF Ts CELLS WHICH PRODUCE ANTIGEN-SPECIFIC TsF

The next fundamental question is how antigen-specific TsF could bind nominal antigen. We suspected that the cell source of TsF is specific for unique epitopes, and determined the epitope specificity of the Ts cells. When we constructed Ts hybridomas from OVA-treated BDF1 spleen cells, we obtained 14 GIF-producing hybridomas. All of these hybridomas produced IgE-binding factor upon stimulation with OVA-pulsed H-2^d or H-2^b macrophages. Among the 14 GIF-producing hybridomas, 8 clones produced OVA-binding GIF upon antigenic stimulation. Determination of the epitope specificity has shown that all of these hybridomas responded to a synthetic peptide representing amino acid residues 307–317 in the OVA molecules in the presence of APC (14). In contrast, all of the hybridomas, which failed to form OVA-binding GIF, failed to respond to the peptide in the context of a MHC product. Some of these hybridomas responded to the major immunogenic determinant corresponding to amino acid 323–339 in OVA molecules, but none of them produced OVA-binding GIF. The results showed that only the hybridomas specific for p307–317 could produce OVA-binding GIF. Another important finding was that the OVA-binding GIF formed by the cells had affinity for the peptide 307–317 (14). Similar findings were obtained on BALB/c-derived Ts hybridomas specific for bee venom phospholipase A$_2$ (PLA$_2$). All of the Ts hybridomas, which produce PLA$_2$-specific GIF upon antigen stimulation, recognize the synthetic peptide representing amino acid 19–34 in the PLA$_2$ molecules in the context of I-A^d product, and the PLA$_2$-specific GIF produced by the cells had affinity for the same peptide (15). This epitope was distinct from the major immunogenic determinant, which is recognized by helper T cells. More importantly, the epitope appears to represent an external structure in the antigen molecule. According to the results of the x-ray analysis, amino acid residues 14–24 form a long loop and 25–34 form α helix (Fig. 1). Thus, the epitope recognized by the Ts hybridomas, i.e., peptide 19–34, consists of a portion of the loop and α helix. Evidence was obtained that this portion of the α helix is essential for the association of this peptide with Ia molecules, while the loop portion is required for recognition of the peptide -Ia complex by T cell receptor (15). Furthermore, this molecular model indicates that residues 19–25 and possibly residues 26 and 27 in the helix are exposed to the surface of the molecule (16). Thus, the epitope recognized by TCR on the Ts hybridomas is an external structure in the antigen molecule. The epitope specificity of TCR on the Ts cells may be related to the fact that these cells and TsF could bind nominal antigen. Furthermore, the common epitope specificity shared by TCR and antigen-specific GIF strongly suggest that this factor is related to TCR.

4. TsF IS A DERIVATIVE OF TCR

Evidence for the relationship between TsF and TCRα chain has been accumulated. Several groups of investigators, including ourselves, found that TsF from various Ts hy-

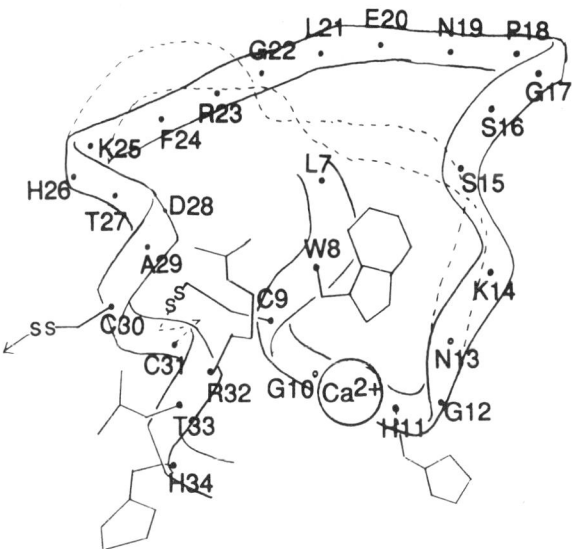

Figure 1. Molecular model of the amino terminal one-third of bee venom PLA$_2$, as compared with bovine pancreatic PLA$_2$ (dotted line).

bridomas and suppressor T cell clones bound to the monoclonal antibody against TCRα chain, H28–710 (14,15,17–19). Furthermore, Douglas Green, at our Institute, found that anti-sense oligonucleotide of TCRα chain mRNA prevents the formation of TsF (20). Finally, Collins, Kuchroo and Dorf from Harvard transfected α chain cDNA of one Ts hybridoma into another Ts hybridoma and obtained TsF from the first hybridoma (21). These findings collectively suggest that TCRαchain gene is being used for the formation of TsF. However, biochemical evidence for the relationship between TCR and TsF was lacking. Since antigen-specific GIF appears to represent TsF, we tried to identify antigen-specific GIF. First of all, OVA-specific Ts hybridoma 231F1 cells and bee venom PLA$_2$-specific Ts hybridoma 3B3 cells were cocultured with antigen-pulsed APC and culture supernatants were fractionated on antigen-coupled Sepharose. As expected, the majority of GIF bioactivity in the original culture supernatant retained in the immunosorbent, and was recovered by acid elution. Analysis of the preparation by SDS-PAGE and immunoblotting with anti-GIF showed a single 55 kDa band which bound anti-GIF (Fig. 2a). Unexpectedly, no 13 kDa GIF was detectable in the preparation even under reducing conditions. In order to determine the nature of the 55 kDa peptide, the 231F1 cells were treated with anti-CD3, and the cells were cultured in protein A-coated dishes for the formation of antigen-binding GIF. Culture supernatants were then fractionated on anti-TCRα chain-coupled Affigel. The acid eluate fraction contained the 55 kDa peptide which bound anti-GIF (Fig. 2b). Further fractionation of the preparation on OVA-Sepharose showed that the acid eluate of the immunosorbent contained the 55 kDa peptide, but this peptide was not de-

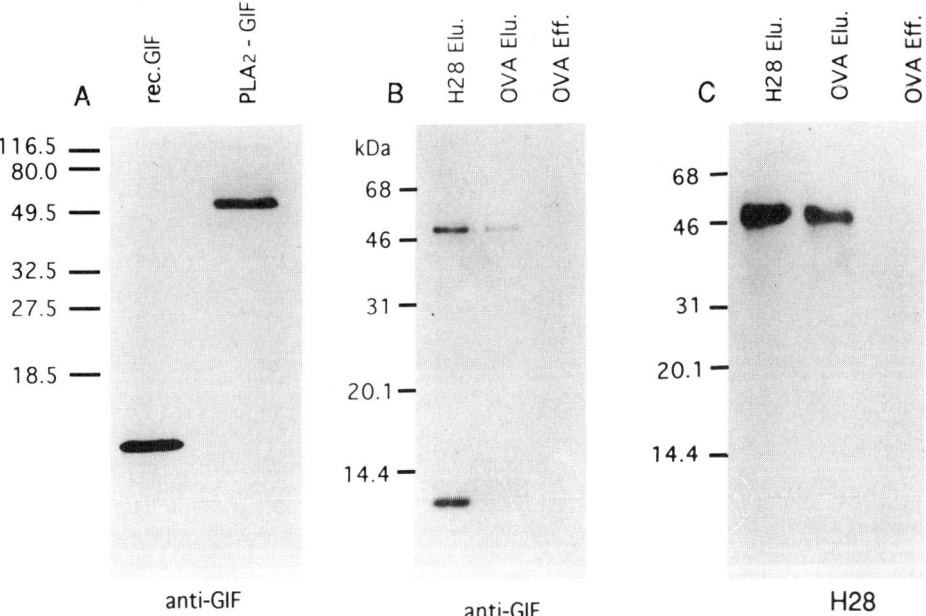

Figure 2. Biochemical characterization of a 55 kDa peptide in antigen-specific GIF. a) Antigen-specific factor in a culture supernatant of antigen-stimulated PLA$_2$-specific Ts hybridoma 3B3 was purified using PLA$_2$-coupled Sepharose. The purified material was analyzed by SDS-PAGE and immunoblotting with anti-GIF. *E.coli*-derived recombinant nonspecific GIF was applied to lane 1 as a control. b) 231F1 cells were stimulated with anti-CD3, and antigen-specific GIF was purified using H28–710 (anti-TCRα)-coupled AffiGel. Proteins retained in the column were recovered (lane 1), and further fractionated on OVA-Sepharose. Each fraction was analyzed by SDS-PAGE, followed by immunoblotting with anti-GIF. c) The same samples were immunoblotted with H28–710.

tectable in the flow through fraction. Another important finding was that the 55 kDa peptide bound not only anti-GIF, but also the monoclonal antibody against TCRα chain in immunoblotting (Fig. 2c).

In order to prove that the 55 kDa peptide is a product of TCRα chain gene, we cloned the cDNA encoding the TCRα chain in the 231F1 cells. Deduced amino acid sequence of the cDNA indicated that TCRα chain from the 231F1 cells consisted of Vα11.3, a unique Jα and complete Cα region. The cDNA was transfected into a T cell line 175.2 which contained CD3 and TCRβ chain mRNA but no detectable TCRα mRNA (22). The 175.2 cells did not express TCR but the stable transfectant expressed both TCRβ chain and CD3, as determined by immunofluorescence. In order to confirm that the TCRα chain is being synthesized in the transfectant, cell lysates of the 175.2 clone and the stable transfectant were fractionated on anti-TCRα (H-28–710)-coupled-Affigel. Analysis of the eluate fraction from the immunosorbent indicated that the stable transfectant contained a 34 kDa peptide which bound the monoclonal anti-TCRα, while the 175.2 cells did not. Thus, we stimulated the stable transfectant with anti-CD3, and culture supernatant was absorbed with the H-28–710-coupled Affigel. However, the supernatant did not contain a peptide which could bind anti-TCRα. We wondered that the formation of the 55 kDa peptide may be unique for Ts cells. Thus, the TCRα cDNA was over-expressed in 231F1 cells. A representative stable transfectant, 211α, was stimulated with anti-CD3 or cultured without stimulation. Analysis of culture supernatant by immunoblotting with anti-TCRα showed that the culture supernatant of the anti-CD3-stimulated transfectant contained the 55 kDa peptide which bound anti-TCRα, while the peptide was not detectable in the cul-

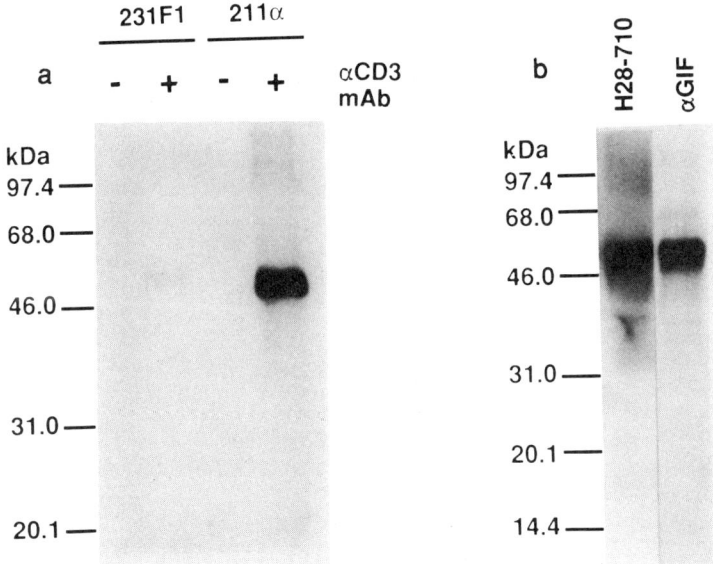

Figure 3. Over-expression of TCRα chain cDNA increases the production of the 55 kDa peptide. a) Untransfected 231F1 cells and a stable transfectant of the cDNA in the 231F1 cells (211α) were stimulated by anti-CD3 (+) or kept unstimulated (-). Culture supernatants were analyzed by SDS-PAGE, and immunoblotting with anti-TCRα (H28–710). The 211α clone produced much more 55 kDa peptide than 231F1 cells upon anti-CD3 stimulation. b) Culture supernatant of the anti-CD3-stimulated 211α cells was absorbed with H28–710-coupled AffiGel, and proteins retained in the column were analyzed by SDS-PAGE followed by immunoblotting with anti-GIF or H28–710. The 55 kDa band bound both anti-GIF and the monoclonal anti-TCRα.

ture supernatant of the unstimulated cells (Fig. 3a). Thus, the culture supernatant of the stimulated cells was fractionated on H-28–710-coupled Affigel, and proteins retained in the immunosorbent were recovered. As expected, the acid eluate fraction contained GIF bioactivity, and the 55 kDa peptide was detected in the preparation. As shown in Fig. 3b, the 55 kDa peptide bound both the anti-TCRα chain and anti-GIF. Another important finding was that the quantity of the 55 kDa peptide formed by the stable transfectant was much more than that released from the untransfected 231F1 cells (Fig. 3a). After purification, we compared the quantities of the peptide formed by 231F1 cells and 211α cells. It appears that the stable transfectant could release about 10 fold more 55 kDa peptide than the 231F1 cells upon antigenic stimulation or cross-linking of CD3.

Definitive evidence for the origin of the 55 kDa peptide was obtained by using the cDNA encoding the TCRα chain containing a peptide of 6 histidine residues at C-terminus (23). A stable transfectant of the TCRα-histidine tag cDNA in the 231F1 cells was stimulated with anti-CD3, and the product of the cDNA was recovered by absorption with Ni^{2+}-nitrilotriacetic acid (Ni-NTA) agarose. Upon stimulation with anti-CD3, the stable transfectant produced the 55 kDa peptide which bound the mAb H-28–710. As expected, the peptide bound to Ni-NTA agarose and was recovered by elution with imidazole. Since the 55 kDa peptide from untransfected 231F1 cells failed to bind to Ni-NTA agarose, the results provided with a clear evidence that the 55 kDa peptide is a product of TCRα chain cDNA.

The 55 kDa peptide has GIF bioactivity, and appears to represent antigen-specific GIF or its subunit. The major problems remain to be solved are the mechanisms involved in the formation of such a peptide, and how this peptide is released from Ts cells upon antigenic stimulation. Nevertheless, we hope that biochemical identification of the peptide will convince the other immunologists for the presence of T cell-derived antigen specific factors, and that such factors could be useful for immune regulation.

ACKNOWLEDGMENT

This work was supported by research grants AI-11202 and AI-14784 from the U.S. H.H.S. This paper is publication number 128 from the La Jolla Institute for Allergy and Immunology.

REFERENCES

1. Jardieu, P., M. Akasaki, and K. Ishizaka. 1987. Carrier-specific suppression of antibody response by antigen-specific glycosylation inhibiting factors. *J. Immunol.* 138: 1494.
2. Ishizaka, K. 1988. IgE-binding factors and regulation of the IgE antibody response. *Ann. Rev. Immunol.* 6: 513.
3. Kronenberg, M., J. Goverman, R. Haars, M. Malissen, E. Kraig, L. Phillips, J. Delovitch, N. Sucin-Fea, and L. Hood. 1985. Rearrangement and transcription of the β chain genes of the T cell antigen receptor in different types of murine lymphocytes. *Nature* 313: 647.
4. Iwata, M., K. Katamura, R. T. Kubo, and K. Ishizaka. 1989. Relationship between T cell receptors and antigen-binding factors. I. Specificity of functional T cell receptors on mouse T cell hybridomas that produce antigen-binding T cell factors. *J. Immunol.* 143: 3909.
5. DeSantis, R., D. Givol, P.-L. Hsu, L. Adorini, G. Doria, and E. Appella. 1985. Rearrangement and expression of the α- and β chain genes of the T cell antigen receptor in functional murine suppressor T cell clones. *Proc. Natl. Acad. Sci., USA* 82: 8638.
6. Kuchroo, V. K., J. K. Steele, P. R. Billings, P. Selvraj, and M. E. Dorf. 1988. Expression of CD3-associated antigen-binding receptors on suppressor T cells. *Proc. Natl. Acad. Sci., USA* 85: 9209.

7. Takata, M., P. K. Maiti, R. T. Kubo, Y. Chen, V. Holford-Strevens, E. S. Rector and A. H. Sehon. 1990. Cloned suppressor T cells derived from mice tolerized with conjugate of antigen and monomethoxy-polyethylene glycol. *J. Immunol.* 145: 2846.

8. Steele, J. K., V. K. Kuchroo, H. Kawasaki, S. Jayaraman, M. Iwata, K. Ishizaka, and M. E. Dorf. 1989. A monoclonal antibody raised to lipomodulin recognizes factors in two independent hapten-specific suppressor networks. *J. Immunol.* 142: 2213.

9. Tagaya, Y., A. Mori, and K. Ishizaka. 1991. Biochemical characterization of murine glycosylation inhibiting factor. *Proc. Natl. Acad. Sci., USA* 88: 9117.

10. Mikayama, T., T. Nakano, H. Gomi, Y. Nakagawa, Y.-C. Liu, M. Sato, A. Iwamatsu, Y. Ishii, W. Y. Weiser, and K. Ishizaka. 1993. Molecular cloning and functional expression of a cDNA encoding glycosyation inhibiting factor. *Proc. Natl. Acad. Sci, USA* 90: 10056.

11. Weiser, W. Y., P. A. Temple, J. S. Wteh-Gianett, H. G. Reynold, S. C. Clark, and J. R. David. 1989. Molecular cloning of a cDNA encoding a human macrophage migration inhibiting factor. *Proc. Natl. Acad. Sci., USA* 86: 7522.

12. Liu, Y.-C., T. Nakano, C. Elly, and K. Ishizaka. 1994. Requirement of post-translational modifications for the generation of biologic activity of glycosylation-inhibiting factor. *Proc. Natl. Acad. Sci., USA* 91: 11227.

13. Liu, Y-C., M. Kawagishi, T. Mikayama, Y. Inagaki, T. Takeuchi, and H. Ohashi. 1993. Processing of a fusion protein by endoproteinase in COS-1 cells for secretion of mature peptide by using a chimeric expression vector. *Proc. Natl. Acad. Sci., USA* 90: 8957.

14. Iwata, M., K. Katamura, R. T. Kubo, H. M. Grey, and K. Ishizaka. 1989. Relationship between T cell receptors and antigen-binding factors. II. Common antigenic determinants and epitope recognition shared by T cell receptors and antigen-binding factors. *J. Immunol.* 143: 3917.

15. Mori, A., P. Thomas, Y. Tagaya, H. Iijima, H. M. Grey, and K. Ishizaka. 1993. Epitope specificity of bee venom phospholipase A_2-specific suppressor T cells which produce antigen-binding glycosylation inhibiting factor. *Intl. Immunol.* 5: 883.

16. Scott, D. L., Z. Otevinowski, M. H. Gelb, and P. B. Sigler. 1990. Crystal structure of bee venom phospholipase A_2 in a complex with a transition-state analogue. *Science* 250: 1564.

17. Fairchild, R. L., R. T. Kubo, and J. W. Moorhead. 1988. Soluble factors in tolerance and contact sensitivity to 2, 4 dinitrofluorobenzene in mice. IX. A monoclonal T cell suppressor molecule is structurally and serologically related to the α/β cell receptor. *J. Immunol.* 141: 3342.

18. Kuchroo, V. K., J. K. Steele, R. M. Ohara, S. Jayaraman, P. Selvara, E. Greenfield, R. T. Kubo, and M. E. Dorf. 1990. Relationships between antigen-specific helper and inducer suppressor T cell hybridomas. *J. Immunol.* 145: 438.

19. Bissonnette, R., H. Zheng, R. T. Kubo, B. Singh, and D. R. Green. 1991. T helper cell hybridoma produces an antigen-specific regulatory activity. Relationship to the T cell receptor by serology and antigenic fine specificity. *J. Immunol.* 146: 2898.

20. Zheng, H., B. M. Sahai, P. Kilgannon, A. Fotedar, and D. R. Green. 1989. Specific inhibition of cell surface T cell receptor expression by antisense oligonucleotides and its effect on the production of an antigen-specific regulatory T cell factor. *Proc. Natl. Acad. Sci., USA* 86: 3758.

21. Kuchroo, V. K., M. C. Byrne, Y. Atsumi, E. Greenfield, J. B. Connolly, M. J. Whitters, R. M. O'Hara, Jr., M. Collins, and M. E. Dorf. 1991. T-cell receptor α chain plays a critical role in antigen-specific suppressor cell function. *Proc. Natl. Acad. Sci., USA* 88: 8700.

22. Ghajchenhans, N., C. Davis, K. Boreschlegel, J. P. Allison, and N. Shastri. 1991. Novel strategy for the generation of T cell lines lacking expression of endogenous α- and/or β chain T cell receptor genes. *J. Immunol.* 146: 2095.

23. Janknecht, R., G. deMartynoff, L. Jueren, R. A. Hipskind, A. Nordheim, and H. G. Stunnenberg. 1991. Rapid and efficient purification of native histidine-tagged protein expressed by recombinant vaccinia virus. *Proc. Natl. Acad. Sci., USA* 88: 8972.

46

IN SITU DETECTION OF CYTOKINES IN ALLERGIC INFLAMMATION

Q. A. Hamid and E. Minshall

Meakins-Christie Laboratories
McGill University
3626 Street Urbain Street, Montreal, Quebec, H2X 2P2

INTRODUCTION

It is now clear that T-cell derived cytokines are important chemical mediators of inflammatory response in allergic diseases. According to their particular mRNA expression and cytokine secretion CD4 positive T lymphocytes were divided into T helper-1 (Th1) and T helper-2 (Th2) type cells (1). Th1 type cell clones produce IL-2, IFNγ and lymphotoxin whereas Th2 type cell clones produce IL-4, IL-5, IL-6, IL-10 and IL-13. Both T cell subtypes produce IL-3, GM-CSF and TNFα. Th1 and Th2 patterns of cytokine expression exhibit reciprocal inhibition via the release of IFNγ and IL-4 respectively. Due to their release of IL-4, Th2 cell clones are involved in immunoglobin production, specifically of the IgE subclass (2). Th2 cytokines are also instrumental in regulating eosinophil differentiation and survival *in vitro* via the actions of secreted IL-5, IL-3 and GM-CSF (3). Such effects *in vivo* may explain the increased tissue survival at the site of allergic inflammation and could also contribute to the inhibition of programmed cell death. It is now clear that T-cells are not the only source of cytokines; eosinophils, mast cells, basophils, macrophages and epithelial cells may also produce cytokines that could be involved in allergic inflammation. Whilst there is growing evidence to suggest that cytokines are playing an important role in initiating and maintaining inflammatory reactions associated with allergic disease in man, to confirm such a role it will be essential to identify the expression of cytokine genes and gene products and to localize cytokine receptors *in vivo* at the level of the tissue. During the last few years we have been using various methods to identify the *in situ* expression of cytokines in tissues obtained from asthmatics, allergic rhinitis and individuals with atopic dermatitis. The most widely used techniques to identify the expression of cytokines within tissues are *in situ hybridization* and immunocytochemistry. In this chapter, the techniques of *in situ hybridization* and immunocytochemistry will be described in the relation to the localization of cytokine genes and gene products. Examples of the application of these techniques to localize cytokines in tissue obtained from the sites of allergic inflammatory reactions will also be discussed.

New Horizons in Allergy Immunotherapy
edited by Sehon et al. Plenum Press, New York, 1996

1. DETECTION OF CYTOKINES USING IN SITU HYBRIDIZATION

In situ hybridization (ISH) has been used extensively to localize cytokine mRNA in tissue sections and cytospin preparations from normal and diseased individuals (4,5,6). This approach is valuable in cytokine research as there is *in vitro* evidence suggesting that cytokines are synthetized *de novo* and released very rapidly. Thus, the chances of detecting their immunoreactivity in lymphocytes or other cells are limited. The localization of cytokine mRNA at the tissue level indicates the expression and activation of the gene and the potential ability of the cell to produce cytokines. *In situ hybridization* in general can be defined as the cellular localization of specific nucleic acid sequences (DNA or RNA), using a labelled complementary strand. The two nucleic acid forms, DNA and RNA, are found in both the nucleus and the cytoplasm and the technical approach to the demonstration of these molecules in each anatomical location is different. ISH was first introduced in 1969 and was used primarily for the localization of specific DNA sequences (7). In more recent years, ISH has been applied to localize mRNA, the intermediate molecule in the transfer of genetic information from genomic DNA to functional polypeptide. The regulation of gene expression through transcriptional activation and inactivation within a cell, is reflected by the cellular content and distribution of the specific message. The demonstration of mRNA within a cell provides valuable information about gene expression and indicates possible synthesis of the corresponding protein. In diseased states, it can be used for temporary studies in relation to physiological, pathological and developmental processes.

2. THE PRINCIPLES OF CYTOKINE mRNA HYBRIDIZATION

The general principle of ISH is based on the fact that labelled single-stranded RNA or DNA containing complementary sequences (probes) are hybridized intracellularly to mRNA under appropriate conditions, thereby forming a stable hybrid. This will be detected according to the type of labelling of the probe (Figure 1). Different probes are available to detect mRNA including double and single stranded DNA, oligonucleotides and single stranded RNA probes. Single stranded RNA probes have been used extensively in recent years for detection of cytokine mRNA by both isotopic and non-isotopic methods. The use of RNA probes has a number of advantages over other types of probes (8). These include the ability to synthesize a probe of relatively constant size, the high stability and affinity of RNA hybrids and the ability of RNase to remove the unhybridized probe

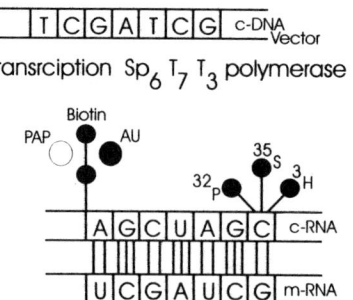

Figure 1. Diagrammatic representation of the principle of mRNA hybridization using a CRNA probe.

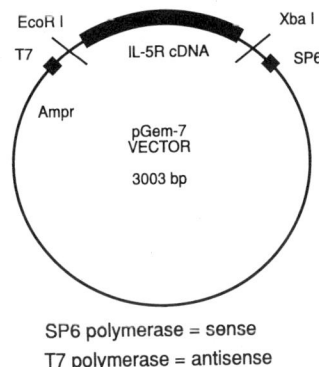

SP6 polymerase = sense
T7 polymerase = antisense

Figure 2. Diagrammatic representation of cDNA subcloning into a pGEM vector.

during the post-hybridization washing stages. All of these favor the high specificity and sensitivity of RNA probes. To construct a labelled RNA probe, the DNA sequences of interest are subcloned into a RNA expression vector (e.g. pGEM), transfected into *E. Coli* bacteria, extracted, and then linearized prior to the *in vivo* transcription (Figure 2).

2.1. In Vivo Transcription and Probe Labelling

To synthesize a single stranded RNA probe, the cDNA which is attached now to promoter side must be transcribed in the presence of labelled nucleotide and the appropriate RNA polymerase (SP67 or T3 polymerase). Following transcription, the labelled probe is extracted from the mixture and the incorporation of the label is assessed. The probe can either be used immediately, stored for a limited time in case of radio-labelled probes or stored for an unlimited time in the case of non-radio-labelled probes. Two types of labelling can be used for RNA probes: isotopic and non-isotopic. Several types of isotopes can be employed for labelling RNA, including 3H, 33P, 32P, and 35S and the hybridization signal is detected using autoradiography. Radio-labelled probes have several advantages including (1) the efficiency of the probes synthesis can be monitored easily; (2) radio-isotopes are readily incorporated into the synthesized RNA; (3) autoradiography represents the most sensitive detection system available. However problems which have occurred with the radio-labelled probes have prompted the development of non-isotopic labelling of RNA probes. Biotin is one of the first non-isotopic labels to be used for RNA hybridization (9). Recently a very sensitive and efficient label has been employed in labelling RNA probes, digoxigenin-11-UTP (10). RNA hybrids obtained by using non-radio-labelled probes are usually detected by immunocytochemical methods. A similar excellent resolution is obtained with the non-isotopic labelled probe and these probes have the advantage that their signals are developed in very short time in comparison to radio-labelled probes. The major limitation of non-isotopic methods is their relatively poor sensitivity for detection of low copy number of mRNA. Most of the cytokines are expressed in a very low copy number and thus this method may not be optimal for use in ISH of cytokine mRNA.

2.2. Tissue Preparation (11)

When performing ISH, it is imperative to keep the tissue RNase free. This entails wearing gloves whenever coming into contact with the tissue since fingertips are a rich source of

RNase. Any procedure involving ISH begins with fixation of the tissue, cytology specimen or cell culture. The fixative must preserve the tissue in a morphologically intact state whilst retaining the maximum accessible mRNA within the cells, particularly in the regular conditions used for ISH. One of the best fixatives commonly used for hybridization is paraformaldehyde which maintains morphological integrity whilst allowing efficient hybridization. Once fixed, the tissue can either be blocked in paraffin, or frozen in liquid nitrogen on the cryostat. Optimal morphological preservation in paraffin-embedded material may be accompanied by substantial reduction in the density of hybridization in comparison to frozen sections. Relatively thick sections (10 μm) are usually employed for ISH and these are placed on poly-L-lysine coated slides to ensure the tissue remains fixed to the slide during the post-hybridization washes. Cytospin preparations can be prepared from body fluids (eg bronchial alveolar lavage fluid) or from cell suspensions. Before starting the hybridization procedure, the tissue preparation must be pretreated to increase the efficiency of hybridization by rendering the target sequences more accessible to the probe. Most of the methods described are directed towards the permeabilization of the fixed cellular protein matrix. These include the use of protease, acid and detergents. Other types of pretreatment are used to reduce background staining. The conditions of hybridization vary to allow the probe sufficient access to the cytoplasmic constituents whilst allowing the appropriate stringency in tissue preservation. For the hybridization of cytokines, the probes should be incubated with the pretreated tissue or cell within optimal incubation conditions, usually overnight, to allow the hybridization between the complementary RNA probe and the cytoplasmic mRNA. However, not all the probes will be hybridized to the mRNA, thus the preparation needs to be stringently washed to remove the background signal. The washing conditions determine the specificity of ISH and degree of background staining, they should allow sufficient diffusion of material trapped in the section and select for a good fit between probe and target mRNA. The availability of RNase to digest the unhybridized probe favours the use of RNA probes for cytokine *in situ hybridization*. The hybridization signals are detected according to the label which has been incorporated into the probe. For radio-labelled probes, autoradiography is performed and the slides are dipped in liquid emulsion. The incubation period will depend upon the radio-labelled probe used and should be standardized beforehand. Once developed, the signal will appear as dark silver granules overlaying the emulsion which covers the cells or sections. For non-radio-labelled probes, the RNA-RNA hybrid is usually detected by immunocytochemical methods in which an antibody (i.e. anti-digoxigenin) is used and developed by chromogens.

2.3. Controls and Specificity of *in Situ Hybridization*

As with any histochemical method, appropriate controls are necessary during every ISH experiment to assess the specificity of the reagents and the procedures used. Proper positive and negative controls for tissue probes and reagents are essential. These include Northern Blot analysis to ensure the specificity of the probe and the signal, treating the sections with sense probe (ie a probe which has a sequence identical to that of the mRNA), and the pretreatment of sections with RNase to degrade the mRNA prior to the application of the complementary RNA probes. Many factors must be carefully considered and controlled if quantitative data are to be collected. These include the section thickness, nucleic acid retention, consistency of hybridization, length of exposure and development conditions. The inclusion of a known standard and the construction of a standard curve are essential. However even under optimal conditions, the quantification of cytokine mRNA at the *in situ hybridization* level is at the best semi-quantitative.

2.4. Localization of mRNA for Cytokine Receptors

Cytokines exert their effects through specific receptors several of which have now been cloned. Although cytokines are a structurally diverse group of glycoproteins, their receptors may be grouped into various families which share structural homology. To support the local role of cytokines in modulating disease processes, the synthesis of cytokine receptors can be detected using ISH (12). Probes coding for cytokine receptor mRNA can be synthesized from the appropriate cDNAs and then processed in a similar way to cytokine ISH to detect the mRNA coding for specific receptors.

2.5. Phenotype of Cells Expressing Cytokine mRNA

Initially, it was generally perceived that most cytokines in allergic inflammation were the products of activated T cells. However, it has been recently demonstrated that other inflammatory cells in man possess the capacity to produce certain cytokines under the appropriate stimulation. For example, eosinophils can produce GM-CSF, IL-3, IL-5, IL-6, and TGFß (13,14,15,16,17,), mast cells produce IL-3, IL-4, IL-5 and TNFα (18,19), whilst epithelial cells, at least *in vitro*, have the ability to generate IL-6, IL-8 and GM-CSF (20). This has created the need to develop a number of techniques specifically to identify the phenotype of cells expressing cytokine mRNA in tissues obtained from the site of allergic inflammation. These techniques include: (1) Simultaneous immunocytochemistry (ICC) and ISH using radio-labelled probes, (2) Simultaneous ICC and non-radio-labelled ISH, (3) Simultaneous ICC and ISH using immunofluorescent probes, (4) The 'flip-flop' technique in which two sections are cut and mounted in such a way that one represents a mirror image of the other. One section will be treated for ISH and the other for ICC for a particular cell marker, these can then be visualized and compared, (5) Serial sectioning, where two adjacent sections are obtained from the cryostat blocks, one section will be treated for ISH and the other for ICC. This latter technique is not applicable to the study of cytokines since many of these are coming from cells which are relatively small compared to the section thickness and the chance of detecting the same cell in two successive sections is remote. For cell cytospins and preparations obtained from body fluids other techniques can be used which include 'flow cytometry in situ hybridization' (FISH) in which the cell suspension can be stained with a surface marker and subsequently hybridized with biotin labelled probe which will be visualized using FITC-conjugated streptavidin allowing the marker and the mRNA can be visualized simultaneously. Other techniques which can be used for cell suspensions include hybridization of cells separated by negative or positive selections using magnetic beads. This is in addition to other methods which are used for the tissue phenotyping of cells expressing mRNA (simultaneous in situ and immunocytochemistry).

2.6. Co-Localization of Multiple Gene Transcripts

More than one cytokine might be produced by the same cell and in some instances it will be important to prove that. The technique which can be utilized for this purpose is called simultaneous *in situ hybridizations*. This technique is usually used to detect more than one mRNA in the same cell, particular in the case of multiple gene expression and alternative supplies. However, it could also be used to identify the phenotype of cell expressing mRNA by combining two probes, one coding for an mRNA in question and the other for mRNA known to be expressed specifically in one type of cells.

3. IMMUNOCYTOCHEMISTRY OF CYTOKINES

Immunocytochemistry is the identification of cellular or tissue constituents by means of an antigen-antibody reaction. The site of interaction is identified by a direct label to the antibody or by the use of a secondary labelling method. This technique allows the precise examination of many aspects of cell function and their relation to our perception of cell and tissue morphology, and such has greatly enhanced our understanding of disease processes. Many methods are available for immunocytochemistry, thus the major criteria for selecting a technique to detect a particular antigen includes the sensitivity, reliability, cost, versatility and safety of the methodology (21). In general, three principle methods are available: (1) *Direct methods*: This is the simplest immunocytochemical method in which a label is directly conjugated to the antibody. This conjugate is then applied to tissue section or preparation in single step. Whilst simple, this technique is not particular sensitive, nor does it utilize the specificity of antibodies used in other methods, (2) *Indirect methods*: The primary antibody is unlabelled and its binding is revealed by a labelled second antibody specific to the immunoglobulin of the species providing the primary antibody. Since at least two secondary antibody molecules can be bound to each primary antibody molecule, this method is more sensitive than the direct method. (3) *Unlabelled antibody enzymatic methods*: An unconjugated bridging secondary antibody is used between the primary antibody and the label detection reagent which is usually an enzyme - anti-enzyme complex or an avidin - biotin complex. Enzymatic methods include the peroxidase and anti-peroxidase (PAP) and the alkaline phosphatase anti-alkaline phosphatase (APAAP) technique. Most of the immunocytochemical techniques are standard and are well-described in other textbooks. For detection of cytokine immunoreactivity few antibodies are available which are optimized for use for tissue ICC, and a number of antibodies are currently being tested by different laboratories. Whilst a particular antibody might be appropriate for use in enzyme-linked immunoassays (ELISA), they may not prove to be equally suitable for ICC. Due to the limited amount of cytokine stored in cells at any particular time, a sensitive method has to be used for detecting cytokine immunoreactivity. The method that is recommended for cytokine detection is the APAAP technique. Due to the similarity between cytokines in general the use of monoclonal antibodies is essential to ensure the specificity of the reaction. The presence of cytokine immunoreactivity in a particular cell does not necessarily indicate that the cell actually synthesized the protein, some cells like macrophages and epithelial cells have the ability to endocytose protein from surrounding media.

4. THE *IN SITU* DETECTION OF CYTOKINES IN ALLERGIC INFLAMMATION

Allergic diseases are characterised by the IgE-dependent release of mast cell derived mediators and cellular infiltration of activated eosinophils and T lymphocytes. The *in situ* detection of cytokines has provided valuable information on the mechanisms responsible for allergic inflammation. Investigating beyond purely the presence of activated cells within the tissues, *in situ* localization has enabled the both the cellular source and relative contribution of cytokines to be assessed, as well as indicating the possible pathways involved. The following examples demonstrate how the techniques eluded to in this chapter have furthered our understanding in the pathogenesis of allergic inflammation.

4.1. Cytokine mRNA in Cutaneous Late Phase Reactions

Cutaneous late phase reactions have been used as a model of allergic inflammation. Biopsies obtained from the skin of atopic individuals after allergen challenge are characterised by infiltration of the dermis with large numbers of chronic inflammatory cells, in particular lymphocytes and eosinophils (22). Using in situ hybridization with probes coding for IL-2, IL-3, IL-4, IL-5, IFNγ and GM-CSF it was possible to show that this type of reaction is associated with the expression of Th2-type cytokines. The expression of IFN-γ and IL-2 (Th1-type cytokines) was not increased following challenge. This has suggested the existence of a human equivalent of the mouse Th-1 and Th2 dichotomy (4). This was supported by the demonstration of predominant expression of Th1-type cytokines (IL-2 and IFNγ) in cutaneous tuberculin reactions (delayed-type hypersensitivity; 23)

4.2. The Expression of Cytokine mRNA in the Nasal Mucosa during the Late Phase Reaction

Eosinophils, mast cells and lymphocytes are present in large numbers in nasal biopsies from allergic rhinitis during seasonal exposure to allergen. Out of season, atopic allergic rhinitis can have similar inflammatory reactions following local antigen challenge (nasal late phase reactions). Although infiltration of activated eosinophils following allergen challenge is a prominent feature of allergic diseases, the mechanisms underlying eosinophil recruitment are largely unknown. Following local allergen provocation, it has been shown that cells from nasal biopsies expressed cytokines such as IL-3, IL-4, IL-5 and GM-CSF but not IFNγ or IL-2. Furthermore, the expression of these Th2-like cytokines, in particular IL-5, was significantly correlated to the infiltration of activated eosinophils, quantified using immunocytochemistry with the EG2 antibody (24).

4.3. Cytokines in the Bronchial Mucosa and BAL fluid of Atopic Asthmatics

Allergic asthma has a similar profile of inflammatory cells as that seen in other allergic disorders. Notably the presence of activated T lymphocytes and eosinophils is a characteristic of this disorder. The cellular localization of interleukin-5 beneath the epithelial basement membrane was achieved by ISH in bronchial biopsy specimens from asthmatic subjects (5). There was a significant correlation between IL-5 mRNA expression and the number of activated lymphocytes and eosinophils suggesting that this cytokine plays an important role in the regulation of eosinophil function within the asthmatic airway. Further evidence to support a role of Th2-type cytokines in the airways of atopic asthmatics was shown in bronchial biopsies after allergen challenge where there was an increase in the numbers of cells expressing mRNA for IL-5, IL-4 and GM-CSF (25). There was no increase in the numbers of cells expressing mRNA for either IL-2 or IFNγ suggesting the Th1-type cytokines are not involved in the allergen-induced late airway responses. These studies have also been performed on BAL cells from atopic asthmatics following allergen provocation using probes for IL-2, IL-3, IL-4, IL-5, GM-CSF and IFNγ (26). The results of this study supported the general hypothesis that cytokines produced by activated Th2-type lymphocytes contribute to the late asthmatic response by mechanisms which include eosinophil accumulation. Glucocorticosteroids are beneficial in the treatment of allergic asthma. A recent study used ISH techniques to determine whether the profile of cytokine mRNA expression in BAL fluid from asthmatics was modulated by prednisolone. Treatment with steroids was associated with the reduction in eosinophil numbers in BAL fluid and a concomitant reduction in the number of cells expressing IL-4 and IL-5 mRNA, whilst the numbers of cells expressing IFNγ was increased (27). Further evidence to suggest the therapeutic action of steroids lies in their ability to modulate cytokine expression is seen in steroid-resistant asthmatics (28), where lack of clinical responsiveness is associated with a dysregulation of the expression of genes encoding for Th1 and Th2-type cytokines in the airways.

4.4. Expression of mRNA for Cytokines in Acute and Chronic Dermatitis

Atopic dermatitis is associated with an intense pruritus, increased serum IgE levels and blood eosinophilia. Due to these characteristic features of allergic inflammation, the profile of cytokine mRNA expression was investigate in acute and chronic forms of the disorder using probes for IL-4 and IL-5, IL-2 and IFN-γ and immunocytochemistry for activated eosinophils (29). Whilst both forms of atopic dermatitis were associated with an increased activation of the IL-4 and IL-5 genes, the maintenance of the chronic form was predominantly associated with an increased expression of IL-5 mRNA and eosinophil infiltration.

ACKNOWLEDGMENTS

The work present in this chapter has been done in collaboration with Drs. Sun Ying, D. Robinson, D. Leung, S. Durham and A.B.Kay. We would also like to thank Mrs. M. Makroyanni for typing the chapter. This work has been supported by the Network of Centres of Excellence and the Montreal Chest Research Institute.

REFERENCES

1. Mosmann TR, Cherwinski H, Bond MW, Gieldin MA & RL Coffman. Two types of murine helper T cell clone. I. Definition according to profiles of lymphokine activities and secreted proteins. J Immunol 1986; 136:2348–2357.
2. Del Prete G, Maggi E, Parronchi P, Chretien I, Tiri A, Macchia D, Ricci M, Banchereau J, De Vries J & S Romagnani. IL-4 is an essential co-factor for the IgE synthesis induced *in vitro* by human T cell clones and their supernatants. J Immunol 1988; 140:4193–4198.
3. Clutterbuck EJ, Hirst EMA & CJ Sanderson. Human interleukin-5 (IL-5) regulates the production of eosinophils in human bone marrow cultures: comparison and interaction with IL-1, IL-3, IL-6 and GM-CSF. Blood 1989; 73:1504–1512.
4. Kay AB, Ying S, Varney V, Durham SR, Moqbel R, Wardlaw A & Q Hamid. Messenger RNA expression of the cytokine gene cluster, IL-3, IL-4, IL-5 and GM-CSF in allergen-induced late-phase cutaneous reactions in atopic subjects. J Exp Med 1991; 173:775–778.
5. Hamid Q, Azzawi M, Ying S, Moqbel R, Wardlaw A, Corrigan C, Bradley B, Durham SR, Collin J, Jeffery P, Quint D & AB Kay. Expression of mRNA for interleukin-5 in mucosal bronchial biopsies from asthma. J Clin Invest 1991; 87:1541–1546.
6. Robinson DS, Hamid Q, Ying S, Tsicopoulos A, Barkans J, Bentley AM, Corrigan C, Durham SR & AB Kay. Predominant T_{H2}-like bronchoalveolar T-lymphocyte population in atopic asthma. New Engl J Med 1992; 326:298–304.
7. Pardue ML & JG Gall. Proc Natl Acad Sci USA 1969; 64:600-
8. Cox KH, DeLeon DV, Angerer LM, Angerer RC. Detection of mRNAs in sea wichin embryos by in situ hybridization using asymmetric RNA probes. Dev Biol 1984; 101:485–502.

9. Giaid A, Hamid Q, Adams C, Trenghi G & JM Polak. Non-isotopic RNA probes; comparison between different labels and detection systems. Histochemistry 1989; 93:191–196.

10. Ying S, Durham SR, Jacobson M, Masuyama M, AB Kay & Q Hamid. Phenotype of cells expressing interleukin-4 (IL-4), IL-5, IL-2 and interferon-gamma (IFNγ) mRNA in the nasal mucosa following allergen provocation. J Allergy Clin Immunol 1994; 93:270-

11. Hamid Q, Wharton J, Terenghi G, Hassall C, Aimi J, Taylor K, Nakazato H, Dixon J, Burnstock G & JM Polak. Localization of atrial natriuretic peptide mRNA and immunoreactivity in rat heart and human atrial appendage. Proc Natl Acad Sci USA 1987; 84:7315–7318.

12. Ploysongsang, M., Humbert, M., Ying S. Yasruel Z, Durham S, Kay, A.B., and Hamid, Q. Increased expression of interleuking-5 receptor gene in asthma. J Allergy Clin Immunol 1995; 95: 279.

13. Kita H, Ohnishi T, Okubo Y, Weiler D, Abrams JS & GJ Gleich. Granulocyte/macrophage colony-stimulating factor and interleukin-3 release from human peripheral blood esoinophils and neutrophils. J Exp Med 1991; 174:745–748.

14. Moqbel R, Hamid Q, Ying S, Barkans J, Hartnell A, Tsicopoulos A, Wardlaw AJ & AB Kay. Expression of mRNA and immunoreactivity for the granulocyte/macrophage colony-stimulating factor in activated human eosinophils. J Exp Med 1991; 174:749–752.

15. Hamid Q, Barkans J, Meng Q, Abrams J, Kay AB & R Moqbel. Human eosinophils synthesize and secrete interleukin-6 in vitro. Blood 1992; 80:1496–1501.

16. Broide DH, Paine MM & GS Firestein. Eosinophils express interleukin-5 and granulocyte macrophage colony-stimulating factor mRNA at sites of allergic inflammation in asthmatics. J Clin Invest 1992; 90:1414–1424.

17. Bradding P, Roberts JA, Britten KM, Montefort S, Djukanovic R, Mueller R, Heusser CH, Howarth PH & ST Holgate. Interleukin-4, -5 and -6 and tumor necrosis factor-α in normal and asthmatic airways: Evidence for the human mast cell as a source of these cytokines. Am J Respir Cell Mol Biol 1994; 10:471–480.

18. Plaut M, Pierce JH, Watson CJ, Hanley-Hyde J, Nordan RP & WE Paul. Mast cell lines produce lymphokines in response to cross-linkage of FcεRI or to calcium ionophores. Nature (London) 1989; 339:64–67.

19. Gordan JR & SJ Galli. Mast cells as a source of both preformed and immunologically inducible TNF-α/cachetin. Nature (London) 1990; 346:274–276.

20. Cromwell O, Hamid Q, Corrigan C, Barkans J, Collins P & AB Kay. Expression and generation of IL-6, iL-8 and GM-CSF by human bronchial epithelial cells and enhancement by IL-1ß and TNF-α. Immunology 1992; 77:330–337.

21. Van Noorden S. Tissue preparation and immunostaining techniques for light microscopy. In: Immunocytochemistry. Modern methods and Applications. Eds, Polak JM & S Van Noorden. 1986. Chapter 3: pp26–53.

22. Frew AJ and Kay AB. The relationship between infiltrating CD4+ lymphocytes, activated eosinophils and the magnitude of the allergen - induced late-phase cutaneous reaction in man. J. Immunol. 1988; 141: 4158–4164.

23. Tsicopoulos, A., Hamid,Q., Varney V, Ying Sun, Moqbel, R., Durham, S.R., Kay, A.B. Preferential messenger RNA expression of Th1-type cells (IFN-γ+, IL-2+) in classical delayed-type (tuberculin) hypersensitivity reactions in human skin. J. Immuno 1992; 148: 2058–2061.

24. Durham S, Ying S, Varney V, Jacobson M, Kay AB & Q Hamid. Cytokine messenger RNA expression for IL-3, IL-4, IL-5 and granulocyte/macrophage-colony stimulating factor in the nasal mucosa after local allergen provocation: Relationship to tissue eosinophilia. J Immunol 1992; 142:2390–2394.

25. Bentley AM, Meng Q, Robinson DS, Hamid Q, Kay AB & SR Durham. Increases in activated T lymphocytes, eosinophils and cytokine mRNA expression for interleukin-5, granulocyte/macrophage colony-stimulating factor in bronchial biopsies after allergen challenge in atopic asthmatics. Am J Respir Cell Mol Biol 1993; 8:35–42.

26. Robinson D, Hamid Q, Bentley A, Ying S, Kay AB & SR Durham. Activation of CD4+ T cells, increased Th2-type cytokine recruitment in bronchoalveolar lavage after allergen inhalation challenge in patients with atopic asthma. J Allergy Clin Immunol 1993; 92:313–324.

27. Robinson D, Hamid Q, Ying S, Bentley A, Assoufi B, Durham S & AB Kay. Prednisolone treatment in asthma is associated with modulation of bronchoalveolar lavage cell interleukin-4, interleukin-5 and interferon-γ cytokine gene expression. Am Rev Respir Dis 1993b; 148:401–406.

28. Leung DYM, Martin RJ, Szefler SJ, Sher ER, Ying S, Kay AB & Q Hamid. Dysregulation of interleukin-4, interleukin-5 and interferon γ gene expression in steroid-resistant asthma. J Exp Med 1995; 181:33–40.

29. Hamid Q, Boguniewicz M & DYM Leung. Differential in situ gene expression in acute versus chronic atopic dermatitis. J Clin Invest 1994; 94:870–876.

47

IS VACCINATION AGAINST IgE POSSIBLE?

Lars Hellman

Department of Medical Immunology and Microbiology
Biomedical Centre, Box 582
University of Uppsala
S-751 23 Uppsala

SUMMARY

A substantial reduction in the levels of both total and antigen specific IgE will most likely result in improved symptom scores in atopic individuals. Based on this assumption we initiated a project to study the possibility of reducing levels of circulating and mast cell bound IgE, by inducing a strong autoimmune antibody response against IgE in the host. Bacterially produced fusion proteins containing constant domains two (CH2) and three (CH3) of rat IgE directly linked to the glutathione-S-transferase (GST) protein from *Schistosoma japonicum* or to the maltose binding protein of *Esherichia coli* were used as the active components of the allergy vaccine. Injection of either of these fusion proteins together with adjuvant led to the induction of a strong autoimmune anti-IgE response in several IgE low or medium responder strains of rats.

Vaccination of ovalbumin sensitised Wistar rats with the GST- C2C3 fusion protein resulted in a profound decrease in serum IgE levels and later in a nearly complete block in histamine release from mast cells and basophils upon challenge with either a cross-linking polyclonal anti-IgE antiserum or a specific allergen. This shows that it is possible to reduce IgE levels in an animal to such an extent that it gives a clear clinical effect. Recent studies with an extended panel of rat strains including four IgE high responder strains, indicate that induction of the autoimmune response is dependent on the plasma concentration of IgE before vaccination. A high concentration of IgE has a negative effect on the induction of autoimmunity, most likely by inducing a B-cell tolerance in the host. Vaccinated subjects with very high IgE concentrations thereby responds poorly to the vaccine. Current studies are aimed at overcoming this potential limitation of the vaccination procedure.

INTRODUCTION

The current treatment of atopic allergies primarily focuses on reducing the effects of compounds released from mast cells or basophils, as exemplified by the use of anti-hista-

New Horizons in Allergy Immunotherapy
edited by Sehon et al. Plenum Press, New York, 1996

337

mines, anti-leukotrienes and β2-adrenergic agonists or more general anti-inflammatory drugs such as corticosteroids. However, several different approaches are presently being studied with the aim of interfering with allergen induced activation of mast cells at a stage prior to the release of granule stored material. Two such strategies focus on reducing levels of circulating and mast cell bound IgE in the atopic subject by directly interfering with the production and accumulation of IgE without affecting other Ig isotypes. One of these strategies is based on intravenous injections of monoclonal antibodies which form immune complexes with circulating IgE thereby clearing it from the circulation (Chang et al., 1990)(Davis et al., 1993)(Presta et al., 1993). Similar methods have been used for in vivo depletion of other Ig isotypes like kappa light chain-containing Ig molecules (Weiss et al., 1984). There are several potential risks connected with injection of monoclonal or polyclonal antibodies for extended periods. Regular injections of purified monoclonal antibodies over several years may lead to the induction of anti-idiotypic responses which may cause life threatening immune complex formation. The risk of this complication occuring will always be present, requiring careful monitoring of the patient's condition after each injection. The injection of very large amounts of a monoclonal antibody may overcome such complications by inducing B cell tolerance against the idiotype by the presence of a high concentration of soluble monoclonal antibody in the patient's circulation. However, this approach may be too expensive for large scale treatment. A second method, which we describe in this paper, is based on the induction of a strong autoimmune response against the IgE of the host. This approach will most likely solve some of the above problems but may also involve some new difficulties. Vaccination induces a polyclonal response against self IgE and the risk for immune complex formation is therefore minimal. However, a potential problem with the vaccination procedure is that it may be difficult to overcome the strong tolerance exhibited towards self molecules to reduce both circulating and mast cell bound IgE to such an extent that it results in a significant clinical effect.

Studies addressing this and related questions have previously been performed by a number of investigators. Chen et al. described an analysis of the effect of injecting monoclonal immunoglobulins of different subclasses during the neonatal period and detected an induction of a class restricted tolerance only for IgE (Chen and Katz, 1983)(Chen et al., 1984). Marshall and Bell presented an extensive study of the effect of immunisation with purified monoclonal rat IgE (Marshall and Bell, 1985)(Marshall and Bell, 1989). They detected an autoimmune anti-IgE response in adult rats of two different strains (Brown Norway (BN) and PVG.RT1), but the observed effect of the immunisation was quite different in these two strains. The response resulted in a reduction in total IgE in the low IgE producing strain (PVG.RT1) but not in the high IgE producing BN strain. In a number of elegant experiments Haba and Nisonoff achieved a prolonged reduction in plasma IgE levels and IgE producing cells in mice injected with syngeneic monoclonal IgE during a short neonatal window of development, from birth to approximately day 10. Injections after the second or third week did not induce an autoantibody response probably because of rising plasma levels of IgE in the animal with subsequent tolerisation (Haba and Nisonoff, 1988)(Haba and Nisonoff, 1990)(Haba and Nisonoff, 1994)(Haba and Nisonoff, 1994). These investigators also observed a strong induction of auto anti-IgE antibodies in adult mice after immunisation with mouse IgE which had been covalently coupled to keyhole limpet hemocyanin (KLH) (Haba and Nisonoff, 1987).

Based on the potential advantages of the vaccination strategy we initiated a project to assess the possibility of inducing a strong autoimmune response in an adult host against the patient's own circulating IgE by using only the receptor binding CH2 and CH3 domains of IgE coupled to a foreign carrier protein, and to study the effects of such a vaccination procedure on an antigen induced and an anti-IgE induced skin reaction in an experimental animal.

RESULTS AND DISCUSSION

Induction of an Autoimmune Anti-IgE Response in an Experimental Animal

In order to minimise the risk of cross linking IgE already bound to the surface of mast cells or basophils and thereby triggering an anaphylactic reaction, the receptor binding region of the IgE molecule was selected as immunogen instead of the entire IgE molecule. The receptor binding region is located in the N-terminal part of the C3 domain (Helm et al., 1988)(Helm et al., 1989). In order to obtain a larger number of surface epitopes, and to have these epitopes in close to native conformation, the entire CH2 and CH3 domains were used instead of only short peptides from the N terminal region of the CH3 domain. The CH2-CH3 region of IgE was covalently linked to a foreign carrier as a fusion protein. This was done with the aim of circumventing the tolerance against the animal's own IgE molecules by the recruitment of a non-tolerized T-cell population which would normally have given help only to B cells directed against the carrier, but which, due to coupling of the receptor binding region to the carrier would also support B cells with specificities directed against the IgE molecules of the vaccinated subject.

The antigen used in our initial experiments was a bacterially expressed fusion protein consisting of the CH2-CH3 domains of rat IgE fused to the *S. japonicum* GST polypeptide. After purification to near homogeneity this fusion protein was used to study the immune response against self IgE in four different rat strains (Hellman, 1994). Four weeks after intraperitoneal injection of the fusion protein in Freunds complete adjuvant, and one week after a booster injection in Freunds incomplete adjuvant, a strong immune response against native rat IgE was detected by ELISA measurements in three out of four strains of rat (Hellman, 1994). The fourth strain did not appear to mount a response to this particular antigen possibly due to an MHC dependent non responder phenomenon. However, more recent experiments with several high responder strains have shown that the lack of induction of an autoimmune response does not depend on the nature of the carrier protein used in the experiment. Thus no, or only minor, differences were found in the anti-IgE response in the different rat strains using either the GST-C2C3 fusion protein or a fusion protein consisting of the *E. coli* maltose binding protein and the CH2-CH3 domains of rat IgE (data not shown). An analysis of the immune response against the carrier protein component alone confirmed this conclusion. In all analysed strains of rats a strong antibody response was detected against the carrier protein, even if no auto anti-IgE response was detected. The anti-IgE response showed instead a correlation with the plasma level of IgE at the time of initiation of the vaccination procedure (data not shown). Thus, a high level of circulating IgE most likely induces a strong tolerance to self IgE making it difficult to induce an anti-IgE response in the vaccinated subject.

Another question of importance was if and how the rising plasma concentration of anti-IgE would affect the different mast cell populations in various tissues. When comparing blank vaccinated animals (which received only adjuvant and phosphate buffered saline (PBS)) with animals having high anti-IgE titres, we were unable to detect any effect on the mast cell number in the skin (mainly connective tissue mast cells) (Hellman, 1994). In contrast Marshall et al. reported an approximately 50% decrease in the number of connective tissue mast cells and a 4 fold increase in the number of mucosal mast cells in skin and tongue in BN rats after induction of a strong autoimmune anti-IgE response by using pure rat IgE (Marshall et al., 1987). This discrepancy may possibly be explained by a difference in the cross linking activity of the in vivo antibody response due to the difference in immunogen used to elicit the response.

Assay of Skin Reactivity in Vaccinated and Control Animals by Evans Blue Administration

Rats sensitized to ovalbumin were used to study the effect of the vaccination on both an allergen and an anti-IgE induced inflammatory reaction. Ricin was used to enhance the sensitization to the allergen according to the protocol of Kemeny and colleagues (Diaz-Sanchez and Kemeny, 1991). Since in our initial experiments we obtained only a relatively modest increase in total IgE levels compared to what had been preported by Kemeny and co-workers, we later performed a more careful titration to determine the optimal ricin concentrations (RCA II) needed to obtain a good sensitizing effect. However, in several experiments with a panel of Lewis and BN rats, we did not detect any effect of co-administration of ricin, even using concentrations approaching a lethal dose. We also tested the less toxic ricin derivative RCA I but again were unable to detect any effect of this lectin. A possible reason for the discrepancy between these studies is that we used relatively pure lectin preparations (RCA I or RCA II from Vector laboratories, CA, USA) rather than partly purified castor bean extract which was used in the former study.

Rats were sensitized for approximately 8 weeks with weekly injections of 1 µg of ovalbumin and 50 ng ricin before initiation of the vaccination, and were then divided into two identical groups of animals one of which was injected with the vaccine and the second of which received only PBS and Freunds adjuvant. Five hundred µg of the fusion protein in 200 µl of Freunds complete adjuvant and PBS (50:50) was administered intraperitoneally at the initiation of the vaccination. Two subsequent booster doses with 100 µg antigen and Freunds incomplete adjuvant were given intraperitoneally 4 and 8 weeks later. After ten weeks of treatment the skin reactivity was assayed by intradermal injections (50 µl) of an allergen solution or a diluted polyclonal cross linking anti-IgE antiserum (rabbit anti-rat IgE). Following these injections, the animals were opened in their jugular vein and a solution containing 2 mg/ml Evans blue in PBS was injected into the bloodstream. The animals were then kept under anaesthesia for an additional 2 hours after which the skin was opened up and the sizes of the inflammatory (blue) zones were measured (Hellman, 1994). Compared to the control group all vaccinated animals showed a profound reduction in inflammatory zones in response to both the allergen and the anti-IgE antiserum. With the latter practically no blue zones were detected in the vaccinated rats. This shows that the vaccine has the capacity to reduce the IgE levels to such an extent that we achieve a significant clinical effect.

IgE Levels in Vaccinated and Control Animals

During vaccination blood samples were taken every three weeks (0, 3, 6 and 9 weeks) and the concentration of IgE was analysed. We found that levels of IgE were decreased in both the vaccinated as well as in the control group (Freund's adjuvant most likely affects the sensitization by favouring a TH1 response which thereby leads to a decrease in plasma IgE levels). However, a marked difference in the reduction of plasma IgE concentrations between the two groups of animals was observed. At nine weeks, the vaccinated animals had IgE levels which were below the detection limit of the assay (approximately 20 ng/ml) while all the control animals had IgE levels of 30–75 ng/ml (Hellman, 1994). In addition, based on the results from the Evans blue skin assay we can conclude that the IgE levels in the vaccinated rats must be far below 20 ng/ml because no inflammatory response was detected in these animals following the injection of a polyclonal anti-IgE antiserum indicating a nearly complete absence of mast-cell bound IgE in these animals.

Future Perspectives

We and others have been able to show that it is possible to induce a strong auto anti-IgE response in several strains of rat and mouse (Marshall and Bell, 1985)(Marshall and Bell, 1989) (Haba and Nisonoff, 1988)(Haba and Nisonoff, 1990)(Haba and Nisonoff, 1994)(Haba and Nisonoff, 1994)(Haba and Nisonoff, 1987)(Hellman, 1994). However, the effect of this anti-IgE response on IgE mediated inflammatory reactions and the amount and binding affinity of the anti-IgE antibodies are quite variable depending on strain and age of the animal studied. It is more difficult to obtain a good clinical effect in adult animals of IgE high responder strains, which have a high IgE titer at the initiation of the vaccination program. In recent experiments with different IgE high responder strains we have been able to induce a strong autoimmune response in two out of four strains while the other two responded relatively poorly to the vaccine (data not shown). In order to increase the immunogenicity of the vaccine and thereby boost the anti-IgE response to such an extent that we also achieve a measurable clinical effect in practically all IgE high responders we are presently studying several new adjuvants and also different modes of administration of the vaccine. However, in order to achieve a substantial reduction of serum IgE also in high responder animals, having a very high IgE concentration at the initiation of vaccination we may have to use a combination of several of the previously described methods. One scenario which we presently favour is the use of monoclonal antibodies for a number of weeks to reduce plasma IgE levels to such an extent that induction of B cell tolerance in newly recruited B-cells from the bone marrow is rendered unlikely. This tolerance or anergy in the B cell compartment is most likely caused by the interaction of membrane Ig on these virgin B cells with soluble IgE (antigen), in the absence of secondary signals like CD40 ligand interaction and interleukins. By initiating the vaccination when the serum levels of IgE are low, we will most likely achieve a strong auto anti-IgE response which will cause a prolonged suppression of the IgE production, without a requirement for further treatment with monoclonal antibodies. Preliminary experiments along this line have already been performed and we have been able to show that the reduction of total IgE levels in BN rats is dependent on the amount of monoclonal antibody administered and on the species of origin of the antibody used for the injections. A heterologous antiserum (rabbit polyclonal antiserum) injected in 250 μg doses three times intramuscularly within a time span of one week did not give any demonstrable effect on total IgE levels in these rats. By contrast, identical injections of 250 μg of a non cross-linking mouse monoclonal antibody directed against rat IgE gave a significant but transient decrease in the two rats analysed. However, with an identical protocol but with injections of only 50 μg at each time point no effect was detected (data not shown). The species dependence is probably caused by the lack of interaction with IgG receptors on phagocytic cells with the heterologous antisera, which is of major importance for clearance of immune complexes and thereby the reduction in the levels of plasma IgE.

We are presently actively persuing these and a few additional potential strategies for the treatment of IgE high responder strains of rats as an animal model for human atopic allergy patients.

ACKNOWLEDGMENTS

This investigation was supported by grants from the Swedish Natural Sciences Research Council. I would like to thank Maria Aveskogh for skilful technical assistance and for fruitful and stimulating discussions, Mats Carlsson, Roger Åkerlund and Molly Vernersson for fruitful collaboration and Stanley Burnett for linguistic revision of the manuscript.

REFERENCES

Chang, T. W., Davis, F. M., Sun, N.-C., Sun, C. R. Y., MacGlashan Jr, D. W., and Hamilton, R. G. (1990). Monoclonal antibodies specific for human IgE-producing B-cells: a potential therapeutic for IgE-mediated allergic diseases. Bio/Technology 8, 122–126.

Chen, S.-S., and Katz, D. H. (1983). IgE class-restricted tolerance induced by neonatal administration of soluble or cell-bound IgE. J. Exp. Med. 157, 722–788.

Chen, S.-S., Liu, F.-T., and Katz, D. H. (1984). IgE class-restricted tolerance induced by neonatal administration of soluble or cell-bound IgE, Cellular mechanisms. J. Exp. Med. 160, 953–970.

Davis, F. M., Gossett, L. A., Pinkston, K. L., Liou, R. S., Sun, L. K., Kim, Y. W., Chang, N. T., Chang, T. W., Wagner, K., Bews, J., Brinkmann, V., Towbin, H., Subramanian, N., and Heusser, C. (1993). Can anti-IgE be used to treat allergy? In Springer Semin. Immunopathol. 15, 51–73.

Diaz-Sanchez, D., and Kemeny, D. M. (1991). Generation of a long-lived IgE response in high and low responder strains of rat by co-administration of ricin and antigen. Immunology 72, 297–303.

Haba, S., and Nisonoff, A. (1994). Effect of syngeneic anti-IgE antibodies on the development of IgE memory and on the secondary IgE response. J.Immunol. 152, 51–57.

Haba, S., and Nisonoff, A. (1988). Immunological responsiveness of neonatal A/J mice to isotypic determinants of syngeneic IgE. J. Exp. Med. 168, 713–724.

Haba, S., and Nisonoff, A. (1987). Induction of high titers of anti-IgE by immunization of inbred mice with syngeneic IgE. Proc. Natl. Acad. Sci. USA 84, 5009–5013.

Haba, S., and Nisonoff, A. (1990). Inhibition of IgE synthesis by anti-IgE: Role of long-term inhibition of IgE synthesis by neonatally administered soluble IgE. Proc. Natl. Acad. Sci. USA 87, 3363–3367.

Haba, S., and Nisonoff, A. (1994). Role of antibody and T cells in the long-term inhibition of IgE synthesis. Proc. Natl. Acad. Sci. USA 91, 604–608.

Hellman, L. (1994). Profound reduction in allergen sensitivity following treatment with a novel allergy vaccine. Eur. J. Immunol. 24, 415–420.

Helm, B., Kebo, D., Vercelli, D., Glovsky, M., Gould, H., Ishizaka, K., Geha, R., and Ishizaka, T. (1989). Blocking of passive sensitization of human mast cells and basophil granulocytes with IgE antibodies by a recombinant human ε -chain fragment of 76 amino acids. Proc. Natl. Acad. Sci. USA 86, 9465–9469.

Helm, B., Marsh, P., Vercelli, D., Padlan, E., Gould, H., and Geha, R. (1988). The mast cell binding site on human immunoglobulin E. Nature 331, 180–183.

Marshall. J. S., and Bell, E. B. (1985). Induction of an auto-anti-IgE response in rats I. Effects on serum IgE concentrations. Eur. J. Immunol. 15, 272–277.

Marshall, J. S., and Bell, E. B. (1989). Induction of an auto-anti-IgE response in rats III. Inhibition of a specific IgE response. Immunology 66, 428–433.

Marshall, J. S., Prout, S. J., Jaffery, G., and Bell, E. B. (1987). Induction of an auto-anti-IgE response in rats II. Effects on mast cell populations. Eur. J. Immunol. 17, 445–451.

Presta, L. G., Lahr, S. J., Shields, R. L., Porter, J. P., Gorman, C. M., Fendly, B. M., and Jardieu, P. M. (1993). Humanization of an antibody directed against IgE. J. Immunol. 151, 2623–2632.

Weiss, S., Lehmann, K., Raschke, W. C., and Cohn, M. (1984). Mice completely suppressed for the expression of immunoglobulin κ light chain. Proc. Natl. Acad. Sci. USA . 81, 211–215.

48

ROLE OF INTERLEUKIN-4 IN THE DEVELOPMENT OF ALLERGIC AIRWAY INFLAMMATION AND AIRWAY HYPERRESPONSIVENESS

M. Wills-Karp,[1] S. H. Gavett,[1] Brian Schofield,[1] and F. Finkelman[2]

[1]Department of Environmental Health Sciences
School of Hygiene and Public Health
Johns Hopkins University
615 N. Wolfe Street, Baltimore, Maryland
[2]Department of Medicine
Uniformed Services University of the Health Sciences
Bethesda, Maryland

Airway inflammation and airway hyperreactivity are consistent features of allergic asthma. The inflammatory response is characterized chiefly by an increase in eosinophils and T cells in bronchial mucosa and bronchoalveolar lavage fluids[1–5]. Furthermore, as therapeutic interventions that reduce airway inflammation ameliorate airway hyperreactivity, inflammation is hypothesized to play a key role in the development of asthma-associated airway hyperreactivity[6,7]. As a primary regulator of the inflammatory cascade, the T lymphocyte has been implicated in the pathogenesis of asthma[8]. Considerable circumstantial evidence has been accumulating to support this hypothesis. For example, increased numbers of activated T cells are found in the bronchial mucosa of asthmatics as compared with control subjects[3]. The degree of peripheral blood T lymphocyte activation correlates with the severity of asthmatic symptoms[9]. In patients with allergic asthma, which is characterized as such by elevated serum IgE levels, allergen challenge induces a selective recruitment of CD4+ T cells into the airways[5]. Moreover, the degree of activation of CD4+ lymphocytes correlates with the number of eosinophils in BAL fluid, with the degree of bronchial hyperreactivity, and with disease severity[10]. CD4+ T cells isolated from bronchoalveolar fluids (BAL) of allergic asthmatics express increased levels of markers of acute and chronic activation[11]. Such lymphocytes demonstrate a specific pattern of cytokine expression, namely, elevated levels of IL-4 and IL-5 mRNA, a pattern consistent with a T-helper 2 (TH2) pattern of differentiation[12]. A possible immunopathogenic role for Th2 CD4+ T lymphocytes in asthma is suggested by the eosinophilia that characterizes asthma in general and the elevated IgE levels associated with allergic

New Horizons in Allergy Immunotherapy
edited by Sehon et al. Plenum Press, New York, 1996

343

asthma. IL-4 is essential for the development of an IgE response[13], while IL-5 in turn promotes eosinophil differentiation[14], recruitment[15], activation[16], and survival[17]. Although considerable descriptive evidence suggest that T lymphocytes may be important in the pathogenesis of asthma, further dissection of the mechanism(s) involved will require development of predictive animal models.

Many animal models of allergen-induced allergic airway responses have been described including the ovalbumin-sensitized and -challenged guinea pig model[18], and the *Ascaris suum* parasite antigen-induced primate model[19]. These models lack a well defined immunological system as well as a wide array of reagents available for the examination of leukocyte subsets and cytokines produced during the reaction. The mouse on the other hand is a particularly suitable species for this type of studies as they are well characterized from an immunologic standpoint and many immunological tools are available for probing single compartments of the immune system. While previous study in mice has been hampered because of limitations in assessing airway function, there have been recent inroads into such assessments, making use of this small mammal a more practical endeavor[20].

Murine models of allergen sensitization and challenge have been recently described in which mice exposed to allergens develop lymphocytic and eosinophilic inflammation and airway hyperresponsiveness typical of that seen in human allergic asthma[20–22]. Another feature of human asthma which has been demonstrated in mice is a dramatic increase in the numbers of goblet cells and their mucus content in the airway epithelium following allergen challenge[23]. Further the importance of CD4+ T cells has been established in this model as the development of antigen-induced airway hyperresponsiveness and eosinophilic inflammation in the mouse is entirely CD4+ T cell dependent[20]. The development of allergic airway responses in this model are also associated with increases in mRNA levels of the Th2 cytokines, IL-4 and IL-5[24]. Thus murine models are likely to prove valuable in the dissection of the role of T cells in the development of allergic airway disease.

The Th2 cytokine, interleukin-4, in addition to its crucial role in the differentiation of Th2 cells, has several other effects which are potentially important in the development of allergic airway disease: the induction of IgE production [13], stimulation of the growth and development of mast cells[25], and induction of VCAM-1 expression on vascular endothelium[26]. Several studies in mice have shown that IL-4 mediates tissue eosinophilia in response to parasite eggs[27], and allergen exposure[28]. In mice sensitized and challenged with allergen, in vivo blockade of the interleukin-4 receptor suppresses not only lung eosinophilia but antigen-induced airway hyperresponsiveness, and increases in goblet cell numbers[23]. In support of this finding, interleukin-4 deficient mice do not develop eosinophilia or airway hyperreactivity when sensitized and challenged with allergen[29]. These studies demonstrate that both allergen-induced eosinophilic inflammation and airway hyperreactivity are interleukin-4-dependent, although the mechanism(s) remain unclear.

One of the characteristics of allergic asthma is the presence of elevated serum IgE levels. IgE crosslinking of high affinity Fc receptors on inflammatory cells induces the release of a variety of bronchoconstrictor mediators which may contribute to the development of airway hyperresponsiveness. IL-4 has clearly been shown to be a key regulator of the synthesis of IgE both in vitro and in vivo[13]. Studies with IL-4 deficient mice support this hypothesis in that after allergen sensitization they do not have increased IgE levels, airway inflammation or airway hyperresponsiveness. These results suggest that IgE and mast cell activation are important in the development of allergic responses. However, when mast cell deficient mice were sensitized to allergen they mounted an inflammatory response equivalent to that of the wild type mice suggesting that mast cell activation is not required for the induction of airway inflammation[28]. Other studies with IgE deficient mice support this conclusion in that these mice become anaphylactic to an intravenous antigen challenge and display pulmonary function changes similar to those seen in wild-type animals[30]. Taken together these data indicate that IgE-independent pathways for allergic reactions exist in mice and that IL-4's role in airway allergic responses may not be due to its effect on IgE production.

Another potential mechanism of IL-4 regulation of allergen-induced eosinophilia is upregulation of vascular cell adhesion molecule-1 (VCAM-1) on endothelial cells. IL-4 has recently been shown to selectively induce VCAM-1 expression on cultured endothelial cells and to increase eosinophil adherence to endothelial cells in vitro[26]. Nakajima et al.[31] showed that blockade of VCAM-1 and VLA-4 prevented antigen-induced eosinophil and T lymphocyte infiltration into the mouse trachea, although IL-4 only partially mediated the expression of VCAM-1 on the vascular endothelium. Thus other cytokines may also regulate VCAM-1 expression following antigenic stimulation. In another study, antibodies to VLA-4 and LFA-1 blocked allergen-induced airway hyperresponsiveness but only antibodies to LFA-1 blocked eosinophilia in rats.[32] Thus it is not clear whether regulation of adhesion molecule expression by IL-4 plays a role in allergic inflammation.

Another possible mechanism by which IL-4 may regulate the inflammatory response to allergen exposure is through its role as the central regulator of the differentiation of Th0 cells into Th2 type cells[33,34] and through mediation of autocrine growth of Th2 cells in vitro and in vivo[35]. Th2 cells respond to antigenic stimuli with the synthesis of several cytokines including IL-4, IL-5, IL-6, IL-9, and IL-10[36]. Interleukin-5 is particularly important in allergic responses as it selectively promotes the chemotaxis[14], activation[16], and survival[17] of eosinophils. In murine models of allergic airway disease, eosinophil infiltration and the development of allergen-induced airway hyperresponsiveness have been shown to be mediated by interleukin-5[21] and CD4+ T lymphocytes[20]. This is consistent with the finding in asthmatics that IL-5 is the predominant eosinophil-active cytokine in the allergen-induced late phase reaction and that exacerbations of asthma are associated with activation of CD4+ T cells and increased serum concentrations of IL-5[37]. Thus, IL-4 may mediate allergic inflammation and airway hyperresponsiveness by regulating Th 2 cell differentiation.

In summary IL-4 is a central mediator of allergic inflammation regulating antigen-induced eosinophil recruitment into the airways and subsequent airway hyperresponsiveness. Further studies are needed to determine the exact mechanisms by which this cytokine directs allergic inflammation. However, the studies outlined here highlight the possibility that antagonism of IL-4 production or function would be a rational therapeutic approach to the treatment of allergic asthma.

ACKNOWLEDGMENTS

This work was supported by a National Heart, Lung and Blood Institute Grant HL43312 , a National Institute for Environmental Health Science Grant ESO3819, and a Center for Indoor Air Grant to M.W.K. and by a Office of Naval Research and Development Command Contract N0007594WR00024 to F.D.K.

REFERENCES

1. Bentley, A.M., G. Menz, C. Storz, D.S. Robinson, B. Bradley, P.K. Jeffrey, S.R. Dunham, and A.B. Kay. 1992. Identification of T lymphocytes, macrophages, and activated eosinophils in the bronchial mucosa in intrinsic asthma. Relationship to symptoms and bronchial responsiveness. Am. Rev. Respir. Dis. 146:500–506.

2. Kelly, C., C. Ward, C.S. Stenton, G. Bird, D.J. Hendrick, and E.H. Walters. 1988. Number and activity of inflammatory cells in bronchoalevolar lavage fluid in asthma and their relation to airway responsiveness. Thorax. 43:684–692.

3. Azzawi, M., B. Bradley, P.K. Jeffrey, A.J. Frew, B. Assiufi, J.V. Collins, S. Durham, and A.B. Kay. 1990. Identification of activated T lymphocytes and eosinophils in bronchial biopsies in stable atopic asthmatics. Am. Rev. Respir. Dis. 142:1407–1413.

4. Metzger, W.J., D. Zavala, H.B. Richerson, P. Moseley, P. Iwamota, M. Monick, K. Sjoerdsma, and G.W. Hunninghake. 1987. Local allergen challenge and bronchoaleolar lavage of allergic asthmatic lungs. Description of the model and local airway inflammation. Am. Rev. Respir. Dis. 135:433–440.

5. Gerblich, A.A., H. Salik, and .R. Schuyler. 1991. Dynamic T-cell changes in peripheral blood and bronchoalveolar lavage after antigen bronchoprovocation in asthmatics. Am. Rev. Respir. Dis. 143:533–537.

6. Snapper, J.R. 1990. Inflammation and airway function: the asthma syndromw. Am. Rev. Respir. Dis. 141:531–533.

7. Alexander, A.G., N.C. Barnes and A.B. Kay. 1992. Trial of cyclosporin in corticosteriod-dependent chronic severe asthma. Lancet. 339:324–328.

8. Rochester, C.L. And J.A. Rankin. 1991. Is asthma T-cell mediated? Am. Rev. Respir. Dis. 144:1005–1007.

9. Corrigan, C.J., and A.B. Kay. 1990. CD4+ T-lymphocyte activation in acute severe asthma: relationship to disease severity and atopic status. Am. Rev. Respir. Dis. 141:970–977.

10. Walker, C., M.K. Kaegi, P. Braun, and K. Blaser. 1991. Activated T cells and eosionphilia in bronchoalveolar lavages from subjects with asthma correlated with disease severity. J. Allergy Clin. Immunol. 88:935–942.

11. Walker, C., E. Bode, L. Boer, T.T. Hansel, K. Blaser, and J.C. Virchow, Jr. 1992. Allergic and nonallergic asthmatics have distinct patterns of T-cell activation and cytokine production in peripheral blood and bronchoalveolar lavage. Am. Rev. Respir. Dis. 146:109–115.

12. Robinson, D.S., Q. Hamid, S. Ying, A. Tsicopoulos, J. Barkans, A.M. Bentley, C. Corrigan, S.R. Durham, and A.B. Kay. 1992. Predominant Th2-like bronchoalveolar T-lymphocyte population in atopic asthma. N. Engl. J. Med. 326:298–304.

13. Finkelman, F.D., I.M. Katona, J.F. Urban, J. Holmes, J. Ohara, A.S. Tung, J.V. Sample, and W.E. Paul. 1988. IL-4 is required to generate and sustain in vivo IgE responses. J. Immunol. 141:2335–2341.

14. Wang, J.M., A. Rambaldi, A. Biondi, Z.G. Chen, C.J. Sanderson, and A. Montovani. 1989. Recombinant human interleukin-5 is a selective eosinophil chemoattractant. Eur. J. Immunol. 19:701–705.

15. Lopez, A.F., C.J. Sanderson, J.R. Gamble, H.R. Campbell, I.G. Young, and M.A. Vadas. 1988. Recombinant human interleukin-5 is a selective activator of human eosinophil function. J. Exp. Med. 167:219–224.

16. Yamaguchi, Y., Y. Hayashi, Y. Sugama, Y. Miura, T. Kasahara, S. Kitamura, M. Torisu, S. Mita. A. Tominaga, K. Takatsu, and T. Suda. 1988. Highly purified murine interleukin-5 (IL-5) stimulates eosinophil function and prolongs in vitro survival: IL-5 as an eosinophil chemotactic factor. J. Exp. Med. 167:1737–1742.

17. Yamaguchi, Y., T. Suda, S. Ohta, K. Tominaga, Y. Miura, and T. Kasahara. 1991. Analysis of the survival of mature human eosinophils: interleukin-5 prevents apoptosis in mature eosinophils. Blood. 78:2542–2547.

18. Iijima, H., M. Ishii, K. Yamauchi, C.L. Chao, K. Kimura, S. Shimura, Y. Shindoh, H. Inoue, S. Mue, and T. Takishima. 1987. Bronchoalveolar lavage and histologic characterization of late asthmatic response in guinea pigs. Am. Rev. Respir. Dis. 136:922–929.

19. Gundel, R.H., C.D. Wegner, and L.G. Letts. 1992. Antigen-induced acute and late-phase responses in primates. Am. Rev. Respir. Dis. 146:369–373.

20. Gavett, S.H., X. Chen, F. Finkelman, and M. Wills-Karp. 1994. Depletion of murine CD4+ T Lymphocytes prevents antigen-induced airway hyperreactivity and pulmonary eosinophilia. Am. J. Respir. Cell Mol. Biol. 10:587–593.

21. Nakajima, H., I. Iwamoto, S. Tomoe, R. Matsumura, H. Tomioka, K. Takatsu, and S. Yoshida. 1992. CD4+ T-lymphocytes and interleukin-5 mediate antigen-induced eosinophil infiltration into the mouse trachea. Am. Rev. Respir. Dis. 146:374–377.

22. Renz, H.R., H.R. Smith, J.E. Henson, B.S. Ray, C.G. Irwin, E. Gelfand. 1992. Aerosolized antigen exposure without adjuvant causes increased IgE production and increased airway responsiveness in the mouse. J. Allergy. Clin. Immunol. 89:1127–38.

23. Gavett, S.H., B.H. Schofield, F.D. Finkelman, and M. Wills-Karp. 1994. Blockade of interleukin-4 receptor prevents pulmonary eosinophilia and airway hyperresponsiveness induced by antigen challenge in mice. Am. J. Respir. Crit. Care Med. 151:A348.

24. Gavett, S.H., D. J. O'Hearn, X. Li, S. Huang, F.D. Finkelman, and M. Wills-Karp. Interleukin-12 inhibits antigen-induced airway hyperresponsiveness, inflammation, and Th2 cytokine expression in mice. J. Exp. Med. In Press.

25. Madden, K.B., J.F. Urban, Jr., H.J. Ziltener, J.W. Schrader, F.D. Finkelman, and I.M. Katona. 1991. Antibodies to IL-3 and IL-4 suppress helminth-induced intestinal mastocytosis. J. Immunol. 147:1387–1391.

26. Schleimer, R.P., Sterbinsky, S. Kaiser, J . 1992. IL-4 induced adherence of human eosinophils and basophils but not neutrophils to endothelium. Association with expression of VCAM-1. J. Immunol. 148:1086–92.

27. Lukacs, N.W., R.M. Strieter, S.W. Chensue, and S.L. Kunkel. 1994. Interleukin-4 dependent pulmonary eosinophil infiltration in a murine model of asthma. Am. J. Respir. Cell Mol. Biol. 10:526–532.

28. Brusselle, G.G., J.C. Kips, J.H. Tavernier, J.G. Van Der Heyden, C.A. Cuvelier, R.A. Pauwels, and H. Bluethmann. 1994. Attenuation of allergic airway inflammation in IL-4 deficient mice. Clin. Exp. Allergy. 24:73–80.

29. Brusselle, G., J. Kips, G. Joos, H. Bluethmann, and R. Pauwels. 1995. Allergen-induced airway inflammation and bronchial responsiveness in wild-type and interleukin4-deficient mice. 12:254–259.

30. Oettgen, H.C., T.R. Martin, A. Wynshaw-Boris, C. Deng, J. Drazen, and P. Leder. 1994. Active anaphylaxis in IgE-deficient mice. Nature. 370:367–370.

31. Nakajiima, H., H. Sano, T. Nishimura, S. Yoshida, and I. Iwamoto. 1994. Role of Vascular Cell Adhesion Molecule 1/Very Late Activation Antigen 4 and Intercellular Adhesion Molecule 1/Lymphocyte Function-associated Antigen 1 Interactions in Antigen-induced Eosinophil and T Cell Recruitment into the Tissue. J. Exp. Med. 179:1145–1154.

32. Laberge, S., H. Rabb, T.B. Issekutz, and J.G. Martin. 1995. Role of VLA-4 and LFA-1 in allergen-induced airway hyperresponsiveness and lung inflammation in the rat. Am. J. Respir. Crit. Care Med. 151:822–829.

33. Swain, S., A. Weinberg, M. English, and G. Hutson. 1990. IL-4 directs the development of Th2-like helper effectors. J. Immunol. 145:3796–3806.

34. Le Gros, G., S. Ben-Sasson, and W. Paul. 1993. Generation of interleukin 4 (IL-4)-producing cells in vivo and in vitro: IL-2 and IL-4 are required for in vitro generation of IL-4-producing cells. J. Exp. Med. 172:921–929.

35. Fernandez-Botran, R., V. Sanders, K. Oliver, Y.W. Chen, P. Krammer, J. Uhr, and E. Vitetta. 1986. Interleukin-4 mediates autocrine growth of helper T cells after antigenic stimulation. Proc. Natl. Acad. Sci. USA. 83:9689–9693.

36. Mosmann, T.R., H. Cherwinski, M.W. Bond, M.A. Gieldin, and R.L. Coffman. 1986. Two types of murine helper T cell clone. I. Definition according to profiles of lymphockine activities and secreted proteins. J. Immunol. 136:2348–2357.

37. Corrigan, C.J., A. Haczku, V. Gemou-Engesaeth, S. Doi, Y. Kikuchi, K. Takatsu, S.R. Durham, and A.B. Kay. 1993. CD4 T-lymphocyte activation in asthma is accompanied by increased serum concentrations of interleukin-5: effect of glucocorticoid therapy. Am. rev. Respir. Dis. 147:540–547.

49

THE ROLES OF CD40 AND CD23 IN IgE REGULATION

Teruhito Yasui,[1] Hiroshi Fujiwara,[1,2,3] Masato Kamanaka,[1] Tsutomu Kawabe,[1] Nobuaki Yoshida,[2] Tadamitsu Kishimoto,[3] and Hitoshi Kikutani[1]

[1]Institute for Molecular and Cellular Biology
Osaka University
Suita, Osaka 565, Japan
[2]Research Institute
Osaka Medical Center for Maternal and Child Health
Izumi, Osaka 590–02, Japan
[3]Department of Medicine III
Osaka University Medical School
Suita, Osaka 565, Japan

1. INTRODUCTION

IgE production is strictly regulated by a number of cytokines and surface molecules. Th2 helper cell-derived IL-4 and IL-13 positively regulate differentiation of B cells to produce IgE while IFN-γ is known to be a negative regulator[1]. IL-4 can induce IgE production in human B cells in the presence of T cells although IL-4 alone is not sufficient. Recently, crosslinkage of CD40 by anti-CD40 or CD40 ligand (CD40L) has been shown to induce IgE secretion of B cells even in the absence of T cells[2,3]. These findings suggest that CD40 may transduce an essential signal to B cells in physical T and B cell interaction. Recently, mutations have been demonstrated in the CD40L gene of patients with X-linked hyper IgM syndrome[4,5,6], indicating that the CD40-CD40L system play an important role in *in vivo* humoral immune responses.

CD23 is known as a low affinity Fc receptor for IgE[7,8]. Certain anti-human CD23 antibodies have been shown to modulate IL-4 induced IgE production *in vitro*[9,10]. It has also been reported that anti-CD23 antibodies can inhibit antigen-specific IgE production of rat *in vivo*[11]. Since CD21, a receptor for C3d fragment of complement, has been identified as a second ligand of CD23[12], CD23-CD21 interaction may transduce a signal required for IgE production in B cells. However, roles of CD23 in IgE regulation are still controversial.

To study roles of CD40 and CD23 in in vivo immune responses including IgE regulation, CD40- and CD23-deficient mice were produced by gene targeting and their immunological phenotypes were analysed[13,14].

New Horizons in Allergy Immunotherapy
edited by Sehon et al. Plenum Press, New York, 1996

349

2. CD40-DIFICIENT MICE

2.1. Humoral Immune Responses in CD40-Deficient Mice

CD40-deficient mice display apparently normal phenotypes and numbers of T and B cells except for that reduced expression of CD23 on B cells has been observed in these mice. This indicates that CD40 is not essential for antigen-independent lymphocyte maturation but necessary for maintenance of CD23 expression. The mutant mice and their wild-type littermates were immunized with T-dependent (TD) antigen, DNP-ovalbumin(DNP-OA), to study a role of CD40 in T-cell dependent antibody responses. The CD40-deficient mice could not mount any detectable IgG, IgA and IgE antibody responses to both DNP and OA after primary and secondary immunizations. However, the mutant mice produced normal or rather higher IgM antibodies to DNP-OA. In contrast to TD antigens, both type 1 T-independent (TI1) antigen (TNP-LPS) and type 2 T-independent (TI2) antigen (TNP-Ficoll) could induce comparable antibody responses of IgG as well as IgM classes in the mutant and wild-type mice. These results suggest that CD40 is indispensable for T cell-dependent Ig class switching but not for T cell-dependent IgM production(Figure 1). Futhermore, T cell independent class switching can take place in the absence of CD40.

Serum levels of each Ig isotype were measured in CD40-deficient and wild type mice. The levels of serum IgG1, IgG2a, IgG2b, IgA and IgE were significantly reduced in

1. T cell-dependent antigens

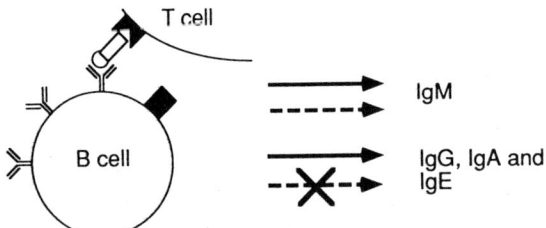

2. Type-1 T-independent antigens

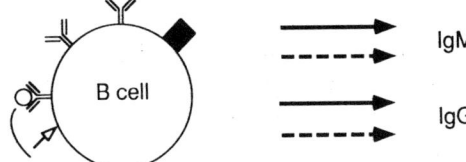

3. Type-2 T-independent antigens

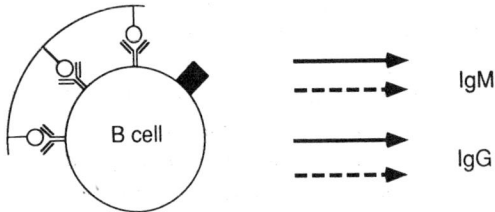

Figure 1. Antibody responses in CD40-deficient mice. The CD40-deficient mice can not mount IgG, IgA and IgE antibody responses to T-dependent antigens while T-dependent IgM responses can be observed. The responses to TI-1 and TI-2 antigens are not affected in the absence of CD40. Solid and dotted lines represent responses in the presence and the absence of CD40, respectively.

CD40-deficient mice while IgM and IgG3 levels mice were normal or a little higher than those of the wild-type mice. The pattern of serum Ig levels may reflect humoral immune responses in CD40-deficient mice. T-dependent IgM production and TI-responses probably contribute to normal levels of serum IgM and IgG3 since IgM and IgG3 are known to be the major isotypes of TI responses[15].

Another important phenotype of CD40-deficient mice is the absence of germinal center formation in secondary lymphoid tissues. Peanut agglutinin (PNA)- positive germinal center cells could not be detected in the follicles of CD40-deficient mice when spleen sections from mice immunized with TD antigen were stained with PNA. Ig class switching, affinity maturation and generation of memory B cells are known to take place in germinal centers[16]. Probably, the absence of germinal centers is closely related to a failure of isotype switching in CD40-deficient mice.

2.2. Cellular Immune Responses in CD40 Deficient Mice

There is some evidence that the CD40-CD40L system may be involved not only in T-B cells interaction but also in the interaction between T cells and other types of cells. In fact, in addition to B cells, macrophages, dendritic cells and epithelial cells express CD40. Furthermore, hyper-IgM patients with mutations in the CD40L gene are known to be susceptible to opportunistic infections such as Pneumocystis carinii, which are characteristic to T cell immunodeficiency[17]. These observations suggest that the CD40-CD40L system may also play a role in cellular immune responses. Hence, we studied the responses of CD40-deficient mice to infection with Leishmania major, one of intracellular bacteria, in resolution of which cellular but not humoral immune responses are essential. The mice were infected by injecting L. major promastigotes into hindfoot pads and then foot pad swelling and numbers of L. major in regional lymphnodes and spleens were analyzed. CD40-deficient mice failed to resolve L major infection while wild-type littermates could recover from infections. This result suggests that CD40 plays an essential role in resolution of L. major infection. There are two possible mechanisms in which CD40 is involved in immunity to L. major infection. First, it has been shown that L. major infection can induce preferentially the development of Th1 helper cells in resistant mice, whereas Th2 helper cells developed in susceptible stains of mice such as BALB/c[18]. Therefore, CD40 may play a critical role in Th1/Th2 development. Alternatively, the physical interaction with helper T cells via CD40 and CD40L may be required for activation of macrophages which directly kill intracytoplasmic parasites. For example, engagement of CD40 with CD40L could induce macrophages to produce NO which is known to be a major effector molecule in L. major infection. Whichever is the case, this observation may imply a possible role of CD40 in cellular immune responses.

3. CD23-DEFICIENT MICE

3.1. Lymphocyte Development in CD23-Deficient Mice

In human and mouse, CD23 expression is known to be restricted to a certain differentiation stage of B cells such as mature IgM/IgD B cells[19,20]. It has been reported that human soluble CD23 has biological activities to induce the growth of B cells[21] and to protect germinal center B cells from apoptosis[22]. Soluble CD23 has also been shown to induce the proliferation of human myeloid precursors[23] and the maturation of human thymocytes[24].

However, surface phenotypes and numbers of white blood cells including B and T cells and myeloid cells were normal when peripheral blood, spleen, lymphnode and thymus cells of CD23-deficient mice were analyzed by FACS. These results suggest that CD23 is not necessary for lymphocyte differentiation and granulopoiesis in mouse.

3.2. A Role of CD23 in IgE Regulation

CD23-deficient mice and their wild-type littermates were infected with Nippostrongirus brasiliensis that was known to induce polyclonal IgE production. There was no detectable difference in serum IgE levels of CD23-deficient and wild-type mice that were infected with N. brasiliensis, suggesting that CD23 may not have a regulatory role in polyclonal IgE antibody responses. To study a role of CD23 in antigen-specific IgE responses, we immunized mice with alum-precipitated-DNP-OA and analyzed DNP-specific IgE after primary and secondary immunization.CD23-deficient mice could mount anti-DNP IgE responses comparable to those of wild-type mice. When mice were immunized with alum-precipitated antigen and Bordetella pertusis, CD23-deficient mice produced several fold increased IgE antibodies compared to wild-type mice. The above experiments were performed using the mice carrying the genetic background of (B6 x 129)F2. Since we used the 129-derived embryonic stem (ES) cell line for targeting of the CD23 gene, we could produce CD23-deficient 129 mice by crossing ES cell-derived chimera mice to 129 mice. Unexpectedly, enhanced IgE responses were not observed in CD23-deficient 129 mice immunized with alum-precipitated antigen + B. pertusis. These results suggests that CD23 may have a role in negative regulation in specific IgE responses although such regulation may be dependent on the genetic background. In addition, our finding may also provide a new insight to the genetic control of atopic diseases.

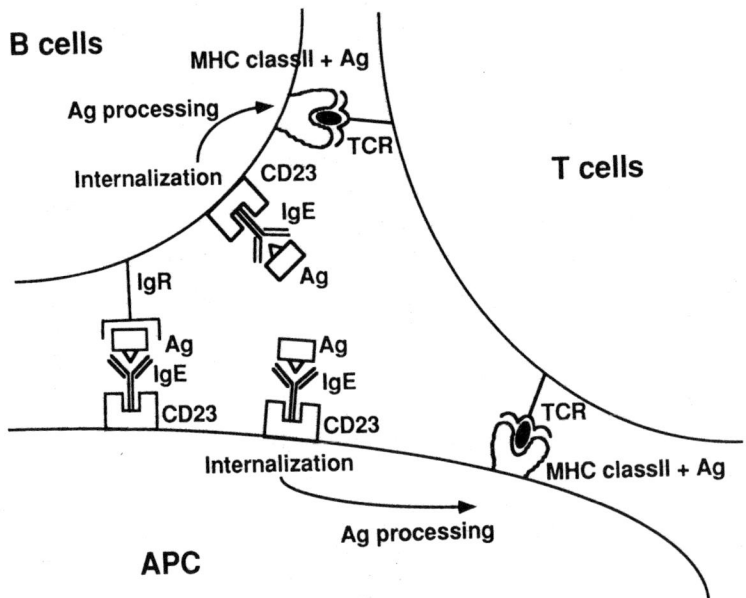

Figure 2. IgE-mediated antigen-focusing and augmentation of specific immune responses.

3.3. The Absence of IgE-Mediated Enhancement of Antibody Responses in CD23-Deficient Mice

CD23 has been shown to be involved in IgE-antibody-mediated antigen focusing of human[25] and mouse B cells[26] and IgE antibody-mediated enhancement of specific immune responses in mouse[27]. When DNP-OA was injected i.v., neither CD23-deficient mice nor wild-type mice could produce appreciable amounts of anti-OA IgG antibodies. Injection of anti-DNP IgE prior to DNP-OA immunization could induce significant anti-OA IgG responses in wild-type mice. In contrast, CD23-deficient mice failed to mount anti-carrier IgG responses even when they received anti-DNP IgE treatment, suggesting that IgE-dependent antigen focusing is hampered in the CD23-deficient mice (Figure 2).

4. CONCLUSION

In CD40-deficient mice, T-dependent Ig class switching and germinal center formation were completely abrogated. These findings directly demonstrate that a signal via CD40 is necessary for differentiation of B cells to IgE producing cells. In addition, we show that CD40 play a critical role in the immune response to L. major infection. At present, we do not know how CD40 is involved in resolution of L. major infection. However, there are two possibilities; 1) CD40 on antigen presenting cells may be required for induction of Th1 helper cells that produce IFN-γ, or 2) engagement of CD40 with CD40L on helper T cells can activate macrophages to kill intracytoplasmic parasites. Both Th1/Th2 development and macrophage activation are important events in cellular responses of atopic diseases. Therefore, the elucidation of CD40 function in cellular immune responses will be of great help to understand atopic immune responses.

Lymphocyte and myeloid development of CD23-deficient mice appear to be normal although human soluble CD23 has been shown to induce the growth of B cells and myeloid precursors and the maturation of thymocyte. Therefore, murine CD23 may not have such functions or its activities on these cells may be compensated by other molecules in the mutant mice. Our results also show that CD23 has a role in negative regulation of IgE responses, which is in good agreement with the finding by Yu et al[28]. This function, however, appears to be dependent on a certain genetic background. Additional function of CD23 is its role in IgE-mediated enhancement of specific antibody responses. This phenomenon may be due to IgE-mediated antigen focusing by antigen presenting cells. In the physiological state, extremely small amounts of allergen or pathogen may not be able to elicit an immune response. In the presence of high concentration of specific IgE antibodies in the airway, gastrointestinal tract, or skin, antigens can be captured or focused by CD23 on antigen presenting cells to T cells, resulting in augmentation of specific immune responses.

REFERENCES

1. Paul, W. E. & Seder, R. Cell 76, 241 (1994)
2. Gascan, H., Gauchat, J. F., Aversa, G., Van Vlasselaer, P. & de Vries, J. E. J. J. Immunol. 147, 8 (1991)
3. Armitage, R. J., Fanslow, W. C., Strockbine, L., Sato, T. A., Clifford, K. N., Macduff, B. M., Anderson, D. M., Gimpel, S. D., Davis-Smith, T., Maliszewski, C. R., Clark, E. A., Smith, C. A., Grabstein, K. H., Cosman, D., & Spriggs, M. K. Nature 357, 80 (1992)

4. Allen, R. C., Armitage, R. J., Conley, M. E., Rosenblatt, H., Jenkins, N. A., Copeland, N. G., Bedell, M. A., Edelhoff, S., Disteche, C. M., Simoneaux, D. K., Fanslow, W. C., Belmont, J., & Spriggs, M. K. *Science* 259, 990 (1993)

5. Aruffo, A., Farrington, M., Noelle, R. J., Ledbetter, J. A., Franke, U., & Ocks, H. D. *Cell* 72, 291 (1993)

6. Disanto, J. P., Bonnefoy, J. Y., Gauchat, J. F., Fischer, A., & de Saint Basile, G. *Nature* 361, 541 (1993)

7. Kikutani, H., Inui, S., Sato, R., Barsumian, E. L., Owaki, H., Yamasaki, K., Kaisho, T., Uchibayashi, N., Hardy, R. R., Hirano, T., Tsunasawa, S., Sakiyama, F., Suemura, M. & Kishimoto, T. Cell 47, 657 (1986)

8. Yukawa, K., Kikutani, H., Owaki, H., Yamasaki, K., Yokota, A., Nakamura, H., Barsumian, E. L., Hardy, R. R., Suemura, M, & Kishimto, T. J. Immunol. 138, 2576 (1987)

9. Bonnefoy, J. -Y., Shield, J., & Mermod, J. J. *Eur. J. Immunol.* 20, 139 (1990)

10. Sarfati, M. & Delespesse, G. *J. Immunol.* 141, 2195 (1988)

11. Flores-Romo, L., Shields, J., Humbert, Y., Graber, P., Aubry, J.-P., Gauchat, J.-F., Ayala, B., Chavez, M., Bazin, H., Capron, M. & Bonnefoy, J.-Y. *Science* 261, 1038 (1993)

12. Aubry, J.-P., Pochon, S., Graber, P., Jansen, K. U. & Bonnefoy, J.-Y. Nature 358, 505 (1992)

13. Kawabe, T., Naka, T., Yoshida, K., Tanaka, T., Fujiwara, H., Suematsu, S., Yoshida, N., Kishimoto, T. & Kikutani, H. *Immunity* 1, 167 (1994)

14. Fujiwara, H., Kikutani, H., Suematsu, S., Naka, T., Yoshida, K., Yoshida, K., Tanaka, T., Suemura, M., Matsumoto, N., Kojima, S., Kishimoto, T. & Yoshida, N. *Proc. Natl. Acad. Sci, USA.* 91, 6835 (1994)

15. Mongini, P. K. A., Stein, K. E. & Paul. W. E. *J. Exp. Med.* 153, 1 (1981)

16. Maclennan, I. C. M., Liu, Y.-J. & Johnson, G. D. *Immunol. Rev.* 126, 143 (1992)

17. Nortarangelo, L. D., Duse, M. & Ugazio, A. G. *Immunodef. Rev.* 3, 101 (1992)

18. Coffman, R. L., Varkila, K., Scott, P. & Chatelain, R. *Immunol. Rev.* 123, 189 (1991)

19. Kikutani, H., Suemura, M., Owaki, H., Nakamura, H., Sato, R., Yamasaki, K., Barsumian, E. L., Hardy, R. R. & Kishimoto, T. *J. Exp. Med.* 164, 1455 (1986)

20. Waldschmidt, T. J., Conrad, D. H. & Lynch, R. G. *J. Immunol.* 140, 2148 (1988)

21. Gordon, J., Carin, J. A., Millisum, M. J., Gillis, S. & Guy, G. R. *Eur. J. Immunol.* 18, 1561 (1988)

22. Liu, Y.-J., Carin, J. A., Holder, M. J., Abbot, S.D., Jansen, K. U., Bonnefoy, J.-Y., Gordon, J. & MacLennan, I. C. M. Eur. *J. Immunol.* 21, 1107 (1991)

23. Mossalayi, M. D., Arock, M., Bertho, J. M., Blanc, C., Dalloul, A. H., Hofstetter, H., Safarti, M., Delespesse, G. & Debre, P. *Blood* 75, 1924 (1990)

24. Mossalayi, M. D., Lecron, J. C., Dalloul, A. H., Safarti, M., Bertho, J. M., Hofstetter, H., Delespesse, G. & Debre, P. *J. Exp. Med.* 171, 959 (1990)

25. Pirron, U., Schlunck, T., Prinz, J. C. & Rieber, E. P. *Eur. J. Immunol.* 20, 1547 (1990)

26. Kehry, M. R. & Yamashita, L. C. *Proc. Natl. Acad. Sci. USA* 86, 7556 (1989)

27. Heyman, B., Tianmin, L. & Gustavsson, S. *Eur. J. Immunol.* 23, 1739 (1993)

28. Yu, P., Kosco-Vilbois, M., Richards, M., Koehler, G. & Lamers, M. C. *Nature* 369 753 (1994)

50

ABSENCE OF MUTATIONS IN THE 6TH EXON OF FcεRI-β

K. A. Deichmann, F. Hildebrandt, A. Heinzmann, S. Schlenther, J. Forster, and J. Kuehr

University Children´s Hospital
Freiburg, Germany

1. INTRODUCTION

In 1989, Cookson et al first reported close linkage between immunoglobulin E responses underlying allergic asthma and rhinitis and a locus on chromosome 11q13[1]. In the following years the same group succeeded in localizing the β-chain of the high affinity IgE receptor (FcεRI-β) in the same chromosomal region, thereby demonstrating close genetic linkage to the atopic state[2]. Their results were marked by the identification of a mutation (Ile181Leu) in the 6th exon of the gene in a region that codes for the 4th transmembrane domain of the protein being associated with positive IgE responses[3]. This mutation could explain about 25% of the subgroup of atopic, symptomatic cases that were shown to be linked to 11q13 in their population. However, transmission of atopy at the 11q13 locus as well as the predictive value of the mutation could only be found through maternally derived alleles[3,4].

The maternally linked inheritance of specific IgE responses corresponded well with population based data of our own previous studies[5]. The analysis of specific IgE immune responses against environmental allergens within 302 nuclear families showed that maternal and not paternal sensitization was predictive for the child´s reactivity in skin prick testing.

Thus we started to examine our population regarding presence of the mutation FcεRI-β/Ile181Leu in order to get more information about its frequency and its relation to atopy in a well defined unselected sample.

2. MATERIAL AND METHODS

2.1. Population

463 randomly contacted families with school children from the area of Freiburg city and a small community in the Black Forest participated in our first study. The status of

New Horizons in Allergy Immunotherapy
edited by Sehon et al. Plenum Press, New York, 1996

355

sensitization of all family members was verified by 3 consecutive skin prick tests (SPT) using standardized test-procedures and standardized aero-allergens (mixture of grass pollens, birch pollens, Dpt, cat dander; ALK). 302 families underwent all 3 SPTs in all family members. Families showing at least one sensitized member were asked for participation in our present study. Sixtyfour (52%) of the target population of 123 families participated.

2.2. Immunology

Specific IgE was detected by immuno chemiluminescence assay against two mixtures of grass pollens, Dpt, Df, cat dander and birch pollens (Magic Lite; ALK). Measurement of total serum IgE was carried out by an enzyme-linked allergosorbent test (Phadezym PRIST; Pharmacia). Atopy was defined as the presence of one or more positive skin prick tests and/or detection of specific IgE against one or more inhalant allergens and/or high total serum IgE concentrations (i.e. above the 75%-level in the population studied).

2.3. Molecular Biology

DNA was extracted by standard methods and column-purified (Quiagen). Sequencing was performed on all children of families presenting with at least one affected child (128 children from 53 families). The region of interest was amplified by PCR from genomic DNA (see figure) followed by asymmetric PCR in order to obtain single-strand DNA suited for direct sequencing. Sequencing by the dideoxy chain termination method was done using DIG-labeled primers and immunologic detection (Boehringer, Mannheim). All doubtful sequencing results have been confirmed by sequencing from both sides of the region of interest. In about a third of the children sequencing spanned all of the 6th exon.

Genotyping and phenotyping were carried out randomised and double blind.

3. RESULTS

The mutation Ile181Leu affecting the 4th transmembrane domain of FcεRI-β was not found in any of the 128 children of 53 unrelated nuclear families investigated. Furthermore, all genotypes studied so far corresponded to the "wildtype" as published by Küster et al. in 1992[6]. We could not find any mutation of the 6th exon of FcεRI-β in any child examined.

4. CONCLUSIONS

Taking in regard the results of Cookson's group we should have expected the mutation Ile181Leu to segregate in about 9 families and to affect about 20 children. However, there was no mutation at all detectable in the 6th exon. The easiest explanation for this finding would be that the mutation Ile181Leu is much rarer in our population. However, technical aspects have to be discussed as well in interpreting these results. The mutation within the 6th exon of FcεRI-β is in close vicinity to a GC tandem repeat, a highly polymorphic region within the 5th intron of the gene. Our PCR product also contained this region (see fig. 1). Under the assumption of linkage disequilibrium of specific alleles of this GC repeat and the mutation one could explain these results as technical artefacts if there

TCCCCTCAAC CCAGGCAAAT TCCTCGGGGT TA<u>AAGTTATC TACTGCAAGT</u>

Amplification Primer 1

<u>GACGATCTCT</u> GGGTTTTTCT GTGCCTGTGT TTGTGTGTGT GTGTGTGTGT

GTGTGTGTGT GTATGTGTCA CTTTAAAAGG ACTGGTCAGA TGGTAGGG<u>AG</u>

<u>ATGAAAACAG GAGATGCTAT AAG</u>AAAATAA ACTTTTGGGG CGAATACCAA

Forward Sequencing Primer

TGTGACTCTT TTTGTTTGTC ATTTGTTGCT GTTCAATAG **G A**<u>**A**</u>**A**<u>**TT**</u>**GTAGT**

AA 181

GATGATGCTG TTTCTCACCA TTCTGGGACT TGGTAGTGCT GTGTCACTA

Exon 6

CAATCTGTGG AGCTGGGGAA GAACTCAAAG GAAACAAG GT AGATAGAAGC

CCGATATAAA ATCTTGAATG ACAG<u>GTTAAC GAATTGGAGC TTTATTCCTT</u>

Reverse Sequencing Primer

AAA<u>ATATGGC CTGGGTTTTC TGAAACATTT C</u>TTCCAGAAA ATAGTTTCTC

Amplification Primer 2

Figure 1. The 6th exon of FcεRI-β and the adjacent genomic sequences; the coding sequence is indicated in bold letters, the primers for amplification and sequencing and the triplet coding for Ile181 are underlined.

were differences in the amplification efficacy of different polymorphic alleles. However, this seems unlikely and it should not account for individuals homozygotic for the mutation. Taking the given frequency in the population examined by Cookson et al, we should have expected 1 or 2 homozygotes.

So we conclude, that the mutation Ile181Leu within the 4th transmembrane domaine of FcεRI-β is not a common finding in our population which is in contrast to the population examined by Cookson et al.

Furthermore, we could not find any other mutation in the 6th exon of FcεRI-β. Provided that FcεRI-β is directly involved in the development of atopy we should expect other variants or mutations of the gene affecting the remaining 6 exons, the splice-sites or the control regions in cis-acting site.

On the basis of the known predictive value of maternal but not paternal sensitization in our population and considering the lack of the mutation Ile181Leu we might expect to find further mutations in the same gene as an explanation for the effect of the predictive parental origin. Alternatively, we might expect other genes to contribute to the maternal effect on phenotype development.

5. ACKNOWLEDGMENTS

We would like to thank Mrs. Ch. Mehl for collecting the blood, Mrs. S. Sparholt from ALK for the data on specific sensitization in all the family members and Mrs. D. Feigl for total IgE testing. Finally, we thank all the families who participated in this study for their support and help. This work is supported by the Deutsche Forschungs Gemeinschaft (DFG), sign De386/2–1.

6. REFERENCES

1. Cookson, W.C.O.M. et al., The Lancet i: 1292–95 (1989)
2. Sandford, A.J. et al., The Lancet i: 332–34 (1993)
3. Shirakawa, T., Nature Genetics: 125–30 (1994)
4. Cookson, W.C.O.M. et al., The Lancet ii: 381–4 (1992)
5. Kuehr, J. et al., Clin Exp Allergy 23: 600–5 (1993)
6. Kuester, H. et al., J Biol Chem. 267: 12782–7 (1992)

51

ROLE OF TYPE 2 T HELPER CELLS (TH2) IN ALLERGIC DISORDERS

P. Parronchi, S. Sampognaro, E. Maggi, and S. Romagnani

Istituto di Medicina Interna e Immunoallergologia
University of Florence, Italy

1. THE TH1/TH2 POLARIZATION

In the last few years evidence has been provided to suggest the existence of functionally distinct subsets of CD4[+] Th cells in both mice and humans (1, 2). At least two polarized forms of the specific Th cell-mediated response, based on their distinct and mutually exclusive pattern of cytokine secretion, have been described. Th1, but not Th2 cells produce IFN-γ and TNF-β, whereas Th2, but not Th1, produce IL-4 and IL-5. Production of other cytokines, such as IL-2, IL-10, and IL-13 is less restricted in humans than in mice, although IL-2 is mainly released by Th1 cells, whereas IL-10 and IL-13 are mainly released by Th2 cells. Different cytokine patterns imply distinct effector functions. Th1 cells, which trigger both cell-mediated immunity and production of opsonizing antibodies mediate phagocyte-dependent defence in response to intracellular infectious agents (3). In contrast, Th2 cells are responsible for IgE and IgG$_4$ antibody production, promote the differentiation and activation of mast cells and eosinophils, but they inhibit several macrophage functions, thus being primarily involved in the phagocyte-independent defence against extra-cellular parasites (3). In addition to cells that fit into the Th1- or Th2-polarized phenotypes, CD4+ Th cells have been identified (Th0 cells), that show a composite profile including production of both Th1- and Th2-type cytokines and mediate effects that depend on the ratio of cytokines produced (3). More recently, human T-cell clones producing Th2 cytokines were found to differ from those producing Th1 cytokines even for the consistent expression of CD30 (4), a member of the TNF-R superfamily (5), as well as for release of its soluble form (sCD30) (4,6).

2. ROLE OF ALLERGEN-SPECIFIC TH2 CELLS IN THE PATHOGENESIS OF ALLERGY

The analysis of cytokine production by T-cell clones specific for different antigens has clearly shown that, in contrast to clones specific for bacterial antigens that show a prevalent

New Horizons in Allergy Immunotherapy
edited by Sehon et al. Plenum Press, New York, 1996

359

Th1/Th0 phenotype, the great majority of allergen-specific T-cell clones generated from peripheral blood lymphocytes of atopic donors express a Th0/Th2 phenotype, with high production of IL-4 and IL-5 and no or low production of IFN-γ (7, 8). Evidence suggesting that Th2-like cells accumulate at level of target organs in different allergic disorders has been provided by using either cloning techniques or *in situ* hybridization. Upon mitogen stimulation, the majority of T-cell clones generated from the conjunctival infiltrates of patients with vernal conjunctivitis (a disease in which an allergic pathogenesis is suspected but not proved) were found to develop into Th2 clones (9). Using *in situ* hybridization, cells showing mRNA for Th2, but not Th1, cytokines were detected at the site of late phase skin reactions in skin biopsies from atopic patients, in mucosal bronchial biopsies or bronchoalveolar lavage (BAL) from patients with asthma (10–12). More importantly, proportions ranging from 14 to 22% of T-cell clones, generated from airway mucosae of grass-allergic patients following inhalation challenge with grass pollen, appeared to be specific for grass allergens and most of them exhibited a definite Th2 profile (13). Since the demonstration that CD30 is preferentially expressed by T-cell clones able to produce Th2-type cytokines (4), CD30 expression was evaluated in circulating CD4$^+$ T cells from six grass pollen-sensitive patients and six nonatopic controls before and during the seasonal exposure to grass pollens. No CD4$^+$CD30$^+$ cells were detected in any of nonatopic donors or the atopic patients examined before the grass pollination season, whereas four out of six grass-sensitive donors examined during the season, when they were suffering from allergic symptoms, showed small proportions of circulating CD4$^+$CD30$^+$ cells (from 0.08 to 0.3%). Circulating CD4$^+$ T cells from these patients were fractionated into CD30$^+$ and CD30$^-$ cells by sorting with an anti-CD30 monoclonal antibody, the two cell fractions expanded by culturing in IL-2, and then assessed for their ability to produce type 1 (IFN-β and TNF-β) or type 2 (IL-4 and IL-5) cytokines and to proliferate in response to Lolium perenne group I (Lol p I) allergen. Only CD30$^+$ cells proliferated in response to Lol p I and exhibited the ability to produce IL-4 and IL-5, whereas production of both IFN-γ and TNF-β was prevalent in the CD30$^-$ cell fractions (4). These findings clearly demonstrate that grass allergen-reactive CD4$^+$CD30$^+$ T cells, inducible to the production of Th2 cytokines, can circulate in the peripheral blood of grass sensitive patients during the *in vivo* natural exposure to grass pollen allergens. More recently, we have found high numbers of CD30+ cells in the skin biopsies of patients with atopic dermatitis (P. Fabbri et al., unpublished results).

3. REGULATORY MECHANISMS OF TH2 DEVELOPMENT

The mechanisms responsible for the preferential development of allergen-reactive Th2 cells in atopic subjects have not yet been completely clarified. Attention has been focused on the possible role of antigen-presenting cells (APC), the T cell repertoire and cytokines present in the microenvironment at the time of allergen presentation. Recently, we have found that CD30 ligation on activated T cells favors their development into Th2-like T-cell clones, whereas blocking of CD30 ligand on APC may shift the *in vitro* differentiation of allergen-specific T cells from the Th0/Th2 to the Th0/Th1 phenotype (14).

The role of the T cell repertoire in determining the development of Th1 or Th2-type responses is still matter of controversies. Evidence for the pivotal role of specific Vβ-expressing T cell subsets in the stimulation of IgE production and increased airways responsiveness induced by ragweed allergen has been reported (15). More recently, we have found a restricted Vβ repertoire in allergen-specific T cell lines, which appeared to be associated with their profile of cytokine production (Parronchi et al., submitted for publication). Thus, it cannot be excluded that the recognition of allergen by the TCR provides a signal or sets of signals that drive the T cells in a certain direction, e.g. to produce IL-4 or alternatively, IFN-γ.

So far, however, the clearest examples of factors affecting the differentiation pathways of both murine and human Th cells appear to be cytokines released by APC and/or other cell types at the time of antigen presentation. Thus, IFN-α, IL-12 and TGF-β produced by macrophages and B cells particularly in response to intracellular bacteria have been shown to play an important role in the induction of Th1 expansion in various systems (16). IFN-γ, which is produced mainly by T cells and NK cells, also promotes the differentiation of Th1 cells (17). Likewise IL-12, a powerful IFN-γ inducer, appears to be the most important natural initiator of Th1 responses by acting either directly or indirectly via the induction of IFN-γ production (18).

The effect of cytokines produced by macrophages and/or B cells on the development of Th2 cells seems to be less critical. IL-10 has been shown to favor the development of Th2 cells both in mouse and man. IL-1 is a selective co-factor for the growth of some murine Th2 clones and can favor the in vitro development of human Th2-like clones (19). However, most striking is the requirement for IL-4 for maturation of Th cells into Th2 cells. In both murine and human systems, IL-4 appears to be the most dominant factor in determining the liklihood for Th2 polarization in cultured cells (17, 20). Accordingly, IL-4-gene-targeted mice fail to generate mature Th2 cells in vivo and to produce IgE antibodies (21), suggesting that early IL-4 production by another cell type must be involved. Possible candidates include a peculiar CD4$^+$ NK1.1$^+$ T-cell subset (22), as well as mast cells and basophils, which have been shown to release stored IL-4 in response to FcεR triggering (23, 24). However, parasites or allergens would be unable to crosslink these receptors prior to a specific immune response that had produced parasite-specific IgG and IgE antibodies. On the other hand, mast cell-deficient mice develop normal Th2 responses (25). Thus, IL-4 production by mast cells triggered by antigen-IgE antibody immune complexes may play a role in amplifying secondary responses to parasites, but cannot account for the Th2 development in primary immune responses. The possibility we favour is that naive Th cells themselves can produce sufficient IL-4 amounts required for the development of Th2 cells. Therefore, the fact that allergens induce Th2-type responses only in selected people suggests that atopic individuals would have genetic disregulation in the production of IL-4 and/or of cytokines exerting regulatory effects on the development and/or function of Th2 cells. The recent demonstration that one or more polymorphisms exist in a coding region or, more probably, in a regulatory region of the IL-4 gene (26) strongly argues in favor of such a possibility.

ACKNOWLEDGMENTS

The experiments reported in this paper have been performed by grants from C.N.R. (Progetto Strategico Citochine) and by EU (Biotech Project)

REFERENCES

1. Mosmann T.R., Cherwinski H., Bond M.W., Giedlin M.A., Coffman R.L. (1986) Two types of murine helper T-cell clone. I. Definition according to profiles of lymphokine activities and secreted proteins. *Journal of Immunology* 136, 2348–2356
2. Romagnani S. (1991) Human Th1 and Th2: doubt no more. *Immunology Today* 12, 256–258

3. Romagnani S. (1994a) Lymphokine Production by Human T Cells in Disease States. *Annual Reviews of Immunology* 12, 227–257

4. Del Prete G.F., De Carli M., Almerigogna F., Daniel C.K., D'Elios M.M., Zancuoghi G., Pizzolo G., Romagnani S. (1995) Preferential Expression of CD30 by Human CD4+ T Cells Producing Th2-type Cytokines. *FASEB Journal* 9, 81–86

5. Smith C.A., Gruss H-J., Davis T., Anderson D., Farrah T., Baker E., Sutherland G.R., Brannan C.I., Copeland N.G., Jenkins N.A., Grabstein K.H., Gliniak B., McAlister I.B., Fanslow W., Alderson M., Falk B., Gimpel S., Gillis S., Din W.S., Goodwin R.G., Armitage R.J. (1993) CD30 Antigen, a Marker for Hodgkin's Lymphoma, Is a Receptor whose Ligand Defines an Emerging Family of Cytokines with Homology to TNF. *Cell* 273, 1349–1360

6. Manetti R., Annunziato F., Biagiotti R., Giudizi M-G., Piccinni M-P., Giannarini L., Sampognaro S., Parronchi P., Vinante F., Pizzolo G., Maggi E., Romagnani S. (1994) CD30 expression by CD8+ T cells producing type 2 helper cytokines. Evidence for large numbers of CD8+CD30+ T cell clones in human immunodeficiency virus infection. *Journal of Experimental Medicine* 180, 2407–2412

7. Wierenga E.A., Snoek M., de Groot C., Chretien I., Bos J.D., Jansen H.M., Kapsenberg M.L. (1990) Evidence for Compartmentalization of Functional Subsets of CD4+ T Lymphocytes in Atopic Patients. *Journal of Immunology* 144, 4651–4656

8. Parronchi P., Macchia D., Piccinni M-P., Biswas P., Simonelli C., Maggi E., Ricci M., Ansari A.A., Romagnani S. (1991) Allergen- and Bacterial Antigen-specific T-cell Clones Established from Atopic Donors Show a Different Profile of Cytokine Production. *Proceedings National Academy of Sciences USA* 88, 4538–4542

9. Maggi E., Biswas P., Del Prete G.F., Parronchi P., Macchia D., Simonelli C., Emmi L., De Carli M., Tiri A., Ricci M., Romagnani S. (1991) Accumulation of Th2-like Helper T Cells in the Conjunctiva of Patients with Vernal Conjunctivitis. *Journal of Immunology* 146, 1169–1174

10. Kay A.B., Ying S., Varney V., Gaga M., Durham S.R., Moqbel R., Wardlaw A.J., Hamid Q. (1991) Messanger RNA Expression of the Cytokine Gene Cluster, Interleukin 3 (IL-3), IL-4, IL-5, and Granulocyte/Macrophage Colony-Stimulating Factor, in Allergen-induced Late-phase Cutaneous Reactions in Atopic Subjects. *Journal of Experimental Medicine* 173, 775–778

11. Hamid Q., Azzawi M., Ying S., Moqbel R., Wardlaw A.J., Corrigan C.J., Bradley B., Durham S.R., Collins J.V., Jeffery P.K., Quint D.J., Kay A.B. (1991) Expression of mRNA for Interleukin-5 in Mucosal Bronchial Biopsics from Asthma. *Journal of Clinical Investigations* 87,1541–1546

12. Robinson D.S., Hamid Q., Ying S., Tsicopoulos A., Barkans J., Bentley A.M., Corrigan C.J., Durham S.R., Kay A.B. (1992) Predominant Th2-like Bronchoalveolar T-lymphocyte Population in Atopic Asthma. *New England Journal of Medicine* 326, 295–304

13. Del Prete G.F., De Carli M., D'Elios M.M., Maestrelli P., Ricci M., Fabbri L., Romagnani S (1993) Allergen Exposure Induces the Activation of Allergen-Specific Th2 Cells in the Airway Mucosa of Patients with Allergic Respiratory Disorders. *European Journal of Immunology* 23, 1445–1449

14. Del Prete G.F., De Carli M., D'Elios M.M., Daniel K.C., Smith C.A., Thomas E., Romagnani S (1995) CD30-mediated signalling promotes the development of human Th2-like T cells. *Journal of Experimental Medicine* (in press)

15. Renz H., Saloga J., Bradley K.L., Loader J.E., Greenstein J.L., Larsen G., Gelfand E.W. (1993) Specific Vβ T Cell Subsets Mediate the Immediate Hypersensitivity Response to Ragweed Allergen. *Journal of Immunology* 151, 1907–1917

16. Romagnani S. (1992) Induction of Th1 and Th2 Responses: a Key Role for the 'Natural' Immune Response ? *Immunology Today* 13, 379–380

17. Maggi E., Parronchi P., Manetti R., Simonelli C., Piccinni M-P., Santoni-Rugiu F., De Carli M., Ricci M., Romagnani S. (1992) Reciprocal regulatory role of IFN- and IL-4 on the in vitro development of human Th1 and Th2 clones. *Journal of Immunology* 148, 2142–2148

18. Manetti R., Parronchi P., Giudizi M-G., Piccinni M-P., Maggi E., Trinchieri G., Romagnani S. (1993) Natural Killer Cell Stimulatory Factor (Interleukin 12) Induces T Helper Type 1 (Th1)-specific Immune Responses and Inhibits the Development of IL-4-producing Th Cells. *Journal of Experimental Medicine* 177, 1199–1204

19. Romagnani S. (1994b) Regulation of Th2 development in allergy. *Current Opinion in Immunology* 6, 838–846

20. Swain S.L. (1993) IL-4 Dictates T-Cell Differentiation. *Research in Immunology* 144, 616–620

21. Kopf M., Le Gros G., Bachmann M., Lamers M.C., Bluthmann H., Kohler G. (1993) Disruption of the Murine IL-4 Gene Blocks Th2 Cytokine Responses. *Nature* 362, 245–248

22. Yashimoto T., Paul W.E. (1994) CD4^{pos}, NK1.1^{pos} T cells promptly produce interleukin 4 in response to in vivo challenge with anti-CD3. *Journal of Experimental Medicine* 179, 1285–1295

23. Bradding P., Feather I.H., Howarth P.H., Mueller R., Roberts J.A., Britten K., Bews J.P.A., Hunt T.C., Okayama Y., Heusser C.H., Bullock G.R., Church M.K., Holgate S.T. (1992) Interleukin 4 Is Localized and Released by Human Mast Cells. *Journal of Experimental Medicine* 76, 1381–1386

24. Brunner T., Heusser C.H., Dahinden C.A. (1993) Human Peripheral Blood Basophils Primed by Interleukin 3 (IL-3) Produce IL-4 in Response to Immunoglobulin E Receptor Stimulation. *Journal of Experimental Medicine* 177, 605–611

25. Wershil B.K., Theodos C.M., Galli S.J., Titus R.G. (1994) Mast cells augment lesion size and persistence during experimental Leishmania major infection in the mouse. *Journal of Immunology* 152, 4563–4571

26. Marsh D.G., Neely J.D., Breazeale D.R., Ghosh B., Freidhoff L.R., Ehrlich-Kautzky E., Schou C., Krishnaswamy G., Beaty T.H. (1994) Linkage analysis of IL-4 and other chromosome 5q31.1 markers and total serum immunoglobulin E concentration. *Science* 264, 1152–1156

52

DIVERSITY OF HUMAN T CELL RECEPTOR SEQUENCES OF T CELL CLONES WITH SPECIFICITY FOR Bet v 1 PEPTIDE/MHC II COMPLEXES

Heimo Breiteneder, Roswitha Hajek, Robert Hüttinger, Christof Ebner, Siegfried Schenk, Dietrich Kraft, and Otto Scheiner

Institute of General and Experimental Pathology
AKH-EBO-3Q, University of Vienna
Waehringer Guertel 18–20, 1090 Vienna, Austria
Tel. +43–1–40400–5102; Fax. +43–1–40400–5130

1. ABSTRACT

T cell clones (TCC) were raised from the peripheral blood of patients suffering from tree pollen allergy. All TCC were restricted by HLA-DR molecules. In order to investigate possible intervention targets in Type I allergic diseases, we have examined T cell receptor (TCR) α– and β-chain nucleotide sequences of several allergen-reactive human CD4$^+$ TCC specific for four frequently found epitopes of Bet v 1, the major birch pollen allergen. In general, TCC specific for the 4 epitopes investigated, used diverse TCRAV and TCRBV gene segments. Moreover, the junctional regions encoding the third complementarity determining regions (CDR3) of the TCR showed striking heterogeneities in length and amino acid composition. A more restricted use of two J gene segments (TCRBJ1S4 and 2S7) was only observed in the β-chain of TCR used by TCC specific for epitope 1. In addition, all TCC specific for epitope 4 showed an arginine residue in the N-terminal region of their TCRBV CDR3 loops despite their sequence diversities. In view of the striking heterogeneities found, therapeutical strategies aimed at the clonal deletion of allergen-specific T cell clones, providing help for IgE synthesis, may not be feasible. Moreover, our results cast a doubt on the theory, that the CDR3 exclusively provides the primary contact with the peptide bound in the major histocompatibility (MHC) groove, and suggest additional interaction with MHC class II.

2. INTRODUCTION

The T-cell antigen receptor (TCR) of mature T lymphocytes recognizes antigens in the form of short peptide fragments bound to major histocompatibility (MHC) molecules on the

New Horizons in Allergy Immunotherapy
edited by Sehon et al. Plenum Press, New York, 1996

365

surface of antigen-presenting cells (APC; Schwartz 1985). Over 90% of peripheral blood T lymphocytes express the TCR in the form of a disulfide linked heterodimer composed of a TCRα– and TCRβ–chain (Haskins et al. 1983; Meuer et al. 1983). Each chain consists of a variable region which confers the specificity of the TCR for the peptide/MHC-complex, and a constant region that attaches this variable region to the cell surface. During thymic matura-tion, unique variable region genes are created by recombination of germ-line-encoded vari-able (V), diversity (D, for the β-chain only) and joining (J) segments. Combinatorial diversity is generated by the joining of unique combinations of these segments as well as the random association of any α-chain with any β-chain. Further diversity of the variable domain is con-tributed by the loss (through nucleotide "nibbling") or template-independent addition of N-re-gion nucleotides at V-(D)-J junctions (Davis and Bjorkman 1988). The structure of the TCR is similar to that of Ig, containing three hypervariable loops that correspond to the complemen-tarity-determining regions (CDR) (Clothia et al. 1988). The CDR1 and CDR2 loops of the TCR are encoded by germ-line V-segment sequences and are believed to interact with the α-helices forming the side walls of the binding groove of the MHC molecules. In contrast, the CDR3 loops are encoded by the V-(D)-J juctional regions and are believed to provide the pri-mary contact with the peptide bound in the MHC binding groove (Davis and Bjorkman 1988; Clothia et al. 1988).

The precise involvement of specific TCR gene products in the recognition of par-ticular MHC molecules or peptide/MHC complexes is still unclear. The same holds true for the extent of diversity of TCR in TCC recognizing an identical peptide presented by the same or different MHC molecules.

In this work, we examined the TCR usage of human CD4$^+$ T cell clones specific for four frequently found T cell epitopes of the major birch pollen allergen, Bet v 1. These epitopes can be considered as a major epitopes of Bet v 1 (Ebner et al. 1993 a, b, c). A detailed charac-terization of TCC recognizing important allergen-derived T cell epitopes is a prerequisite for the development of therapeutic measures aimed at the deletion of specific TCC.

3. MATERIALS AND METHODS

3.1. Birch Pollen-Allergic Volunteers

The TCC studied in this paper were obtained from birch pollen-allergic patients. They all showed typical case histories, positive skin tests, and their sera displayed IgE-binding to Bet v 1, the major birch pollen allergen.

3.2. Bet v 1 and Bet v 1 Peptides

Recombinant Bet v 1 was expressed in *E. coli* as a non-fusion protein and purified as described (Ferreira et al. 1993). A panel of 75 overlapping peptides was synthesized ac-cording to the Bet v 1 sequence and used for epitope mapping of TCC as described (Ebner et al. 1993 a).

3.3. Bet v 1-Specific T Cell Clones

Short term T cell lines (TCL) were generated by incubating PBMC of birch pollen-allergic donors with Bet v 1. The specificity of TCC was assessed and epitope mapping was performed as previously described (Ebner et al. 1993 a).

3.4. HLA-Typing and Restriction

HLA-DR typing of patients was performed according to methods described (Fischer et al. 1992). Using the antibody L243, which recognizes a determinant common to all DR molecules, proliferation in response to stimulation with Bet v 1 could be blocked in all TCC in a dose dependent manner, indicating restriction by HLA-DR molecules.

3.5. Isolation of RNA, cDNA Synthesis, and PCR

Total RNA was prepared from 1×10^6 cells by the a single step guanidinium-isothio-cyanate-phenol-chlorofom extraction method (Chomczynski and Sacchi 1987). Single-stranded cDNA synthesis was carried out on 1.2 - 1.8 µg of total RNA. PCR was performed by amplification of TCRα and β cDNA with oligonucleotide primers complementary to TCR V and C region sequences (Panzara et al. 1992; Genevée et al. 1992).

3.6. Cloning and Sequence Analysis of Amplified TCR Gene Products

The PCR reaction products were cloned and sequenced. For each of the TCRα- and β-chains studied three independent subclones were sequenced. Sequences were compared with gene data bank entries and to available published TCR J segments (Klein et al. 1987; Yoshikai et al. 1986; Kimura et al. 1987; Roman-Roman et al. 1991; Concannon et al. 1986; Kimura et al. 1986; Toyonaga et al. 1985).

4. RESULTS

4.1. T Cell Clones and HLA Typing

TCC were established from the peripheral blood of birch pollen allergic donors. HLA typing revealed the following MHC class II types for the donors. XPAA: DRB1*13, 13; DRB3. XPAS: DRB1*07, 14; DRB3, DRB4. XPBE: DRB1*07, 07; DRB4. XPBP: DRB1*11, 16; DRB3, DRB5. XPHC: DRB1*07, 11; DRB3, DRB4. XPMS: DRB1*04, 13; DRB4, DRB5. XPSZ: DRB1*07, 15; DRB4, DRB5. XPTF: DRB1*07, 15; DRB4, DRB5. XPWD: DRB1*07, 07; DRB4; XPRR: DRB1*07, 16; DRB4, DRB5. All clones revealed the helper cell phenotype (CD3$^+$, CD4$^+$) and expressed the TCRαβ.

4.2. Peptide Specificity of Bet v 1-Specific T Cell Clones

The panel of TCC derived from allergic donors could be divided into four groups. Each group was composed of TCC recognizing the same frequently occurring Bet v 1 peptide in the context of HLA-DR molecules. Six TCC were responsive to Bet v 1 epitope 1 spanning aa positions 77–92 (TNFKYNYSVIEGGPIG), 4 TCC were specific for epitope 2 with the sequence aa 93–108 (DTLEKISNEIKIVATP), 5 TCC were reactive to epitope 3 spanning aa 113–126 (ILKISNKYHTKGDH), and 5 TCC were responsive to epitope 4 with the sequence aa 144–154 (LRAVESYLLA) as shown in Table 1.

Table 1. TCR usage in recognition of four Bet v 1 epitopes

patient	TCC	TCRAV	TCRAJ	TCRBV	TCRBJ
epitope 1	^{77}TNFKYNYSVIEGGPIG^{92}				
XPHC	5 I	12S1	4S1	5S1	1S4
	8 III	8S1	16S1	5S2/3	2S7
XPSZ	11 II	17S1	17S11	6S2/3	2S7
	31 II	8S2	9S7	12S2	1S4
	31 II	12S1	14S3		
XPBP	53 I	2S2	1S1	2S3	1S4
	173 I	2S1	17S6	2S3	1S4
epitope 2	^{93}DTLEKISNEIKIVATP^{108}				
XPHC	2 III	5S1	26S7	6S2/3	1S1
XPSZ	97 III	18S1	9S5	5S2/3	2S1
				5S2/3	2S1
XPMS	2 I	2S1	9S16	12S2	1S2
XPTF	1 I	8S1	17S7	5S1	2S3
epitope 3	^{113}ILKISNKYHTKGDH^{126}				
XPHC	33 I	6S1	9S6	13S2	2S7
	46 IV	2S1	17S1	13S3	1S2
	46 IV	11S1	3S2		
XPAS	16 I	8S2	14S3	6S2/3	2S7
	27 I	8S2	9S15	13S5	1S1
XPAA	4 I	13S1	9S10	14S1	1S4
epitope 4	^{144}LRAVESYLLA^{154}				
XPBE	15 I	11S1	15S3	24S1	2S2
XPSZ	10 IV	2S3	17S7	17S1	2S3
XPWD	25 II	5S1	16S7	2S3	1S5
XPRR	4 I	8S1	9S5	15S1	2S5
XPTF	10 I	8S2	9S15	2S3	2S4
	10 I	9S1	9S3		

4.3. Epitope Specific TCC Use Multiple TCR V and J Genes

TCRα- and β-chain sequences of TCC reactive with Bet v 1 were analyzed according to the following criteria: use of TCRAV and BV genes (Tab. 1), use of TCRJ gene segments (Tab. 1), length of the CDR3 (data not shown for epitopes 1–3, Fig. 1A and 1B), selection for amino acid residues especially through N-region additions (data not shown for epitopes 1–3, Fig. 1 and 1B).

Epitope 1 (Tab. 1). The data for the TCRα-chain revealed a diverse use of V and J genes in the human response against this epitope peptide. No preferential TCR gene usage was detectable. Jα segment usage was diverse, each TCC used a different Jα segment. The sequences of the CDR3 loops were quite heterogeneous and there was no conservation in their length (8–15 aa; data not shown). TCC XPSZ 31 II yielded transcripts for two α-chains (Tab. 1). On the contrary, for the β-chains of the same TCC, the selection was much narrower. The J segment usage was restricted to 1S4 (2 TCC) and 2S7 (4 TCC) with most of their germline sequence still present (Tab. 1). The length of the CDR3 was quite uniform (9–10 aa, data not shown).

Epitope 2. TCR junctional region sequences of TCC specific for this epitope did not show selection for specific gene segments, sequence motifs or certain amino acid residues. There was no conservation in the length of the α-chain CDR3 (9–13 aa, data not shown). Only the β-chain CDR3 showed a more uniform length of 9–10 aa residues (data not shown). Interestingly, TCC XPSZ showed the presence of two TCRB transcripts coding for two different β chains.

Epitope 3. With the exception of TCRAV8S2 for TCC XPAS 16 I and 27 I A, a biased use of gene segments was not detected in the α– chains (Tab. 1). The TCC XPHC 46 IV showed two mRNAs coding for two different α-chains. Although the β-chains used the TCRBV family 13 in 3 of 5 TCC, they did not display the uniform length of their CDR3, which now ranged from 7–10 aa (Tab. 1).

Epiotope 4. Two of the TCC expressed the closely related TCRAV8S1 and 8S2 gene segments (XPRR4 and XPTF10, respectively, Fig. 1A). All other TCRAV gene segments were drawn from different families. Two transcripts for α-chains were detected for TCC XPF10. The use of TCRBV2S3 was revealed in two (XPWD 25 II and XPTF10 I) of the 5 TCC, each of the other three TCC expressed a different TCRBV family member (Fig. 1B). Each TCC used an AJ and BJ segment different from the ones found in the other TCC (Tab. 1). The diverse J region gene usage and variability in sequences used was reflected in the heterogencity of CDR3 regions of both α– and β–chain. Their lengths varied greatly, with 8–12 aa for the α CDR3, and 6–14 aa for the β CDR3 (Fig. 1A and B). Interestingly, a positively charged basic residue (R, boxed) was observed in the amino-terminal portion of the TCRBV CDR3 loops of all TCC investigated (Fig. 1B).

5. DISCUSSION

One of the key roles in the development of allergies is played by the T cell an its receptor. In a first reaction step, the TCR interacts with the allergenic peptide presented by the MHC II molecule on the surface of the antigen presenting cells. This interaction initi-

A

144LRAVESYLLA154

T cell clone	TCRA gene segments	TCRAV	CDR3 (8-12)	TCRAJ	TCRAC
XPBE15	AV11S1J1S3C	GAGGCAGAATGCTGCTGTTACTACTGTGCT E A D A A V Y Y C A	GTGGGGCTGCATCAGGAGGAAGCTACATACCTACA V G A A S G G S Y I P T	TTTGGAAGAGGAACCAGCCTTATTGTTCATCCG F G R G T S L I V H P	TATATCCAG Y I Q
XPS210	AV2S3J17S7C	CTCAGTGATTCAGCCACCTACCTCTGTGTG L S D S A T Y L C V	GTGAACACTGCCAGTAAACTCACC V N T A S K L T	TTTGGGACTGGAACAAGACTTCAGTCACGCTC F G T G T R L Q V T L	GATATCCAG D I Q
XPWD25	AV5S1J16S7C	AATGCAGACTCAGCTACCTACCTCTGTGCT N A D S A T Y L C A	CTAGTGGGAACTTCAACAAATTTAC L V G N F N K F Y	TTTGGGATCTGGGACCAAACTCAATGTAAAACCA F G S G T K L N V K P	AAATCCAG N I Q
XPRR4	AV8S1J9S5C	CCTGAAGACTCGGCTGTCTACTTCTGTGCA P E D S A V Y F C A	GCAAGTAACGGCCAGGCAGGAACTGCTCTGATC A S N G Q A G T A L I	TTTGGGAGGGAACTCCTTATCACTGAGTTCC F G K G T T L S V S S	AAATCCAG N I Q
XPTF10	AV8S2J9S15C	CCTGGAGACTCAGCTGTCTACTTTTGTGCA P G D S A V Y F C A	GAGATGATGAATTCAGGATACAGCACCCTCACC E M M N S G Y S T L T	TTTGGGAGGGGACTATGCTTCTCTAGTCTCTCCA F G K G T M L L V S P	GATATCCAG D I Q
XPTF10	AV9S1J9S3C	GAGGAAGACTCAGCCATGTATTACTGTGCC E E D S A M Y Y C A	TCTAAGAGTAGTGGAGGTAGCAACTATAAACTGACA S K S S G G S N Y K L T	TTTGGAAAAGGAACTCTCTTAACCGTGAATCCA F G K G T M L L V S P	AAATCCAG N I Q

XPE: DRB1*07, 07; DRB4; DRB5
XPZ: DRB1*07, 15; DRB4; DRB5
XPD: DRB1*07, 07; DRB4
XPR: DRB1*07, 16; DRB4; DRB5
XPF: DRB1*07, 15; DRB4; DRB5

B

T cell clone	TCRB gene segments	TCRBV	TCRBD	CDR3 (6-14)	TCRBJ	TCRBC
XPE15	BV24S1D1J2S2C2	GCCATGTACCTGTGTGCCACCAGC A M Y L C A T S	AGTCGGGCAGCCAACACCGGGGAGCTGTTT S [R] A A N T G E L F		TTTGGAGAAGGCTCTAGGCTGACCGTACTG F G E G S R L T V L	GAGGACCTG E D L
XPZ10	BV17S1D1J2S3C2	GCTTTCTATCTCTGTGCCAGTAGT A F Y L C A S S		AGGGATCCAGATACGGCAGTAT [R] D P D T Q Y	TTTGGCCCAGGCACCCGGCTGACAGTGCTC F G P G T R L T V L	GAGGACCTG E D L
XPD25	BV2S3D1J1S5C1	AGCTTCTACATCTGCAGTGCTAGA S F Y I C S A [R]	GGAAATGGGGGACAGGGTCTAATAAGCAATCAGCCCCAGCAT G N G G Q G L I S N Q P Q H		TTTGGTGATGGGACTCGACTCTCCATCCTA F G D G T R L S I L	GAGGACCTG E D L
XPR04	BV15S1D1J2S5C2	GCTCTTTACTTCTGTGCCACCAGT A L Y F C A T S	GTCACCAGGGGGAGAAGACCCAGTAG V T [R] G R K T Q Y		TTCGGGCCAGGCACGCGGCTCCTGGTGCTC F G P G T R L L V L	GAGGACCTG E D L
XPF10	BV2S3D2J2S4C2	AGCTTCTACATCTCCAGTGCTAGA S F Y I C S A [R]		GAGGGACAAGATTCAGTAC E G Q I Q Y	TTCGGGCCCGGGACCCGGCTCTCAGTGCTG F G A G T R L S V L	GAGGACCTG E D L

Figure 1. A and B. TCR α (A) and β (B) cDNA junctional nucleotide sequences of independent epitope 4-specific TCC. The deduced amino acid sequence is shown under each corresponding nucleotide sequence. V gene segments were classified according to family designations outlined by Wilson et al. 1988. TCRAJ germline sequences were assigned as described by Moss et al. 1993. TCRBD, BJ, and BC elements were assigned according to Toyonaga et al. 1985. For each clone, only the last 7 – 10 V gene residues are shown, followed by the presumed Ig - like loops (CDR3) defined according to Clothia et al. 1988 and by the first three residues of the C region.

ates a cascade of immunological events that result in IgE synthesis causing the symptoms of Type I allergic diseases. In order to find out about a possible interference with the first step of the cascade, this study was designed to investigate the diversity of TCR usage by CD4$^+$ T cells in atopic individuals sensitized to Bet v 1.

We have examined the TCR expression of clones specific for four frequently found epitopes of Bet v 1. Twenty CD4$^+$ TCC were isolated from the peripheral blood of 11 different birch pollen-allergic individuals. For all TCC the recognition of these peptides was restricted by HLA-DR molecules.

Sequence analysis of TCRα– and β–chain derived PCR products from these TCC revealed diversity in V (D) and J gene segments in both chains. The junctional regions of both chains appeared to be quite diverse in both, length and amino acid composition, although some restriction was observed in the TCRBV CDR3 of TCC specific for epitopes 1 and 4. For epitope 1, the TCRBJ usage was restricted to two different gene segments (1S4 and 2S7). For epitope 4, a basic charged residue (R) was found in the β-chain CDR3 for all five clones. This amino acid was present exclusively at the BV - BJ junction of the clones. Although this arginine residue was contributed by the BV2 gene segments in clones XPWD 25 II and XPTF 10 I, it may well have been selected for recognition of the peptide - MHC complex. CDR3 regions of the α– and β–chain are believed to be rearranged independently of thymic MHC molecules and are believed to represent the particular parts of the TCR which come in contact with the antigenic peptide. It was therefore tempting to speculate that this region might display a certain degree of homology in TCC recognizing identical peptides. However, again no similarity, neither in length nor in the amino acid composition, could be observed in the sequences. It is therefor highly possible that the CDR3 loops do not exclusively contact the peptide.

In accordance with our findings, a study examining the T cell response to an influenza virus hemagglutinin determinant, HA 255–270, in the context of HLA-DQ and -DR molecules also showed a diverse selection of TCRAV and J gene segments that contributed to the junctional heterogeneity of the TCR. TCRBV9 and BV13 gene segments seemed to be preferentially used by these TCC. CDR3 sequences of both the α– and β-chain were heterogeneous (Jones et al. 1994). TCC reactive with a tetanus toxin-derived peptide (tt830–844) presented by HLA-DR molecules showed a preferential TCRBV gene usage. TCRAV gene use was more heterogeneous. Again, a striking heterogeneity was found in the junctional regions of both α– and β–chains (Boitel et al. 1992). TCC specific for mycobacterial 65 kDa heat shock proteins showed restricted TCR expression, also in this case CDR3 sequence conservation was not apparent (Henwood et al. 1993). TCC involved in the human autoreactivity to myelin basic protein with a defined peptide specificity and HLA-DR restriction also expressed multiple TCR (Giegerich et al. 1992).

Conservation of amino acid residues, a more restricted use of V gene families or J gene segments was only found in the TCRβ– chains. Overall, the TCRα-chain sequences displayed a striking heterogeneity in all their characteristics. Therefor, the TCRβ-chains may be the ones that are much more involved in the interaction with the peptide. In the light of these diverse findings, we come to the conclusion that the hypervariable regions of these TCC may not be able to serve as targets for the elimination of Bet v 1-specific TCC.

6. ACKNOWLEDGMENT

This work was supported by Grants S06704-MED and S06707-MED of the "Fonds zur Förderung der Wissenschaftlichen Forschung".

7. REFERENCES

Boitel, B., Ermonval, M., Panina-Bordignon, P., Mariuzza, R. A., Lanzavecchia, A., and Acuto, O. Preferential Vβ gene usage and lack of junctional sequence conservation among human T cell receptors specific for a tetanus toxin-derived peptide: Evidence for a dominant role of a germline-encoded V region in antigen/major histocompatibility complex recognition. *J Exp Med* 175: 765–777, 1992

Chomczynski, P. and Sacchi, N. Single-step method of RNA isolation by acid guanidinium thiocyanate-phenol-chloroform extraction. *Anal Biochem.* 162:156–159, 1987

Clothia, C., Boswell, D. R., and Lesk, A.M. The outline structure of the T-cell αβ receptor. *EMBO J* 7: 3745-3755, 1988

Concannon, P., Pickering, L., Kung, P., and Hood, L. diversity and structure of human T-cell receptor β-chain variable regions. *Proc Natl Acad Sci USA* 83: 6598–602, 1986

Davis, M. M. and Bjorkman, P. J. T-cell antigen receptor genes and T-cell recognition. *Nature* 334: 395–402, 1988

Ebner, C., Szépfalusi, Z., Ferreira, F., Jilek, A., Valenta, R., Parronchi, P., Maggi, E., Romagnani, S., Scheiner, O., and Kraft, D. Identification of multiple T cell epitopes on Bet v I, the major birch pollen allergen, using specific T cell clones and overlapping peptides. *J Immunol* 150: 1047–1054, 1993

Ebner, C., Schenk, S., Szépfalusi, Z., Hoffmann, K., Ferreira, F., Willheim, M., Scheiner, O., and Kraft, D. multiple T cell specificities for Bet v I, the major birch pollen allergen, within single individuals. Studies using specific T cell clones and overlapping peptides. Eur J Immunol 23: 1523–1527,1993

Ebner, C., Ferreira, F., Hoffmann, K., Szépfalusi, Z., Hirschwehr, R., Schenk, S., Parronchi, P., Romagnani, S., Scheiner, O., and Kraft, D. T-cell clones specific for Bet v I, the major birch pollen allergen, cross-react with the major allergens of hazel, Cor a I and alder, Aln g I. *Mol Immunol* 30: 1323–1329, 1993

Ferreira, F., Hoffmann-Sommergruber, K., Breiteneder, H., Pettenburger K., Ebner, C., Szépfalusi, Z., Steiner, R., Bohle, B., Rumpold, H., Kraft, D., and Scheiner, O. Purification and characterization of recombinant Bet v I, the major birch pollen allergen. *J Biol Chem* 268: 19574–19580, 1993

Fischer, G. F., Faé, I., and Pickl, W. F. Distribution of polymorphic HLA-DR and -DQ alleles as determined by restriction fragment length polymorphism analysis in an Austrian population. Vox Sang 62: 236–241, 1992

Genevée, C., Diu, A., Nierat, J., Caignard, A., Dietrich, P.-Y., Ferradini, L., Roman-Roman, S., Triebel, F., and Hercend T. An experimentally validated panel of subfamily-specific oligonucleotide primers (V$_α$1-w29/V$_β$1-w24) for the study of human T cell receptor variable V gene segment usage by polymerase chain reaction. *Eur J Immunol* 22: 1261–1269, 1992

Giegerich, G., Pette, M., Meinl, E., Epplen, J. T., Wekerle, H., and Hinkkanen, A. Diversity of T cell receptor α and β chain genes specific for similar myelin basic protein peptide/major histocompatibility complexes. *Eur J Immunol* 1992. 22: 753–758, 1992.

Haskins, K., Kubo, R., White, J., Pigeon, M., Kappler, J. and Marrack, P. The major histocompatibility complex restricted antigen receptor on T cells. I. Isolation with a monoclonal antibody. *J Exp Med* 157: 1149 - 1169, 1983

Henwood, J., Loveridge, J., Bell, J. I., and Gaston, J. S. H. Restricted T cell receptor expression by human T cell clones specific for mycobacterial 65-kDa heat-shock protein: selective *in vivo* expansion of T cells bearing defined receptors. *Eur J Immunol* 23: 1256–1265, 1993

Jones, C. M., Lake, R. A., Lamb, J. R., and Faith, A. Degeneracy of T cell receptor recognition of an influenza virus hemagglutinin epitope restricted by HLA-DQ and -DR class II molecules. *Eur J Immunol* 24: 1137–1142, 1994

Kimura N., Toyonaga B., Hoshikai Y., Triebel F., Debre, P., Minden, M.D., and Mak, T.W. Sequences and diversity of human T cell receptor β chain variable region genes. *J Exp Med* 164: 739–750, 1986

Kimura, N., Toyonaga, B., Yoshikai, Y., Du, R.-P., and Mak, T.W. Sequences and repertoire of the human T cell receptor α and β chain variable region genes in thymocytes. *Eur J Immunol* 17: 375–383, 1987

Klein, M. H., Concannon, P., Everett, M., Kim, L. D. H., Hunkapiller, T., and Hood, L. Diversity and structure of human T-cell receptor α-chain variable region genes. *Proc Natl Acad Sci USA* 84: 6884–6888, 1987

Meuer, S. C., Fitzgerald, K. A., Hussey, R. E., Hodgdon, J. C., Schlossman, S. F., and Reinherz, E. L. Clonotypic structures involved in antigen-specific human T cell function. Relationships to the T3 molecular complex. *J Exp Med* 157: 705–719, 1983

Moss, P. A. H., Rosenberg, W. M. C., Zintzaras, E., and Bell, J. I. Characterization of human T cell receptor α-chain repertoire and demonstration of a genetic influence on Vα usage. *Eur J Immunol* 23: 1153 - 1159, 1993

Panzara, M. A., Gussoni, E., Steinman, L., and Oksenberg, J. R. Analysis of the T cell repertoire using the PCR and specific oligonucleotide primers. *BioTechniques* 12: 728–735, 1992

Roman-Roman, S., Ferradini, L., Azocar, J., Genevée, C., Hercend, T., and Triebel, F. Studies on the human T-cell receptor α/β variable region genes. I. Identification of 7 additional $V_α$ subfamilies and 14 $J_α$ gene segments. *Eur. J. Immunol.* 1991. 21: 927.

Schwartz, R.H. T-lymphocyte recognition of antigen in association with gene products of the major histocompatibility complex. *Annu Rev Immunol* 3: 237–261, 1985

Toyonaga, B., Yoshikai, Y., Vadasz, V., Chin, B., and Mak, T.W. Organization and sequences of the diversity, joining, and constant region genes of the human T-cell receptor β chain. *Proc Natl Acad Sci USA* 82: 8624–8628, 1985

Wilson, R. K., Lai, E., Concannon, P., Barth, R. K., and Hood, L. E. Structure, organization and polymorphism of murine and human T-cell receptor α and β chain gene families. *Immunol Rev* 101: 149–172, 1988.

Yoshikai, Y., Kimura, N., Toyonaga, B., and Mak, T.W. Sequences and repertoire of human T cell receptor α chain variable region genes in mature T lymphocytes. *J Exp Med* 164: 90–103, 1986.

53

IDENTIFICATION OF DIFFERENTIALLY EXPRESSED GENES IN CD19+ve B LYMPHOCYTES IN ALLERGIC ASTHMA

Roslan B. Harun, Alexander F. Markham, and John F. J. Morrison

Molecular Medicine Unit
Clinical Sciences Building
St James's University Hospital
Beckett Street, Leeds, United Kingdom. LS97 TF

INTRODUCTION

Allergic asthma is one of the important clinical manifestation of atopy, which has both environmental and genetic components. Atopy is characterized by abnormal IgE responses to common allergens which results in high total or specific serum IgE levels, and positive skin tests to common aeroallergens. The regulation of IgE production is controlled by many factors including cytokines, cognate and noncognate interactions between B and T lymphocytes, and the low affinity IgE receptor, CD23.

IgE synthesis involves germline transcription of the $C\varepsilon$ gene in B cells followed by switch recombination to produce the translated ε mRNA and selective clonal expansion of IgE committed B lymphocytes. There are two main signals that are required for isotype switching to IgE. The first signal is provided by IL-4 which can only induce germline $C\varepsilon$ transcripts but not productive ε mRNA in purified mIgE- B cells (1). The B cells require an additional signal for switch recombination. This second signal can be provided by activated T helper cells (2,3), Epstein-Barr virus (4), anti-CD40 monoclonal antibodies (5,6) and hydrocortisone (7).

The physical interaction of T and B cells is essential for the modulation of IgE synthesis. There are two types of T and B cell interaction: a) cognate and, b) noncognate interaction. Cognate interaction occurs when the specific T cell receptor (TCR)/CD3 complex on CD4+ T helper cell recognizes a processed peptide in association with MHC class II on B cells. This results in activation of both B and T cells (8).

Non-cognate interaction involves the CD40 ligand (CD40L) on activated T cells and CD40 on B cells. The CD40-CD40L binding induces IgE synthesis (9) and promotes B cell proliferation (10). Recently, another adhesion molecules complex, LFA-3 (CD58) on B cells and CD2 on T cells has been shown to induce IgE synthesis in the absence of CD40 stimulation (11). T cell clones from an X-linked hyper-immunoglobulinaemia

New Horizons in Allergy Immunotherapy
edited by Sehon et al. Plenum Press, New York, 1996

375

(IgM) patient which have defective or no CD40 ligands are capable of inducing IgE synthesis in the presence of IL-4 (12) . Other surface molecules may be involved in the induction of IgE synthesis and T-B cell interactions.

B cells from atopic patients produce IgE spontaneously *in vitro*, whereas normal B lymphocytes require additional signals provided by IL-4 and T lymphocytes to produce IgE (13). There may be differences in the responses of the B cells of atopic asthmatics and normal individuals to these regulatory factors which contribute to the aberrant IgE production. The abnormalities may involve surface or adhesion molecules, signal transduction proteins or transcription factors.

In this study, we analyse the molecular mechanisms which may account for the differences in IgE secretion between normal and atopic asthmatic subjects using differential display technology.

METHODS

1. Isolation of B Lymphocytes

Peripheral blood mononuclear cells from atopic asthmatic and normal subjects were isolated by Ficoll-Hypaque density gradient centrifugation and B lymphocytes were positively selected using Dynabeads M-450 (Dynal) coated with anti-CD 19 mAb as described previously (14). The B cells were then detached from the immunomagnetic beads by using anti-Fab antiserum (DETACHaBEAD, Dynal) (15) . The isolated B cells were consistently > 98% pure as revealed by flow cytometry analysis and > 97% viable (data not shown).

2. Differential Display

2.1. RNA Isolation and Reverse Transcription. Differential display was performed using a total of 75 different combinations of random decamers and anchored oligo(dT) primers as previously described, with some modifications (16). Total RNA was extracted from B cells using the acid guanidinium thiocyanate/ phenol-chloroform RNA extraction method (17). DNase I (Pharmacia) and RNase inhibitor (Promega) were added to total RNA in 1 x PCR buffer (see below) and incubated at $37°$ C for 30 minutes. Reverse transcription was done in four independent reactions for each total RNA sample using anchored oligo(dT) primers: $T_{12}MG$, $T_{12}MA$, $T_{12}MT$, and $T_{12}MC$ (where M is a degenerate base G, A or C in equimolar concentrations). For each reaction (20μl) , 0.2μg of DNA-free total RNA was primed with 1 μM anchored oligo(dT) primer in x μl DEPC-treated distilled water at $65°$ C for 10 minutes and then immediately chilled on ice for 1 minute. A master mix containing reverse transcription buffer [25mM TrisHCl (pH 8.3), 37.5mM KCl, 1.5 mM $MgCl_2$], 10 mM dithiothreitol, and mixed dNTPs (Pharmacia) containing 20 mM each of dATP, dGTP, dCTP and dTTP at neutral pH was added. After incubation at $42°$ C for 10 minutes, 200 U of MMLV reverse transcriptase (Gibco/BRL) were added and the reactions were continued for 1 hour. The reactions were terminated by heating at $95°$ C for 5 minutes. Control reactions were performed in the absence of reverse transcriptase.

2.2. Polymerase Chain Reaction (PCR). PCR was performed in 0.5 mL tubes (Eppendorf) containing 1x PCR buffer [10mM Tris-HCl (pH 8.3), 50 mM KCl, 1.5 mM $MgCl_2$], 2 μM dNTP mixture, 1.0 μM anchored primer $T_{12}MN$, 0.2 μM random decamer,

0.1 vol of cDNA, 1 µCi ^{35}S-dATP (1200 Ci/mmole) (Amersham) and 1 U Taq DNA polymerase (Promega). PCR was done initially at 94° C for 5 minutes with 40 cycles at 94° C for 30 sec, 42° sec for 2 min, 72° C for 30 sec, followed by 72° C for 10 minutes.

2.3. Electrophoresis. The PCR products were displayed on 6 % denaturing polyacrylamide urea gels. After electrophoresis, the gel was dried without fixation and exposed to X-ray film for 48 hours. cDNA bands of interest were identified. The differential display was repeated using several samples from atopic asthmatic and normal subjects to confirm the findings.

3. Reamplification, Cloning, and Sequencing

The differentially displayed bands were cut out and DNA was eluted by boiling. After ethanol precipitation, the DNA was reamplified using the same set of anchored oligodT primers and random decamers which produced the cDNA fragment of interest using the same cycle parameters. PCR was carried out in 40 mL reactions using 20 mM of dNTP mixes without addition of radioactive isotope. Reamplified PCR products were cloned into a TA cloning vector (Invitrogen) according to the manufacturer's protocol. The cDNA fragments were sequenced with Taq DyeDeoxy Terminator cycle sequencing (Applied Biosystems). An homology search was done for the nucleotide sequences using BLAST or FASTA programs from the GenBank and EMBL data bases.

RESULT

Figures 1 shows the 4 bands which were consistently differentially displayed. A total of 7 clones with inserts were sequenced (Table 1). One of the partial cDNA sequences was identical to the signal transduction protein SHC and another to the human proto-oncogene protein tyrosine kinase (abl). The other sequences had no homology to recognized sequences.

DISCUSSION

These results showed that there were differences in gene expression in peripheral CD 19+ve B cells of atopic asthmatic and non-atopic normal individuals.The strength of the differential display method is that it allows the isolation and identification of new candidates genes that are potentially involved in the regulation of IgE synthesis. One of the transcribed genes which was identified produces SHC mRNA which encodes SHC protein. SHC protein is one of the upstream regulators of p21ras in the ras -mitogen activated protein kinase (MAPK) mitogenic pathway which is important for cell growth (18). SHC gene expression was seen in atopic asthmatic B cells but not in normal B cells. Most of the B cell lines used in previous studies on SHC are tumour cell lines such as Burkitt lymphoma cells. These cells are oncogenic and have rapid cell growth. The expression levels of the SHC gene in mature normal B lymphocytes are unknown. Crosslinking of B cell receptor (BCR) by anti-IgM antibodies induces tyrosine phosphorylation of SHC protein which facilitates binding to the SH2 domain of the Grb-2 protein (19,20). However, BCR stimulation does not increase SHC gene expression (20) .

Several cytokines such as IL-2, IL-3, IL-6, granulocyte-macrophage colony stinulating factor (GM-CSF), Steel factor (SLF), and colony stimulating factor-1 (CSF-1) induce

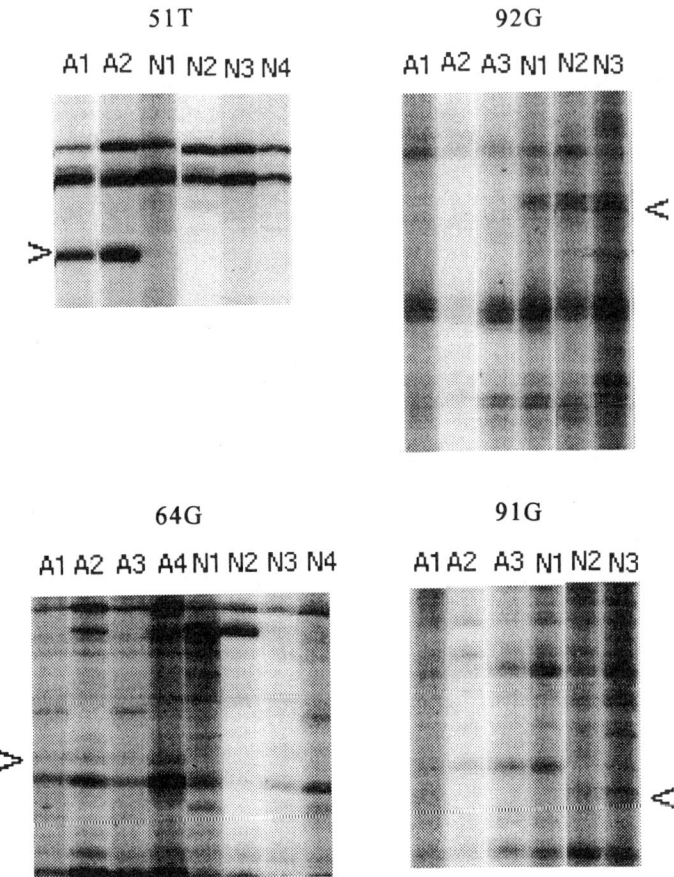

Figure 1. Differential display of four differentially expressed genes. 51T was identical to SHC protein gene and 64G was identical to human proto-oncogene protein tyrosine kinase (*abl*). The other two cDNA fragments had no homology to recognized sequences. (A = Atopic asthma N = Normal).

phosphorylation of SHC protein in murine mast cells (21). These cytokines may also use the ras-MAPK pathway to induce cell proliferation in B lymphocytes. Although IL-4 does not induce SHC protein phosphorylation in mast cells, its effect in B cells has not been studied. Recently, it has been shown that activation of protein tyrosine kinase, but not protein kinase C or protein kinase A, may be involved in the IL-4 and the CD40 signalling pathways in IgE isotype switching in B cells (22).

Table 1. Analysis of differentially expressed cDNA fragments

Bands	Clones	Source	Sequence homology
51T	515T	Asthma	SHC protein
	516T	Asthma	SHC protein
61G	614G	Asthma	Human proto-oncogeneprotein tyrosine kinase *abl*
91G	911G	Normal	Unknown
	913G	Normal	Unknown
92G	922G	Normal	Unknown
	923G	Normal	Unknown

Clone 614G found only in atopic asthma was identical with the human proto-onco-gene, protein tyrosine kinase (ABL) gene. c-Abl is a tyrosine kinase mainly localized in the nucleus but which may be found in the cytoplasm in transformed cells (23) . Recently, c-Abl has been shown to inhibit cell growth in fibroblasts (24) , in contrast to the onco-genic Abl fusion proteins. A cDNA, encoding a protein 3BP-1 has been demonstrated to bind to the SH3 domain of c- Abl which is important in the negative regulation of trans-formation (25). This protein has similar sequence to guanosine triphosphatase-activating protein (GAP)-rho. The SH3 region of Abl may be involved in the negative regulation of cell growth induced by the ras-MAPK mitogenic pathway by binding to the 3BP-1 protein or other Ras-related proteins. c-Abl regulates the protein binding activity of c-Crk which contains SH2 and SH3 domains. c-Abl binds to the first Crk SH3 domain and phosphory-lates a tyrosine residue in the spacer region between the Crk SH3 domains. The precise function of c-Crk is unknown, but the presence of SH2/SH3 domains suggests its involve-ment in signal transduction (26).

Further work to characterize the two currently unknown genes is underway. It is in-teresting to note that these unknown genes are primarily expressed in B lymphocytes from non-atopic subjects.

REFERENCES

1. Jabara HH, Schneider LC, Shapira SK, et al. Induction of germ-line and mature C epsilon transcripts in hu-man B cells stimulated with rIL-4 and EBV. J Immunol 1990;145:3468–73.
2. Gascan H, Gauchat J-F, Aversa G, Vlasselaer PV, de Vries JE. Anti-CD40 monoclonal antibodies or CD4+ T cell clones and IL-4 induce IgG4 and IgE switching in purified human B cells via different signaling pathways. J Immunol 1991;147:8–13.
3. Gascan H, Gauchat J-F, Roncarolo MG, Yssel H, Spits H, de Vries JE. Human B cell clones can be induced to proliferate and to switch to IgE and IgG4 synthesis by interleukin 4 and a signal provided by activated CD4+ T cell clones. J Exp Med 1991;173:747–50.
4. Thyphronitis G, Tsokos GC, June CH, Levine AD, Finkelman FD. IgE secretion by Epstein-Barr virus in-fected purified human B lymphocytes is stimulated by interleukin 4 and suppressed by interleukin-gamma. Proc Natl Acad Sci USA 1989;86:5580–4.
5. Jabara HH, Fu SM, Geha RS, Vercelli D. CD40 and IgE: synergism between anti-CD40 monoclonal anti-body and IL-4 in the induction of IgE synthesis by highly purified B cells. J Exp Med 1990;172:1861–4.
6. Rousset F, Garcia E, Banchereau J. Cytokine-induced proliferation and immunoglobulin production of hu-man B lymphocytes triggered through their CD40 antigen. J Exp Med 1991;173(3):705–10.
7. Jabara HH, Ahern DJ, Vercelli D, Geha RS. Hydrocortisone and IL-4 induce IgE isotype switching in hu-man B cells. J Immunol 1991;147:1557–60.
8. Vercelli D, Jabara HH, Arai K, Geha RS. Induction of human IgE synthesis requires interleukin 4 and T-B cell interaction involving the T cell receptor/CD3 complex and MHC class II antigens. J Exp Med 1989;169:1295–307.
9. Parronchi P, Tiri A, Macchia D, et al. Noncognate contact-dependent B cell activation can promote IL-4 dependent in vitro human IgE synthesis. J Immunol 1990;144:2102–8.
10. Clark EA, Lane PJ. Regulation of human B-cell activation and adhesion. Ann Rev Immunol 1991;9:97–127.
11. Diaz-Sanchez D, Chegini S, Zhang K, Saxon A. CD58(LFA-3) stimulation provides a signal for human iso-type switching and IgE production distinct from CD40. J Immunol 1994;153:10–20.
12. Life P, Gauchat JF, Schnuriger V, et al. T cell clones from an X-linked hyper-immunoglobulin (IgM) pa-tient induce IgE synthesis in vitro despite expression of nonfunctional CD40 ligand. J Exp Med 1994;180(5):1775–84.
13. Katona IM, Urban JF, Kang JrSS, Paul WF, Finkelman FD. IL-4 requirements for the generation of secon-dary in vivo IgE response. J Immunol 1991;146:4215–21.
14. Funderud S, Erikstein B, Asheim HC, et al. Functional properties of CD19+ B lymphocytes positively se-lected from buffy coats by immunomagnetic seoaration. Eur J Immunol 1990;20:201–6.

15. Rasmussen A-M, Smeland EB, Erikstein BK, Caignault L, Funderud S. A new method for detachment of Dynabeads from positively selected B lymphocytes. J Immunol Methods 1992;146:195–202.

16. Liang P, Averboukh L, Pardee AB. Distribution and cloning of eukaryotic mRNAs by means of differential display: Refinements and optimization. Nucleic Acids Res 1993;21:3269–75.

17. Chomczynski P, Sacchi N. Single-step method of RNA isolation by acid guanidium thiocyanate-phenol-chloroform extraction. Anal Biochem 1987;167:157–9.

18. Pelicci G, Lanfrancone L, Grignani F, et al. A novel transforming protein (SHC) with an SH2 domain is implicated in mitogenic signal transduction. Cell 1992;70:93–104.

19. Saxton TM, van Oostveen I, Bowell D, Aebersold R, Gold MR. B cell antigen receptor cross-linking induces phosphorylation of the p21ras oncoprotein activators SHC and mSOS1 as well as assembly of complexes containing SHC, GRB-2, mSOS1, and a 145- kD tyrosine phosphorylated protein. J Immunology 1994 ; 153:623–36.

20. Smit L, de Vries-Smits AMM, Bos JL, Borst J. B cell antigen receptor stimulation induces formation of a Shc-Grb2 complex containing multiple tyrosine-phosphorylated proteins. J Biol Chem 1994;269:20209–12.

21. Welham MJ, Duranio V, Leslie KB, Bowtell D, Schrader JW. Multiple hemopoietins,with the exception of interleukin-4, induce modification of Shc and mSos1, but not their translocation. J Biol Chem 1994;269:21165–76.

22. Loh RK, Jabara HH, Ren CL, Fu SM, Geha RS. Role of protein tyrosine kinases in CD40/interleukin-4-mediated isotype switching to IgE. J Allergy Clin Immunol 1994;94(4):784–92.

23. Van Etten RA, Jackson P, Baltimore D. The mouse type IV c-abl gene product is a nuclear protein,and activation of transforming ability is associated with cytoplasmic localization. Cell 1989;58:669–78.

24. Sawyers CL, McLaughlin J, Goga A, Havlik M, Witte O. The nuclear tyrosine kinase c-Abl negatively regulates cell growth. Cell 1994;77:121–31.

25. Cicchetti P, Mayer BJ, Theil G, Baltimore D. Identification of a protein that binds to the SH3 region of Abl and is similar to Bcr and GAP-rho. Science 1992;257(5071):803–6.

26. Feller SM, Knudsen B, Hanafusa H. c-Abl kinase regulates the protein binding activity of c-Crk. EMBO J. 1994;13: 2341–51.

54

NON RANDOM USAGE OF T CELL RECEPTOR α GENE EXPRESSION IN ATOPY USING ANCHORED PCR

A. H. Mansur,[1] C. M. Gelder,[2] D. Holland,[1] D. A. Campell,[1] A. Griffin,[1] W. Cunliffe,[1] A. F. Markham,[1] and J. F. J. Morrison

[1]Molecular Medicine Unit
St. James's University Hospital
Leeds, United Kingdom
[2]Department of Immunology
St. Mary's Hospital
London, United Kingdom

1. ABSTRACT

The T cell receptor (TCR) αβ heterodimer recognises antigenic peptide fragments presented by Class II MHC. This interaction initiates T cell activation and cytokine release with subsequent recruitment of inflammatory cells. Previous work from our group suggests a qualitative difference in variable α gene expression in atopy as compared to non atopic controls. In this study we examine TCR α repertoire using anchored PCR to provide a quantitative assessment of the Vα and Jα repertoire. One atopic (DRB1*0701,DRB1*15: DRB4*0101, DRB5*01: DQB1* 0303, DQB1*601/2) and one non-atopic (DRB1*0701,DRB1*03011/2: DRB4*01, DRB3*0×: DQB1* 0303, DQB1*0201/2) control were studied. Variable gene usage was markedly limited in the atopic individual. Vα 1, 3, 8 accounted for 60% and Jα 12, 31 30% of the gene usage. There was evidence of preferential Vα-Jα gene pairing and clonal expansion. We conclude that there is a marked non random TCR α gene distribution in atopy using both Vα family and anchored PCR. This may be due in part to antigen driven clonal expansion.

2. INTRODUCTION

Asthma and Atopy are common conditions affecting respectively 10% and 30% of the population in UK[1]. They are generally recognised to be inflammatory diseases with an immunological basis[2]. Though the exact cause and the cell type primarily responsible remain controversial, the CD4+ T- lymphocyte is likely to be of pivotal importance[3]. CD4+

New Horizons in Allergy Immunotherapy
edited by Sehon et al. Plenum Press, New York, 1996

381

T-Lymphocytes play a key role in the regulation of the immune system and in particular control of IgE responsiveness[4], which is strongly correlated to the presence of atopy and asthma[5,6]. There are increased numbers of T lymphocytes in affected tissues in atopy, which have increased expression of activation markers and cytokine production.

Antigen is processed by macrophages or other antigen presenting cells. Class II MHC presents antigenic fragments to the T cell receptor. The TCR is a heterodimer consisting ofα and β, or γ and δ subunits. The TCR αβ receptor is present on 95% of T cells in peripheral blood. The TCR confers antigen specificity through the use of different variable (Vα, Vβ) , diversity (Dβ), and junctional (Jα and Jβ) gene segments. These undergo somatic rearrangement during thymocyte development[7]. The insertion or deletion of junctional nucleotides creates further diversity[8]. Structural consideration suggests that the resulting V-(D)-J junction, which corresponds to the CDR3 region of immunoglobulins, directly binds to antigenic peptides in the MHC peptide binding site[9].

The T-cell receptor repertoire is shaped by interaction between developing thymocytes and thymic stroma. Both positive and negative selection involve clonotypic TCR and MHC molecules carrying self peptides. This is further shaped in the periphery through antigen driven clonal expansion. Previous studies on TCR gene usage in disease have reported oligoclonality in multiple sclerosis[10,11], auto-immune thyroid disease[12], rheumatoid arthritis[13,] myasthenia gravis[14], and diabetes mellitus[15]. In addition, analysis of the αβ repertoire in house dust mite sensitive T cell clones in an atopic subject, showed dominant expression of TCR Vβ 3 and Vα 8 genes[16]. Previous studies on TCR α repertoire have shown that the Vα is indistinguishable between identical twins, suggesting a major genetic influence on the Vα usage[17.] Moreover, one study has reported a linkage of antigen specific IgE responses to Vα-δ region on chromosome 14 [18.]

To further explore the relationship between the genetic and environmental influences shaping the TCR Vα gene repertoire in asthma and allergy we have analysed the gene repertoire using both qualitative and quantitative PCR methodologies. Here we report in vivo non random use of Vα gene segments in atopy, primarily as a consequence of T cell clonal expansion.

3. MATERIALS AND METHODS

3.1. Qualitative Vα Gene Family PCR

Peripheral blood monocytes were obtained from 8 non-atopic non-asthmatic, 8 atopic asthmatic, 8 non-atopic asthmatic, and 8 atopic non-asthmatic subjects, using Ficoll Hypaque density centrifugation. All the atopic subjects were sensitive to House Dust Mite. RNA was extracted using the acid guanidium thiocyanate-phenol-chloroform protocol[19]. Reverse transcription{1 μg RNA, 0.4 μg oligo dT, in 30 μl of water, 65°C for 5 minutes, followed by the addition of 4 μl deoxynucleotides(10 mM each), 4 μl 10x RT buffer, 1 μl rRNAase inhibitor(Promega), and 1 μl Reverse Transcriptase HC (Promega), incubated at 42 °C for 1 hour, and 72 °C for 10 minutes}. This was followed by 35 cycles of Polymerase chain reaction carried out in microtitre plates using a Techne Thermal Cycler (PHC-3) { 1 μl cDNA, 25.7 μl primer mix (2.5 μmolar each primer, 2 mM each deoxynucleotide), 3 μl 10x buffer, 0.3 μl Taq Polymerase (Promega), denatured at 95°C for 5 minutes, followed by 35 cycles of 95 °C 30 seconds denaturing, 55 °C 30 seconds annealing, and 72 °C 60 seconds extension, followed by final extension 72 °C 5 minutes}. 1 μl PCR products were then used as a template for a further 35 cycles. PCR products were size fractionated on 3 % agarose gel containing ethidium bromide, and directly viewed under UV light.

Primers. 18 forward primers specific for Vα gene families (1.....18), and a single reverse primer to the Vα constant region were used[20]. Primers specific for Transfer RNA Synthetase, whose product spanned a small intron were used as a control for genomic DNA contamination, and normal pooled peripheral blood lymphocytes were used as a positive control. Product specificity was confirmed by sequencing the PCR products.

3.2. Anchored PCR, and Cloning

Peripheral blood monocytes were obtained as in 3.1 from one house dust mite sensitive atopic non asthmatic subject with class II MHC haplotype(DRB1*0701, DRB1* 15: DR B4*0101, DRB5*01: DQB1*0303, DQB1, 601/2), and one non atopic non asthmatic individual with a haplotype (DRB1*0701,DRB1* 03011/2: DRB4*01, DRB3*0×: DQ B1*0303, DQB1* 0201/2).

RNA extraction and reverse transcription were performed as in 3.1. The product was purified by Geneclean to remove excess primer and nucleotides. ss cDNA was 3' tailed with dGTP using terminal deoxytransferase according to manufacture's instructions (Boehringer Mannheim), and again the product was cleaned using Geneclean to remove excess dGTP. Vα gene segments were amplified by PCR using a forward primer (5' CAG CCG CGG CCG CAA GCT TCC CCC CCC CCC CCC), and a Vα constant region reverse primer (5' GTC TGT GAT ATA CAC ATC AGA A). The reaction conditions were as follows: 95°C one cycle for 5 min, followed by 30 cycles of 55°C for 45 sec, 72 °C for 90 sec, and 95°C for 45 sec, with a final extension period of 10min at 72 °C. Products were size separated on 3% agarose gel, purified using Geneclean, ligated into the Promega pGEM-T vector according to the manufacture's instructions, and transformed into E coli, using high efficiency JM109cells (Promega). After plating in the presence of ampicillin (75 µl / ml), 5-bromo-4-chloro-3-indolyl β-D-thiogalactopyranside (X-gal) and isopropyl-β-D-galactopyranoside (IPTG) and incubation at 37°C, individual positive white colonies were picked and glycerol stocks made for later plasmid preparation and sequencing.

3.3. Plasmid Extraction and Sequencing

Plasmids were extracted using a modified alkaline lysis procedure. Bacteria from individual colonies were incubated at 37°C in 10ml Luria Broth with ampicillin. Bacterial pellets were redissolved in 200µl GTE buffer(50mM glucose, 25mM Tris pH8.0, 10mM EDTA pH 8.0), lysed using 400µl of freshly made 0.2N NaOH /1.0%SDS, and incubated on ice for 5 min. Solutions were neutralised by adding 300µl of 3.0M potassium acetate PH 4.8, and incubated on ice for 10 minutes. Plasmids were precipitated by adding one volume100% isopropanol, washed in 70% alcohol, and dissolved in 50µl RNAase containing distilled H_2O.

Plasmids were sequenced in both directions using M13 primers and Taq Dye DeoxyTerminator Cycle Sequencing, on an Applied Biosystems Model 373A machine. A 20 µl final PCR volume was prepared as follows {9.5µl premix(4µl 5x TACS buffer, 1 µl dNTP mix [7.5µM dITP,1.5 µM dATP, 1.5 µM dTTP, 1.5 µM dGTP], 1 µl A DyeDeoxy Terminator, 1 µl T DyeDeoxy Terminator, 1 µl C DyeDeoxy Terminator, 1µl G DyeDeoxy Terminator, 0.5 µl AmpliTaq DNA Polymerase), 3.2 pM of each M13 primers, 1 µg of plasmid solution, made up to final volume of 20 µl with distilled H_2O}. 25 PCR cycles were performed using Perkin Elmer Cetus Model 480. The reactions conditions were as follows: denaturing at 96 °C for 30 seconds, annealing at 50 °C for 30 seconds, and extension at 60 °C for 4 minutes. Excess dye terminators were removed from PCR reactions prior to gel loading using the CTAB precipitation method according to manufacture's protocol. Sequence was analysed using ABI 373A software and ambiguities were resolved by resequencing. The determined sequences were compared to available published Vα-Jα gene segments.

4. RESULTS

4.1. Family PCR

Using ethidium fluorescence, normal and non-atopic asthmatic subjects expressed a mean of 16 and 15 Vα families respectively (figure 1a). Analysis of individual gene segment use showed random gene usage. In contrast the atopic and atopic asthmatic subjects

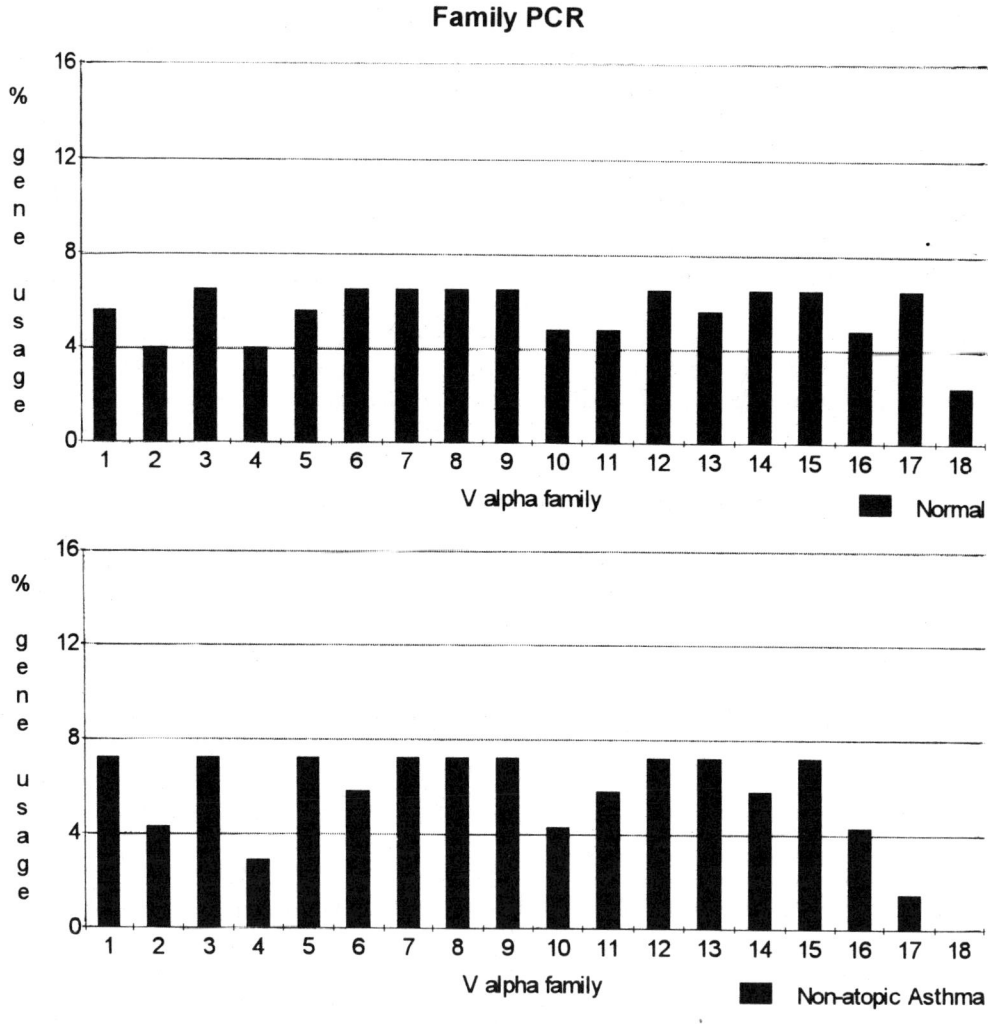

Figure 1. a: (Top graph)This figure illustrates the random TCR V alpha gene segment expression in peripheral blood obtained from normal individuals. (Lower graph) Showing a random expression of TCR V alpha gene families in peripheral blood obtained from non-atopic asthmatic individuals.

expressed a mean of only 7 and 9 gene families respectively. An excess of Vα 3, 8 and 15 was seen (figures 1b). This implies that the differences seen gene family usage reflect atopy rather than asthma.

4.2. Anchored PCR

4.2.1. TCR Vα and Jα Gene Expression. Of the 84 individual V-J-C α clones analysed for each subject, approximately 75% were in frame. The data analysis is based on these clones. Analysis of the TCR Vα gene expression in peripheral T cells in the atopic

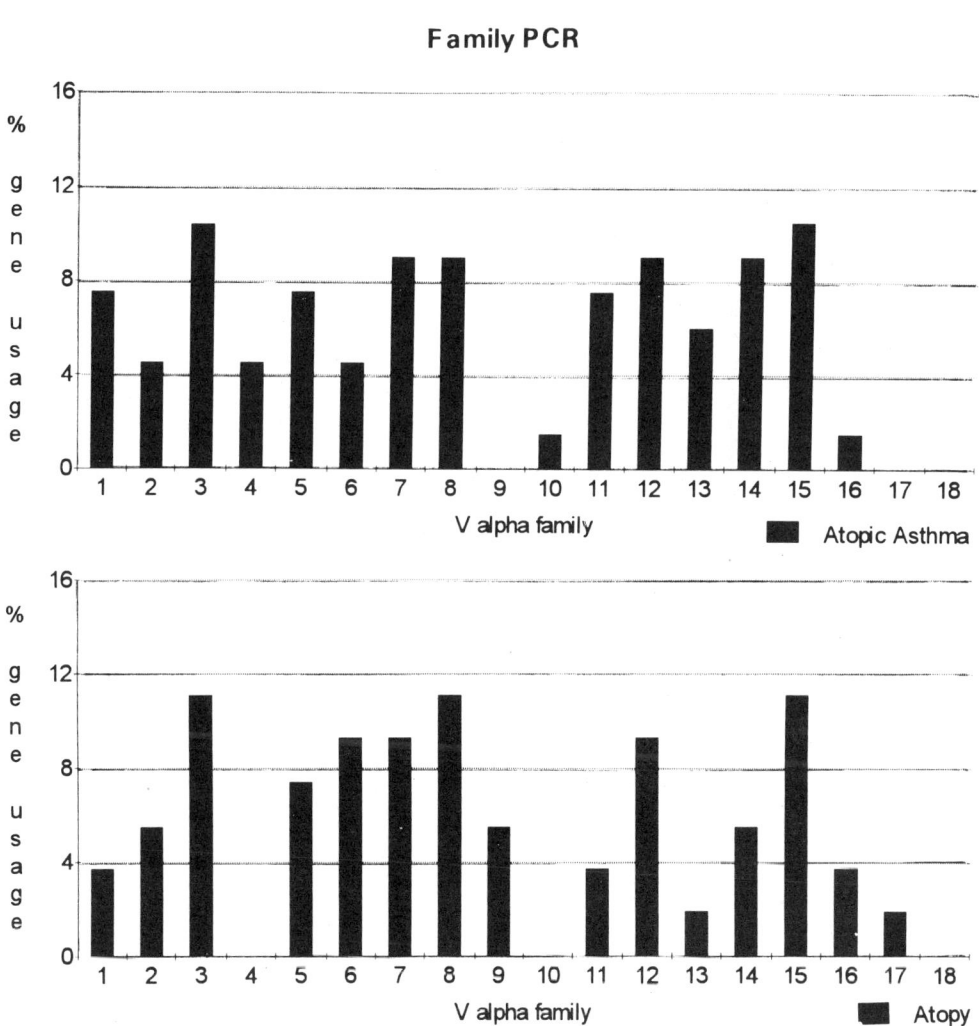

Figure 1. b: (Top graph)This graph demonstrates the restricted TCR V alpha gene expression in the peripheral blood obtained from atopic asthmatic individuals. (lower graph): Showing a restricted expression of TCR V alpha gene families in the peripheral blood obtained from atopic individuals. It also demonstrates the predominant expression of V alpha families 3, 8, and 15.

subject showed marked non random gene usage (figure 2a). Vα 1, 3, and 8 were predominantly expressed and accounted for about 60% of the whole gene expression. The TCR Jα gene expression showed an excess use of Jα12 and 31, which accounted for about 30% of the total gene usage (figure 2b). These finding contrasted with the even and random distribution of both Vα And Jα gene usage in the normal control.

4.2.2. TCRα Gene Rearrangement and Evidence of Oligoclonality in Atopy. T h e r e was preferential V-Jα gene pairing in the predominately expressed genes. Vα 1.5 was paired to Jα31 in 60% of cases. Vα3.0 was paired to Jα 20 in all of cases observed, while Vα 8.2 was paired to Jα12 in 70% of cases and to Jα 48 in 30% of cases.

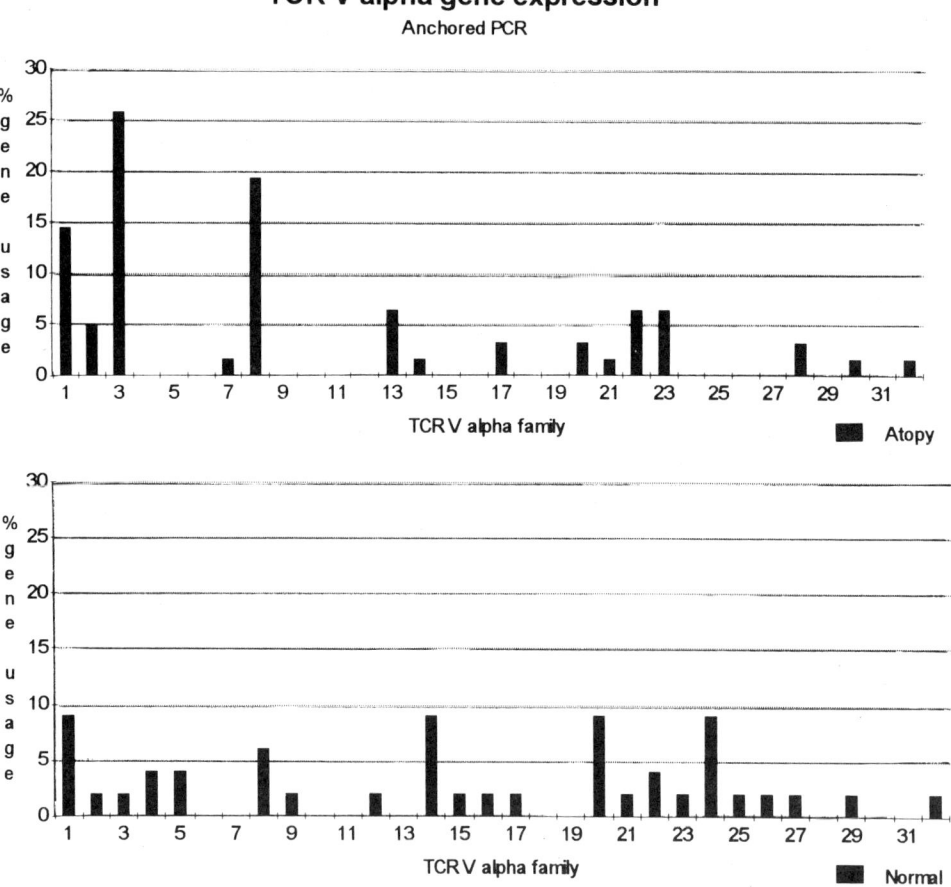

Figure 2. a: (above); The percentage of TCR V alpha families gene expression, in peripheral blood obtained from an atopic individual. There is marked non random gene expression. V alpha 1, 3,and 8 accounted for about 60% of the total TCR V alpha gene expression in this individual. (below); The percentage of TCR V alpha gene families expression in peripheral blood obtained from non-atopic (normal) individual. There is a random expression of TCR V alpha gene families.

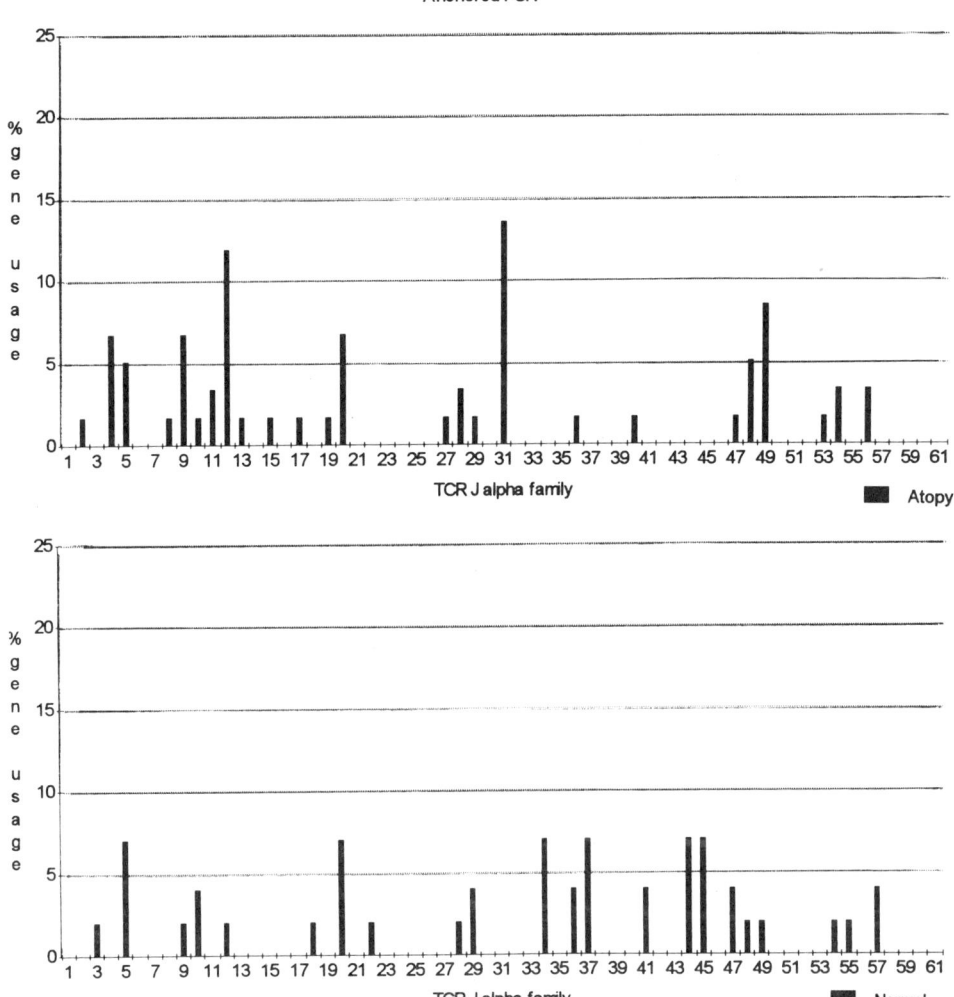

Figure 2. b: (above); The percentage of total gene expression of TCR J alpha families in the peripheral blood obtained from an atopic individual. There is an excess use of TCR J alpha 12, and 31, in which both accounted for about 30% the total TCR J alpha gene expression in this subject. (below); The percentage of total TCR J alpha gene expression in peripheral blood obtained from a non-atopic (normal) individual. This graph demonstrates a random distribution of J alpha gene usage in this individual.

Examination of the CDR3 region of those clones showing preferential pairing (Vα 1.5/Jα 31, Vα 3.0/Jα 20, Vα 8.2/Jα 12,48) showed preservation of (N) region sequences, which indicates the expansion of particular T cell clones. These individual T cell clones accounted for about 25% of the total TCR α gene usage in the atopic subject.

5. DISCUSSION

Qualitative analysis of the TCR Vα repertoire in peripheral blood using family PCR showed evidence of non-random Vα gene expression in atopy but not in asthma. These observations were confirmed by anchored PCR in one-atopic and one non-atopic subjects. These individuals shared 50 % of MHC class II alleles. There was a clear difference in the frequency of Vα gene usage using both anchored and family PCR in atopy. In addition, there was evidence of preferential pairing between certain Vα and Jα genes. Examination of the CDR3 insertions of these Vα-Jα pairings revealed evidence of clonality, which is presumably secondary to antigen stimulation. These T cell clones account for around 25% of the total TCR α gene usage in this subject. In contrast, the non-atopic subject showed a random use of Vα and Jα, gene segments with no evidence of clonality.

Wedderburn and colleagues have shown dominance of Vα 1, 8, and 15 in HDM specific T cell clones from an individual with perennial rhinitis[16]. This was not associated with Jα repertoire skewing. In our study we observed dominant expression of V α 1, 3, and 8 in a subject who was allergic to HDM. This may be evidence of in vivo clonal expansion to HDM epitopes.

In twin studies the Vα repertoire has been shown to be influenced by genetic control[17]. In addition, data from Moffat and colleagues[18] suggest that there may be a locus in the α/δ locus on chromosome14q which may influence antigen-specific IgE responses. Our data suggests that antigen driven clonal expansion is a major component of the non random Vα and Jα repertoire seen in atopy. However, this does not exclude a genetic influence on this phenomenon.

Finally, whether these results represent activated clones of T cells producing increased levels of mRNA or whether a true clonal expansion of T cells has occurred is uncertain. The absence of Vα monoclonal antibodies to the TCR Vα segments 1, 3, 8 makes this impossible to examine at this time.

6. ACKNOWLEDGMENT

Work in the authors laboratory is supported by the MRC, Wellcome Trust, National Asthma Campaign, Northern and Yorkshire Regional Health Authority and the West Riding Medical Research Trust.

7. REFERENCES

1. Burney, P.G., Chinn, S. Rona, R.J. (1990). Br. Med. J. 300: 1306–10.
2. Barnes, P.J. (1989). J. Allergy Clin. Immunol. 83: 1013–26.
3. Corrigan, C.J. , Kay, A.B. Brit Med. Bull. 48: 72–84.
4. Okumura, K. Tada, T. (1971). J. Immunol 106: 1012–18.
5. Lebovitz, M.D., Barbee. R., Burrows, B. (1984).J Allergy Clin Immunol.73:259–64.
6. Hopp, J., Bewtra, A.K. ,Watt, G.D. (1984). J. Allergy Clin Immunol.73: 265–70.

7. Wilson, R. K. ,Lai, E. , Concannon, P. , Barth, R. K. & Hood, L.E. (1988) Immunol. Rev. 101, 149–172.

8. Hedrick, S. M. , Engel, I., McElligott, D. L., Fink, P.J., Hsu, M. L., Hansburg, D. & Matis, L. A. (1988) Science 239, 1541–1544.

9. Jorgensen, J. L., P. A. Reay, E. W. Ehrich, and M. M. Davis. 1992. Molecular components of T cell recognition. Annu. Rev. Immunol 10:835.

10. Oksenberg, J. R., Stuart, S., Begovich, A.B, Bell, R.B., Erlich, H.A. , Steinman, L., Bernard, C.C.A. (1990) . Nature 345: 344–347.

11. Ben-Nun, A., Liblau, R.S., Cohen. L., Lehmann., Tournier-Lasserve.E., Rosenzweig, A., Jingwu, Z., Raus, J.C.M., Bach, M.A. (1991). Proc. Nati. Acad. Sci. USA 88: 2466–2470.

12. Davies, T.F., Martin, A., Conception, E.S. ,Graves, P., Cohen, L. ,Ben-Nun. A. (1991). N. Engl. J. Med. 325: 238–44.

13. Palliard, X. , West, S.G. , Lafferty, J.A., Clements, J.R., Kappler, J. W, Marrack, P., Kotzin, B.L. (1991). Science 253:325.

14. Wucherpfenning, K.W., Bewcombe, J., Li, H., Keddy, C., Cuzner, M.L., Hafler, D.A. (1992) J. Exp. Med. 175:993–1002.

15. Kontianen S. et al (1991) Clin Exp Immunol 83:347–51.

16. Wedderburn, L. R., O'Hehir R. E., Hewitt C. R., Lamb J. R., Owen M. J. (1993) Proc. Natl. Acad. Sci. USA Vol. 90, pp. 8214–8218.

17. Moss P. A. H., Rosenberg W. M.C., Bell J. I., (1992) Annu Rev Immunol.10:71–96.

18. Moffat M F, Hill M R, Hopkin J M, Cookson W O C M, (June 25 1994), Vol.343, 1597–1599.

19. Chomczynski, P.& Sacchi, N. (1987) Anal. Biochem.162, 156–159.

20. Davies, T.F., Martin, A., Conception, E. S., Graves, P., Cohen, L., Ben-Nun. A. (1991). N. Engl. J. Med. 325: 238–44.

55

REDUCTION OF IgE ANTIBODY BINDING TO rDer p 2 VARIANTS GENERATED BY SITE-DIRECTED MUTAGENESIS

Alisa M. Smith and Martin D. Chapman

Asthma and Allergic Diseases Center
Department of Medicine
University of Virginia
Charlottesville, Virginia 22908

1. INTRODUCTION

Our studies have focused on the 14 kD Group 2 allergens of *D. pteronyssinus* which are potent immunogens and elicit humoral and cellular responses in 80–90% of mite allergic individuals. Previous studies have shown that the B cell epitopes are heat and pH resistant, but are destroyed upon reduction and alkylation, suggesting that these determinants are dependent on the tertiary structure of the protein (1). This conclusion is supported by studies that showed a low prevalence of IgE Ab binding to polypeptide fragments produced from truncated Der p 2 cDNA (2,3). Synthetic peptides spanning the entire Der p 2 sequence have also been used to map Ab binding regions, however, only one peptide, amino acids 65–78, retained IgE Ab binding, confirming that the majority of epitopes are conformational (4). Taken together, these studies suggested that an alternative approach was required to further map the conformational determinants on Group 2 allergens.

Site-directed mutagenesis has been used successfully for epitope mapping of antigens of known three dimensional structure (5–7). Since the tertiary structure of Der p 2 was not known, this provided an opportunity to investigate whether secondary structural predictions could be used to identify potential antigenic sites. Therefore, we used predictive algorithms to target surface residues (8,9). Variants were generated at lysine at position 100 and at three residues (asparagine-glutamine-asparagine) at position 44–46. Additional variants were generated to systematically disrupt each of the three disulfide bonds (Cys8–119, Cys21–27, and Cys73–78) to evaluate the contribution of each bond to the antigenic structure of the protein (10). The variants were evaluated by competitive binding ELISA using murine monoclonal antibodies and sera from dust mite allergic patients as well as intradermal skin testing.

New Horizons in Allergy Immunotherapy
edited by Sehon et al. Plenum Press. New York. 1996

391

2. RESULTS AND DISCUSSION

2.1. Contribution of Predicted Surface Residues to Antigenic Determinants

Since the three dimensional structure of Der p 2 was not known, surface residues were predicted using hydrophilicity and flexibility profiles from the primary amino acid sequence. The primary peak of hydrophilic sequence corresponded to Asn44-Gln45-Asn46, with a secondary peak at Lys100. Two variants at Asn44–46 were evaluated by competitive inhibition assays. Conservative substitutions Gln-Thr-Thr (N44Q) gave comparable inhibition curves to rDer p 2 for mAb αDpX, 7A1, 13A4, and for IgE Ab, using a serum pool from seven house dust mite allergic patients. However, this variant had reduced antigenicity for mAb 15E11, suggesting that this region is important to the epitope defined by this mAb. By contrast, the Pro-Pro-His (N44P) substitution, predicted to introduce a "helix breaker" motif, failed to bind most mAb and IgE Ab suggesting that this substitution has effects on several epitopes.

Two variants generated at Lys100 were evaluated. The arginine substitution is conservative, maintaining the positively charged side chain, while the threonine substitution removes this charge and introduces a less hydrophilic side chain. The substitutions at Lys100 gave overlapping inhibition curves with rDer p 2 for mAb αDpX and IgE Ab. The other mAb showed distinct binding patterns. The mAb 13A4 was inhibited by <10% using either substitution, suggesting that the epitope defined by mAb 13A4 "maps" to lysine 100. Inhibition of binding of mAb 15E11 reached 55% and 60% with Lys100Thr and Lys100Arg, respectively at the maximum concentration tested, indicating that this amino acid may contribute to the 15E11 epitope. Inhibition of binding of mAb 7A1 was slightly reduced for Lys100Arg but reached only 30% for Lys100Thr, thus the positive charge of the side chain at position 100 is critical for mAb 7A1 binding. These results strongly suggest that Lys100, a residue predicted to be on the surface of Der p 2, is important for epitopes defined by three mAb. Table I summarizes the binding studies of the variants at surface residues.

2.2. Contribution of Disulfide Bonds in Maintaining Antigenic Structure

Using our mutagenesis strategy, one cysteine from each pair was replaced by another amino acid, preventing the disulfide from forming at that position. The ability of the

Table 1. ELISA inhibition profiles of rDer p 2 variants[a]

Inhibitor	% Inhibition of Antibody Binding				
	αDpX	7A1	15E11	13A4	IgE[b]
rDer p 2	80	85	80	85	90
N44Q	75	85	**40**	85	90
N44P	**<20**	**50**	**<10**	**<20**	**40**
K100T	80	**30**	55	**<10**	90
K100R	80	75	60	**<10**	90

[a]Maximal inhibition of Ab binding in ELISA using 100μg/ml rDer p 2 or variant.
[b]Serum pool from seven house dust mite allergic patients.

variants to inhibit binding of IgE Ab or mAb to rDer p 2 was evaluated by comparing the amount of variant required to give inhibition of Ab binding with the positive control, rDer p 2. The Cys21Ser, Cys27Gly, Cys8Gly and Cys119Tyr variants showed comparable reactivity with αDpX, however, the Cys73Arg and Cys78Gly variants gave <20% inhibition of αDpX binding at the highest inhibitor concentration tested. The Cys73Arg variant also failed to inhibit the binding of two additional mAb, 13A4 and 15E11. The mAb 7A1 reacted with all six variants; Cys119Tyr showed reactivity equivalent to rDer p 2, while the Cys21Ser, Cys27Gly and Cys8Gly variants had slightly reduced antigenicity and required up to ten-fold more antigen to give 50% inhibition. The Cys73Arg and Cys78Gly variants gave 50% inhibition of mAb 7A1 binding at 10 to 15-fold higher antigen concentration than rDer p 2. The reactivity of mAb 7A1 with Cys73Arg and Cys78Gly indicates that this variant is not totally denatured. Thus while all 4 mAb gave unique binding profiles, the Cys73 and Cys78 variants consistently showed the greatest reduction in antigenicity.

The inhibition of binding of IgE Ab was assessed for 13 individual sera and for the serum pool, from 7 additional patients. All of the individual sera were inhibited by Cys119Tyr at concentrations comparable to rDer p2. The Cys21Ser variant gave overlapping inhibition curves with rDer p2 for two sera, but required 2 to 11-fold more antigen for the other 11 sera. Maximum inhibition by Cys73Arg ranged from 11% to 48% for 12 sera and only one serum gave 50% inhibition (at 12.5-fold higher concentration than rDer p 2). Six sera were from patients with atopic dermatitis and seven were from asthmatics, however, no significant differences in inhibition patterns by the variants were seen among these patients. Figure 1 shows the inhibition curves for 2 representative sera. All 13 sera tested gave the same pattern as seen with the mAb binding to the disulfide variants: the Cys73Arg variant showed the greatest reduction in antigenicity, the Cys21Ser variant showed slightly reduced antigenicity, and the Cys119Tyr variant showed reactivity comparable to rDer p 2.

To correlate the *in vitro* reactivity with *in vivo* IgE binding, quantitative intradermal skin testing was preformed, comparing reactivity of rDer p 2 with Cys78Gly. Four patients with allergic rhinitis or asthma were skin test positive (8 x 8 mm wheal) to rDer p 2 at dilutions of 10^{-1} to 10^{-2} μg/ml. Three of the four patients showed a one log decrease in the dose of Cys78Gly giving a comparable response and one patient showed a two log decrease. Three non-allergic controls did not react to rDer p 2 and Cys78Gly at 1 μg/ml.

In summary, this study demonstrates the contribution of the three disulfide bonds of Der p 2 to the antigenic structure of the protein. In addition, the bonds make different con-

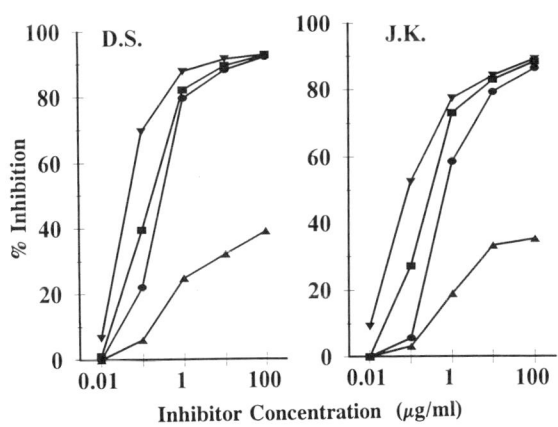

Figure 1. Inhibition of IgE Ab binding to rDer p 2 using the cysteine variants. Binding of IgE Ab to rDer p 2 was inhibited using rDer p 2 (■), Cys21 (●), Cys73 (▲), or Cys119 (▼) over a 4 log range of concentrations. Results are shown for 2 representative sera (D.S. has atopic dermatitis and J.K. has asthma). In the absence of inhibitor, using PBS as a control, maximum binding in the ELISA system was O.D.$_{405}$ = 1.4–1.6, using 1/4 - 1/16 serum dilutions.

tributions to maintaining this structure as shown by the IgE Ab binding curves for each variant. Residues predicted to be surface exposed are involved in epitopes defined by mAb, but variants at these positions did not distinguish a population of IgE Ab epitopes. Variants with reduced IgE binding, such as Cys73Arg or Cys78Gly, may provide an alternative strategy for immunotherapy. The use of complete recombinant proteins with reduced IgE Ab binding, but with a full complement of T cell epitopes, may offer an alternative approach to immunotherapy, which could potentially be applicable to any cloned allergen.

3. ACKNOWLEDGMENTS

Dr. Hirokazu Okudaira, Tokyo, and Dr. Rob C. Aalberse, Amsterdam, kindly provided some of the monoclonal antibodies used in this study. We thank Dr. Lisa M. Wheatley for help with the skin testing and Ms. Nicolle Couture for help with DNA sequence analysis.

4. REFERENCES

1. Lombardero M., Heymann, P. W. , Platts-Mills, T. A. E. , Fox, J. W. and Chapman, M. D., *J. Immunol.* 1990. *144:*1353.
2. Chua, K.Y., Doyle, C.R., Simpson, R. J., Turner, K. J., Stewart, G. A. and Thomas, W. R., *Int. Arch. Allergy Appl. Immunol.* 1990. *91:*118.
3. Chua, K. Y., Greene, W. K. , Kehal, P. and Thomas, W. R., *Clin. Exp. Allergy* 1991. *21:*161.
4. van't Hof, W., Drieduk, P. C. , van den Berg, M., Beck-Sickinger, A. G., Jung, G. Aalberse, R. C., *Mol. Immunol.* 1991. *28:*1225.
5. Smith A. M., Woodward, M. P., Hershey, C. W., Hershey, E. D. and Benjamin, D. C., *J. Immunol.* 1991. *146:*1254.
6. Smith A. M. and Benjamin, D. C., *J. Immunol.* 1991. *146:*1259.
7. Dudler T., Schneider, T., Annand, R., Gelb, M. and Suter, M., *J. Immunol.* 1994. *152:*5514.
8. Hopp T. and Woods, K., *Proc. Natl. Acad. Sci. USA* 1981. *78:*3824.
9. Karplus P., and Schultz, G., *Naturwissenschaften* 1985. *72:*212.
10. Nishyama, C., Yuuki, T., Takai, T., Okumura, Y. and Okudaira, H., *Int. Arch. Aller Immunol.* 1993. *101:*159.

56

EXPRESSION OF THE HOUSE DUST MITE ALLERGEN Der p2 AND MUTANTS IN THE BAKER'S YEAST *Saccharomyces cerevisiae*

G. A. J. Hakkaart, R. C. Aalberse, and R. van Ree

Department of Allergy
Central Laboratory of the Netherlands
Red Cross Blood Transfusion Service and
Laboratory for Experimental and Clinical Immunology
University of Amsterdam
Plesmanlaan 125, 1066 CX Amsterdam, The Netherlands

The aim of our study was to express the house dust mite allergen Der p2 in *E. coli* and *S. cerevisiae*. The immunological and biological activities were compared to the native, mite-derived allergen molecule. Mutagenesis of the Der p2 cDNA was carried out in order to construct allergen variants with diminished IgE binding. These mutant molecules will be used to investigate the minimal requirements to induce histamine release from basophilic leukocytes. (Also IgG binding will be studied). Mutant allergen molecules with diminished biological activity might eventually be applicable in immunotherapy.

EXPRESSION OF Der p2 IN *E. coli*

In first instance the Der p2 cDNA (1) was cloned into the plasmid pQE10 (2). This *E. coli* transformant produces the allergen as an urea-resoluble fusion protein with an 11 amino-acid residues leader sequence attached to the N-terminus. This tag contains a histidine sextette which enables the purification of the recombinant allergen by means of nickel-chelate chromatography.

The purified recombinant allergen showed a substantial Der p2-like reactivity. We were able to induce proliferation of Der p2 specific T-cell lines and clones (3) and induced IgE-mediated histamine release from basophilic leukocytes. Furthermore, the allergen showed reactivity with human IgE and a number of Der p2 specific mAb's. Discrepancies with natural Der p2 were, however, also detected. 11/22 mAb's did not show reactivity with the recombinant allergen. Furthermore, Der p2 specific IgE from one human serum (no. 54) out of 29 did not show reactivity with the *E. coli* derived allergen.

New Horizons in Allergy Immunotherapy
edited by Sehon et al. Plenum Press, New York, 1996

395

EXPRESSION OF Der p2 IN YEAST

In order to obtain a better-folded recombinant allergen the Der p2 was expressed in the baker's yeast *Saccharomyces cerevisiae*. The Der p2 cDNA was cloned into the expression plasmid pSY1 (4,5). The yeast transformants were secreting the allergen as a water soluble protein into the growth medium. Der p2 was produced with an additional vector encoded alanine residue attached to the N-terminus. This recombinant allergen also lacked reactivity with the 11 non-reactive mAB's and the single non-reactive serum.

RECOMBINANT VERSUS NATIVE Der p2

The discrepancies in reaction pattern between the two recombinant allergens and the native counterpart were explained by the following experimental data.

Serum 54: Reactive with Breakdown Product?

SDS-PAGE of mite extract followed by immuno-blotting did not show an IgE reactivity with the expected 14kd band, but with a lower MW band. Therefore mite-extract was gel-filtrated. Der p2 reactivity in the fractions was measured by means of an indirect RAST. mAb αdpX was the catching antibody, detection took place with IgE from a pool serum with Der p2 reactivity or from serum 54. The IgE pool was showing reactivity with the 14kd protein, whereas IgE from serum 54 was reactive with a compound of a lower molecular weight, possibly a breakdown product of the 14kd allergen.

mAb's Reactive with the N-Terminus

Both recombinant allergens contained additional amino acid residues attached to the N-terminus (11 residues for the *E. coli* Der p2, one single alanine residue for the yeast derived allergen). It was investigated whether these residues might disturb a particular antigenic determinant. For this purpose a yeast expression plasmid was constructed encoding a mature allergen molecule, without any extra amino-acid residues, resulting in a recombinant Der p2 which is sequence-identical to the mite derived allergen. This recombinant allergen showed reactivity with 4/11 unreactive mAbs, e.g. 10E11. Inhibition studies were carried out. The Der p2 RAST with mAb 10E11 was inhibited with the two allergen molecules. Ala-Der p2 did not inhibit the Der p2 RAST for 10E11.

Iso-Form Specific mAbs

Recently Dr. K.Y. Chua has isolated the cDNA encoding an isoform of Der p2 differing in 3 amino-acids residues from the initially cloned Der p2 (1). The recombinant isoform demonstrated different IgE binding than the initial recombinant Der p2 (K.Y. Chua, pers. comm.). To investigate the role of the particular amino acid substitutions, we constructed three Der p2 variants each harboring one of these substitutions. These cDNA's were expressed in yeast and the binding with the mentioned mAb's was studied. The remaining 7/11 mAbs showed reactivity with variant (asp114→asn).

MUTAGENESIS OF Der p2

An antigenicity plot was made by means of MacVector, based on predictions according to Chou-Fasman and Robson-Garnier. Mutations were made in the predicted antigenic sites on the protein. These mutant allergens were expressed in yeast. Their antibody binding capacities were studied in inhibition RASTs with IgE as well as monoclonal antibodies. From these studies we concluded that these mutations resulted in a decrease in binding with IgE and with mAbs 2B12B3 and αdpX. Furthermore, the decrease in IgE binding varied among patients.

In conclusion, we expressed Der p2 in the baker's yeast *S. cerevisiae*. This allergen can be isolated as a water soluble protein, without the requirement of denaturing steps. Furthermore, *E. coli* produces toxic and pyrogenic cell wall components, whereas *S. cerevisiae* has, during long time use in food industry, proven to be non-pathogenic to man and therefore has been granted official GRAS (Generally Recognized As Safe) status. For this reason, the baker's yeast might be preferred over *E. Coli* when *in vivo* applications are aimed. Altogether yeast is the preferred host to express Der p2. This yeast derived allergen, possesses a substantial Der p2 reactivity.

Of the 22 mAbs tested with the recombinant protein, 4 are only reactive with the allergen without additional amino acid residues attached to the N-terminus, 7 mAbs are only reactive with a variant of Der p2 differing in only one amino acid residue. These two findings have implications for the use of N-terminally fused recombinant Der p2 (in epitope-studies) and monoclonal antibodies (in standardization and environmental control measurements).

Furthermore, by means of site directed mutagenesis (and expression of a N-terminally fused allergen), the epitopes of three mAbs could be determined. The particular mutant molecules also showed a decrease in IgE binding. This decrease varied among patient.

ACKNOWLEDGMENT

The authors like to thank Dr. W. Thomas and Dr. K.Y. Chua for providing the Der p2 cDNA and the sequence of the isoform, Dr. M. Chapman (Charlottesville) for providing a set of mAbs, and Dr. J.W. Chapman (Vlaardingen, The Netherlands) for providing the vector pSY1.

This research was financially supported by the Netherlands Asthma Foundation (Grant No. 90.33).

REFERENCES

1. Chua, K.Y., Doyle, C.R., Simpson, R.J., Turner, K.J., Stewart, G.A., and Thomas W.R.: Isolation of cDNA coding for the major mite allergen Der pII by IgE plaque immunoassay. Int Arch Allergy Appl Immunol 1990; 91:118–123.

2. Stüber, D., Matile, H., Garotta, G.: System for high level production in *E. coli* and rapid purification of recombinant proteins: Application to epitope mapping, preparation of antibodies and structure-function analysis. Immunological Methods, 4th ed. 1990, I. Lefkovits and B. Pernis, eds. Academic Press, New York, p 121–152.

3. Van Neerven, R.J.J., Van't Hof, W., Ringrose, J.H., Jansen, H.M., Aalberse, R.C., Wierenga, E.A., and Kapsenberg, M.L.: T cell epitopes of house dust mite major allergen Der p 2. J Immunol 1993; 151:2326–2335.

4. Verbakel, J.M.A.: Heterologous gene expression in the yeast *Saccharomyces cerevisiae.* PhD thesis, 1991, Rijksuniversiteit Utrecht, The Netherlands.
5. Harmsen, M.M.: Heterologous protein secretion by the yeast *Saccharomyces cerevisiae.* PhD thesis, 1995, Vrije Universiteit, Amsterdam, The Netherlands.

57

THE FUNCTION OF ALLERGENS MAY DETERMINE ALLERGENICITY

A. Bufe,[*] G. Schramm, A. Petersen, M. Schlaak, and W. -M. Becker

Forschungsinstitut Borstel
Molecular Allergology
Parkallee 21, D-23845 Borstel, Germany

1. INTRODUCTION

Allergenicity of an antigen in terms of Type-1 allergy has always been described as the ability of a given protein to bind to specific IgE antibodies and the potency of these allergens to crosslink cellbound IgE to induce mediator release like histamine in basophils or mast cells. Whether the ability of allergens to induce a primary sensitization by switching B-cells to produce specific IgE antibodies is linked to a special feature of the allergens is unknown. In this context it is argued that the function of an allergen itself contributes to the allergenicity either by representing a specific structure or by influencing the process of presentation. Recently evidence was presented that cysteine protease *Der p* 1, the major house dust mite allergen, increases the permeability of bronchial epithelium for albumin by its functional ability of protein cleavage and may thus facilitate its own penetration (1). Furthermore enzymatically intact phospholipase A1 was able to induce an IgE mediated immune response in an animal model whereas the inactive mutant did not lead to IgE but IgG1 production (2). Finally it was proposed that a number of allergens with high homology to protease inhibitors, which can bind directly to cell membranes of antigen presenting cells, influence their endocytosis by being protease inhibitors (3).

Among the identified allergens from plants, animals and foods in only a part the functions have been discovered and described. In Tab. 1 most known functions are summarized and correlated to the main entrance they usually find into the human body. It seems as if all the enzymes and enzyme-inhibitors are preferable introduced through the nasal and bronchial mucosa whereas the transport- and storage proteins mainly enter via the gastrointestinal tract. While in only a small number of allergens the function has now been explained this interpretation of Tab. 1 could lead to a rather simplified view. In the biological system it is always a mixture of proteins which is presented to the mucosa. But

---

[*] Communication to: Albrecht Bufe, Forschungsinstitut Borstel, Molecular Allergology, Parkallee 22, D-23845 Borstel, Germany. Tel.: 04573/10314; FAX: 04537/10404.

New Horizons in Allergy Immunotherapy
edited by Sehon et al. Plenum Press, New York, 1996

Table 1. Functions of a number of different allergens in relation to their usual entrance into the human body. 1 = nasal mucosa, 2 = bronchial mucosa, 3 = gastrointestinal, 4 = subcutaneously. Data taken from Stewart et al. (3) and King et al. (18)

Function	Allergen	Entrance
Enzymes		
Cysteine protease	*Der p* 1	1,2
Other protease	*Brom p* 1	4
Trypsin	*Der p* 3	1,2
Chymotrypsin	*Der p* 6	1,2
Amylase	*Der p* 4, Yeast	1,2
RNascs	*Phl p* 5, *Bet v* 1	1,2
Cytochrome C	Grasses	1,2
Phospholipase A2	*Api m* 1	4
Hyaluronidase	*Api m* 2	4
Lysozymc	*Gal d* 4	3
Protease inhibitor		
Wheat, barley:	Cm 16, NMAI 1, CM b, BMAI-1	3
Mustard seed	*Ric c* 1	3
Castor bean	*Sin a* 1	3
Structural proteins		
Profilin	Tree- and Grass pollen	1,2
Tropomyosin	*Pen a* 2	3
Melitin	*Api m* 4	4
Storage protein		
Vicilin	*Ara h* 1, Soybean	3
Ovalbumin	*Gal d* 2	3
Conalbumin	*Gal d* 3	3
Albumin	*Bra g* 1, *Sin a* 1	3
Transport protein		
Hemoglobin	*Chi t* 1	3

Data taken from Stewart et al. (3) and King et al. (18)

recent data reveals that the enzymes which are allergens may play an important role in facilitating their presentation and it is known that many enzymes are relatively resistant and stabile proteins thus possibly behaving as competent allergens in the mucosa.

In the following a newly discovered group of enzymes in grass and birch pollen is discussed and some data on the influence of this function in correlation to allergenicity is critically reviewed.

2. MAJOR GRASS POLLEN ALLERGEN Phl p 5b IS A RIBONUCLEASE

First hints that group 5 allergens in grass pollen are transported into starch granules, the so called amyloplast, came from Singh et. al. (4) when he was able to show that the major allergen of rye-grass pollen (*Lol p* 5) is intracellularly targeted to this structure. Knox then demonstrated the release of the starch granules into the environment under certain conditions, like changes of humidity in the air (5). Nothing was known about the actual function of these proteins and the reason for this transport. Sequence comparison of a number of cloned group 5 allergens in the different grass pollen species demonstrated that the sequences spanning the central region of all group 5 allergens were highly constant whereas the C-terminal and N-terminal regions were highly variable (7). These proteins seemed to be similar enough among the different species to show a degree of immunological identity, but they were sufficiently diverse in other sites to explain individually different IgE immunoreactivity of allergic patients (8). Years ago it was shown that pollen wall proteins of ragweed interacted with pollen stigma as recognition substances and these proteins were identified as allergens by binding to IgE containing serum (6). Like group 5 allergens they exist as relatively variable isoforms of the same protein family. It is still speculation that group 5 allergens may be involved in recognition processes between pollen and stigma considering that sequence identity and homology to other proteins of known function especially to incompatibility genes were not found. But looking for functional homologies we were able to show that a protein released from the mother plant of timothy grass pollen after stimulation with salicylic acid, a signal hormone of plant resistance (8), is highly cross-reactive with group 5 pollen allergens (7). This strongly indicated that a group 5 allergen equivalent could be involved in host pathogen interaction although we did not demonstrate direct pathogen induced activation. Some host pathogenically induced proteins may be evolutionary and functionally related to plant RNases (9), which lead us to analyze whether group 5 allergens show ribonuclease activity. We could clearly demonstrate that natural *Phl p* 5a and highly purified recombinant *Phl p* 5b acted as RNases although compared to pancreatic RNase A their activity was significantly weaker (7). This indicated the different specificities of the pollen RNases. But it could have been influenced by the purification procedure, by refolding conditions of the recombinant protein, and perhaps by unknown posttranslational differences between the bacterial and the natural protein.

3. INFLUENCE OF RNase FUNCTION ON THE ALLERGENICITY

Like in other pollen which RNases have been extensively analyzed (10) timothy grass pollen contains a number of different ribonucleases of which group 5 allergens are only one. In birch pollen we demonstrated the same situation whereas it turned out that *Bet v* 1, the major birch pollen allergen with homology to plant resistance genes (11) and a ginseng RNase (12) shows RNase activity as well (13). Thus looking at the influence of enzyme activity on allergenicity one has always to take into account that there are more RNases in pollen which are not defined as allergens and which still might have an effect on the mucosa. It was already seen (7) that recombinant *Phl p* 5b in the RNase assay had build complexes with the RNA and an placental RNase inhibitor. This was confirmed in gel shift experiments where the interaction of the RNase inhibitor with the allergen and the RNA was studied (14). This complex of the inhibitor with the RNase did not influence significantly the IgE binding of recombinant *Phl p* 5b. We then demonstrated dose dependant IgE production of mononuclear cells of an allergic patient in vitro induced by *Phl p* 5b. IgE production was significantly inhibited by RNase inhibitor. Histamine release of basophils taken from the same patient and also induced by *Phl p* 5b was reduced in a dose dependant manner by RNase-inhibitor. With this data it was suggested that the interaction of the enzyme inhibitor with the RNase *Phl p* 5b has influenced the allergenicity of this protein. This indicated that the enzyme activity as well as IgE binding depended on the protein structure of the allergen and this seemed to influence antigen presentation and processing as shown by the in vitro IgE production assay. There is no evidence yet that RNA degradation itself may be involved in this process and facilitate or influence presentation of allergens. But in this context it is interesting to note that human eosinophil cationic protein which participates in the destruction of parasites and the bronchial endothelium in bronchial asthma shows ribonuclease activity (15).

In summary it becomes more and more evident that the function of allergens may be involved in their allergenicity in different ways as mentioned above. Whether this phenomenon is an important part of the pathomechanism which allergens can induce in allergic patients and whether this knowledge can be used for future therapeutic concepts is still an open question.

4. REFERENCES

1. Herbert, C.A., King, C.M., Ring, P.C., Holgate, S.T., Stewart, G.A., Thompson, P.J., Robinson, C. (1995) Augmentation of permeability in the bronchial epithelium by house dust mite allergen Der p1. Am J Respir Cell Mol Biol; 12:369–378
2. Kolbe, L., Dudler, T., Suter, M., Kölsch, E. (1993) Parameters influencing the immunogenicity of phospholipase A_2 (PLA$_2$), the major allergen of bee venom. Abstract; Immunobiol;189:145
3. Steward, G.A., Thompson, P.J., McWilliam, A.S. (1993) Biochemical properties of aeroallergens: contributory factors in allergic sensitization ? Pediatr Allergy Immunol; 4:163–172.
4. Singh,M.B., Hough,T., Theerakulpisut,P., Avjioglu,A., Davies,S., Smith,P.M., Taylor,P., Simpson,R.J., Ward,L.D., McCluskey,J., Puy,R., Knox,R.B. (1991) Isolation of cDNA encoding a newly identified major allergenic protein of rye-grass pollen: intracellular targeting to amyloplast. Proc Natl Acad Sci; 88:1384–1388
5. Knox,R.B., (1993) Grass pollen, thunderstorms and asthma. Clin Exp Allergy, **23**, 354–359.
6. Knox,R.B., (1973) Pollen wall proteins: pollen-stigma interactions in ragweed and cosmos (compositae) J Cell Sci; 12:421–443
7. Bufe, A., Schramm, G., Keown, M.B., Schlaak, M., Becker, W.-M. (1995) Major allergen Phl p Vb in timothy grass is a novel pollen RNase. FEBS Letter; 363:6–12
8. Bufe A, Becker W-M, Schramm G, Petersen A, Mamat U, Schlaak M (1994) Major allergen *Phl p* Va (timothy grass) bears at least two different IgE-reactive epitopes. J Allergy Clin Immunol.,94:173–181
9. Gaffney,T., Friedrich,L., Vernooij,B., Negrotto,D., Nye,G., Uknes,S., Ward,E., Kessmann,H., Ryals,J. (1993) Requirement of salicylic acid for induction of systemic acquired resistance. Science; 261:754–756
10. Dickinson, H. (1994) Simply a social disease. Nature; 367:517–18
11. Yen, Y., Green, P.J. (1991) Identification and properties of the major ribonucleases of arabidopsis thaliana. Plant Physiol; 97:1487–93
12. Breiteneder,H., Pettenburger,K., Bito,A., Valenta,R., Kraft,D., Rumpold,H., Scheiner,O., Breitenbach,M. (1989) The gene coding for the major birch pollen allergen Bet v I, is highly homologous to a pea disease resistance response gene. EMBO J; 8:1935–1938.
13. Moiseyev GP, Beintema JJ, Fedoreyeva LI, Yakovlev GI (1994). High sequence similarity between a ribonuclease from ginseng calluses and fungus-elicited proteins from parsley indicates that intracellular pathogenesis-related proteins are ribonucleases. Planta,193:470–472
14. Bufe, A., Kahlert, H., Schlaak, M., Becker, W.-M. (1995) Major birch pollen allergen Bet v 1 shows ribonuclease activity. (submitted)
15. Bufe, A., Schramm, G., Haas, H., Schlaak, M., Becker, W.-M. (1995) Influence of enzyme activity of major allergen Phl p 5b on its allergenicity. (submitted)
16. Rosenberg, H.F., Ackerman, S.J., Tenon, D.G. (1989) Human eosinophil cationic protein; molecular cloning of a cytotoxin and helminthotoxin with ribonuclease activity. J Exp Med; 170:163
18. King, T.P., Hoffman, D., Lowenstein, H., Marsh, D.G., Platts-Mills, T.A.E., Thomas, W. (1994) Allergen Nomenclature. Int Arch Allergy Immunol; 105:224–233

58

DIFFERENTIAL GENE EXPRESSION FOR INTERLEUKIN-13 AND OTHER CYTOKINES IN THE SKIN OF ATOPIC DERMATITIS PATIENTS AND HEALTHY SUBJECTS

I. Van der Ploeg[1], M. Tengvall Linder[1], Ö. Hägermark[2], C. -F. Wahlgren,[2] and A. Scheynius[1]

[1]Department of Clinical Immunology
[2]Department of Dermatology
Karolinska Hospital
S-171 76 Stockholm, Sweden

T helper cells are thought to be of importance in the pathogenesis of atopic dermatitis (AD)[1,2]. Most patients with (AD) have elevated serum IgE levels[2–4]. Allergens stimulate a certain population of T helper cells, the Th2-cells, that produce high amounts of interleukin-4 (IL-4), and relative low amounts of interferon-γ (IFN-γ)[5]. IL-4 stimulates B-cells to IgE production[6]. Bacteria and viruses induce the activation of Th1-cells, resulting in IFN-γ production and as a result we see a delayed hypersensitivity reaction (e.g.).[7]

Our purpose was to study the role of cytokines in the pathogenesis of AD. More specifically we wanted to investigate what cytokines are involved in atopic eczema and we were especially interested in the recently described cytokine IL-13 that like IL-4 stimulates to the production of IgE from B cells[8, 9]. Since IL-2 induces the production of other cytokines, we also used IL-2 injection as a tool to enhance the cytokine mRNA production in the skin of patients with AD and healthy controls.

The method we have used is a semi-quantitative reverse transcription PCR (RT-PCR) method. We have taken punch skin biopsy specimens (3 mm) from 6 healthy individuals and of 5 patients with AD, both from non-lesional (uninvolved) skin and from chronic lichenified lesional skin. RNA was extracted from the biopsies, and specific complementary DNA was amplified for the cytokines IFN-γ, IL-2, IL-4, IL-5, IL-13 and GM-CSF. β-actin that is expressed in all cells was used as a positive control. As a negative control we had no RNA in the RT-PCR reaction, and as a positive control RNA from lymphocytes whose T-cell receptors were stimulated for 6 h with an antibody against the CD3 receptor, and which therefore produced many cytokines.

Interestingly, we could detect much more IL-13 gene expression in non-lesional AD skin than in normal skin, and still more IL-13 mRNA in chronic lesional skin. We ob-

New Horizons in Allergy Immunotherapy
edited by Sehon et al. Plenum Press, New York, 1996

403

served a tendency of lower gene expression for IFN-γ in non-lesional skin compared to the levels detected in the skin of the healthy controls. This is what one would expect for a Th-2 cell like cytokine profile. We detected a higher gene expression for IFN-γ in lesional skin, and this corresponds to what others have found in late patch test reactions, namely a shift from a Th2- to a Th1 cell like cytokine profile (T. Thepen, personal communication). We did not detect IL-2, IL-4 and IL-5 gene expression, probably because very little of mRNA is expressed, or it is produced during a short time interval. GM-CSF is both expressed by Th1 and Th2-like cells, and we did not see any differences between AD patients and healthy individuals for this cytokine.

We used IL-2 induced T cells proliferation to enhance the signals for cytokine gene expression. An intradermal injection of 20 μg of IL-2 in 8 AD patients (non-lesional skin) and in 8 healthy individuals caused a T-cell infiltrate at 24 h, in both groups. This was assessed with an antibody to the T cell receptor and APAAP staining. After IL-2 injection we observed an increased gene expression for all cytokines except for IL-2 itself, indicating that IL-2 may downregulate its own production. We observed lower IFN-γ levels in the skin of the AD patients than in the skin of the healthy controls, and a tendency for a higher gene expression for IL-4, IL-5 and IL-13 in the AD skin.

We can draw the conclusion that non-lesional AD skin shows a Th2 cells cytokine profile, with elevated IL-4, IL-5 and IL-13 levels, and low IFN-γ levels. We observed, on the contrary, elevated IFN-γ levels in chronic lesional skin, indicating a switch to a Th1-cells cytokine profile. Considering that IL-13 gene expression is higher in atopic eczema patients compared to healthy controls, and higher in lesional than in non-lesional skin IL-13 expression might be used as a marker in skin inflammation. Whether IL-13 gene expression is also altered in other skin diseases has still to be investigated and will determine if IL-13 is or is not a specific marker for AD.

REFERENCES

1. Kapsenberg, M.L., Jansen, H.M., Bos, J.D., and Wierenga, E.A., Role of type 1 and type 2 T helper cells in allergic diseases. *Curr Opin Immunol* **4**, 788–793, 1992.
2. Cooper, K.D., Atopic dermatitis: Recent trends in pathogenesis and therapy. *J Invest Dermatol* **102**, 128–137, 1994.
3. Öhman, S., and Johansson, S.G.O., Immunoglobulins in atopic dermatitis. *Acta Derm Venereol (Stockh.)* **54**, 193–202, 1974.
4. Hanifin, J.M., and Rajka, G., Diagnostic features of atopic dermatitis. *Acta Derm. Venereol. Suppl. (Stockh.)* **92**, 44–47, 1980.
5. Romagnani, S., Human TH1 and TH2 subsets: regulation of differentiation and role in protection and immunopathology. *Int Arch Allergy Immunol* **98**, 279–285, 1992.
6. Del Prete, G., Maggi, E., Parronchi, P., Chrétien, I., Tiri, A., Macchia, D., Ricci, M., Banchereau, J., de Vries, J., and Romagnani, S., IL-4 is an essential factor for the IgE synthesis induced in vitro by human T cell clones and their supernatants. *J Immunol* **140**, 4193–4198, 1988.
7. Tsicopoulos, A., Hamid, Q., Varney, V., Ying, S., Moqbel, R., Durham, S.R., and Kay, A.B., Preferential messenger RNA expression of Th1-type cells (IFN-gamma+, IL-2+) in classical delayed-type (tuberculin) hypersensitivity reactions in human skin. *J Immunol* **148**, 2058–2061, 1992.
8. Minty, A., Chalon, P., Derocq, J.-M., Dumont, X., Guillemot, J.-C., Kaghad, M., Labit, C., Leplatois, P., Liauzun, P., Miloux, B., Minty, C., Casellas, P., Loison, G., Lupker, J., Shire, D., Ferrara, P., and Caput, D., Interleukin-13 is a new human lymphokine regulating inflammatory and immune responses. *Nature (Lond.)* **362**, 248–250, 1993.
9. Punnonen, J., Aversa, G., Cocks, B.G., McKenzie, A.N.J., Menon, S., Zurawski, G., de Waal-Malefyt, R., and de Vries, J.E., Interleukin 13 induces interleukin 4-independent IgG4 and IgE synthesis and CD23 expression by human B cells. *Proc Natl Acad Sci USA* **90**, 3730–3734, 1993.

59

PEPTIDE INDUCED ANERGY OF HUMAN ALLERGEN-SPECIFIC T CELLS

Hans Yssel, Stephan Fasler, Gregorio Aversa, and Jan E. de Vries

Human Immunology Department
DNAX Research Institute for Molecular and Cellular Biology
901 California Avenue
Palo Alto, California 94304

INTRODUCTION

A common feature of allergic disorders is the presence of allergen-specific antibodies of the IgE isotype which bind to high affinity receptors on mast cells and basophils. Upon interaction of the mast cell-bound IgE antibody with allergen, soluble mediators, like histamine and leukotriens, are released which cause allergic reactions in the various target organs. In house dust mite-induced allergy IgE antibodies that react with a variety of allergens are detected; the predominant IgE response however is directed at the *Dermatophagoides pteronyssinus* group I (*Der p* I) and group II (*Der p* II) allergens(1).

Since the synthesis of IgE in human is tightly regulated by cytokines, helper T cells play a central role in the regulation of the IgE response. Most allergen-specific human T cell clones, generated from skin biopsies or peripheral blood of atopic patients belong to the T helper type 2 (Th2) subset, in that they produce high levels of IL-4 and IL-5 and low levels of IFN-γ, respectively, upon activation with allergen. In addition, *Der p* I-specific Th2 T cell clones have been found to produce IL-13, although the production of this cytokine does not seem to be restricted to the Th2 subset of T cell clones (2). Importantly, co-cultivation of activated *Der p* I-specific Th2 T cell clones with purified B cells resulted in the production of IgE which could partially be inhibited by the addition of neutralizing anti-IL-4 or anti-IL-13 mAbs (3). The latter findings indicate that IL-4 and IL-13 play a major role in the induction of IgE synthesis *in vitro*, although the relative contribution of both cytokines to this process has yet to be determined. It is likely however that due to the central role of allergen-specific T cells in the synthesis of IgE, inhibition of IL-4 and IL-13 production by these cells may provide an efficient way to block allergen-induced IgE synthesis and treat IgE-mediated allergic diseases.

New Horizons in Allergy Immunotherapy
edited by Sehon et al. Plenum Press, New York, 1996

405

INDUCTION OF NON-RESPONSIVENESS IN
ALLERGEN-SPECIFIC Th2 CELLS

Early studies, using human and mouse T cell clones, have shown that interaction of the TCR with Antigen (Ag) in the absence of costimulation does not result in activation of the cells, but rather leads to a state of non-responsiveness or anergy, during which the cells do no longer proliferate or produce IL-2 following stimulation with Ag and Antigen presenting cells (APC) (4,5). Using a similar model system, we have demonstrated recently that allergen-specific T cell clones can be rendered functionally non-responsive to subsequent antigenic stimulation. The results of this study which will be discussed in this chapter are summarized in Table 1. *Der p* I-specific T clones, incubated for 16 h with peptides, representing two minimal T cell activation inducing epitopes on the *Der p*I-molecule, did no longer proliferate or produce IL-2, IL-4, IL-5 or IL-13, following stimulation with *Der p* I, presented by autologous- or HLA-matched APC. It is of interest to note that during the peptide-mediated induction of anergy the T cell clones produced high levels of IL-4, IL-5, IL-13, GM-CSF and TNF-α, suggesting that the cells went through a state of activation prior to becoming non-responsive.

In view of the above mentioned capacity of activated allergen-specific Th2 cells to provide help to B cells for the synthesis of IgE, the effect of anergy induction on this Th2 helper activity was investigated. *Der p* I-specific, T cell clones, rendered anergic following incubation with specific peptides in the absence of APC, failed to induce the synthesis of IgE and IgG_4 when cocultured with purified B cells, even in the presence of exogenous

Table 1. Functional and phenotypic characterization of anergic allergen-specific
T helper type 2 clones

	Stimulation condition of T cell clones [a]		
	Resting	**Optimally activated**	**Anergic**
CD3 expression	High	Decreased	Decreased
CD80/CD86 expression	Dim/High	High	High
CD40L expression	No	Induced	Induced
Help for IgE synthesis	No	Yes	No
Cytokine production	No	Yes	Yes
Upon restimulation [b]			
Proliferation	Yes	Yes	No
Ca^{2+} flux	Yes	Yes	No
Cytokine production	Yes	Yes	No

[a] T cell clones were cultured in medium only (Resting), in the presence of 1 µg/ml of the *Der p* I derived peptide p94-104 and autologous APC (Optimally activated) or in the presence of 50 µg/ml p94-104 (Anergic). After 24 h of incubation, the cells were washed and analyzed for function and phenotype.

[b] T cell clones were restimulated with 1 µg/ml p94-104 / autologous APC and analyzed.

recombinant (r)IL-4 or rIL-13. Interestingly, levels of CD40L expression were comparable between anergic *Der p* I-specific T cell clones and T cell clones that had been optimally stimulated with *Der p* I-derived peptide, presented by APC, which were able to provide efficient B cell help (3). These results indicate that CD40L expression on anergic T cell clones by itself is insufficient to induce IgE synthesis and furthermore suggest that additional, yet to be determined, signals are required for productive T-B cell interaction, resulting in Ig isotype switching and IgE production. It is of note to mention that in one study a lack of correlation was found between the levels of CD40L expression on murine T cell clones and the ability of these cells to induce B cell proliferation (6). This observation led to the proposal that either post-translational modification of CD40L or its interaction with other cell surface molecules might be responsible for productive T-B cell interaction. With respect to the latter hypothesis, it is likely that these putative surface molecule(s), expressed on optimally activated T cell clones, are downregulated or not expressed at all on T cell clones rendered anergic by stimulation with allergen-derived peptides.

The anergic T cell clones expressed functional CD25 and were highly responsive to the growth promoting effects of rIL-2, which is in agreement with results obtained in many murine and human anergy models described to date (7–9). Importantly, addition of rIL-2 was found to reverse the peptide-mediated anergic state of *Der p* I-specific T cell clones, by partially restoring their helper activity for the induction of IgE and IgG$_4$ synthesis by B cells (3). Moreover, combinations of rIL-2 and rIL-4 or rIL-2 and rIL-13, respectively, had synergistic effects on the induction of IgE and IgG$_4$ synthesis and resulted in levels of these isotypes that were even higher than those obtained with optimally activated T cell clones. The capacity of rIL-2 to reverse the anergic state suggests that the anergic T cells fail to respond only when triggered via the TCR/CD3-complex, but that signal-transduction pathways circumventing this complex are unaffected.

One explanation for the defective Ag-induced responses of the anergic T cell clones may be the decreased expression of the TCR/CD3 complex which was generally observed following induction of non-responsiveness. This down-regulation of the TCR/CD3 complex *in vitro* was also reported on human T cell clones that had been rendered unresponsive by stimulation with influenza virus peptide (10). Down-regulation of the TCR however does not seem to be a hallmark of anergic T cells *per se*, since this phenomenon was also observed, to the same extent, on T cell clones that were optimally stimulated with *Der p* I and APC. More importantly, decreased expression of the TCR/CD3 complex cannot account by itself for the inability of the anergic T cells to respond to specific Ag, since the down-regulation TCR/CD3 complex on anergic, as well as peptide/APC-stimulated, T cell clones was found to be only partial. In addition, TCR/CD3 expression on one of the T cell clones returned to normal levels after culturing the cells for an additional 3 days, while these cells were still unresponsive to Ag-specific stimulation (3).

In order to confirm the notion that peptide-mediated non-responsiveness may result in part from impaired signaling via the TCR, rather than from a reduced number of TCR molecules on the cell surface, the capacity of anergic T cells to mobilize intracellular Ca^{2+} ($[Ca^{2+}]_i$) following Ag-specific stimulation was analyzed. In contrast to resting T cell clones or T cell clones that had been optimally stimulated with *Der p* I and APC and cultured in medium for three days, anergic T cell clones were not able to mobilize $[Ca^{2+}]_i$ from internal stores when triggered with Ag or crosslinked anti-CD3 antibodies, irrespective of the expression of the TCR/CD3 complex (3). In contrast, elevated $[Ca^{2+}]_i$ levels were readily demonstrated after activation of the anergic T cells with calcium ionophore, which acts via a pathway independent from signaling through the TCR/CD3 complex.

Moreover anergic T cell clones were able to produce high levels of IL-2, IL-4, IL-5, IL-13 and IFN-γ after stimulation with the phorbol ester TPA and calcium ionophore (3). Comparable results have been described by LaSalle et al.(8) who showed that anergic myelin basic protein-specific T cell clones could proliferate and express cytokine mRNA following stimulation with phorbol ester and ionomycine. Taken together, these data suggest that the signaling defect in anergized cells seems to occur before protein kinase C activation and $[Ca^{2+}]_i$ release. Recently, evidence for the latter notion has been provided by a study which showed that anergy induced in mouse T cell clones was associated with altered phosphorylation of the TCR/CD3 complex ζ chain and subsequent lack of association of the tyrosine kinase Zap70 with this complex (11).

Results obtained in experimental murine models have fueled the notion that induction of T cell effector function generally requires two sets of signals: TCR ligation by antigenic peptide-MHC complexes and non-cognate, costimulatory signals, mediated mainly by interactions between CD28 on T cells (12) and their ligands CD80 (13), or CD86 (14) expressed on APC. It has been proposed that engagement of the TCR in the absence of CD28-mediated signals leads to a non-responsive state in mouse T cells, as a result of rapid degradation of IL-2 transcripts and lack of IL-2 production (reviewed in (15)). Most human T cell clones express functional CD80 (16, 17) and CD86 (Yssel, et al unpublished) molecules on their surface, which are able to trigger CD28-mediated signal transduction events in these cells. It was found however that human T cell clones become anergic following incubation with relevant peptides, regardless of the presence of CD28, CD80 and CD86 on their surface (3). The reason for the discrepancy observed between different experimental system is not clear yet, but our results suggest that signal transduction pathways other than those mediated by CD28 and CD80/CD86, respectively, may be involved in providing the costimulatory signal(s) necessary for T cell activation.

PEPTIDE VACCINATION OF ALLERGIC PATIENTS

At present little information is available about the possibility of allergen-derived peptides to induce non-responsiveness in allergen-specific Th2 cells in human *in vivo*. It has been reported by several groups using animal models that immunization with peptides, representing dominant T cell epitopes, can induce Ag-specific non-responsiveness and can be used successfully to treat autoimmune diseases (18, 20) demonstrating the tolerogenic activity of synthetic peptides *in vivo*. Based on the results derived from such studies, it is tempting to speculate that peptide-induced, allergen-specific, T cell non-responsiveness may have potential use in successful immunotherapy. According to the present information, allergen-derived peptides, containing T cell activation-inducing epitopes, should be administered ideally at high concentrations in order to bypass professional APC and to render allergen-specific T cell directly anergic. Allergen-derived peptides, containing minimal T cell epitopes, seem to be ideal tools for the induction of specific tolerance *in vivo*, since they are unable to bind IgE antibodies on sensitized mastcells and basophils and therefore do not induce the release of histamine and other mediators which cause anaphylactic reactions.

There are however some potential problems using synthetic allergen-derived peptides in the treatment of allergic disorders. Epitope mapping of recombinant allergens has shown that most allergens contain multiple T cell activation-inducing epitopes (21–24). Furthermore, the recognition of peptides representing these epitopes is restricted by different MHC class II antigens (21, 22), including HLA-DRβ3 and HLA-DRβ4 gene products (25), which underscores the heterogeneity of T cell responses to allergens. Finally, although mouse studies have indicated that total T cell responses to complex native proteins can be limited to a few immunodominant epitopes (26–28), T cells can escape tolerance induction because of the presence of other, non-immunodominant, T cell epitopes which become available after *in vivo* processing of the native Ag (29). Collectively, this information implies that optimal immunotherapy for each patient requires the mapping of all individual T cell epitopes, as well as precise HLA typing. This approach is presently impractical for large scale treatment of allergies, but the principle of this type of immunotherapy could be explored in selected individual patients. Based on results obtained with experimental mouse models, which showed that subcutaneous immunization with immunodominant peptides of the major cat allergen *Fel d* I could successfully induce a state of tolerance (30), a clinical trial with cat-allergic atopic patients are currently in progress (see Norman, P.S. Chapter 66). The outcome of this clinical trial will provide more information about the efficacy and safety of this type of therapy. In conclusion, allergen-derived peptides have been found to induce non-responsiveness in human allergen-specific Th2 cell resulting in the failure of these cells to provide B cell help for the synthesis of IgE synthesis *in vitro*. Since short allergen-derived peptides do not react with IgE antibodies and therefore are unable to induce anaphylactic reactions, they seem to be of promising value for the treatment of IgE-mediated atopic diseases.

ACKNOWLEDGMENT

DNAX Research Institute for Molecular and Cellular Biology is supported by Schering-Plough Corporation.

REFERENCES

1. Platts-Mills, T. A. and M. D. Chapman. 1987. Dust mites: immunology, allergic disease, and environmental control. *J. Allergy Clin. Immunol. 80: 755.*
2. de Waal Malefyt, R., J. S. Abrams, S. Mohan-Peterson, B. F. Bennett, J. S. Silver, P. V. Schneider, J. E. de Vries and H. Yssel. 1995. Differential regulation of IL-4 and IL-13 expression by human T cell clones and EBV-transformed B cells. *Int. Immunol. In press:*
3. Fasler, S., G. Aversa, S. Terr, K. Thestrup-Pedersen, J. E. de Vries and H. Yssel. 1994. Peptide-induced anergy in allergen-specific Th2 T cells results in lack of cytokine production and B-cell help for IgE synthesis: reversal by IL-2, not by IL-4 or IL-13. J. Immunol. In press:
4. Lamb, J. R., B. J. Skidmore, N. Green, J. M. Chiller and M. Feldmann. 1983. Induction of tolerance in influenza virus immune T lymphocyte clones with synthetic peptides of influenza haemagglutinin. J. Exp. Med. 157: 1434.
5. Jenkins, M. K. and R. H. Schwartz. 1987. Antigen presentation by chemically-modified splenocytes induces antigen-specific T cell unresponsiveness *in vitro* and *in vivo. J. Exp. Med. 167: 302.*
6. Castle, B. E., K. Kishimoto, C. Stearns, M. L. Brown and M. R. Kehry. 1993. Regulation of expression of the ligand for CD40 on T helper Lymphocytes. *J. Immunol. 151: 1777.*
7. Essery, G., M. Feldmann and J. R. Lamb. 1988. Interleukin-2 can prevent and reverse antigen-induced unresponsiveness in cloned human T lymphocytes. *Immunology 64: 413.*
8. La Salle, J. M., P. J. Tolentino, G. J. Freeman, L. M. Nadler and D. A. Hafler. 1992. Early signaling defects in human T cells anergized by T cell presentation of autoantigen. *J. Exp. Med. 176: 177.*
9. Sloan-Lancaster, J., B. D. Evavold and P. Allen. 1994. Th2 cell clonal anergy as a consequence of partial activation. *J. Exp. Med. 180: 1195.*
10. Zanders, E. D., J. R. Lamb, M. Feldmann, N. Green and P. C. Beverley. 1983. Tolerance of T-cell clones is associated with membrane antigen changes. *Nature 303: 625.*
11. Sloan-Lancaster, J., A. S. Shaw, J. B. Rothbard and P. Allen. 1994. Partial T cell signalling: altered phospho-ζ and lack of Zap-70 recruitment in APL-induced T cell anergy. *Cell 79: 913.*

12. Linsley, P. S., W. Brady, L. Grosmaire, A. Aruffo, N. K. Damle and J. A. Ledbetter. 1991. Binding of the B cell activation antigen B7 to CD28 costimulates T cell proliferation and interleukin 2 mRNA accumulation. *J. Exp. Med. 173: 721.*

13. Freeman, G. J., A. S. Freedman, J. M. Segil, G. Lee, J. F. Whitman and L. M. Nadler. 1989. B7, a new member of the Ig superfamily with unique expression on activated and neoplastic B cells. *J. Immunol. 143: 2714.*

14. Azuma, M., D. Ito, H. Yagita, K. Okumura, J. H. Phillips, L. L. Lanier and C. Somoza. 1993. B70 antigen is a second ligand for CTLA-4 and CD28. *Nature 366: 76.*

15. Schwartz, R. H. 1990. A cell culture model for T lymphocyte clonal anergy. *Science 248: 1349.*

16. Sansom, D. M. and N. D. Hall. 1993. B7/BB1, the ligand for CD28 in expressed on repeatedly activated human T cells *in vitro. Eur. J. Immunol. 23: 295.*

17. Azuma, M., Y. H., J. H. Phillips, H. Spits and L. L. Lanier. 1993. Functional expression of B7/BB1 on activated T lymphocytes. *J. Exp. Med. 177: 845.*

18. Wraith, D. C., D. E. Smilek, D. J. Mitchell, L. Steinman and H. O. McDevitt. 1989. Antigen recognition in autoimmune encephalomyelitis and the potential for peptide-mediated immunotherapy. *Cell 59: 247.*

19. Gaur, A., B. Wiers, A. Liu, J. Rothbard and C. G. Fathman. 1992. Amelioration of autoimmune encephalomyelitis by myelin basic protein synthetic peptide-induced anergy. *Science 258: 1491.*

20. Critchfield, J. M., M. K. Racke, J. C. Zúñiga-Pflücker, B. Cannella, C. S. Raine, J. Goverman and M. J. Lenardo. 1994. T cell deleltion in high antigen dose therapy of autoimmue encephalomyelitis. *Science 263: 1139.*

21. Yssel, H., K. E. Johnson, P. V. Schneider, J. Wideman, A. Terr, R. Kastelein and J. E. de Vries. 1992. T cell activation inducing epitopes of the house dust mite allergen *Der p* I. Induction of a restricted cytokine production profile of *Der p* I-specific T cell clones upon antigen-specific activation. *J. Immunol. 148: 738.*

22. Verhoef, A., J. A. Higgins, C. J. Thorpe, S. G. Marsh, J. D. Hayball, J. R. Lamb and R. E. O'Hehir. 1993. Clonal analysis of the atopic immune response to the group 2 allergen of Dermatophagoides spp.: identification of HLA-DR and -DQ restricted T cell epitopes. *Int. Immunol. 5: 1589.*

23. van Neerven, J. R., W. van t'Hof, J. H. Ringrose, H. M. Jansen, R. C. Aalberse, E. A. Wierenga and M. L. Kapsenberg. 1993. T cell epitopes of house dust mite major allergen Der p II. *J. Immunol. 151: 2326.*

24. Carballido, J. M., N. Carballido-Perrig, M. K. Kagi, R. H. Meloen, B. Wuthrich, C. H. Heusser and K. Blaser. 1993. T cell epitope specificity in human allergic and nonallergic subjects to bee venom phospholipase A2. *J. Immunol. 150: 3582.*

25. O'Hehir, R. E., B. Mach, C. Berte, R. Greenlaw, J. M. Tiercy, V. Bal, R. I. Lechler, J. Trowsdale and J. R. Lamb. 1990. Direct evidence for a functional role of HLA-DRB1 and -DRB3 gene products in the recognition of Dermatophagoides spp. (house dust mite) by helper T lymphocytes. *Int. Immunol. 2: 885.*

26. Gammon, G., N. Shastri, J. Cogswell, S. Wilbur, S. Sadegh-Nasseri, U. Krzych, A. Miller and E. Sercarz. 1987. The choice of T-cell epitopes utilized on a protein antigen depends on multiple factors distant from, as well as at the determinant site. *Immunol. Rev. 98: 53.*

27. Adorini, L., E. Appella, G. Doria and Z. A. Nagy. 1988. Mechanisms influencing the immunodominance of T cell determinants. *J. Exp. Med. 168: 2091.*

28. Perkins, D. L., G. Berriz, T. Kamradt, J. A. Smith and M. L. Gefter. 1991. Immunodominance: intramolecular competition between T cell epitopes. *J. Immunol. 146: 2137.*

29. Gammon, G. and E. Sercarz. 1989. How some T cells escape tolerance induction. *Nature 342: 183.*

30. Briner, T. J., M. C. Kuo, K. M. Keating, B. L. Rogers and J. L. Greenstein. 1993. Peripheral T-cell tolerance induced in naive and primed mice by subcutaneous injection of peptides from the major cat allergen Fel d I. *Proc. Natl. Acad. Sci USA 90: 7608.*

60

NATURAL AND RECOMBINANT ANTI-IgE AUTOANTIBODIES

Beda M. Stadler, Martin Stämpfli, Monique Vogel, Michael Rudolf,
Adrian Zürcher, and Sylvia Miescher

Institute of Immunology and Allergology, Inselspital
University of Bern
Bern, Switzerland

1. INTRODUCTION

Since the first description of anti-IgE autoantibodies by Williams et al. in 1972[1], these antibodies have remained a much disputed subject. Most immunologists considered such natural autoantibodies as low affinity antibodies of no importance. Despite the fact that Manning et al. described only 4 years later that repeated injections of a rabbit anti-Ig antiserum to neonatal mice suppressed not only IgM but also IgG, IgA and IgE synthesis[2], it was still not generally accepted that anti-IgE autoantibodies may have the same profound effect as heterologous anti-IgE antisera. Subsequent animal experiments, showing that anti-IgE antibodies are strongly immunoregulatory and lead to the suppression of IgE synthesis in vivo have not been associated with the possibility to use such antibodies for therapy[3,4], or to postulate that such antibodies may represent a normal physiological control. Only recently, both possibilities have become feasible. Here we demonstrate that anti-IgE antibodies, isolated from the human genome, as recombinant antibodies, may possess the necessary fine specificity for future therapeutic application.

1.1. Detection of Natural Anti-IgE Autoantibodies

There are numerous reports documenting that anti-IgE autoantibodies exist in the sera of patients suffering from allergic disorders or from other diseases with high levels of IgE[5–7]. Nevertheless, it was always puzzling that anti-IgE antibodies also exist in normal individuals[8]. One of the major problems for the determination of anti-IgE autoantibodies in serum was the fact, that IgE and anti-IgE autoantibodies co-exist in approximately equimolar concentrations, leading to immune complexes[9,10]. Clearly, this hampered the detection of anti-IgE antibodies and is one of the reasons why still nowadays it is not possible to precisely quantify these antibodies.

New Horizons in Allergy Immunotherapy
edited by Sehon et al. Plenum Press, New York, 1996

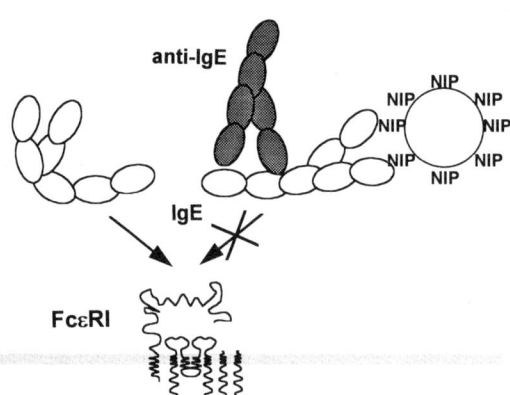

Figure 1. Importance of IgE conformation for the binding to FcεRI. The incubation of NIP coupled BSA with NIP-specific IgE leads to a formation of complexes that can no longer bind to FcεRI; thus, immune complexes consisting of allergen and allergen specific IgE may undergo a conformational change preventing sensitization of basophils and mast cells. Sensitization can also be prevented by adding antibodies directed against binding structures of the IgE molecule for FcεRI. However, also antibodies that do not directly intefere with the binding can induce a similar conformational change like the antigen, also preventing sensitization of FcεRI expressing cells.

Recently we have shown that antigen binding to IgE leads to a conformational change in the IgE molecule, preventing anti-IgE antibodies from detecting such immune complexes[11]. This may be one of the reasons why some IgE may always remain uncomplexed in a free form[12,13]. More importantly, the conformational change induced by the antigen produces an IgE that is no more capable of binding to FcεRI (Figure 1).

1.2. Pathophysiological Role of Anti-IgE Antibodies

One of the most striking findings concerning anti-IgE and IgE-complexes in vivo was the report by Ritter et al.[8] We could show that in non-atopic asthmatic children the levels of IgE within immune complexes corresponded to the levels of free IgE in the individuals with atopic asthma. We speculated that anti-IgE antibodies may eventually neutralize the IgE, or alternatively, that IgE within these immune complexes may still be active, namely that it would be capable of binding to FcεRI[14].

When we used monoclonal anti-IgE antibodies, we found that these anti-IgE antibodies could be grouped according to their biological function. Using mediator release from human basophils, it was clear that some antibodies were anaphylactogenic, and others were not. Interestingly, we found a non-anaphylactogenic antibody that was even capable of slowly removing surface IgE from human basophils. This clearly suggests that there are anti-IgE antibodies that may have a pathophysiological role[14].

A similar approach has been chosen by two different companies that reported their results at this symposium, namely that non-anaphylactogenic murine anti-IgE antibodies were humanized and then used for human therapy (Jardieu et al.; Heusser et al.; Davies et al.) These therapeutic approaches will be crucial for the understanding of allergic disease. On the one hand, they may revolutionize the therapy of atopic disease if these clinical approaches are successful. On the other hand, if this kind of therapy is not successful, it would mean that the role of IgE in atopic disease has to be redefined, or that the selected anti-IgE antibodies for therapy did not have an appropriate epitope specificity and thus lacked the desired biological activity.

We could show that anti-IgE antibodies cannot only be grouped according to the capacity to release mediators, but also according to their capacity to inhibit in vitro IgE synthesis[15]. Again, some of the antibodies did not have an inhibitory activity, while others were very potent inhibitors of IgE synthesis exceeding even the in vitro effect of TGF-β.

Based on the previous literature, one might assume to find anti-IgE antibodies that may even induce IgE synthesis. Indeed, some antibodies were found that had a weak capacity to enhance IgE synthesis in the presence of IL-4. However, these antibodies lost this "stimulatory" capacity if they were tested on purified B-cell populations, suggesting an indirect effect[15]. The precise mechanisms for the inhibition of IgE synthesis is not yet known, but based on our findings that Bcl-2 expression was downregulated in anti-IgE treated, purified B-cells, one might assume that cross-linking of surface IgE may lead to apoptosis (unpublished observation).

When we further analyzed the inhibitory effect of anti-IgE antibodies on human IgE synthesis, by using either complete, Fab, or F(ab)2 antibodies, we found that only the divalent antibodies were capable of inhibiting IgE synthesis[15]. These experiments cause a theoretical problem, namely the widely accepted concept that an immunoglobulin cross-linking on the surface of B cells will lead to an induction of proliferation. Our experiments indicate the opposite, but may also provide an explanation for the negative selection procedure of human B cells (Figure 2). Namely autoreactive B cells may indeed recognise several antigenic determinants on cell surfaces leading to a cross-link and a final elimination of these B cells. The soluble antigen or allergen, on the other hand, as long as it is not aggregated or has multiple and repeated epitopes will normally result in a univalent recognition. Thus, one may assume that this univalent recognition together with the action of co-factors, such as CD40 and CD40 ligand, may represent the positive signal.

1.3. Isolation of Anti-IgE Antibodies

The isolation of IgE from serum is a difficult task, as we have shown earlier, because IgE is often associated with IgG[10]. Furthermore, to obtain pure serum IgE in its native form, will always remain a quantitative problem. Anti-IgE antibodies in serum are

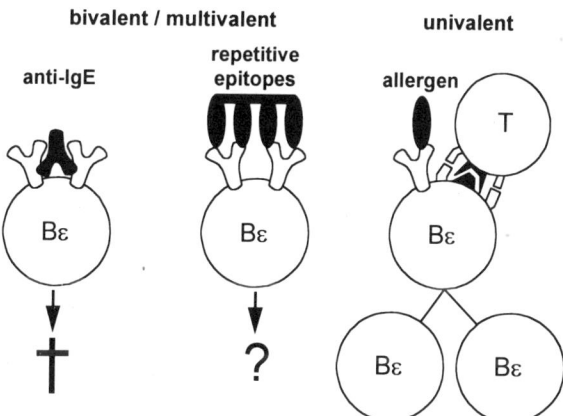

Figure 2. Triggering of Bε+ cells. Anti-IgE antibodies that inhibit IgE synthesis are only inhibitory if used as divalent antibody molecules (complete antibody or F(ab)2). The same antibodies in the form of Fab are non inhibitory. These data suggest that antigens with repeated epitopes, such as self antigens on body surfaces, may also lead to the distruction of Bε cells (clonal deletion). So far, divalent (complete antibodies) were only stimulatory for B cells at low concentrations and in the presence of T cells and antigen presenting cells, suggesting that the univalent stimulation resulting from allergens without repetitive epitopes is strictly dependent on accessory cells.

usually present in lower concentrations then IgE, except in cord blood where they are in excess, rendering the task practically impossible to isolate the necessary quantities of anti-IgE autoantibodies for in vitro experimentation.

Thus, we chose an approach to isolate the immunoglobulin genes encoding for anti-IgE autoantibodies from the human genome in order to produce anti-IgE autoantibodies[16].

2. RESULTS AND DISCUSSION

2.1. Generation of Recombinant Antibodies

A recently described technology to isolate human antibodies now offers the tools to isolate natural antibodies, autoantibodies or antibodies from immunized individuals, based on mRNA from peripheral B cells[17]. This method represents to a certain degree an approach similar to the immune system in vivo. The first crucial step was the finding that the immunoglobulin repertoire can be cloned by PCR. The next crucial step was an expression system that allowed the co-expression of heavy and light chains on the surface of a filamentous phage, thereby forming an "organism" that in analogy to the B cell can bind to the antigen. While the B cell will clonally expand in vivo, phages recognizing the antigen are isolated and are then amplified in bacteria. Phages carrying the Fab molecules can again be applied on to the antigen on a solid support and re-isolated during several rounds of expansion by a process called biopanning, resembling the boosting effect on B cells in vivo.

We and others have shown that the resulting antibodies resemble very much the naturally occurring antibodies in serum. For example, we isolated anti-tetanus toxoid antibodies that showed the same oligoclonal distribution, the same affinity, and the same protective activity as the antibodies found in the serum after immunization[16].

The same patient that was immunized with tetanus toxoid and used to generate the Fab expressing phage display library had also anti-IgE antibodies in his serum, and thus we were able to isolate antibodies that recognized IgE from this library, although with a somewhat lower frequency than the antibodies that recognized tetanus toxin[16].

2.2. Anti-Idiotype versus Anti-Isotype Antibodies

The frequency of anti-IgE antibodies that we isolated was still higher than we ever expected. We used five different myeloma IgE-proteins to isolate anti-IgE specific phages. When these phages were then analyzed at the clonal level, we realized that the majority of the anti-IgE phages actually only recognized the corresponding myeloma IgE we used to pan the phages. Thus, it became clear that most of the anti-IgE phages were directed against the variable part of the IgE myelomas and therefore can be regarded as anti-idiotypic antibodies.

On the one hand this opens the possibility to study questions related to anti-idiotypes because this methodology clearly is a very simple way to isolate anti-idiotypic antibodies. This finding also supports our view that the detection and measurement of anti-IgE antibody is an estimation and that the conclusions that can be drawn from results obtained by the measurement of "anti-IgE antibodies" may be only of relative importance.

2.3. Specificity of Isotype Specific Anti-IgE Antibodies

Nevertheless, we also isolated antibodies against the constant part of the IgE molecule, and some of these antibodies were analyzed at the clonal level. Interestingly, the clones that were derived from an atopic individual were specific for the second domain of the IgE molecule. Based on our earlier work on murine monoclonal anti-IgE antibodies that were typed for their epitope specificity, we have to conclude that these recombinant anti-IgE autoantibodies would most likely not have a beneficial effect in vivo. Namely, we could show that antibodies against this domain are frequently anaphylactogenic. In the case of IgE-binding to CD23 we even found an enhanced binding of IgE to this receptor-like structure[18]. Furthermore, antibodies that recognized the second domain had no activity or were only weakly inhibitory for human IgE synthesis[15].

2.4. Characterization of IgE Epitopes

From this work we concluded that the idiotypic determinants were the most "immunogenic" parts for phage display libraries, and that it would be more favorable to present only the relevant epitopes of IgE to Fab expressing phages, so that only antibodies are selected that may also have a beneficial effect.

One antibody that we believe would be a possible candidate for in vivo use, is termed BSW17. This antibody recognizes the third domain of the IgE molecule and is strongly inhibitory for human IgE synthesis[15]. More importantly, the antibody is non-anaphylactogenic and is capable of slowly removing surface IgE either bound to FcεRI or CD23[14]. The mechanism of this removal is still unknown, as the antibody recognizes surface IgE. In the moment the IgE/BSW17 complex is dissociated from the cell, it is no longer capable of re-sensitizing basophils[14]. Thus, this anti-IgE antibody can also be regarded as a neutralizing antibody.

Next we isolated peptides randomly generated from the gene of the constant part of the IgE molecule and expressed them on a filamentous phage, in order to detect the actual epitope that is recognized by BSW17. However, these IgE based random libraries did not contain any sequences that could be recognized by the monoclonal anti-IgE antibody BSW17. As we knew that BSW17 does not recognize heat denatured IgE, it must be a conformational epitope that is recognized and that cannot be generated by small peptides, representing basically linear sequences of the ε constant domains.

Thus we used random nonapeptide libraries either in a linear or circular form, provided by Dr. Felici[19,20]. Again, the linear, random nonapeptide library, containing approximately 10^8 different phages, did not contain any peptide-carrying phages that were recognized by BSW17. However, the random, circular phage peptide library was specifically and quickly enriched for the BSW17 antibody. Most of the isolated clones had exactly the same sequence, and the residual clones that were isolated showed the same sequence motifs, suggesting that the actual IgE epitope recognized by BSW17 was found. However, the sequences we obtained did not occur in the primary sequence of the IgE molecule, which again points in the direction that the BSW17 epitope is conformational. Therefore, epitopes that are isolated from a random circular library are often also called "mimotopes" as they mimic conformational epitopes.

3. CONCLUSION

The cloning of human anti-IgE autoantibodies has clearly demonstrated that such antibodies are not immunological artifacts. However, most of the antibodies that reacted with IgE were actually not isotype specific but were anti-idiotypic antibodies. While this shows that anti-idiotypic antibodies can now easily be isolated, it became clear that phage display libraries enriched on such complicated antigens as antibodies, may always favor determinants of the idiotype. For this purpose, it is mandatory that the most relevant IgE epitopes are characterized in order to isolate useful anti-IgE autoantibodies that may then represent "follow-up" antibodies of those that are presently used in clinical trials.

4. REFERENCES

1. Williams RC, Griffiths RW, Emmons JD, Field RC. 1972. Naturally occurring human antiglobulins with specificity for gamma-E. *J. Clin. Invest.* 51: 955.
2. Manning DD, Manning JK, Reed ND. Suppression of reaginic antibody (IgE) formation in mice by treatment with anti-μ antiserum. *J Exp Med* 1976; 144:288
3. Haba S, Nisonoff A. Inhibition of IgE synthesis by anti-IgE: Role in long-term inhibition of IgE synthesis by neonatally administered soluble IgE. Proc Natl Acad Sci USA 1990;87:3363–3367.
4. Marshall JS, Bell EB: Induction of an auto-anti-IgE response in rats. III. Inhibition of a specific IgE response. Immunology 1989;66:428–433.
5. Carini C, Brostoff J: An antiglobulin: IgG anti-IgE. Occurrence and specificity. Ann Allergy 1983;51:251–4.
6. Inganäs M, Johansson SG, Bennich H: Anti-IgE antibodies in human serum: occurrence and specificity. Int Arch Allergy Appl Immunol 1981;65:51–61.
7. Nawata Y, Koike T, Hosokawa H, Tomioka H, Yoshida S: Anti-IgE autoantibody in patients with atopic dermatitis. J Immunol 1985;135:478–82.
8. Ritter C, Bättig M, Kraemer R, Stadler BM: IgE hidden in immune complexes with anti-IgE autoantibodies in children with asthma. J Allergy Clin Immunol 1991;88:793–801.
9. Vassella CC, de Weck AL, Stadler BM: Natural anti-IgE auto-antibodies interfere with diagnostic IgE determination. Clin Exp Allergy 1990;20:295–303.
10. Jensen-Jarolim E, Vogel M, de Weck AL, Stadler BM: Anti-IgE autoantibodies mistaken for specific IgG. J Allergy and Clinical Immunol 1992;89:31–43.
11. Martin R. Stämpfli, Michael Rudolf, Sylvia Miescher, J.M. Pachlopnik and Beda M. Stadler. Antigen specific inhibition of IgE binding to the high affinity receptor. J. Immunol. in press, 1995.
12. Czech, W., Stadler, B.M., Schöpf, E. and Kapp. A. IgE antibodies in atopic dermatitis - occurence and different antibodies against the CH3 and the CH4 epitope of IgE. Allergy . 50: 243–248.1995.
13. Yu, Yan, de Weck, A.L., Stadler, B.M. and Müller. U. IgE Anti-IgE autoantibodies and bee sting allergy. Eur. J. of Allergy and Clin. Immunol. in press. 1994.
14. Stadler BM, Stämpfli MR, Miescher S, Furukawa K, Vogel M: Biological activities of anti-IgE antibodies. Intern. Arch. Allergy. Immunol. 1993, 102:121–126.
15. Stämpfli MR, Miescher S, Aebischer I, Stadler BM: Modulation of IgE synthesis by anti-IgE antibody. Eur J Immunol. 1994; 24:2161–2167.
16. Vogel M, Miescher S, Stadler BM, Human anti-IgE antibodies by repertoire cloning. Eur J Immunol. 1993;24;1200–1207.
17. Clackson T, Hoogenboom HR, Griffiths AD, Winter G. 1991. Making antibody fragments using phage display libraries. Nature 352:624.
18. Miescher S, Vogel M, Stämpfli MR, Holzner ME, Wasserbauer E, Kricek F, Vorburger S, Stadler BM: Domain specific anti-IgE antibodies interfere with IgE binding to FcεRII. Int. Archives of Allergy and Immunology. 1994;105:75–82.
19. Felici F., Castagnoli L., Musacchio A., Jappelli R., and Cesareni G.: Selection of antibody ligands from a large library of oligopeptides expressed on a multivalent exposition vector. J. Mol. Biol. 222:301–310, 1991.
20. Luzzago A., Felici F., Tramontano A., Pessi A. and Cortese R. Mimicking of discontinuous epitopes by phage-displayed peptides, I. Epitope mapping of human H ferritin using a phage library of constrained peptides. Gene 128:51–57, 1993.

61

MODULATION OF ANTI-ALLERGEN IMMUNE RESPONSES BY ALLERGEN-ANTIBODY COMPLEXES

Jean-Marie R. Saint-Remy

Allergy and Clinical Immunology Unit
International Institute for Cellular and Molecular Pathology
Hippocrate Avenue, 74, 1200, Brussels, Belgium

Inducing a state of tolerance to allergens has been the aim of a number of studies, which were initiated soon after the identification of IgE as the antibody responsible for anaphylactic reactions. The advantages of such an approach are obvious: high selectivity and lack of possibly detrimental interference with other functions of the immune system. Early work on the subject, including the use of allergens coupled to isologous gammaglobulins (1, 2), had shown that IgE immune responses were amenable to tolerance induction in animals. Derivatives of allergens made by coupling with monomethoxy-polyethylene glycol have also demonstrated their capacity to prevent or down-regulate an IgE response (3).

An allergen-specific approach has its place in the treatment of allergic diseases. Suppressing the production of IgE antibodies as a whole might have unexpected consequences on the host immune system, as IgE could have important immunological functions unrelated to allergic reactions, such as antigen presentation (4) or defence against parasites. On the other hand, it is not entirely sure that even if the whole IgE isotype is suppressed, this would be sufficient to eliminate all risks of allergic reactions. There is indeed evidence showing that anaphylaxis can occur in the absence of IgE antibodies (5).

1. CONCEPT

Some years ago we decided to design a therapy for IgE-mediated diseases based on the use of antibodies. The idea was to induce a state of tolerance to allergens which would be specific for a given allergen, but would involve all antibody isotypes. Antibodies have indeed the property of regulating their own production by at least two mechanisms. The first one is related to the immunogenicity of the variable part (idiotype) of the antibody. Anti-idiotypic antibodies are part of the normal immune response to an antigen and their function, at least under certain experimental conditions, is to reduce the production of the

New Horizons in Allergy Immunotherapy
edited by Sehon et al. Plenum Press, New York, 1996

417

antibodies carrying corresponding idiotypes (6). That IgE-mediated immune responses were amenable to suppression by anti-idiotypic antibodies had already been nicely demonstrated by Blaser and de Weck (7). Secondly, antibodies can interfere with the intracellular processing of antigens in such a way as to alter the presentation of peptides to T cells and their subsequent activation (8). The hope was therefore to block Th2 cell activation by masking allergen epitopes with specific antibodies. Lastly, the addition of a specific antibody to an allergen can divert the antigen processing to cells bearing a surface receptors for IgG. This could provide a further advantage in favour of using antibodies, as the type of APC can have a determining effect on the subset of T cells that is activated. In an attempt to exploit these antibody properties, we designed a system in which pre-formed allergen-antibody complexes were used for administration to allergic patients.

Antigen-antibody complexes have been used in a number of experimental models, with sometimes contradictory results: enhancement or reduction of immune responses. However, complexes prepared in excess of antibodies and containing isologous antibodies usually have immunosuppressive properties. More specifically, the possible regulation of IgE antibody production in experimental animals by the use of antigen-antibody complexes has been described. Thus, rats pre-treated with complexes made from egg albumin and specific antiserum were unable to mount a primary or secondary IgE immune response towards egg albumin, provided the complexes were made at equivalence or, better, in antibody excess; in this latter case, however, the total production of antibodies to egg albumin is reduced (9). Guinea-pigs can develop anaphylaxis together with bronchial hyperreactivity in response to an inhalation challenge with ovalbumin; pre-treatment by regular injections of ovalbumin-anti-ovalbumin complexes has a transitory preventive effect on the induction of anaphylaxis, but this effect is not superior to that obtained with injections of ovalbumin alone (10). The IgE response to the same antigen can be inhibited in mice receiving intravenous injections of antigen-antibody complexes made at equivalence, provided these complexes are made of whole isologous antibodies and administered prior to the antigen (11).

We therefore opted for a treatment in which polyclonal antibodies of autologous origin only were used. Polyclonal antibodies offered the additional advantage of covering a maximum number of epitopes, therefore avoiding to boost an immune response towards unmasked determinants (12). In addition, if a suppression was exerted at the level of idiotypes, the use of polyclonal antibodies was thought to minimise the risk of inducing a shift in idiotype expression (13). However, preparing complexes exclusively made of IgE antibodies was not feasible, due to the very low concentration of IgE antibodies even in the serum of atopic patients. We therefore used specific IgG antibodies, which share most of their idiotopes with IgE (14).

2. SOURCE AND PREPARATION OF MATERIAL FOR TREATMENT

To satisfy the above-described conditions, we had to prepare allergen-specific antibodies from the serum of each single patient to be treated. This was carried out using conventional methods of salt precipitation, gel filtration chromatography and affinity-chromatography on insolubilised allergens. The volume of serum necessary to prepare a sufficient amount of antibodies (see below) varied between 5 and 20 ml, as the concentration of allergen-specific antibodies varied from 6 to 35 µg/ml, with the highest titres being found in atopic dermatitis.

It however appeared with time that obtaining an appropriate preparation of specific antibodies by these methods was difficult, and in particular the adsorption step itself. It is indeed essential, for the therapy to be successful, that complexes contain antibodies representative of the whole antibody response of the patient. Clinical failures have been systematically related to either incomplete antibody adsorption on insolubilised allergens, or to difficulties in recovering specific antibodies from the immunosorbent. Alternatives to avoid such difficulties will be discussed at the end of the present paper. Along the same line, it is worth noting that all antibody subclasses should be present in complexes. For instance, treatment of antibody samples with a reducing agent such as dithiothreitol, which destroys IgM, IgE and a variable proportion of IgG3 and IgG4, results in antibody preparations that are not clinically effective.

Allergens were obtained from commercial suppliers, dialysed and concentrated by conventional methods. Antibodies and allergens were mixed at ratios comprised between 4/1 and 10/1, which corresponds to a 1/1 to 3/1 molar ratio, depending on the allergens used.

3. CLINICAL STUDIES

Two diseases of atopic origin were studied: allergic bronchial asthma and atopic dermatitis. All studies in bronchial asthma were carried out by Dr. Jacques Machiels (Ottignies, Belgium) and those in atopic dermatitis by Dr. Bernard Leroy (Brussels, Belgium).

Initially, our aim was to develop a therapy that would be useful to severely ill patients; if the treatment proved to be beneficial to such patients, and provided that it was simple and free of side-effects, it could of course be later extended to moderately ill patients. However, in the category of patients selected here, asthma or dermatitis could obviously be exacerbated by a number of factors quite distinct from allergen sensitivity. Most asthmatics also suffered from asthma due to non-specific irritants. Moreover, the majority of patients presented a sensitivity to several allergens, unrelated to the single one used for the treatment. In atopic dermatitis, it was assumed that airborne allergens played a role in the triggering or exacerbation of symptoms. The patients participating in grass-pollen hypersensitivity trials were those with intractable nasal symptoms and, for a majority of them, also suffering from seasonal asthma.

The patients were treated by regular intradermal injections of complexes made of their own anti-allergen antibodies and the corresponding allergens. Clinical studies were designed as placebo-controlled double-blind trials. Depending on the condition treated, injections were administrated for a few weeks (seasonal asthma) or a few months (perennial asthma and atopic dermatitis). In some cases, however, significant improvement was already observed after 3 to 4 weeks. Alternative treatment regimens are possible, such as the administration of 5 or 6 injections within a few hours, followed by one monthly injection. The cumulative amount of material injected varied between 20 to 300 µg specific antibodies, with some variations from one clinical condition to the other; the highest amount of material is required for the treatment of atopic dermatitis patients.

We have conducted a series of clinical trials involving a total of about 400 patients. They suffered from either perennial asthma (with or without rhinitis) due to hypersensitivity to *Dermatophagoides pteronyssinus* (*Dp*), seasonal asthma with rhinitis in relation to hypersensitivity to grass pollens (15, 16, 17), or atopic dermatitis and *Dp*-hypersensitivity (18, 19). At the present time, the salient features of these studies can be summarised as follows.

3.1. Safety of the Treatment

The injection of allergen-antibody complexes seems to be completely innocuous; no systemic or even significant local side-effects were observed in a total of about 3,000 injections.

3.2. Clinical Efficacy

Dp-hypersensitive patients showed a significant reduction in symptoms of asthma already after a few weeks after the beginning of treatment and their clinical condition continued to improve progressively thereafter. The treatment completely prevented the appearance of bronchial asthma related to pollen exposure, whereas in atopic dermatitis, both the intensity of the skin lesions and the affected body surface area began to show improvement after a few weeks. Within 2 to 3 months, 50% of the lesions had disappeared, together with pruritus. At longer term, 80 % of patients had an average improvement of 85 %. Together with symptomatic improvement, the patients were able to progressively reduce their medication intake. In bronchial asthma, for example, none of the patients had to use systemic corticosteroids during a 4-year follow-up and a third of the patients could even do without any regular medication at all.

3.3. Reduction of Allergen Reactivity

A significant reduction in skin test and bronchial reactivity was observed during the trials. For example, the concentration of *Dp* that, after inhalation, induced a 35 % fall in specific airway conductance gradually increased over time to reach a mean of 70-fold the initial value. In fact, a third of the patients became completely unresponsive to allergen bronchial challenges.

3.4. Reduction in the Non-Specific Bronchial Reactivity

One of the most convincing results we observed during these studies was the progressive reduction in the non-specific bronchial reactivity. Challenges were carried out using acetyl-choline at concentrations up to 10 mg/ml. At the end of the third year of therapy, and even one year after the end of the injection schedule, half of the treated patients had completely lost their reactivity to acetyl-choline inhalation.

4. BIOLOGICAL STUDIES

A finding which was repeatedly made concerns the reduction in the level of specific antibodies. In studies with patients hypersensitive to *Dp*, a significant reduction in specific IgE, but also in IgG and IgA antibodies, was observed within a few months after the start of the therapy, without change in the levels of total antibodies (16, 20). It usually took longer in atopic dermatitis than in bronchial asthma. In grass pollen hypersensitivity, the treatment suppressed the increase in anti-pollen IgE usually observed during the season, even when injections were started as late as one month prior to the start of pollen exposure. In addition, specific IgE levels progressively declined afterwards to values significantly lower than prior to therapy (15). Interestingly enough, clinical improvement correlated best with the reduction of IgG levels, and not with those of IgE. Failure to respond to the therapy was associated with either no change or an increase in specific antibodies.

In atopic dermatitis, in which the amount of material used for treatment was higher than for the treatment of asthma, we observed that IgE antibodies were induced towards allergen components that were not initially recognised by the patient, and were therefore present in an free form in the material used for injections (20). This could simply represent an immune response towards determinants to which the patient is not exposed in natural conditions and should therefore not be harmful.

The suppression of anti-allergen antibody production is not only specific for the allergen, but even restricted to antibodies that are present in the complexes used for treatment. This epitope-specific mechanism was demonstrated by taking advantage of the partial cross-reactivity between *Der pI* and *Der fI*. Patients treated with *Der pI* -anti-*Der pI* complexes showed a reduction in the level of antibodies to *Der fI*, but only of those antibodies directed to epitopes shared between the two allergen molecules (20).

Although these findings confirm that injection of allergen-antibody complexes can produce a highly specific down-regulation of antibody production, it could represent a disadvantage, i.e., to render inevitable the use of polyclonal anti-allergen antibodies. An alternative would be to identify dominant epitopes on allergen molecules, which would offer the possibility of making allergen-antibody complexes with one or a limited number of antibodies. Whether such epitopes exist is however far from certain. This question is now addressed in our laboratory thanks to the production of human monoclonal antibodies.

We have also demonstrated that injections of allergen-antibody complexes boost the production of corresponding anti-idiotypic antibodies (20). The analysis was however limited to anti-idiotypic antibodies able to inhibit the binding of specific antibodies to allergens, which are the only ones that can be reliably measured in a system in which polyclonal anti-allergen antibodies are used. Whether the latter play a determining role in the reduction in antibody production observed in our studies is not entirely clear at this stage. The same holds true *a fortiori* for the relationship between anti-idiotypic antibodies and clinical improvement: only a loose correlation between levels of anti-idiotypic antibodies and clinical improvement was found. On the other hand, anti-idiotypic antibodies can interact with specific IgE antibodies located at the surface of basophils or mastocytes (21), and might therefore block cell degranulation. These issues should be resolved by using human monoclonal antibodies.

5. ADVANTAGES AND LIMITATIONS

We think that the present therapy represents a novel approach for the treatment of IgE-mediated diseases, at least in its concept. It is therefore worthwhile to briefly review the advantages over other forms of immunotherapy, as well as the problems and difficulties we are facing.

5.1. Safety

It is reasonable to assume that allergen-antibody injections do not carry a significant risk of local or systemic anaphylactic reactions. Indeed, the amount of allergen present in the complexes is at least two orders of magnitude lower than in conventional hyposensitization and, in addition, allergen epitopes are masked by specific antibodies, which prevent the binding of allergens to mast cell-bound IgE antibodies.

5.2. Efficiency

The therapy has demonstrated its efficacy in the treatment of moderate to severe asthma and of atopic dermatitis, two conditions in which other forms of immunotherapy are considered as poorly effective or contraindicated, respectively. However, the most significant effect is the reduction in bronchial or cutaneous non-specific hyperreactivity, which can be maintained without further treatment for at least two years, namely, the time-period during which the patients were followed. Whether this effect results from a reduction in bronchial or cutaneous inflammation (22) is not formally demonstrated yet. Practically, however, it could offer an alternative to the daily drug usage required by most patients.

5.3. Material Used for Injection

It is of interest to compare the amount of material which was used during the clinical trials reported here with that used for conventional hyposensitization. The total quantity of allergen administered in the form of complex with specific antibodies is 100 to 350-fold less than that which would have been used for allergen alone, and even this does not take into account the maintenance treatment which usually follows the induction phase of conventional hyposensitization. The amount of specific antibodies administered during the treatment does not exceed 20 µg in asthma and 300 µg in atopic dermatitis. These values correspond to the quantity of antibodies contained in an average serum volume of 10 ml.

5.4. Rapidity

Conventional hyposensitization usually requires several months of treatment before showing the first signs of clinical benefit. For instance, a treatment for grass-pollen hypersensitivity takes a mean of two years before being fully effective. A prominent advantage of the current therapy is the rapidity with which the results can be obtained. As was indeed the case in our studies of grass-pollen hypersensitivity, the treatment can be applied during the pollen season itself, while achieving its full efficacy within a few weeks.

5.5. Indications

- bronchial asthma: this therapy was initially developed primarily for the treatment of severe allergic bronchial asthma and all *Dp*-hypersensitive patients treated so far belonged to this category. We have therefore no formal proof yet that it would be efficient in mild asthma, in which bronchospasm may be more prominent than inflammation.
- rhinitis: although no controlled clinical evaluation has been made with allergic rhinitis patients, the observations we made in pollinosis indicate that the treatment is likely to be efficient.
- atopic dermatitis: evidence for efficacy has been presented for patients with mild and severe atopic dermatitis associated to hypersensitivity to either *Dp* or grass pollens
- children: the results obtained so far in children show a rapid and significant improvement, in particular in atopic dermatitis. On the other hand, some children respond poorly for reasons that are not clearly identified. This question awaits further studies.

5.6. Biological Alterations

The selective and parallel reduction of both specific IgE and IgG antibodies suggests that allergen-antibody complexes selectively suppress the production of anti-allergen antibodies *in vivo*. Whether the reduction in specific IgE is sufficient to explain the clinical benefit of the treatment is disputable. We nevertheless favour the idea that the reduction of specific IgG - and IgA - antibodies is more relevant than that of IgE. Specific IgG antibodies can modulate the anti-allergen immune response in a number of ways, such as the modulation of the IgE-dependent degranulation of mast cells (23).

6. PERSPECTIVES

The preparation of polyclonal anti-allergen antibodies from the serum of each individual is cumbersome and, to some extent, difficult to standardise. It is therefore obvious that the preparation ought to be simplified and automated prior to envisaging broader applications of the therapy. One particular concern relates to the necessity to treat patients with complexes containing the whole repertoire of specific antibodies they produce. As noted above, subtle changes in the preparation procedure can result in an absence of significant clinical benefit.

Two alternatives are now pursued. The first possibility is to use pooled gammaglobulins as the source of specific antibodies. However, using such antibodies could result in inducing an anti-allotypic immune response. To avoid such risk, we have recently conducted a study in which specific antibodies were used in the form of $F(ab')_2$ fragments instead of whole antibody molecules (24). The success of this study, carried out with autologous antibodies, enables us to start a trial in which $F(ab')_2$ fragments of specific antibodies prepared from pooled gammaglobulins are used. A second possibility would be to use human monoclonal antibodies to produce complexes. This is currently under study in our laboratory.

It is however already envisaged to use the same type of approach in clinical conditions in which conventional desensitisation cannot be used. Some allergens are too dangerous to be used in free form: examples of this are food allergens, such as ovalbumin or peanut, and drug allergens, such as penicillin. Atopic dermatitis due to food hypersensitivity will be studied in the forthcoming months.

Lastly, the fact that allergen-antibody complexes suppress the production of IgG antibodies opens the perspective of using a similar approach in IgG-mediated diseases in which the relevant antigen is identified. Some auto-immune diseases, such as myasthenia gravis, are obvious candidates for an experimental trial.

We believe that this approach of immunomodulation of the anti-*Dp* immune response is worth pursuing. Its present form should be considered as a first step in a series of developments that should lead to a treatment by which tolerance to allergens should be rendered feasible.

ACKNOWLEDGMENTS

The author thanks Marc Jacquemin for collaboration, Thérèse Briet, Yves Delmarcelle, Monique Schroeder for expert technical assistance, and Brigitte Firket for editorial help.

REFERENCES

1. Borel Y, Kilham L, Hyslop V, Borel H. Isologous IgG-induced tolerance to benzyl penicilloyl. *Nature* 1976; 261: 49–50.
2. Filion LG, Lee WY & Sehon AH. Suppression of the IgE antibody response to ovalbumin in mice with a conjugate of ovalbumin and isologous gamma-globulins. Cell Immunol 1980; 54: 115–128.
3. Sehon AH. Suppression of antibody responses by chemically modified antigens. Int Arch Allergy Appl Immunol 1991; 94: 11–20.
4. Mudde GC, Hansel TT, Reijsen FCV, Osterhoff BF, and Bruijnzeel-Koomen CAFM. IgE: an immunoglobulin specialized in antigen capture? Immunol Today 1990; 11: 440–443.
5. Oettgen HC, Martin TR, Wynshaw-Boris A, Deng C, Drazen JM, & Leder P. Active anaphylaxis in IgE-deficient mice. Nature 1994; 370: 367–370.
6. Eichmann K. Idiotype suppression. I. Influence of the dose and of the effector functions of anti-idiotypic antibody on the production of an idiotype. Eur J Immunol 1974; 4: 296.
7. Blaser K, de Weck AL. Regulation of the IgE antibody response by idiotype-anti-idiotype network. Prog Allergy 1982; 32: 203–264.
8. Watts C and Lanzavecchia A. Suppressive effect of antibody on processing of T cell epitopes. J Exp Med 1993; 178: 1459–1463.
9. Hall EP, Gault EA. Regulation of rat IgE responses by immune complexes. Immunology 1987; 61: 415–419.
10. Poulsen LK, Lundberg L, Sondergaard I, Weeke B. Allergen-containing immune complexes used for immunotherapy of allergic asthma. Allergy 1988; 44: 132–142.
11. da Costa PS, de Macedo MS, Perini A. Suppression of mouse IgE response by immune complexes. J Allergy Clin Immunol 1990; 86: 496–502.
12. Coulie PG & Van Snick J. Enhancement of IgG anti-carrier responses by IgG2 anti-hapten antibodies in mice. Eur J Immunol 1985; 15: 793.
13. Rajewsky K & Takemori T. Genetics, expression, and function of idiotypes. Ann Rev Immunol 1983; 1: 569–607.
14. Saint-Remy JMR. Idiotypic network and immediate hypersensitivity. *in* Idiotypic network and diseases. Eds. Hiernaux J and Cerny J. American Society of Microbiologists, 1990 pp 139–173.
15. Machiels JJ, Somville MA, Lebrun PM, Jacquemin MG, and Saint-Remy JMR. Allergen-antibody complexes can efficiently prevent seasonal rhinitis and asthma in grass pollen hypersensitive patients. Allergy 1991; 46: 335–348.
16. Machiels JJ, Somville MA, Lebrun PM, Lebecque SJ, Jacquemin MG, and Saint-Remy JMR. Allergic bronchial asthma due to D. pteronyssinus hypersensitivity can be efficiently treated by inoculation of allergen-antibody complexes. J Clin Invest 1990; 85: 1024–1035.
17. Machiels JJ, Lebrun P, Jacquemin MG, and Saint-Remy JMR. Significant reduction of nonspecific bronchial reactivity in patients with *Dermatophagoides pteronyssinus*-sensitive allergic asthma under therapy with allergen-antibody complexes. Am Rev Resp Disease1993; 147: 1407–1412.
18. Leroy B, Lachapelle JM, Somville MM, Jacquemin MG, and Saint-Remy JMR. Injection of allergen-antibody complexes is an effective treatment of atopic dermatitis. Dermatologica 1991; 182: 98–106.
19. Leroy BP, Boden Griet, Lachapelle JM, Jacquemin MG, and Saint-Remy JMR. A novel therapy for atopic dermatitis using antigen-antibody complexes: a double-blind placebo-controlled study. J Am Acad Dermatol 1993; 28: 232–239.
20. Jacquemin M, and Saint-Remy JMR. Specific down-regulation of anti-allergen IgE and IgG antibodies in man associated with injections of allergen-specific antibody complexes. Therapeutic Immunol 1995; *in press*.
21. Weyer Anne, Le Mao Joëlle, Etievant M, David B, Guinnepain Marie-Thérèse, and Saint-Remy JMR. Human auto-anti-idiotypic antibodies to mite-specific IgE can degranulate human basophils in vitro. Clin Exp Allergy 1995; 25: *in press*.
22. Platts-Mills TAE. Allergen-specific treatment for asthma: III. Am Rev Respir Dis 1993; 148:553–555.
23. Daëron M, Malbec O, Latour S, Arock M, Fridman WH. Regulation of high-affinity IgE receptor-mediated mast cell activation by murine low-affinity IgG receptors. J Clin Invest 1995; 95: 577–585.
24. Leroy BP, Jacquemin MG, Lachapelle JM, and Saint-Remy JMR. Allergen-sensitive atopic dermatitis is improved by injections of allergen combined to F(ab')$_2$ fragments of specific antibodies. Br J Dermatol 1995; 132: *in press*.

62

CHARACTERIZATION OF ALLERGENIC DETERMINANTS ON THE C-TERMINAL REGION OF THE r-Lol p 1

P. Lamontagne,[1] Y. , Boutin,[1,2] C. Brunét,[2] J. Boulanger,[2] J. Berton,[2] and J. Hébert[1,2]

[1]Centre de Recherche en Immunologie et Rhumatologie
Le Centre de Recherche du Centre Hospitalier de l'Université Laval
Sainte-Foy, Québec, Canada
[2]Immunova Ltd.
Sainte-Foy, Québec, Canada

1. INTRODUCTION

Current forms of allergy diagnosis and therapies are based on the use of natural allergenic extracts. Such extracts represent mixtures of more than 50 different molecules, mostly proteins. Despite strong evidence that higher therapeutic efficacy may be achieved with purified extracts, the purification of multiple allergic components from a given extract is a fastidious and sometimes an impossible task. However, the use of recombinant allergens may be an alternative to overcome this problem. To date, cDNA from several allergic proteins have been cloned and the corresponding recombinant allergens have been synthesized. The characterization of these allergens by cDNA technology provides important information about the primary structure of allergens and about the similarities with already known proteins. In the case of ryegrass pollen (*Lolium perenne*), which is responsible for a large portion of grass pollen allergies worldwide, at least three major classes of allergenic proteins (Lol p 1, Lol p 2 and Lol p 3)(1–5) have been isolated and characterized. The major allergen, Lol p 1, is a glycoprotein of about 32 kDa and represents the major IgE-binding protein, as 85–90% of ryegrass sensitive patients react against this protein. Moreover, elevated levels of Lol p 1-specific IgE have been detected in the sera of up to 95% of grass pollen sensitive patients. Recently, the cDNA of two isoforms of Lol p 1 have been sequenced and found to encode a protein of the same size (240 residues). However a lack of information still persists about the IgE-binding epitopes on the Lol p 1. The present study has therefore further characterized the IgE binding epitopes on the rLol p 1 using recombinant technology, mAbs, and synthetic peptides.

New Horizons in Allergy Immunotherapy
edited by Sehon et al. Plenum Press, New York, 1996

2. RESULTS

2.1. Cloning of the Recombinant Lol p 1

In this study, the gene cloning technology was pursued in order to express rLol p 1 in the bacteria *E. coli* TB1. The complete gene encoding the Lol p 1 was amplified by polymerase chain reaction directly from the genomic DNA using oligoprimers designed from the primary structure of the Lol p 1 protein, as previously described. The amplified Lol p 1-product was cloned into the Bluescript KS- vector and then subcloned into the expression vector pMALc. The rLol p 1 was then expressed as a fusion protein in association with a 45 kDa-carrier protein, maltose binding protein (MBP) in the cytoplasm of the bacteria. Using this pMALc vector, it was possible to produce up to 20 mg/liter of purified rLol p 1 protein, following a stimulation with IPTG. Also, rLol p1 could be cleaved from the carrier protein using the Factor Xa and then affinity-purified by amylose resin column.

2.2. Immunological and Biological Properties of rLol p1

In order to verify that the rLol p 1 shares the same immunological and biological properties with its natural counterpart, comparative studies between the rLol p 1 and the native Lol p 1 were carried out. We demonstrated a lack of significant differences in the capacity of rLol p 1 and native Lol p 1 to inhibit the binding of specific IgG or IgE to native Lol p 1. Also, the rLol p 1 induced a release of histamine from basophils and a skin test reactivity comparable to those observed with native Lol p 1. Finally, the rLol p 1 induced the proliferation of T-cells in mice at a level comparable to that observed with the native protein. Together, these results suggest that the rLol p 1 shares similar B and T-cell epitopes with its natural counterparts.

2.3. Production of Recombinant Fragments

To define the allergenic epitopes on Lol p 1, we produced a panel of ten recombinant fragments either by PCR amplification or restriction enzyme which were then expressed as fusion proteins in association with the MBP, as shown in Fig 1. These overlapping recombinant fragments spanning the entire molecule were detected in the lysate of transformed bacteria and corresponded to a molecular weight varying from 45 to 70 kDa as determined by SDS-PAGE.

2.4. Immunoreactivity Patterns of Individual Patients

By immunoblot, we assessed the ability of human IgE from pooled sera to bind to our overlapping recombinant fragments. It was observed that human IgE from atopic do-

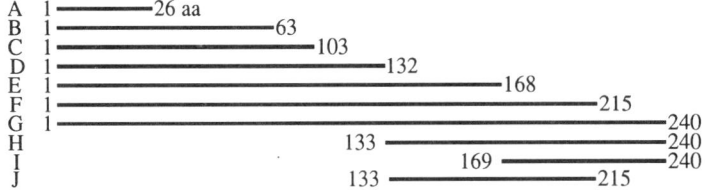

Figure 1. Overlapping recombinant fragments of Lol p 1.

Table 1. Immunoreactivity patterns

Recombinant Fragments							
A	B	C	D	E	F	G	1
			D	E	F	G	1
				E	F	G	6
					F	G	11
					F		4
1	1	1	2	8	23	19	Patients n=23

nors bound to all fragments whereas the sera from non atopic donors did not react with any of these fragments. Thus, these results suggest that IgE-reactive epitopes could be found at any location along the Lol p 1 molecule. However, these data did not permit to appreciate the relative importance of each of these epitopes in allergic diseases. In order to clarify this point, the direct binding of human IgE from 23 different grass-sensitive patients to recombinant fragments was assessed by immunoblot: Table 1 shows that at least five different patterns of reactivity were found.

All the atopic sera reacted against one or more epitopes found on the C-terminal region of Lol p 1, corresponding to the amino acids 133 to 240. It is noteworthy that the fragments A, B, and C corresponding to the N-terminal were recognized by a weak proportion of grass-sensitive subjects. These data also clearly indicate that the C-terminal region represents a major IgE-binding region.

2.5. Identification of IgE-Binding Sites of Lol p 1

To further characterize the IgE-binding sites of Lol p 1, we analyzed the capacity of each overlapping recombinant fragments to inhibit the binding of human IgE to rLol p 1. It was found that rLol p 1 inhibited completely the IgE binding to rLol p 1, while the negative control MBP did not. Also, it was observed that the binding was significantly inhibited by the fragment corresponding to the amino acids 133 to 240.

2.6. Epitope Mapping of rLol p 1 Using mAbs

To better define the allergenic determinants of rLol p 1, a panel of murine anti-Lol p 1 mAbs were screened for their capacity to inhibit the IgE binding of human IgE to solid phase rLol p 1. As shown in Figure 2, three mAbs (290A167, 6D1 and 4F7) inhibited significantly the IgE binding to rLol p 1. Using direct binding assays on a panel of synthetic peptides of 15 amino acids overlapping by ten residues (6, 7) and spanning different regions on Lol p 1, we were able to localize the binding site of each anti-Lol p 1 mAbs. The mAb 290A167 recognized a region corresponding to the amino acids 25 to 40 and inhibited up to 70% the IgE-binding of each individual patient in this study. Two other mAbs

Table 2. IgE binding-inhibition capacity of recombinant fragments

r-fragments	A	B	C	D	E	F	G	H	I	J	MBP
% IgE binding-inhibition to rLol p 1	7	8	6	4	17	32	98	96	51	30	7

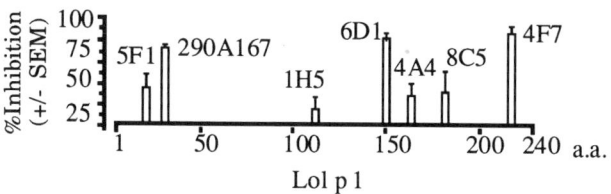

Figure 2. IgE binding-inhibition to rLol p 1 by mAbs in relation to their binding on rLol p 1.

(6D1 and 4F7) recognized regions corresponding to the amino acids 133 to 168 and 216 to 230, respectively. They inhibited the IgE-binding to Lol p 1 from 85 to 95%.

2.7. Fine Epitope Mapping Using Synthetic Peptides

The results of IgE binding-inhibition studies by recombinant fragments and direct assays of anti-Lol p 1 mAbs on synthetic peptides suggest that the C-terminal region contains most of IgE-binding sites. To better define the C-terminal allergenic determinants, synthetic peptides spanning the region 133 to 240 of the Lol p 1 were used in their ability to inhibit the binding of IgE to rLol 1. Only three synthetic peptides corresponding to the region 151–165, 206–220, and 226–240 inhibited significantly the IgE binding. Since these peptides did not overlap, we conclude that there are at least 3 different IgE-binding sites on the C-terminal region of Lol p 1.

3. DISCUSSION

Rapid progress in allergen characterization has been made with the advent of molecular biology. Cloning and expression of allergens with recombinant DNA have greatly facilitated the identification, characterization and analysis of their B- and T-cell epitopes. However, the use of recombinant allergen for diagnostic and therapeutic purposes requires more information about their IgE-binding properties. This study was undertaken to characterize the repertoire of allergenic determinants on a Lol p 1.

Using pooled sera from atopic patients, we demonstrated that, even in denaturing conditions, specific IgE recognized all the recombinant fragments. Moreover, we have found heterogeneity in specific IgE immunoreactivity to Lol p 1. Indeed, we observed that the NH$_2$-terminal region bears some allergenic epitopes but a small portion of the population recognized this region, while the C-terminal region corresponding to the amino acids 133 to 240 bears major IgE epitopes.

To further characterize the IgE binding sites on the C-terminal part of the rLol p 1, we assessed the capacity of anti-Lol p 1 mAbs, overlapping recombinant fragments, and overlapping synthetic peptides to inhibit the binding of IgE to Lol p 1. The figure 3 illustrates the regions on C-terminal portion of Lol p 1 which most likely bear IgE-binding sites. As previously reported by other investigators (8–10), the region 216 to 240 is a major IgE-binding site. Our results confirm these finding; however, we found that this site is in fact composed of two IgE-binding regions which correspond to amino acids 206–220 and 226–240. Furthermore, we demonstrated that an additional allergenic determinant on the amino acid region 151–165 may also represent a major IgE binding site.

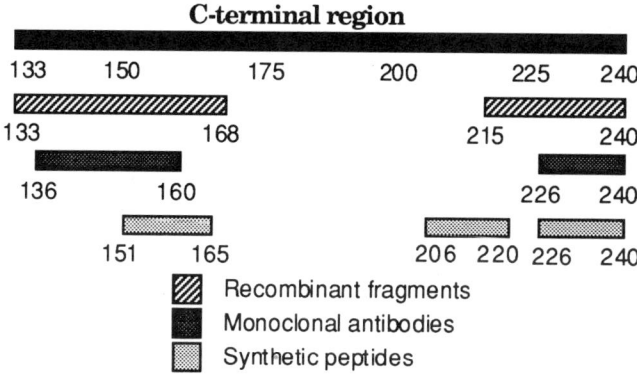

Figure 3. Summary of the results obtained for the epitope mapping of the Lol p 1.

In conclusion, using mAbs, recombinant fragments and synthetic peptides we demonstrated that the C-terminal region of Lol p 1 bears the most important IgE-binding sites and that this region contained at least 3 distinct allergenic determinants.

4. REFERENCES

1. Perez, M, Ishioka, GY, Walker, LE and Chesnut, RW, J Biol Chem, 265: 16210, 1990
2. Griffith, IJ, Smith, PM, Pollock, J, Theerakulpisut, P, Avjioglu, A, Davies, S, Hough, T, Singh, MB, Simpson, RJ, Ward, LD et al. Febs Lett, 279: 210, 1991
3. Ansari, AA, Shenbagamurthi, P and Marsh, DG, J Biol Chem, 264: 11181, 1989
4. Ansari, AA, Shenbagamurthi, P and Marsh, DG, Biochemistry, 28: 8665, 1989
5. Sidoli, A, Tamborini, E, Giuntini, I, Levi, S, Volonte, G, Paini, C, De, LC, Siccardi, AG, Baralle, FE, Galliani, S et al. J Biol Chem, 268: 21819, 1993
6. Geysen, HM, Meloen, RH and Barteling, SJ, Proc. Natl. Acad. Sci. USA, 81: 3998, 1984
7. Geysen, HM, Rodda, SJ, Mason, TJ, Tribbick, G and Schoofs, PG, J. Immunol. Methods, 102: 259, 1987
8. Esch, RE and Klapper, DG, Mol Immunol., 26: 557, 1989
9. Esch, RE and Klapper, DG, Journal of Immunology, 142: 0179, 1989
10. van, RR, van, LW, van, den, Berg, M, Weller, HH and Aalberse, RC, Allergy, 49: 254, 1994

63

ANTI-IDIOTYPIC ANTIBODIES IN THE TREATMENT OF ALLERGIES

Jacques Hébert and Yvan Boutin

Centre de Recherche en Immunologie et Rhumatologie
Le Centre de Recherche du Centre Hospitalier de l'Université Laval
Sainte-Foy, Québec, Canada G1V 4G2

1. REGULATION OF IgE ANTIBODY SYNTHESIS

An increased IgE synthesis and local inflammatory response are the hallmarks of the atopic immune response. Therefore a better understanding of the mechanisms regulating the IgE production and multiple events or factors leading to the inflammation is needed to define strategies of treatment targeting the abnormal response.

A growing body of evidence supports the concept of the genetic control of the antibody response [1–5] as well as its regulation at B and T cell levels by a number of regulatory molecules such as cytokines, [6] isotype-specific factors [7] or anti-idiotypic (aId) antibodies [8, 9].

1.1. Regulation of IgE Antibody Response by Idiotypic Network

A given antibody molecule is specific for one target antigen, and its specificity is determined by the structure of the variable (V) regions of the antibody. Variable regions as well as constant regions bear immunogenic sites, and antibodies can be induced against these determinants. Within the V regions, antigenic determinants are known as idiotopes, and they collectively define the idiotype (Id) of the molecule [10]. Idiotypes are unique and specific for each antibody molecule in the same way fingerprints are unique and specific for individuals. It has been established that an animal can be immunized with autologous antibody molecules to produce antibodies against the Id and referred to as anti-Id (aId) antibodies [10]. These observations suggested that the self-idiotope determinants are indeed recognized by the immune system. In 1974 Nils Jerne postulated that the interaction between Id and aId constituted a regulatory network important in the control of antibody production [11]. According to this concept, an antigenic epitope induces the production of antibody (Ab1), recognizing the epitope through its paratope and expressing an Id, so called Id_1. Id_1 induces Ab2, which possesses Id_2 and recognizes Id_1. In its turn the Id_2 induces Ab3, and so on.

New Horizons in Allergy Immunotherapy
edited by Sehon et al. Plenum Press, New York, 1996

1.1.1. Regulation of Immune Responses in Animals by Idiotypic Network. For obvious reasons, there is an interest in assessing the potential ways to manipulate the immune response in an antigen-specific manner. In some cases, such as in organ transplantation, autoimmune diseases or allergic hypersensitivities, specific suppression would be desirable, while for other purposes, such as vaccinations or tumor rejection, a stimulation of the immune defense mechanisms is rather required. According to Jerne's network theory, aId antibodies might be involved in a normal event that modulates the degree and the duration of immune response. Therefore, aId reagents could be used to regulate an immune response to a specific antigen.

The idiotypic regulation of primary mouse IgE response has been studied mainly by the group of De Weck [8, 9, 12]. BALB/c mice were inoculated by subcutaneous (s.c.) or intraperitoneal (i.p.) route with purified isologous anti-benzylpenicilloyl (BPO) coupled with ovalbumin (OVA) in Freund's adjuvant. Active production of specific aId antibodies was detected after 6 weeks. In these mice, further immunization with BPO-OVA failed to induce IgE production, even on repeated immunizations with antigen [9]. Suppression of IgE production was specific for the hapten, since the response to OVA was not affected [9]. These data have been partly confirmed in study with PC [8], in that a partial reduction of IgE production was obtained in mice that produced antibodies to T15, a major Id of the anti-PC response.

Passive transfer of aId antibodies has been also shown to suppress IgE response in animals. In various studies, isologous and heterologous have been used. Intravenous (i.v.) administration of anti-T15 isologous antiserum completely prevented the formation of IgE antibodies to PC. Suppression was specific to T15$^+$ Id since aId raised to T15$^-$ anti-PC myeloma proteins had no effect [8].

The suppression of an ongoing IgE response is much more difficult to achieve. Repeated transfers of isologous aId antibodies or use of heterologous aId antibodies has usually been successful [13–15]. However, the state of suppression remained transient in most cases, since subsequent boosts with antigen usually restore IgE production.

1.1.2. Regulation of IgE Antibody Response in Human by Idiotypic Network.
Repeated immunizations with antigen led to the production of auto-aId as described in tetanus toxoid model by Geha et al. [16, 17]. Allergic diseases involved repeated stimulation by natural antigen. Thus the presence of auto-aId antibodies to allergen-specific antibodies in humans would be expected. Auto-aId has been described in allergic patients receiving immunotherapy [18, 19]. Presence of auto-aId was also reported in normal subjects and in patients allergic to ragweed [20] and to grass pollen [19]. Furthermore, in allergic subjects treated with immunotherapy, the level of auto-aId appeared to go up to the normal range [20]. These results suggested that decreased production of auto-aId in allergic subjects allows the escape of IgE antibody synthesis from immunoregulatory influences.

It was demonstrated that rabbit aId antibodies could elicit a Prausnitz-Küstner reaction in normal skin previously sensitized with IgE antibodies from an allergic donor [21] or they induced release of histamine when added to IgE-coated basophils isolated from peripheral blood of patients hypersensitive to grass pollens [22]. More directly, a regulatory role for aId antibodies in the production of IgE antibodies has been suggested by Geha and co-workers [23, 24]. Addition of rabbit aId antibodies raised to anti-tetanus toxoid IgG antibodies to peripheral-blood B cells resulted in the suppression of IgE production. Taken together these data strongly suggest a role of aId antibodies in the regulation of the allergic response.

2. STUDY OF THE REGULATION OF IMMUNE RESPONSE TO Lol p 1 BY IDIOTYPIC NETWORK IN ANIMALS

2.1. Lol p 1

For the last decade we have been particularly interested to study the role of aId-Id interactions in the modulation of immune response to allergens in the animal and human. To achieve that, we studied the IgE response to a particular allergen: Lol p 1 [25–27], the major allergenic component of ryegrass pollen that is widely distributed throughout the world particularly in temperate zones. It is the major IgE-binding protein and approximately 90% of ryegrass sensitive patients had positive skin tests to Lol p 1 [28]. Moreover, elevated levels of Lol p 1-specific IgE have been detected in sera of up 95% of grass pollen allergic individuals [28]. Knowledge of antigenic structure of allergens is critical for a better understanding of their biological activities and may help to find answers about human allergic responses. Therefore, using different anti-Lol p 1 monoclonal antibodies (mAb) (290A-167, 539A-6, 348A-6 and P3B2), we identified four different and non overlapping epitopes on Lol p 1 [25, 26, 29]. They were used to confirm cross-reactivity between grasses [25, 30] and to purify, by affinity chromatography, Lol p 1 in a biologically active form.

Since the complete amino acid sequence of Lol p 1 was deduced from cDNA sequence analysis [31, 32], we have produced recombinant Lol p 1 (see in these proceedings). This recombinant Lol p 1 shares the same biological and immunological properties as its natural counterpart. The deduced amino acid sequence had also permitted us to identify major allergenic epitopes using overlapping synthetic peptides and recombinant polypeptidic fragments.

Finally, we also demonstrated that the Id borne by one of our anti-Lol p 1 (290A-167) and shared by IgE was a public Id since it was expressed in 80% of grass-sensitive patients [22]. These data suggested that the Id 290A-167 might be a preferential target for selective immunomodulation.

2.2. Production of mAb against a Cross-Reactive Id

To study the regulation of immune response to Lol p 1 by Id network, we produced and characterized aId mAb [33] directed against an anti-Lol p 1 mAb representing a major cross-reactive idiotype (290A-167). Monoclonal aId antibody bore internal image properties as assessed by its direct binding to Id and its capacity to inhibit the binding of Id to Lol p 1. This aId mAb (A7H2) also inhibited the binding of human IgE to Lol p 1 [34]. It induced, in a dose-dependent fashion, histamine release by leukocytes from grass-sensitive patients. The inhibition of this histamine release by the addition of the Id (290A-167) confirmed the specificity of the reaction. Finally, we demonstrated that this aId mAb elicited an anti-Lol p 1 response in naive animals [33]. Together these data confirmed that our aId mAb could biologically and functionally mimic the original antigen.

2.3. Effects of aId mAb Pretreatment on Subsequent Lol p 1 Immune Response

The effects of pretreatment with the aId mAb bearing the internal image of Lol p 1 before immunization with the antigen have been examined [35]. The aId mAb or unrelated

Table 1. Titer of IgE anti-Lol p 1 in mice pretreated with either aId mAb
or control mAb

	Titre of IgE anti-Lol p 1	
	aId-pretreated	Control mAb-pretreated
Before Lol p 1 immunization	< 50	< 50
After the third boost with Lol p 1	250	6250

Mice weekly received aId mAb or control mAb during 8 weeks. After the pretreatment the animals were immunized at two-week interval with Lol p 1 adsorbed onto alum.

mAb was weekly given for 8 weeks (i.p). Then mice received Lol p 1 adsorbed onto alum. Serum anti-Lol p 1 antibodies (IgG or IgE) and specific idiotypic responses were measured. Anti-Lol p 1 IgG antibodies could be detected before immunization with Lol p 1 only in mice pretreated with aId mAb. Immunization with Lol p 1 induced an anti-Lol p 1 IgG response in both groups, but this response was higher in mice that received aId mAb. Similar profiles were seen for specific IgE antibodies and idiotypic responses. Surprisingly, idiotypes borne by other anti-Lol p 1 mAb (539A-6 and 348A-6) had also been enhanced after pretreatment with the anti-290A-167 mAb. These observations suggested that the modulation of immune response by an aId mAb is not restricted to the respective Id, but modulates the expression of other Id.

2.4. Effects of Id mAb Pretreatment on Subsequent Lol P 1 Immune Response

In our system, aId administration led to an enhancement of immune response. However to achieve a suppression of immune response, more encouraging results were produced in experiments in which Ab1 rather than Ab2 was used for pretreatment in other antigenic system.

Mice were treated with an anti-Lol p 1 mAb (290A-167) [36]. This resulted in the production of aId antibodies, as evidenced by their ability to bind to the Fab fraction of 290A-167, and to inhibit the binding of rabbit polyclonal aId antibodies to 290A-167. The animals were then immunized with Lol p 1 adsorbed onto alum and the immune response to the protein was analyzed. Antigen specific IgG1 and IgE responses were strongly suppressed as measured by immunoassay. Suppression of anti-Lol p 1 IgE antibodies was confirmed by a reduction of end point titers measured by passive cutaneous anaphylaxis. The suppression of antigen specific antibody was accompanied by a reduction of anti-Lol p 1 antibody-producing spleen cells. These data indicate that pretreatment with 290A-167 can strongly down-regulate the IgE response to the main allergen of rye grass pollen,

Table 2. PCA titer of IgE anti-Lol p 1 in mice pretreated with either Id mAb
or control mAb

	PCA titre of IgE anti-Lol p 1	
	Id-pretreated	Control mAb-pretreated
Before Lol p 1 immunization	< 40	< 40
After the third boost with Lol p 1	350	5120

Mice weekly received Id mAb or control mAb during 8 weeks. After the pretreatment the animals were immunized at two-week interval with Lol p 1 adsorbed onto alum.

which is associated with increase in aId antibodies. This approach could provide rapid and long-standing hyposensitization in patients with grass pollen allergy.

3. STUDY OF THE REGULATION OF IMMUNE RESPONSE TO BEE VENOM BY IDIOTYPIC NETWORK IN HUMAN

Passive infusion of beekeeper's plasma was shown to protect patients against systemic reactions occurring during active immunotherapy [37]. However the mechanisms involved in a such protection are still unknown. It is tempting to speculate that a low production of aId led in patients sensitive to bee venom to a specific IgE production whereas non atopic subjects exposed to bee venom and having high levels of aId antibodies develop no symptoms.

We had the opportunity to evaluate a patient highly allergic to honeybee venom who experienced systemic reactions to injection therapy [38]. Since she did not tolerate sufficient amounts of venom to achieve protection against bee stings, beekeeper's plasma rich in aId antibodies was administered to the patient. After transfusion of plasma, she was immunized with increased doses of bee venom. Clinical and immunological parameters were measured along the combined immunotherapy protocol.

Immediately after beekeeper's plasma transfer, a decrease of skin sensitivity and basophil histamine release induced by bee venom was observed. Her tolerance to bee venom was also improved since she could receive 100μg without reactions. No differences in specific IgG and IgE were observed. Following the modified rush immunotherapy, increased levels of aId antibodies in the serum of the patient were associated with a diminution of specific antibodies (IgG and IgE) to honeybee venom. These results suggest a dual role for aId: 1) an immediate action on clinical sensitivity along with a decrease of skin mast cell and basophil sensitivity and 2) an immunoregulatory role on specific antibody production.

4. CONCLUSION

Several interacting factors contribute to the regulation of IgE. Although considerable evidence has accumulated on the regulation of a protective immune response by an Id-aId network, studies on allergen-specific responses are few but supported this concept. In animal, aId antibodies can be produced through repeated conventional immunization with specific antibodies. We and others have demonstrated that animals producing aId antibodies are unable to mount a specific IgE immune response upon subsequent immunization with alum-adsorbed proteins or hapten-carrier conjugates [8, 9, 12, 36].

Table 3. Clinical parameters after and before passive transfer of beekeeper's plasma

	Passive transfer	
	Before	After
Tolerated dose (μg of bee venom)	25	100
End point titration skin test (μg/ml of bee venom)	0.1	1
Basophil histamine release (%)	85	45

Table 4. Measurement of aId activity in bee-sensitive patient's serum

	aId activity* (%)
Before plasma transfer	< 5
After plasma tranfer	15
76 weeks after initiation of rush immunotherapy	33

* The aId activity is the percentage of the inhibition of specific IgE to bee venom by patient'serum depleted of anti-bee venom antibodies.

In human, the levels of aId antibodies are associated with the severity of allergic symptoms. Levels of aId antibodies are more elevated in normal subjects and patients under specific immunotherapy than allergic patients. The exact role of aId antibodies is still unknown. It was suggested that this suppression of specific IgE response by aId antibodies was due to the activation of Ts cells [39]. Furthermore, since the balance between the T helper subsets (Th1 and Th2) is an important feature of the allergic contidion, it might be interesting to speculate that aId antibodies can interact in this balance. Obviously, it is also concievable that aId antibodies act directly on B cells. However all these hypotheses remain to be clarified.

5. REFERENCES

1. Benacerraf B and McDevitt HD. Science:**175**, 273,1972.
2. Katz DH and Benacerraf B. Transplant Rev:**22**, 175,1975.
3. Ansari AA, Shinomiya N, Zwollo P and Marsh DG. Immunogenetics:**33**, 24,1991.
4. Huang SK and Marsh DG. Ann Allergy:**70**, 347,1993.
5. Huang SK, Yi M, Kumai M and Marsh DG. Adv Exp Med Biol:**347**, 11,1994.
6. Vercelli D and Geha RS. J Allergy Clin Immunol:**88**, 285,1991.
7. Ishizaka K. Annu Rev Immunol:**2**, 159,1984.
8. Blaser K, Geiser M and de Weck AL. Eur J Immunol:**9**, 1017,1979.
9. Blaser K, Nakagama T and De Weck AL. J Immunol:**125**, 24,1980.
10. Oudin J and Michel M. C R Hebd Séance Acad Sci Ser D Sci Nat:**257**, 805,1963.
11. Jerne NK. Ann Immunol (Paris):**125C**, 373,1974.
12. Blaser K and de Weck AL. Prog Allergy:**32**, 203,1982.
13. Blaser K, Nakagawa T and de Weck AL. Inter Arch Allergy Appl Immunol:**64**, 42,1981.
14. Geczy AF, de Weck AL, Geczy CL and Toffler O. J Allergy Clin Immunol:**62**, 261,1978.
15. Malley A, Brandt CJ and . Immunology:**45**, 217,1982.
16. Geha RS. J Immunol:**129**, 139,1982.
17. Geha RS. J Immunol:**130**, 1634,1983.
18. Bose R, Marsh DG and Delespesse G. Clin Exp Immunol:**66**, 231,1986.
19. Hébert J, Bernier D and Mourad W. Clin Exp Immunol:**80**, 413,1990.
20. Castracane JM and Rocklin RE. Int Arch Allergy Appl Immunol:**86**, 288,1988.
21. Geha RS. J Clin Invest:**69**, 735,1982.
22. Mécheri S, Mourad W, Lapeyre J, Jobin M, David B and Hébert J. Immunology:**64**, 11,1988.
23. Geha RS and Comunale M. J Clin Invest:**71**, 46,1983.
24. Geha RS and Weinberg RP. J Immunol:**121**, 1518,1978.
25. Mourad W, Pelletier G, Boulet A, Islam N, Valet J-P and Hébert J. J Immunol Methods:**89**, 53,1986.
26. Mourad W, Mécheri S, Peltre C, David B and Hébert J. J Immunol:**141**, 3486,1988.
27. Ford D and Baldo BA. Int Arch Allergy Appl Immunol:**81**, 193,1986.
28. Friedhoff L, Ehrlich-Kautzky E, Grant JH, Meyers DA and Marsh DG. J Allergy Clin Immunol:**78**, 1190,1986.
29. Mourad W, Bernier D and Hébert J. Mol Immunol:**26**, 1051,1989.
30. Lin ZW, Ekramoddoullah AK, Kisil FT, Hebert J and Mourad W. Int Arch Allergy Appl Immunol:**87**, 294,1988.
31. Perez M, Ishioka GY, Walker LE and Chesnut RW. J Biol Chem:**265**, 16210,1990.

32. Griffith IJ, Smith PM, Pollock J, *et al.* FEBS:**279**, 210,1991.
33. Hébert J, Bernier D, Boutin Y, Jobin M and Mourad W. J Immunol:**144**, 4256,1990.
34. Boutin Y, Jobin M, Bernier D and Hébert J. Inter Arch Allergy Appl Immunol:**102**, 10,1993.
35. Boutin Y and Hébert J. Clin Exp Immunol:**96**, 350,1994.
36. Boutin Y and Hébert J. J Allergy Clin Immunol:**95**, 751,1995.
37. Bousquet J, Fontez A, Aznar R, Robinet-Levy M and Michel F-B. J Allergy Clin Immunol:**79**, 947,1987.
38. Boutin Y, Jobin M, Bédard P-M, Hébert M and Hébert J. J Allergy Clin Immunol:**In press**, 1994.
39. Malley A and Dresser DW. Immunology:**46**, 653,1982.

64

ENHANCED PRODUCTION AND GENE EXPRESSION OF IL-5 IN BRONCHIAL ASTHMA

Possible Management of Atopic Diseases with IL-5 Specific Gene Transcription Inhibitor

Akio Mori, Matsunobu Suko, Osamu Kaminuma, Yoko Nishizaki, Toshifumi Nagahori, Tadashi Mikami, Takeo Ohmura, Akihiko Hosino, Yumiko Asakura, and Hirokazu Okudaira

Department of Medicine and Physical Therapy
Faculty of Medicine
University of Tokyo 7–3–1 Hongo
Bunkyo-ku, Tokyo 113 Japan

1. INTRODUCTION

Infiltration of various inflammatory cells into the bronchial mucosa and submucosa is a prominent pathological feature of bronchial asthma.[1-3] Persistent mucosal inflammation, particularly epithelial damage caused by eosinophil-derived products, is believed to contribute to the pathogenesis of bronchial hypersensitivity.[4-7] Inhalation of a relevant allergen results in an early asthmatic reaction (EAR) that subsides within 1 to 2 hours. In 40–60% of patients, this early reaction is followed after 6 to 10 hours by a late asthmatic reaction (LAR), which usually subsides during the next 1 to 2 days.[8] Accumulating evidence suggests that LAR is a consequence of eosinophilic inflammation in the lung induced by a T cell cytokine, interleukin 5 (IL-5).[9-15]

CD4+ T cells and T cell cytokines have been strongly implicated in chronic bronchial asthma[16], and the involvement of IL-5 in the pathophysiology of asthma has been elucidated recently. For example, bronchoalveolar lavage (BAL) fluid of atopic and non-atopic asthma patients showed increased concentrations of IL-5.[17] Serum IL-5 concentration was elevated in symptomatic asthmatics and decreased after oral prednisolone therapy[18.] Activated T cells expressing IL-5 mRNA were detected in the bronchial mucosa in chronic asthmatics [12] and increased after allergen challenge.[19] The degree of IL-5 mRNA expression correlated well with the degree of eosinophil infiltration, whereas those of IL-3 and GM-CSF did not[20]. IL-5-producing T cells were also demonstrated in the late phase cutaneous lesions of atopic dermatitis.[21] IL-5 seems to be one of the key mediators involved in the pathogenesis of allergic diseases characterized by eosinophilic inflammation.

New Horizons in Allergy Immunotherapy
edited by Sehon et al. Plenum Press, New York, 1996

Our previous report indicated that IL-5 production by CD4$^+$ T cells is enhanced in both atopic and non-atopic asthmatics.[22] Glucocorticoids (GCs) and immunosuppressants, FK506 and cyclosporin A (CsA), suppressed IL-5 synthesis by PBMC of asthmatic patients in vitro. Clinical improvement of asthma after inhaled corticosteroid therapy was accompanied with a clear reduction of IL-5 production by peripheral CD4$^+$ T cells.[23] Reduction of IL-5 production was also observed in patients with severe atopic dermatitis treated with topical FK506.[24] Control of IL-5 production by activated T cells may be a beneficial approach to manage allergic diseases characterized by eosinophilic inflammation. To delineate the cellular and molecular mechanisms of IL-5 production by human CD4$^+$helper T cells, and explore possible interventions to control IL-5 production, we established allergen-specific T cell clones and T cell hybridomas from peripheral blood lymphocytes of atopic asthmatics, and analyzed the molecular mechanisms of human IL-5 gene transcription.

2. ENHANCED IL-5 PRODUCTION IN ALLERGIC DISEASES

2.1. D.f. Mite Extract Induced IL-5 Production by PBMC of Atopic Asthmatics but Not of Healthy Controls

Peripheral blood mononuclear cells (PBMC) from atopic asthmatics and healthy controls were incubated with *Dermatophagoides farinae (D.f.)* mite extract and the resulting supernatants were assayed for IL-5. All of the atopic patients were sensitive to house dust mite in this series of experiments. Figure 1 shows that PBMC of atopic asthmatics produced significantly higher amounts of IL-5 in response to *D.f.* mite allergen than those of healthy controls (66.733.9 pg/ml in atopic asthmatics, 1.70.6 pg/ml in healthy controls). Similar results were obtained when antigen was added at 0.1 or 10 g/ml in the culture. IL-5 production was totally abolished by the depletion of CD4$^+$ cells from the original PBMC using anti-CD4 mAb-coated magnetic beads (Dynal, NY), suggesting that IL-5 was produced by CD4$^+$ helper T cells.

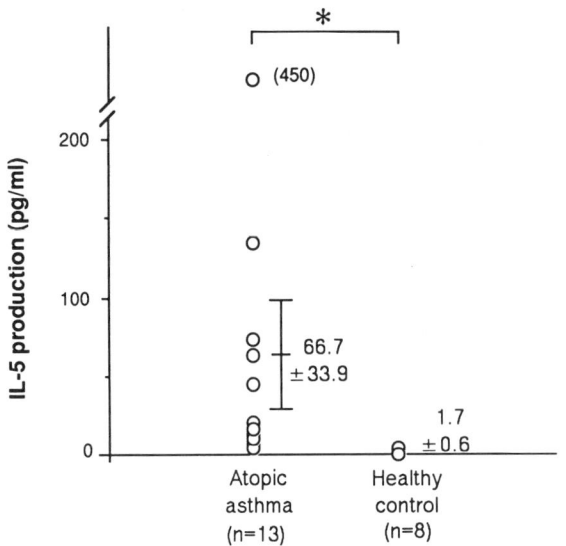

Figure 1. IL-5 is produced by PBMC of mite-sensitive atopic asthmatics in response to D.f. mite allergen. PBMC (2$\cdot$10^6/ml) were incubated with D.f. mite allergen extract (1 μg/ml) for 6 days. IL-5 content in the supernatants was assayed by ELISA. Data are presented as the mean result of triplicate cultures. Values of p<0.05 by Wilcoxon signed-ranks test (*) are considered to be statistically significant.

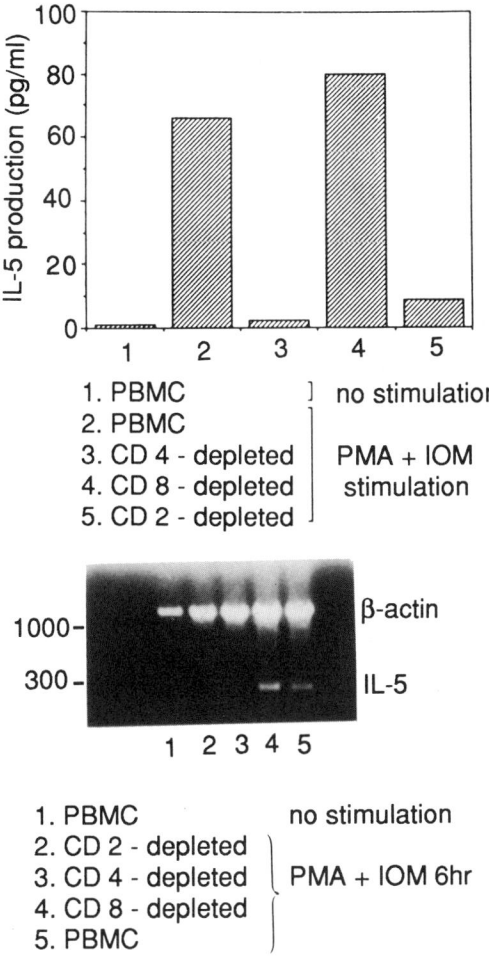

Figure 2. IL-5 is produced by CD4+ T cells. CD2-, CD4- or CD8-positive cells were depleted from PBMC using immunomagnetic beads. Each population (210^6 U/ml) and original unfractionated PBMC (210^6 U/ml) were stimulated with PMA (20 nM) and IOM (1 M) for 24 hours (a) or 8 hours (b). IL-5 production was measured by sandwich ELISA (a). Data are presented as the mean result of triplicate cultures. Cytoplasmic RNA was extracted, reverse transcribed and amplified by PCR using IL-5 and β-actin primers sets (b). The 294 bp products and 1128 bp products correspond with the expected size of IL-5 and β-actin amplification products, respectively.

2.2. Enhanced IL-5 Production by CD4$^+$ T Cells in Allergic Diseases

In order to delineate the signal requirements for IL-5 production, PBMC of atopic asthmatics were incubated with either phorbol 12-myristate 13-acetate (PMA) or ionomycin (IOM) or both. IL-5 production was induced only with the combined stimuli of PMA and IOM, suggesting that both protein kinase C (PKC) activation and Ca^{2+} influx were required for IL-5 synthesis, as well as for IL-2 synthesis by T cells. When CD2-, CD4- positive cells were depleted from the original PBMC, IL-5 production and IL-5 mRNA expression were abolished (Figure 2), clearly indicating that CD4$^+$ T cells are the principal source of IL-5 in atopic PBMC.

PBMC obtained from atopic asthmatics, non-atopic asthmatics and control subjects were stimulated with PMA plus IOM for 24 hours (Figure 3). No significant difference was observed among the three groups in the amounts of IL-2, IL-3, IL-4, GM-CSF and IFN-γ produced. In contrast, significant IL-5 production was observed in atopic asthmatics and non-atopic asthmatics, but not in healthy controls (p<0.05). The results indicate that T

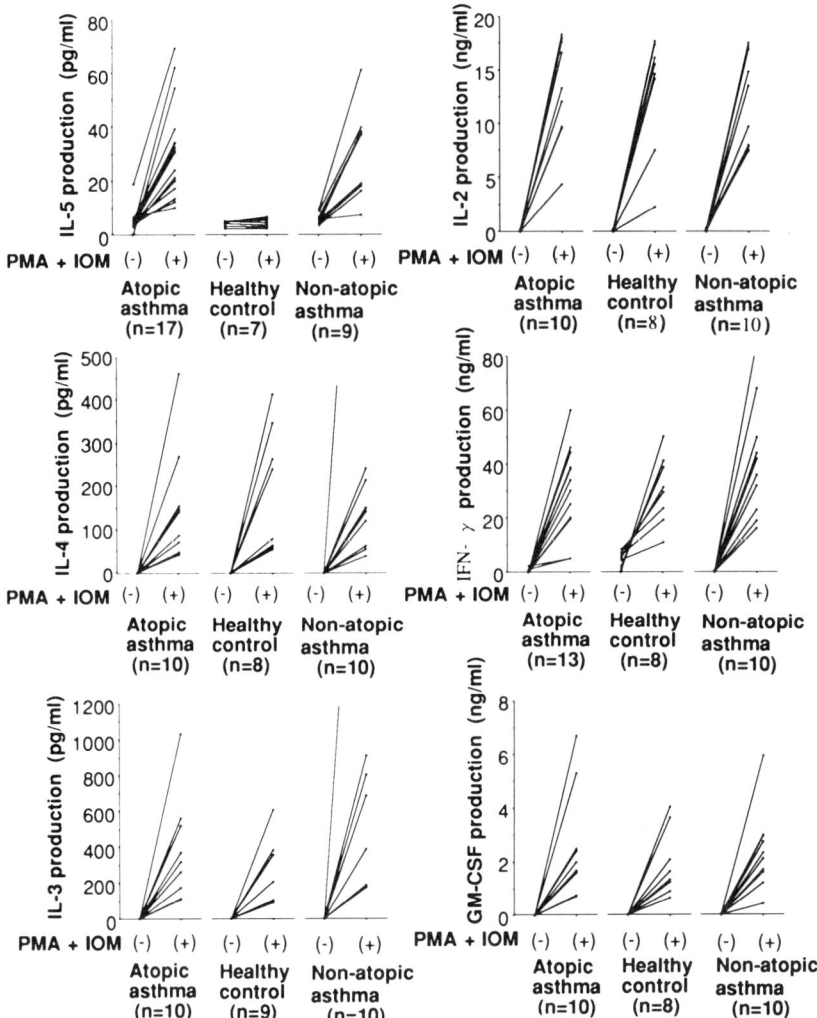

Figure 3. Comparison of IL-2, IL-3, IL-4, IL-5, GM-CSF and IFN-γ production by PBMC obtained from atopic asthmatics, non-atopic asthmatics and healthy controls. PBMC ($2 10^{6}$/ml) were stimulated with PMA (20 nM) and IOM (1 μM) for 24 hours. Supernatants were assayed for IL-2, IL-3, IL-4, IL-5, GM-CSF and IFN-γ by specific ELISAs. The numbers of donors included in each study are shown in the parentheses. IL-5 production upon stimulation was 37.6 7.1, 3.6 0.4, 25.7 5.5 pg/ml in atopic asthmatics, healthy controls and non-atopic asthmatics, respectively (mean standard error). IL-2 production upon stimulation was 139.2 16.0, 123.4 13.0, 137.3 18.1 ng/ml. IL-3 production was 385.086.3, 229.160.9, 1051.3404.1 pg/ml. IL-4 production upon stimulation was 146.0 41.2, 190.8 48.6, 266.5 117.2 pg/ml. GM-CSF production was 2514.8609.6, 1786.0393.1, 2208.8450.3 pg/ml. IFN-γ production upon stimulation was 29.9 4.4, 27.4 2.0, 28.7 6.2 ng/ml. IL-5 production in atopic and non-atopic asthmatics was significantly greater than that in healthy controls (p<0.05). No significant difference was observed among the three groups in the amounts of IL-2, IL-3, IL-4, GM-CSF and IFN-γ produced.

cells that produce IL-5 upon PMA plus IOM stimulation exist in the peripheral blood of atopic and non-atopic asthmatics, but not of healthy subjects, suggesting that *so-called non-atopic asthmatics are actually hypersensitive at the level of T cells.* The major T cell allergen(s) of non-atopic asthmatics are unknown at present, but some of the patients (2 of 8 examined) significantly responded to *D.f.* allergen.

IL-5 production by PBMC was also observed in atopic dermatitis which is another atopic disease accompanied by eosinophilia. It is reported that PBMC of helminth-infected patients produce IL-5 upon stimulation with PMA plus IOM. [25] The existence of IL-5-producing T cells in peripheral blood seems to be a common feature of diseases associated with eosinophilic inflammation.

3. CELLULAR MECHANISMS OF IL-5 PRODUCTION IN ALLERGIC DISEASES

GC, FK506 and CsA inhibited IL-5 synthesis by $CD4^+$ T cells in vitro.[22] Clinical improvement of both asthmatic patients treated with inhaled corticosteroids and atopic dermatitis patients treated with topical application of FK506 was accompanied by a clear reduction of IL-5 production.[23, 24] These findings strongly implicate a role of IL-5 in the pathogenesis of allergic diseases, and prompted us to investigate the precise mechanisms of human IL-5 production in the search for a possible therapeutic intervention.

3.1. IL-5 Production by T Cell Clones Is Dependent on IL-2

T cell clones specific for *Der f* II, a major allergen of the house dust mites, were established from PBMC of asthmatic donors by the antigenic stimulation with recombinant *Der f* II (r*Der f* II) protein, followed by the limiting dilution. Cytokine production was analyzed in culture supernatants obtained from T cell clones treated with antigenic, immobilized anti-CD3 monoclonal antibody (OKT3) or PMA plus IOM stimulation. More than 60 clones tested so far all produced both IL-2 and IL-4 (Th0 phenotype). As shown in Figure 4, IL-5 was clearly produced by T cell clones stimulated with immobilized OKT3. Addition of anti-IL-2 monoclonal antibody to the culture totally abrogated IL-5 production, suggesting that IL-5 synthesis by the T cell clones is dependent on endogenously produced IL-2. IL-4 production was not affected by the addition of the antibodies. The presence of anti-IL-4 antibody did not affect IL-5 synthesis. Moreover, IL-5 production of concanavalin A-stimulated PBMC obtained from asthmatic patients was also completely blocked by the anti-IL-2 neutralizing antibodies, suggesting that IL-2 is commonly required for IL-5 production by human peripheral T cells.

3.2. IL-2 Induced Gene Expression and Protein Synthesis of IL-5 by T Cell Clones

T cell clone YA5 which produced IL-2, IL-4 and IL-5 upon activation clearly produced IL-5 in response to human recombinant IL-2. IL-4 neither induced IL-5 production, nor was produced by IL-2 stimulation. All of the T cell clones that produced IL-5 upon antigenic stimulation produced IL-5 upon IL-2 stimulation. RT-PCR analysis revealed that IL-5 mRNA in T cell clones increased 3 hours after IL-2 stimulation and reached a maximum at 6 hours.

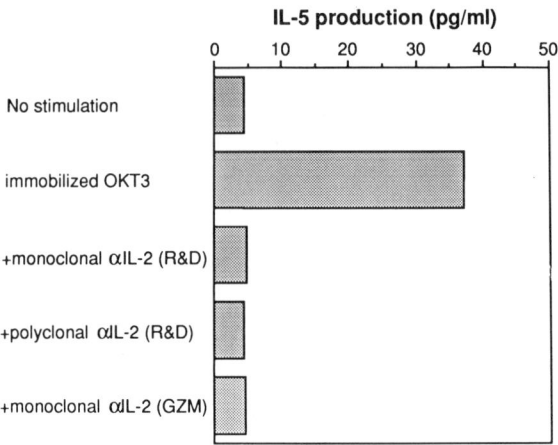

Figure 4. IL-2-dependent production of IL-5. 96-well culture plates were coated with anti-CD3 monoclonal antibody (10 μg/ml). T cell clone (YA 5) (10^5 cells/well) was cultured for 24 hours and the resulting supernants were assayed for IL-5 by a specific ELISA. Anti-IL-2 monoclonal antibody (10 μg/ml) was included in some cultures. The mean result of triplicate cultures is shown in the figure.

Pretreatment of T cell clones with calphostin-C, a protein kinase C inhibitor, suppressed IL-5 production by T cell clones stimulated with IL-2 in a dose-dependent manner. Herbimycin A and genistein, tyrosine kinase inhibitors, also suppressed IL-2-induced IL-5 production. It has been known that the proliferative response induced by IL-2 is mainly mediated by γ chain-associated Jak3, β chain-associated Jak1 and lck.[26] Our findings suggest that these tyrosine kinases would also be essential for cytokine synthesis, as well as proliferation of T cells, induced by IL-2.

Although Th2-like cytokine production has been observed in allergic diseases such as asthma and atopic dermatitis,[27, 28] some reports pointed out that IL-2 protein or IL-2 mRNA-expressing T cells were increased in bronchoalveolar lavage fluid of asthmatics[17, 29, 30] and in the late phase cutaneous reactions of atopic patients.[21] These findings and our results suggest that locally produced IL-2 may contribute to eosinophilic inflammation by inducing IL-5 production by T cells in vivo.

4. TRANSCRIPTIONAL REGULATION OF IL-5 PROMOTER/ENHANCER GENE IN HUMAN T CELLS

4.1. Human IL-5-Luciferase Analysis in T Cell Clones

Cytokine genes, including the IL-5 gene, remain quiescent in resting T cells. Upon antigenic stimulation, various activation signals are transduced into the cytoplasm via membrane receptors and finally initiate transcription of several genes. Various signal transducing molecules, such as tyrosine kinsaes, protein kinase C, protein kinase A, calmodulin, and phosphatases, are involved in the processes. IL-2 synthesis is mainly controlled at the transcriptional level.[31] Gene transcription of human IL-2 is controlled

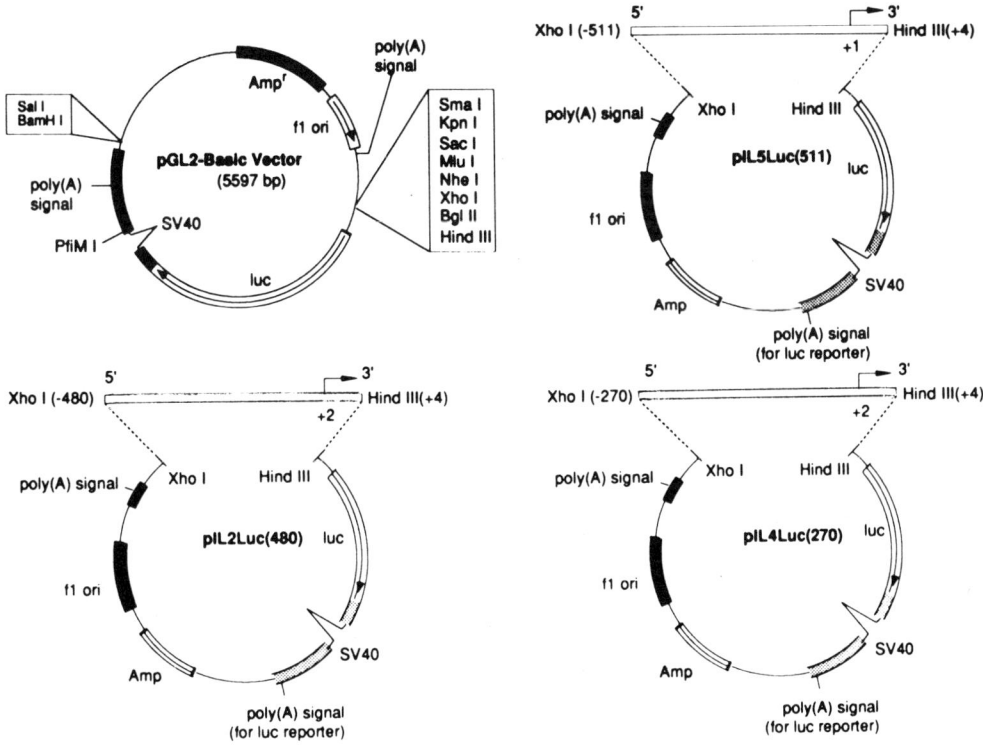

Figure 5. Plasmid maps.

primarily by a 300 bp region that lies 5' upstream of the transcription initiation site.[32] To analyze the mechanisms of human IL-5 gene transcription, we constructed a human IL-5 promoter/enhancer-luciferase reporter gene construct (Figure 5). As shown in Figure 6, IL-5-producing T cell clone YA5 clearly transcribed pIL-5Luc upon stimulation with PMA plus IOM or IL-2 (100 U/ml), indicating that the 500 bp human IL-5 promoter/enhancer is functionally sufficient to mediate activation-dependent gene transcription in human T cells. In contrast, the non-IL-5-producing clone YA10 did not transcribe pIL-5Luc. Transfection efficiency determined by β-galactosidase activity in the cell lysates was comparable between each transfection (A574 /μg protein; 0.462 in YA5 versus 0.470 in YA10). The findings that pIL-5Luc was effectively transcribed by IL-5-producing clones, but not by non-IL-5-producing clones, suggest that transcriptional control is also important in IL-5 synthesis, as well as in IL-2 synthesis. Those cells unable to transcribe pIL-5Luc may lack some transcription factors (tentatively NF-IL-5) expressed in IL-5-producing T cell clones, or may express some repressor factors that actively interfere with IL-5 gene transcription.

IL-2 stimulation resulted in a 7-fold increase in the induction of luciferase activity compared to that in unstimulated cells. β-Galactosidase activity derived from pCMV—gal did not differ significantly between stimulated and unstimulated T cell clones, clearly indicating that IL-2 induced gene transcription and protein synthesis of IL-5 by human helper T cells, and the 515 bp promoter/enhancer segment was sufficiently responsive to IL-2 stimulation in human T cells.

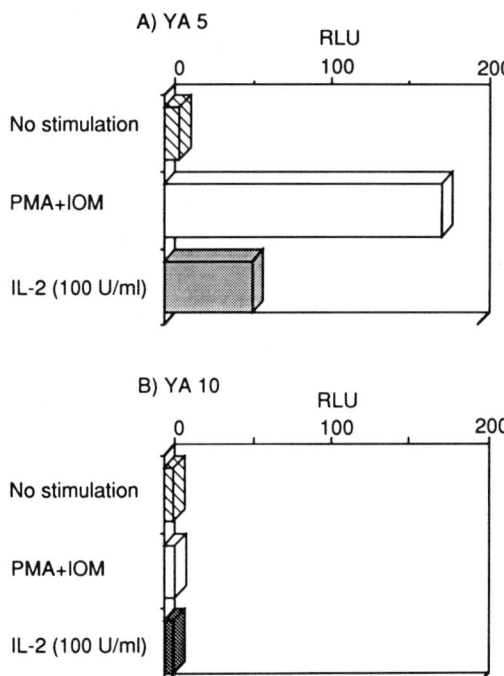

Figure 6. Analysis of IL-5 promoter activity in T cell clones stimulated with PMA plus IOM or IL-2. IL-5-producing (YA5) and non-producing (YA10) T cell clones were transiently transfected with pIL-5Luc (50 μg) + pCMV-β-gal (10 μg), and then stimulated with PMA (20 nM) and IOM (1 μM) or human recombinant IL-2 (100 U/ml). After 24 hours, cell lysates were prepared and tested for luciferase and β-galactosidase activity.

4.2. IL-5 Promoter Activity in IL-5 Gene-Expressing and Non-Expressing-Transformed T Cell Lines

In order to analyze human IL-5 promoter more extensively, T cell clones YA5 and YA10 were fused with human a transformed T cell line (BUC). IL-5 mRNA was clearly induced upon stimulation with PMA plus IOM in the resulting hybridoma, S-1 cells derived from YA5 clone, but not in S-4 cells derived from YA10, BUC or Jurkat cells. An approximately 250-fold increase in luciferase activity was induced in S-1 cells transfected with pIL-5Luc when stimulated with PMA plus IOM (Figure 7). In contrast, S-4 cells or BUC cells showed only a 30-fold increase, which was comparable to that observed when S-1, S-4 or BUC cells were transfected with pGL2 basic vector which contained no promoter segments. Jurkat cells, known to produce IL-2 and IL-4 but not IL-5 upon stimulation, did not induce any luciferase activity upon stimulation when transfected with pIL-5Luc. Nonetheless, Jurkat cells did transcribe pIL-2Luc which contained human IL-2 promoter (-480 to +2) upon PMA plus IOM or immobilized anti-CD3 plus soluble anti-CD28 stimulation. The findings that the gene transcription mediated by the 500 bp human IL-5 promoter/enhancer segment was only initiated in IL-5-gene-expressing hybridomas when stimulated with PMA plus IOM, and not in non-IL-5-gene-expressing hybridomas or Jurkat cells, well reflect the transcriptional regulation observed in T cell clones.

EMSA (electrophoretic mobility shift analysis) revealed that nuclear factors, NF-AT, AP-1 and NF-kB, were actually induced and Oct-1 was constitutively expressed in both IL-5 gene-expressing and non-expressing T cells, further implicating the possible involvement of NF-IL-5 in IL-5 gene transcription.

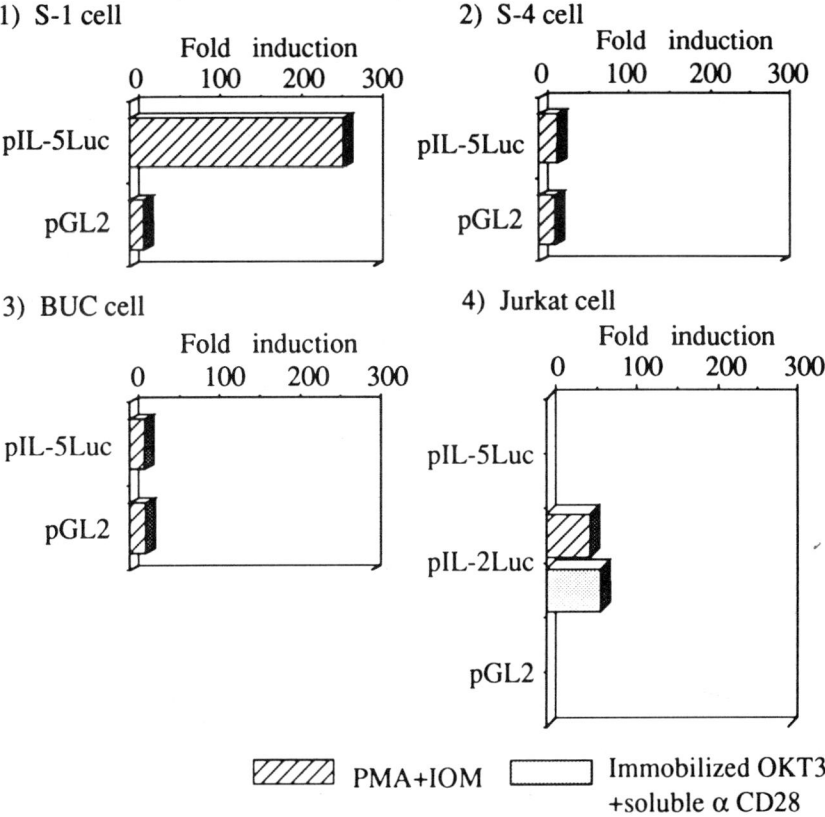

Figure 7. Analysis of IL-5 and IL-2 promoter activity in T cell hybridomas, BUC and Jurkat cells stimulated with PMA plus IOM. IL-5 gene-expressing (S-1) and non-expressing (S-4) T cell hybridomas, BUC cells and Jurkat cells were transiently transfected with pIL-5Luc or pIL-2Luc, and then stimulated with PMA (20 nM) and IOM (1 μM). Jurkat cells were also stimulated with immobilized OKT3 (10 μg/ml) plus soluble anti-CD28 antibody (1 μg/ml). After 24 hours, cell lysates were prepared and tested for luciferase and β-galactosidase activity.

4.3. IL-5 Gene Transcription Can Be Regulated Independently from Il-2 and Il-4

FK506 and CsA exert immunosuppressive effects through binding to their respective cellular ligands, FK-binding protein (FKBP) and cyclophilin.[33] FK506-FKBP complex and CsA-cyclophilin complex inhibit the Ca^{2+}-calmodulin-dependent phosphatase, calcineurin, which is essential for a T cell-specific transcription factor, nuclear factor of activated T cells (NF-AT), which undergoes translocation into the nucleus for the initiation of IL-2 gene transcription. [34] On the other hand, GCs and their receptor form a complex which competitively inhibits the activity of another transcription factor, activating protein-1 (AP-1), to bind to the enhancer element (TPA responsive element: TRE) of cytokine genes.[35, 36] Both AP-1 and NF-AT play critical roles in IL-2 gene transcription.[35] Our previous findings that GCs, FK506 and CsA suppressed human IL-5 production and gene expression suggest the importance of AP-1 and NF-AT in IL-5 gene transcription.

GCs possess a wide range of pharmacological actions not only on immune systems but also on various other tissues and organs.[37] FK506 and CsA have a more restricted target speci-

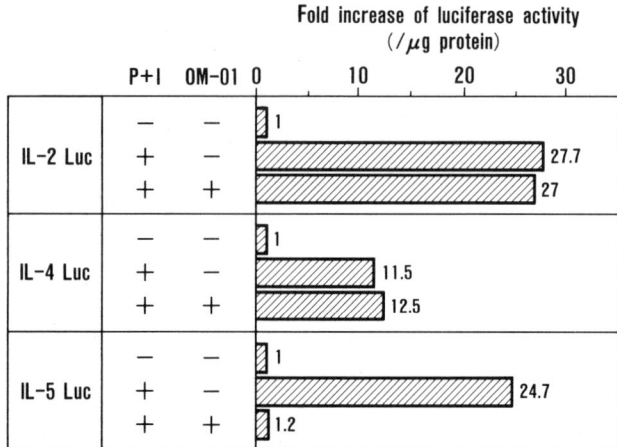

Figure 8. Selective regulation of human IL-5 gene transcription. 5·10⁶ cells of IL-5 gene-expressing hybridoma (S-1) were transiently tranfected with 10 μg of either pIL-5Luc, pIL-2Luc, or pIL-4Luc, followed by PMA + IOM stimulation. Compound OM-01 was included in the culture from the beginning. After 24 hours, cells were harvested and lysates were assayed for luciferase activity.

ficity compared to GCs, but still interfere with too many functions of T cells, thereby causing general immune suppression. The findings described above suggest that an agent capable of interfering with NF-IL-5 activity could selectively suppress IL-5 production without affecting IL-2 or IL-4 production. Such agents would be an ideal therapeutic modality to ameliorate eosinophilic inflammation, without general immune suppression.

We have found such a substance (OM-01) that suppressed IL-5 synthesis of T cells without any effects on IL-2 and IL-4 synthesis. OM-01 inhibited IL-5 gene expression and also suppressed the induction of luciferase activity mediated by the approximately 2 kb human IL-5 promoter/enhancer gene segment (Figure 8). On the other hand, neither IL-2 nor IL-4 promoter/enhancer activity was affected. The results clearly indicate that the gene transcription of IL-5 can be regulated differentially from IL-2 or IL-4, and further implicate the existence of a distinct transcription factor (NF-IL-5) that is required for IL-5 gene transcription. OM-01 administered in vivo inhibited the late phase recruitment of eosinophils into the bronchial mucosa in murine experimental asthma. We might expect that the agent can open up a new era for a therapeutic strategy of specific gene transcription inhibition to manage human disorders.

5. CONCLUDING REMARKS

We have investigated IL-5 production by CD4⁺ T lymphocytes of asthmatic patients and obtained the following findings:

1. IL-5 production by CD4⁺ T cells from atopic and non-atopic asthmatics was significantly enhanced compared to that from control subjects. IL-2, IL-3, IL-4, GM-CSF and IFN-γ production were not significantly different among the three groups.
2. FK506, CsA and dexamethasone inhibited IL-5 production by activated T cells in a dose-dependent mannor. FK506 reduced IL-5 mRNA level in activated T cells.

3. Topical application of FK506 in patients with severe atopic dermatitis resulted in marked amelioration accompanied by a clear reduction of IL-5 production by CD4$^+$ T cells.

4. IL-5 production by activated human CD4$^+$ T cells is dependent on IL-2.

5. IL-2 induced gene transcription, gene expression and protein synthesis of IL-5 by human CD4$^+$ T cell clones.

6. The 515 bp segment of human IL-5 promoter/enhancer (-511 to +4 relative to the transcription initiation site) confers tissue-specific and activation- dependent gene transcription.

7. Transcriptional control regulates IL-5 production by human CD4$^+$ T cells.

8. Transcription factor(s) other than NF-AT, AP-1 and NF-kB may be essential for human IL-5 gene transcription.

9. IL-5 gene transcription may be differentially regulated from IL-2 and IL-4 gene transcription.

10. OM-01, a specific IL-5 gene transcription inhibitor, offers a potential new therapeutic modality for allergic diseases.

REFERENCES

1. Azzawi, M., Bradley, B., Jeffery, P. K., Frew, A. J., Wardlaw, A. J., Knowles, G., Assoufi, B., Collins, J. V., Durham, S., and Kay, A. B. 1990. Identification of activated T lymphocytes and eosinophils in bronchial biopsies in stable atopic asthma. *Am. Rev. Respir. Dis.* 142:1410.

2. Dunnill, M. S. 1960. The pathology of asthma with special reference to changes in the bronchial mucosa. *J. Clin. Pathol.* 13:27.

3. Wardlaw, A. J., Dunnette, S., Gleich, G. J., Collins, J. V., and Kay, A. B. 1988. Eosinophils and mast cells in bronchoalveolar lavage in mild asthma: relationship to bronchial hyperreactivity. *Am. Rev. Respir. Dis.* 137:62.

4. Gleich, G. J., and Adolphson, C. R. 1986. The eosinophilic leukocyte: structure and function. *Adv. Immunol.* 39:177.

5. Jeffery, P. K., Wardlaw, A. J., Nelson, F. C., Collins, J. V., and Kay, A. B. 1989. Bronchial biopsies in asthma: an ultrastructural, quantitative study and correlation with hyperreactivity. *Am. Rev. Respir. Dis.* 140:1745.

6. Kay, A. B. 1992. "Helper" (CD4) T cells and eosinophils in allergy and asthma. *Am. Rev. Respir. Dis.* 145:S22.

7. Kirby, J. G., Hargreave, F. E., Gleich, G. J., and O'Byrne, P. M. 1987. Bronchoalveolar cell profiles of asthmatic and non-asthmatic subjects. *Am. Rev. Respir. Dis.* 136:379.

8. Dohi, M., Okudaira, H., Sugiyama, H., Tsuramachi, K., Suko, M., Nakagawa, H., and Miyamoto, T. 1990. Bronchial responsiveness to mite allergen in atopic dermatitis without asthma. *Int. Arch. Allergy Appl. Immunol.* 92:138.

9. Coffman, R. L., Seymour, B. W., Hudak, S., Jackson, J., and Rennick, D. 1989. Antibody to interleukin-5 inhibits helminth-induced eosinophilia in mice. *Science* 245:308.

10. De Monchy, J. G., Kauffman, H. F., Venge, P., Koeter, G. H., Jansen, H. M., Sluiter, H. J., and De Vries, K. 1985. Broncho-alveolar eosinophilia during allergen-induced late asthmatic reactions. *Am. Rev. Respir. Dis.* 131:373.

11. Durham, S. R., and Kay, A. B. 1985. Eosinophils, bronchial hyperreactivity and late asthmatic reactions. *Clin. Allergy* 40:411.

12. Hamid, Q., Azzawi, M., Sun Ying Moqbel, R., Wardlaw, A. J., Corrigan, C. J., Bradley, B., Durham, S. R., Collins, J. V., Jeffery, P. K., Quint, J., and Kay, A. B. 1991. Expression of mRNA for interleukin-5 in mucosal bronchial biopsies from asthma. *J. Clin. Invest.* 87:1541.

13. Kaliner, M. 1984. Hypotheses on the contribution of late-phase allergic responses to the understanding and treatment of allergic diseases. *J. Allergy Clin. Immunol.* 73:311.

14. Okudaira, H., Nogami, M., Matsuzaki, G., Dohi, M., Suko, M., Kasuya, S., and Takatsu, K. 1991. T-cell-dependent accumulation of eosinophils in the lung and its inhibition by monoclonal anti-interleukin-5. *Int. Arch. Allergy Appl. Immunol.* 94:171.

15. Nogami, M., Suko, M., Okudaira, H., Miyamoto, T., Shiga, J., Ito, M., and Kasuya, S. 1990. Experimental pulmonary eosinophilia in mice by ascaris suum extract. *Am. Rev. Respir. Dis.* 141:1289.

16. Corrigan, C. T., and Kay, A. B. 1992. T cells and eosinophils in the pathogenesis of asthma. *Immunol. Today* 13:501.

17. Walker, C., Bode, E., Boer, L., Hansel, T. T., Blaser, K. and Virchow, J. C. 1992. Allergic and non-allergic asthmatics have distinct patterns of T cell activation and cytokine production in peripheral blood and bronchoalveolar lavage. *Am. Rev. Respir. Dis.* 146:109.

18. Corrigan, C. J., Haczku, A., Gemou-Engesaeth, V., Doi, S., Kikuchi, Y., Takatsu, K., Durham, S. R., and Kay, A. B. 1993. CD4 T-lymphocyte activation in asthma is accompanied by increased serum concentrations of interleukin-5. Effect of glucocorticoid therapy. *Am. Rev. Respir. Dis.* 147:540.

19. Robinson, D., Hamid, Q., Bentley, A., Ying, S., Kay, A. B., and Kurham, S. R. 1993. Activation of CD4+ T cells, increased Th2-type cytokine mRNA expression, and eosinophil recruitment in bronchoalveolar lavage after allergen inhalation challenge in patients with atopic asthma. *J. Allergy Clin. Immunol.* 92:313.

20. Huang, S. K., Krishnaswamy, G., Suz, S. N., Marsh, D. G., and Liu, M. 1993. Analysis of cytokine transcripts in the broncho-alveolar lavage cells of patients with asthma. *J. Immunol.* 150:138A. (AAI meeting, Abstr.)

21. Kay, A. B., Ying, S., Varney, V., Gaga, M., Durham, S. R., Moqbel, R., Wardlaw, A. J., Hamid, Q. 1991. Messenger RNA expression of the cytokine gene cluster, interleukin 3 (IL-3), IL-4, IL-5 and granulocyte/macrophage colony-stimulating factor, in allergen-induced late-phase cutaneous reactions in atopic subjects. *J. Exp. Med.* 173:775–778.

22. Mori, A., Suko, M., Nishizaki, Y., Kaminuma, O., Kobayashi, S., Matsuzaki, G., Yamamoto, K., Ito, K., Tsuruoka, N., and Okudaira, H. 1995. Interleukin-5 production by CD4+ T cells of asthmatic patients is suppressed by glucocorticoids and the immunosuppressants FK506 and cyclosporin A. *Int. Immmol.* 7:449.

23. Okudaira, H., Mori, A., Suko, M., Etoh, T., Nakagawa, H., and Ito. K., 1994. Enhanced production and gene expression of IL-5 in bronchial asthma - management of atopic diseases with agents that down regulate IL-5 gene transcription. *ACI News* 6:19

24. Mori, A., M. Suko, N. Tsuruoka, T. Etoh, H. Nakagawa, O. Kaminuma, K. Ito, and H. Okudaira. 1994. Atopic diseases and eosinophilic inflammation - Possible management with downregulation of IL-5 gene transcription. *Environ. Dermatol.* 1:42.

25. Steel, C., and Nutman, T. B. 1993. Regulation of IL-5 in onchocerciasis - a critical role for IL-2. *J. Immunol.* 150:5511.

26. Minami, Y., Kono, T., Miyazaaki, T., and Taniguti, T. 1993. The IL-2 receptor complex: Its structure, function, and target gene. *Annu. Rev. Immunol.* 11:245

27. Robinson, D. S., Ying, S., Bentley, A. M., Meng, Q., North, J., Durham, S. R., Kay, A. B. and Hamid, Q. 1993. Relationships among number of bronchoalveolar lavage cells expressing messenger ribonucleic acid for cytokines, asthma symptoms, and airway methacholine responsiveness in atopic asthma. *J. Allergy Clin. Immunol.* 92:397.

28. Robinson, D., Hamid, Q., Bentley, A., Ying, S., Kay, A. B., Durham, S. R., 1993. Activation of CD4+ T cells, increased Th2-type cytokine mRNA expression, and eosinophil recruitment in bronchoalveolar lavage after allergen inhalation challenge in patients with atopic asthma. *J. Allergy Clin. Immunol.* 92:313.

29. Robinson D. S, Hamid Q., Ying S., Tsicopoulos A., Barkans J., Bentley A. M., Corrigen C., Durham S. R., Kay A. B.: Predominant Th2-like bronchoalveolar T-lymphocyte population in atopic asthma. *N Engl J Med* 1992;326:298–304.

30. Broide, D. H., Lots, M., Cuomo, A. J., Coburn, D. A., Federman, E.C., and Wasserman, S. I. 1992. Cytokines in symptomatic asthma airways. *J. Allergy Clin. Immunol.* 89:958.

31. Crabtree, G. R. 1989. Contingent genetic regulatory events in T lymphocyte activation. *Science.* 243:355.

32. Durand, D. B., Morgan, M. R., Weiss, A., Crabtree. G. R., 1987. A 257 basepair fragment at the 5' end of the interleukin 2 gene enhances expression from a heterologous promotor in response to signals from the T cell antigen receptor. *J. Exp. Med.* 165:359.

33. Sigal, N. H., and Dumont, F. J. 1992. Cyclosporin A, FK506 and rapamycin: pharmacologic probes of lymphocyte signal transduction. *Annu. Rev. Immunol.* 10:519.

34. Schreiber, S. L., and Crabtree, G. R. 1992. The mechanism of action of cyclosporin A and FK506. *Immunol. Today* 13:136

35. Vacca, A., Felli, M. P., Farina, A. R., Martinotti, S., Maroder, M., Screpanti, I., Meco, D., Petrangeli, E., Frati, L., and Gulino, A. 1992. Glucocorticoid receptor-mediated suppression of the interleukin 2 gene expression through impairment of the cooperativity between nuclear factor of activated T cells and AP-1 enhancer elements. *J. Exp. Med.* 175:637.

36. Weinberger, C., Hollenberg, S. M., Ong, E. S., Harmon, J. M., and Brower, S. T., Cidlowski, J., Thompson, E. B., Rosenfeld, N. G., and Evans, R. H. 1985. Identification of human glucocorticoid receptor complementary DNA clones by epitope selection. *Science* 228:740.

65

PEPTIDE MEDIATED REGULATION OF ALLERGEN SPECIFIC IMMUNE RESPONSES

Jonathan R. Lamb[1,2] and Robyn E. O'Hehir[2]

[1]Infection and Immunity Section
Department of Biology and
[2]Department of Immunology
Imperial College of Science,Technology & Medicine
Prince Consort Road
London, United Kingdom SW7 2BB

1. INTRODUCTION

The exposure of susceptible individuals to environmental allergens induces enhanced levels of specific IgE antibodies, which bind to high affinity receptors on mast cells and basophils. Cross linking of receptor-bound IgE occurs, mediators are released and the immediate allergic reactions develop. Increased vascular permeability and the production of cytokines and chemokines cause polymorphonuclear granulocytes and lymphocytes to migrate into the site of allergic reactions and the late phase reaction is established. This illustrates that the cellular and cytokine networks activated in the pathogenesis of allergic inflammation are complex and involve many different cell types. However, the regulation of allergic immune responses in atopic individuals is mediated by cytokines characteristic of the Th2 functional phenotype (IL-4, IL-5, IL-10 and IL-13).[1-5] In non-atopic individuals Th1 cells, which produce IL-2 and IFN-γ, but not IL-4 or IL-5, are activated and regulate immune responses to allergens.[6,7] However, from clonal analysis it is evident that Th0 cells, which have the potential to produce both Th1 and Th2 cytokines, form a major component of the allergen specific repertoire in atopic individuals. Therefore, the ability to modify qualitative aspects of immune responses to allergens in atopic individuals by inhibiting the release of Th2 cytokines, and/or promoting the production of Th1 cytokines may alter the clinical phenotype of some patients. The approach of immunotherapy mediated by peptides and designed to target allergen reactive CD4+ T cells are discussed in this report.

New Horizons in Allergy Immunotherapy
edited by Sehon et al. Plenum Press, New York, 1996

451

2. RESULTS AND DISCUSSION

2.1. Competitor Peptides

Although individual MHC class II molecules may bind many antigenic peptides,[8–10] the potential of peptides with high affinity for a particular MHC class II molecule to inhibit *in vivo* T cell responses restricted by that MHC allele has been considered for immunotherapy. The rationale for this approach is based on evidence for linkage between certain HLA haplotypes and specific diseases and, the observation that T cell function *in vivo* and *in vitro* can be inhibited through competition for antigen presentation.[11–14] In terms of the therapeutic potential it has been demonstrated that non-immunogenic, non-self peptides administered at high doses are able to prevent experimental autoimmune encephalomyelitis (EAE) in a rodent model of multiple sclerosis induced by immunisation with myelin basic protein.[13,14] Applying this strategy to allergy requires identification of MHC class II molecules associated with allergen specific responsiveness and the T cell epitopes involved in the initiation of the allergic response. For house dust mite (HDM) specific responses genetic epidemiological studies have failed to demonstrate a MHC class II disease association and analysis of T cell recognition has emphasized the heterogeneity of HLA class II gene usage (HLA-DR, -DQ and -DP) in the presentation of HDM derived peptides.[15,16] However, it was observed that a non-immunogenic peptide analogue derived from the carboxyl terminus of influenza virus haemagglutinin (HA; residues 306–318), in which tyrosine had been replaced with serine at position 308, inhibited the proliferative response of HDM reactive human CD4+ T cells.[17] The mode of action of the peptide was at the level of peptide binding to MHC class II molecules and inhibited, both DRB1 and DRB3 gene product restricted T cell recognition of HDM derived allergens. To date no information is available on the ability of competitive peptides to inhibit *in vivo* T cell responses to HDM in experimental models. However, as discussed above, there is heterogeneity in the HLA class II restriction specificity of T cell responses to HDM allergens both between individuals and within the same individual. For example, T cell clones specific for the same epitope (*Der p* II, residues 22–40) and restricted by either -DQ or -DR class II molecules have been isolated from the peripheral blood of the same subject.[16] Therefore, competitive inhibition may not be the most viable method with which to regulate HDM specific responses *in vivo*.

2.2. Allergen-Derived Peptides

From analysis of the response of polyclonal and monoclonal T cell populations epitope maps of *Der p* I and *p* II have been constructed and demonstrate that multiple epitopes are located through the entire sequence of both proteins, with the pattern of reactivity and magnitude of responsiveness of each individual being determined by the HLA class II phenotype and level of allergen exposure. At face value the diversity in antigen specificity would argue against the use of peptides as a potential means of immunotherapy for HDM induced atopic disease. However, on repeated screening over a period of over two years it was noted that the pattern of epitope recognition remained constant for a particular individual,[16] unlike T cell responses to autoantigens where the phenomenon of determinant spreading has been observed.[18] The lack of plasticity in T cell recognition of HDM derived allergens is also reflected in the analysis of the human T cell repertoire, which has revealed a bias both in the TcR-Vα and -Vβ gene segment usage, as well as the existence *in vivo* of long-lived T cell clones.[19] Therefore, theoretically the ability to inactivate or physically eliminate selected clones of allergen reactive T cells may alter the clinical phenotype of some patients. This prompted us to develop an *in vitro* model using human T cells with which to investigate the immunological basis of peptide-mediated T cell desensitisation.

CD4+ T cells, irrespective of their HLA class II restriction specificity, when exposed to supraoptimal concentrations of HDM peptides, in the presence or absence of APCs, become refractory to rechallenge with their specific ligand and fail to proliferate or provide B cell help, even though their responsiveness to IL-2 is enhanced.[15] The loss of functional activity is accompanied by complex phenotypic changes and, in general, these parallel those observed during activation.[20] After exposure to peptide there is downregulation of the TcR/CD3 complex and concomitant upregulation of both CD2, CD25 and adhesion molecules, such as LFA-1. In contrast, while the levels of CD28, the co-stimulatory receptor, are upregulated during T cell activation, the induction of anergy results in the loss of membrane expression and rapid decay of CD28 specific mRNA.[21] Furthermore, it has been reported that CD4 may form a structural component of the TcR complex[22] and we have observed for some but not all T cells that CD4 is comodulated with the TcR.

The restoration of anergic phenotype to that of untreated T cells is not accompanied by recovery of function and this finding implies that anergy does not arise merely as a result of receptor modulation. It appears that the immunological basis of the loss of antigen induced responsiveness is mediated by the dysregulation of cytokine production.[20,23] During the induction phase of anergy cytokine specific mRNA levels are enhanced,[24] although this is not necessarily reflected in the levels of soluble product and is well illustrated by the comparison of IL-8 mRNA levels and soluble protein during activation and anergy induction. However, when the anergic T cells are restimulated with their natural ligand they fail to secrete IL-4 and IL-5, although IFN-γ production remains unaltered.[20] This change in the functional phenotype from the Th2 to the Th1 pathway would favour a reduction in allergen specific IgE, based on the premise that IL-4 and IFN-γ have antagonistic effects on IgE synthesis.[25]

In order to determine if peptides can modulate the function of HDM specific T cells *in vivo*, T cell recognition of *Der p* I was investigated in H-2[b] mice.[26] Intranasal delivery of peptide was chosen as the route of administration in view of its potential clinical application. Following the inhalation of peptide containing a major T cell epitope of *Der p* I (residues 111–139) inhibition of responses to both peptide and intact *Der p* I was observed when the T cells were restimulated with antigen *in vitro*. In addition to their ability to proliferate only weakly to antigen, T cells isolated from the tolerant mice produced low levels of IL-2, IL-4 and IFN-γ and failed to provide cognate help for the production of *Der p* I specific antibodies. Although resulting in the induction of antigen specific non-responsiveness, the intranasal administration of peptides induces a marked but transient T cell activation that is observed in the draining lymph nodes at 2 days and, which then spreads parenterally to the spleen. However, despite T cell activation and the production of cytokines the intranasal delivery of peptides fails to elicit effector immune responses, in that not only low levels of peptide specific IgM, but of IgG1 or IgG2a are induced. In a murine model of the response to *Fel d* I it has been reported that the subcutaneous administration of a dominant peptide diminished the production of IL-2, IL-4 and IFN-γ, suggesting that Th1 and Th2 cells were being tolerised.[27]

Environmental exposure to HDM leads to the induction of chronic inflammatory responses, therefore, potential therapeutics in the treatment of HDM allergy must be effective in the downregulation of established immune responses. In order to test this activity mice were primed with *Der p* I to the intranasal administration of peptide. The results of these experiments demonstrated that both ongoing and long-term immune responses to HDM derived allergens could be inhibited, establishing that peptide mediated immunotherapy is effective in the regulation of chronic immune responses.[26]

2.3. TcR-Vβ Derived Peptides

In rodent models of EAE it has been demonstrated that the encephalitogenic T cells, namely those capable of transferring the disease, express predominantly TcR-Vβ8.2 genes. Immunisation with a synthetic peptide corresponding to the CDR2 sequence of TcR-Vβ8.2 was able to modulate MBP specific responses and both prevent the onset and reverse ongoing disease.[28–30] Detailed analysis of TcR gene usage by the HDM reactive T cell repertoire demonstrated for an atopic individual that TcR-Vβ3 gene elements may form a major component of the T cell repertoire.[19] Based on these observations we investigated the ability of a peptide derived from the CDR2 region of the TcR-Vb3 gene segment to modulate HDM induced T cell responses. The results of these experiments established that the TcR peptide inhibited polyclonal T cell responses of both atopic and non-atopic donors to HDM, and that this effect was specific because it required the presence of Vb3+ T cells.[31] Depletion of CD8+ T cells abolished peptide mediated inhibition of CD4+ T cell proliferation to HDM, suggesting that a regulatory subset of CD8+ cells are induced by the CDR2 peptide. Furthermore, it appears that these cells mediate their regulatory effects through the production of TGF-β1.

3. CONCLUDING COMMENTS

There is accumulating evidence from clinical trials that successful desensitisation of allergic individuals is accompanied by a reduction in the IL-4 to IFN-γ ratio. Whether this results from either tolerising Th2 cells, inducing T cells of the Th1 functional phenotype or a combination of both remains to be clarified. Although both human and murine Th2 cells can be tolerised *in vitro* evidence to support that this can achieved *in vivo* is divided. However, peptides can be administered *in vivo* under conditions that downregulate antigen-dependent cytokine production, including IL-4 when rechallenged with antigen. The induction of non-responsiveness appears not to be a failure to activate T cells, since transient activation and cytokine production precedes the development of anergy. If this occurs during desensitisation it is unclear what the clinical effects would be. On the subject of peptide-mediated non-responsiveness it is worth emphasising that tolerance to intact allergenic proteins may be induced by the administration of a single peptide, which has the advantage that T cell epitopes distinct from antibody binding sites may be selected for therapy.

Perhaps rather than needing to induce anergy in the Th2 population all that is required for successful immunotherapy is to induce the production of Th1 cytokines. It is documented that immunisation with proteins whose physicochemical structure has been modified may selectively induce Th1 type responses.[32] Likewise, stimulating T cell clones with peptides in which the TcR contact residues have been substituted can dissociate the effector function.[33] Whether or not ligands such as these can mediate the same effects *in vivo* has not been tested but if they can they offer considerable opportunities for immunotherapy.

4. ACKNOWLEDGMENTS

This work was funded by grants from the Wellcome Trust and Medical Research Council. Robyn O'Hehir is the recipient of a Wellcome Senior Clinical Fellowship.

5. REFERENCES

1. Wierenga, E. A., Snoek, M., de Groot, C., Chretien, I., Bos,. J. D., Jansen, H. M. and Kapsenberg, M. L. Evidence for compartmentalisation of functional subsets of CD4+ T lymphocytes in atopic patients. *J. Immunol.*, 144, 4651, 1990.

2. Parronchi, P., Macchia, D., Piccini, M-P., Biswas, P., Simonelli, C., Maggi, E., Ricci, M., Ansari, A. and Romagnani, S. Allergen and bacterial antigen specific T cell clones established from atopic donors show a different production profile of cytokine production. *Proc. Natl. Acad. Sci. USA.*, 88, 4538, 1991.

3. Yssel, H., Johnson, K. E., Schneider, P. V., Wideman, J., Terr, A., Kastelein, R. and de Vries, J. E. T cell activation inducing epitopes of the house dust mite allergen *Der p* I. Induction of a restricted cytokine profile of *Der p* I specific T cell clones upon antigen specific activation. *J. Immunol.*, 148, 738, 1992.

4. Varney, V. A., Hamid, Q. A., Gaga, M., Ying, S., Jacobson, M., Frew, A. J., Kay, A. B. and Durham S. R. Influence of grass pollen immunotherapy on cellular infiltration and cytokine mRNA expression during allergen induced late phase cutaneous responses. *J. Clin. Invest.*, 92, 644, 1993.

5. Punnonen, J. and de Vries, J. E. IL-13 induces proliferation, Ig isotype switching and Ig synthesis by immature human foetal B cells. *J. Immunol.*, 152, 1094, 1994.

6. Halvorsen, R., Bosnes, V. and Thorsby, E. T cell responses to *Dermatophagoides farinae* allergen preparations in allergics and healthy controls. *Int. Arch. Allergy Appl. Immunol.*, 80, 62, 1986.

7. O'Hehir, R. E., Garman, R. D., Greenstein, J. L. and Lamb, J. R. The specificity and regulation of T cell responsiveness to allergen. *Ann. Rev. Immunol.*, 9, 76, 1991.

8. Babbitt, B. P., Matsueda, G., Haber, E., Unanue, E. R. and Allen, P. M. Antigenic competition at the level of Ia binding. *Proc. Natl. Acad. Sci. USA.*, 83, 4509, 1986.

9. Buus, S., Sette, A., Colon, S. M., Miles, C. and Grey, H. M. The relation between major histocompatibility complex (MHC) restriction and the capacity of Ia to bind immunogenic peptides. *Science*, 235, 1353, 1991.

10. Rudensky, A. Y., Preston-Hulburt, P., Hong S-C., Barlow, A. and Janeway, J. A. Sequence analysis of peptides bound to MHC class II molecules. *Nature*, 353, 622, 1991.

11. Werdelin, O. Chemically related antigens compete for presentation by accessory cells to T cells. *J. Immunol.*, 129, 1883, 1982.

12. Adorini, L., Muller, S., Cardinaux, F., Lehmann, P. V., Falcioni, F. and Nagy, Z. A. *In vivo* competition between self peptides and foreign antigens in T cell activation. *Nature*, 334, 623, 1988.

13. Lamont, A. G., Sette, A., Fujinami, R., Colon, S. M. Miles, C. and Grey, H. M. Inhibition of experimental autoimmune encephalomyelitis induction in SJL/J mice by using a peptide with high affinity for IA^s molecules. *J. Immunol.*, 145, 1687, 1990.

14. Wraith, D. C., Smilek D. E., Mitchell, D. J., Steinman, L. and McDevitt, H. O. Antigen recognition in autoimmune encephalomyelitis and the potential for peptide mediated immunotherapy. *Cell*, 59, 247, 1989.

15. Higgins, J. A., Lamb, J. R., Hayball, J. D., Marsh, S., Tonks, S., Rosen-Bronson, S., Bodmer, J. A. & O'Hehir, R. E. Peptide-induced non-responsiveness of HLA-DP restricted human T cells with *Dermatophagoides* spp. (house dust mite). *J. Aller. Clin. Immunol.*, 90, 749, 1992.

16. Verhoef, A., Higgins, J. A., Thorpe, C., Marsh, S. G. E., Hayball, J. D., Lamb, J. R. and O'Hehir, R. E. Clonal analysis of the atopic immune response to the group 2 allergen of *Dermatophagoides* spp: identification of HLA-DR and -DQ restricted T cell epitopes. *Int. Immunol.*, 5, 1589, 1993.

17. O'Hehir, R. E., Busch, R., Rothbard, J. B. and Lamb, J. R. An *in vitro* model of peptide-mediated immunomodulation of the human T cell response to *Dermatophagoides* spp. (house dust mite). *J. Aller. Clin. Immunol.*, 87, 1120, 1991.

18. Lehmann, P. V., Forsthuber, T., Miller, A., Sercarz, E. E. Spreading of T cell autoimmunity to cryptic determinants to an autoantigen. *Nature*, 358, 155, 1992.

19. Wedderburn, L. R., O'Hehir, R. E., Hewitt, C. R. A., Lamb, J. R. and Owen, M. J. *In vivo* clonal dominance and limited T cell receptor usage in human CD4+ T cell recognition of house dust mite allergens. *Proc. Natl. Acad. Sci. USA.*, 90, 8214, 1993.

20. O'Hehir, R. E., Yssel, H., Verma, S., de Vries, J. E., Spits, H. and Lamb, J. R. Clonal analysis of differential lymphokine production in peptide and superantigen induced T cell anergy. *Int. Immunol.*, 3, 819, 1991.

21. Lake, R. A., O'Hehir, R. E., Verhoef, A. and Lamb, J. R. CD28 mRNA rapidly decays when activated T cells are functionally anergised with specific peptide. *Int. Immunol.*, 5, 461, 1993.

22. Dianzani U., Shaw, A., Al-Ramadi, B. K., Kubo, R. T. and Janeway, C. A. Physical association of CD4 with the T cell receptor. *J. Immunol.*, 148, 678, 1992.

23. Yssel, H., Fasler, S., Lamb J. R. and de Vries, J. E. Induction of non-responsiveness in human allergen specific Th2 cells. *Curr. Opin. Immunol.*, 6, 847, 1994.

24. Schall, T. J., O'Hehir, R. E., Goeddel, D. V. and Lamb, J.R. Uncoupling of cytokine mRNA expression and protein secretion during the induction phase of T cell anergy. *J. Immunol.*, 148, 381, 1992.

25. Snapper, C. M. and Paul, W. E., Interferon-g and B cell stimulatory factor-1 reciprocally regulate Ig isotype production. *Science*, 236, 944, 1987.

26. Hoyne, G., O'Hehir, R. E., Wraith, D. G., Thomas, W. R. and Lamb, J. R. Inhibition of T cell and antibody responses to house dust mite allergen by inhalation of the dominant T cell epitope in naive and sensitised mice. *J. Exp. Med.*,178, 1783, 1993.

27. Briner, T. J., Kuo, M-C., Rogers, B. R., Keeting, K., Fleishell, M. L., O'Brien, M. M., Bollinger, B. K., Craig, S. and Greenstein, J. L. Inhibition of allergen-specific murine T cell responses after subcutaneous injection of T cell epitope-containing peptide. *Proc. Natl. Acad. Sci. USA*, 90, 7608, 1993.

28. Vandenbark, A. A., Hashim, G. A. and Offner, H. Immunisation with a synthetic T cell receptor V-region peptide protects against experimental autoimmune encephalomyelitis. *Nature*, 341, 541, 1989.

29. Gaur, A., Haspel, R., Mayer, J. P. and Fathman, C. G. Requirement for CD8+ cells in T cell receptor peptide induced clonal unresponsiveness. *Science*, 259, 91, 1993.

30. Offner, H., Hashim, G. A. and Vandenbark, A. A. T cell receptor peptide therapy triggers autoregulation of experimental encephalomyelitis. *Science*, 251, 430, 1991.

31. Jarman, E. R., Hawrylowicz, C. M., Panagiotopolou, E., O'Hehir, E. R. and Lamb, J. R. Inhibition of human T cell responses to house dust mite allergens by a T cell receptor peptide. *J. Allergy Clin. Immunol.*, 94, 844, 1994.

32. HayGlass, K. T. and Stefura, W. P. Anti-interferon-γ treatment blocks the ability of glutaraldehyde polymerised allergens to inhibit specific IgE responses. *J. Exp. Med.*, 173, 279, 1991.

33. Evavold B. D., Sloan-Lancaster J. and Allen P. M. Tickling the TCR: selective T-cell functions stimulated by altered peptide ligand. *Immunol. Today*,14, 602, 1993.

66

CLINICAL EXPERIENCE WITH TREATMENT OF ALLERGIES WITH T CELL EPITOPE CONTAINING PEPTIDES

Philip S. Norman[*]

Johns Hopkins Asthma and Allergy Center
Johns Hopkins University School of Medicine
Baltimore, Maryland 21224

1. STANDARD IMMUNOTHERAPY

Immunotherapy by repeated subcutaneous injections of increasing doses of crude extracts of allergens redirects allergic immunologic responses. At first IgE antibodies increase but then they decline slowly. Serum IgG antibodies rise markedly, and secretory antibodies increase modestly. Serum IgG and secretory IgA and IgG antibodies can block in vitro antigen stimulated mediator release by IgE antibody sensitized mast cells and basophils[1]. After immunotherapy, allergic subjects show reduced immediate responses to allergen challenges to the nasal or bronchial mucosa[2].

1.1. T Cell Role

Patients receiving immunotherapy also have a reduction of several antigen driven in vitro activities attributable to T cells. Furthermore, after immunotherapy, late phase responses to allergen challenges, by both clinical observations and measurements of local mediator release, are reduced[3]. The potential role of downregulation of T cell activity in the immunologic management of allergic conditions is therefore being studied in man. The information obtained could lead to improvements in immunotherapy that would lessen the risk of allergic reactions to parenterally administered allergens and improve efficacy.

2. CONTROLLING T CELL REACTIVITY

The recognition that the level of IgE antibody depends on T cell regulation leads to consideration of how to alter or downregulate T cell stimulation of the B cells that synthe-

---

[*] Correspondence: Philip S. Norman, M.D., Johns Hopkins Asthma and Allergy Center, 5501 Hopkins Bayview Circle, Baltimore Maryland 21224.

New Horizons in Allergy Immunotherapy
edited by Sehon et al. Plenum Press, New York, 1996

size antibody. This is reinforced by the realization that the T cells that appear to play a direct role in allergic inflammation are probably the same CD4+ cells. Downregulation of these cells could at the same time reduce IgE synthesis and limit inflammatory responses to allergens.

2.1. T Cell Epitopes

T cells and antibodies interact with different ligands on allergens. IgE antibodies attach to complex B cell epitopes that require intact tertiary structures. T cell receptors, on the other hand, respond to short peptides from the allergen imbedded in surface mixed histocompatibility molecules on antigen presenting cells (APC). T cell activation occurs when presentation is accompanied by pro-inflammatory second signals[4]. These events usually engender immunity against foreign antigens, but can cause pathologic immune reactions such as allergies or autoimmune diseases.

The identification of T cell epitopes on allergens is now progressing rapidly. A number of major allergens have been cloned, sequenced and expressed. These include proteins from honey bee venom, cat, ragweed, rye grass and the house dust mites, *D. pteronyssinus* and *D. farinae*. Knowing the full peptide sequence of an allergen allows the synthesis of a series of overlapping peptides or generation of a series of deletion mutants that can be used as test materials for T cell stimulation.

2.2. T Cell Tolerance

Induction of tolerance (anergy) of T cells has been studied extensively in vitro and in vivo. This type of tolerance is to be distinguished from clonal deletion in the thymus. The T cells survive but their reactivity is down regulated. Of greatest interest therapeutically is tolerization of T cells with peptides derived from disease producing antigens. Such tolerization may be achieved in vitro by exposure of T cells to peptide fragments bound to class II MHC molecules without costimulatory activity from APC[5]. Tolerization of two clones of T cells from a *D. pteronyssinus* sensitive patient was also achieved in vitro by exposing them to high concentrations of the clone specific peptide in the absence of APC. During such exposure, however, there was considerable production of IL-2, IL-4 and IFN-γ. Subsequent cultures of tolerized cells with APC and peptide showed inhibition of IL-4 production while still producing IFN-γ [6]. To quote the authors: "This information may be relevant in the design of immunomodulatory agents for potential use in the treatment of allergic or autoimmune diseases."

Preliminary study of T cell lines from patients with ragweed allergy shows that a degree of T cell tolerance can be induced in vivo by standard immunotherapy. The T cell lines were grown in the presence of ragweed allergen Amb a 1, along with IL-2 and IL-4, rested and then restimulated by allergen in the presence of irradiated mononuclear cells as APC. Cell lines from untreated patients regularly showed proliferation, whereas lines from patients receiving ragweed extract immunotherapy showed much less proliferation. In some cell lines there was no proliferation post treatment. Furthermore production of IL-2, IL-3 and IL-4 during restimulation was reduced in the treated individuals[7]. These results confirm that T cell anergy can be induced in man.

2.2.1. Costimulatory Signals. In vivo tolerization with peptides or proteins depends on administration in such a way as to preclude a costimulatory signal. This has been done in mouse strains susceptible to autoimmune encephalomyelitis (EAE) induced by immunization with myelin basic protein (MBP) in complete Freund's adjuvant (CFA). Intraperitoneal administration of either intact MBP or synthetic peptides (Ac 1–11 and 35–47) which correspond to the major immunodominant epitopes emulsified in incomplete Freund's adjuvant (IFA) tolerizes the animal to subsequent induction of EAE by immunization. More relevant to eventual therapeutic use is that animals can be immunized for EAE and at the first sign of disease be given the tolerizing regimen. The progression and severity of disease are blocked. Such treatment either before or after immunization induces anergy in proliferative, antigen-specific T cells[8].

2.2.2. Animal Models of Tolerance

A murine model for tolerance to an antigen important in human allergic disease, i.e., the principal allergen of cat hair and dander, Fel d 1, has been developed. The two peptide chains of this allergen (chain 1 and 2) have been cloned, sequenced and expressed[9]. Mapping of the human T cell epitopes for Fel d 1 has demonstrated that the majority of the T cell response is specific for a broad area of the protein contained within two 27 member peptides, IPC-1 and IPC-2 from Fel d 1 chain 1 (a 70 member peptide). Injections of IPC-2 subcutaneously were given before an immunizing dose of IPC-2 in CFA. IPC-2 specific production of IL-2, IL-4 and IFN-γ was decreased in the peptide tolerized animals in comparison with saline treated controls. In animals with a preexisting immune response induced by Fel d 1 in IFA, IPC-2 subcutaneously resulted in tolerization of T cells as evidenced by decreased IL-2 production when spleen cells were cultured with IPC-2. In another experiment, a combination of IPC-1 and IPC-2 produced as complete tolerance to subsequent immunization with chain 1 as did chain 1 itself[10]. These results indicate that tolerance can be achieved without administering all possible T cell epitopes.

Indeed, tolerance to an allergen such as ragweed pollen that contains several allergenic proteins may be possible without epitopes from each protein. We showed many years ago that immunization with a single purified protein from ragweed, Amb a 1, would induce as useful a clinical tolerance as treatment with the whole extract containing many proteins[11].

3. CLINICAL DEVELOPMENT OF T CELL TOLERIZING PEPTIDES

Successful induction of tolerance to allergens in man depends on the development of peptides that do not interact with antibodies and thereby trigger immediate allergic responses. A survey of sera from cat sensitive humans has found no detectable interactions of IPC-1 or IPC-2 with IgE antibodies. A mix of these two peptides has therefore been proposed for human use. The goal would be achievement of T cell tolerance and the consequent downregulation of inflammatory responses on natural exposure to cats. Eventual decline of IgE antibodies to Fel d 1 might also be seen. Administration of potentially efficacious amounts of these substances has been started in cat sensitive patients.

3.1. Safety Study

In a preliminary safety study 19 cat sensitive patients underwent intradermal tests with each peptide in concentrations up to 1500 µg/mL without an allergic response. Sixteen patients were started on increasing doses weekly of the two peptides given separately subcutaneously. Doses were 7.5, 75, 250, 750, and 1500 µg of each, the final dose being 500 nmoles. In comparison, cat extract equivalent to 2.5 nmoles of Fel d 1 is the usual maximum tolerated dose for immunotherapy. The treatment was well tolerated. One asthmatic patient noted asthma after allergen skin testing and after the first injection and dropped out. After the 750 µg dose another asthmatic patient had an asthma attack at 6 hours and hives at 11 hours. A subsequent 250 µg dose was well tolerated. By ELISA, 2 patients developed low titers of IgE to peptides, but had had no allergic reaction to treatment. There was no change in IgE or IgG antibody titer to Fel d 1.[12]

3.2. Clinical Trial

In a study of the dose required for clinical efficacy, we divided 95 cat sensitive patients at random into four groups: Placebo, 7.5 µg, 75 µg, and 750 µg. Each group received a mix of both peptides by subcutaneous injection once a week for four weeks. We evaluated efficacy by exposure under controlled conditions in a room inhabited by live cats. Nose, eye and lung symptoms were rated on a 6 pt scale every 5 minutes up to 1 hour unless the patient asked to leave the room. Exposures were carried out before treatment and 1 and 6 weeks after the last injection. A linear trend analysis of differences between before and after treatment showed a dose response effect on lung and nose scores at 6 weeks. The 750 µg dose was significantly different from placebo at 6 weeks but the 7.5 µg dose was the same as placebo while 75µg dose showed an intermediate result. In 35 patients, the treatment injections induced mild symptoms consisting of stuffy runny nose, itchy eyes or chest tightness starting at about 1 to 3 hours and lasting several hours. They were either not treated or responded readily to a bronchodilator inhalation or an antihistamine. An earlier reaction occurred in one additional patient. These post treatment symptoms occurred in a few placebo patients. In treated patients their frequency was related to dose and decreased with each subsequent dose. At the time of clinical evaluations, IgE and IgG antibodies to cat extract were not changed. ALLERVAX- CAT downregulated early responses to allergens without significantly altering antibodies.[12] To examine the duration of laboratory and clinical responses we have followed 38 patients distributed among the dose groups for more than 12 months. Of the 5 patients who had developed evidence of anti-peptide IgG at 6 weeks after treatment, 3 no longer had detectable antibodies 5 months after treatment. Of the 4 patients with detectable anti-peptide IgE at six weeks post treatment, 3 no longer had measurable antibody by 5 months. In the 750 mg group (n=9), at 8 months post treatment, 4 patients maintained or improved benefit, 2 patients maintained some benefit, and 2 patients lost benefit. We gave 32 patients a repeat dose of blinded study medication at 12 months. All patients have tolerated the dose well[13].

Further studies with treatent peptides for cat and a mix of peptides designed to represent T cell epitopes of the prinicipal allergen of ragweed has been developed for clinical trial.

ACKNOWLEDGMENT

Supported by contracts with ImmuLogic Pharmaceutical Corporation, Waltham MA, and grant AI 33079 from the National Institute of Allergy and Infectious Diseases, Bethesda MD.

REFERENCES

1. Norman PS. Immunotherapy for nasal allergy. J Allergy Clin Immunol 1988;81:992–996.
2. Creticos PS, Marsh DG, Proud D, et al. Responses to ragweed-pollen nasal challenge before and after immunotherapy. J Allergy Clin Immunol 1989;84(2):197–205.
3. Iliopoulos O, Proud D, Adkinson NF, Jr., et al. Effects of immunotherapy on the early, late and rechallenge nasal reaction to provocation with allergen: Changes in inflammatory mediators and cells. J Allergy Clin Immunol 1991;87:855–866.
4. Neefjes JJ, Mombouafg F. Cell biology of antigen presentation. Curr Opin Immunol 1993;5:27–34.
5. O'Hehir RE, Garman RD, Greenstein JL, et al. The specificity and regulation of T-cell responsiveness to allergens. Annual Review of Immunology 1991;9:67–95.
6. O'Hehir RE, Yssel H, Verma S, et al. Clonal analysis of differential lymphokine production in peptide and superantigen induced T cell anergy. Int Immunol 1991;3:819–26.
7. Greenstein JL, Morgenstern JP, LaRaia J, et al. Ragweed immunotherapy decreaes T cell reactivity to recombinant Amb a I. J Allergy Clin Immunol 1992;89:322.
8. Gaur A, Wiers B, Liu A, et al. Amelioration of autoimmune encephalomyelitis by myelin basic protein synthetic peptide-induced anergy. Science 1992;258:1491–94.
9. Morgenstern JP, Griggith IJ, Brauer AW, et al. Determination of the amino acid sequence of *Fel d* I, the major allergen of the domestic cat: Protein sequence analysis and cDNA cloning. Proceedings of The National Academy of Sciences 1991;88:9690–96.
10. Briner TJ, Kuo M-C, Keating KM, et al. Peripheral T-cell tolerance induced in naive and primed mice by subcutaneous injection of peptides from the major cat allergen Fel d I. Proc Natl Acad Sci USA 1993;90:7608–12.
11. Norman PS, Winkenwerder WL, Lichtenstein LM. Immunotherapy of hay fever with ragweed antigen E: comparisons with whole pollen extract and placebos. J Allergy 1968;42(2):93–108.
12. Norman PS, Ohman JL, Long AA, et al. Early clinical experience with T cell reactive peptides from cat allergen Fel d 1. J Allergy Clin Immunol 1994;93:231 Abstract.
13. Norman PS, Ohman JL, Long AA, et al. Follow on study of the first clinical trial with T cell defined peptides from cat allergen Fel d 1. J Allergy Clin Immunol 1995;95:259 Abstract.

67

CLINICAL USE OF RECOMBINANT ALLERGENS AND EPITOPES

Jean Bousquet,[*] Anne Des Roches, and Louis Paradis

Clinique des Maladies Respiratoires and CJF-INSERM 92–10
Hopital Arnaud de Villeneuve
Centre Hospitalier Universitaire
34295-Montpellier-Cedex 5, France

The most recent advances in the characterization of allergens using molecular biology techniques has lead to the development of recombinant allergens (RA) (1), epitopes (2, 3) and peptides including several overlapping epitopes (4). Studies using RA, epitopes and peptides are of importance for the understanding of cellular and molecular basis of allergogy and other relevant scientific fields but, more importantly, these basic advances in technology are likely to improve the management of allergic patients for both the diagnosis and the treatment (5, 6).

1. RECOMBINANT ALLERGENS

1.1. Requirements of RA

The strategy of expressing allergens in vectors as recombinant proteins requires that IgE-binding epitopes are mainly protein structures and carbohydrate moieties participate to a minor extent in IgE-binding. RAs used for *in vitro* diagnosis should have the same *IgE binding activity* as their natural counterparts. The question whether a single RA accounts for a high percentage of specific IgE in allergic individuals needs to be tested by different *in vitro* assays such as ELISA (7, 8) or related tests, IgE immunoblotting (9) or histamine release assay (10) and is of particular interest for therapeutic purposes. Only a few RA have been synthetized and their IgE-binding capacity may be less than that of the corresponding natural allergens. It has been observed that the IgE reactivity of some RA

* Correspondence to: Pr. J Bousquet, Clinique des Maladies Respiratoires, Hopital Arnaud de Villeneuve, Avenue du doyen G Giraud, 34295 Montpellier-Cedex 5, France. Telephone: 33–67–33–61–04; Telefax: 33–67–04–27–08.

New Horizons in Allergy Immunotherapy
edited by Sehon et al. Plenum Press, New York, 1996

463

was very high in some (7) but not all studies (11–14) Moreover, differences in IgE-binding activity were shown to be variable according to the patient's reactivity (11).

RAs used for *in vivo* diagnosis should have the additional following properties:

- Purity,
- Lack of toxicity,
- Stability,
- Biological activity: e.g. enzymatic activity of the natural allergens,
- Skin test reactivity: RAs should be tested in a representative sample of allergic patients.

For safety reasons the starting dose of RA should be carefully determined and always low. Prick tests should be used first (15–17). A Der pII RA has been tested in mite allergic subjects and was found to be almost as active as the purified native allergen in stimulating immediate hypersensitivity reactions (18). As much as possible, the consistency on a molecular basis between RA and its natural counterpart (when available in a pure state) should be tested. In case of many minor allergens and some major allergens, this comparison cannot be made because natural allergens have not been purified or prepared in sufficient quantities.

1.2. Diagnosis of Allergic Diseases

1.2.1. Advantages. In a representative number of patients it has been demonstrated in pollen, mite, cat, mould or venom allergy that RAs share IgE-binding epitopes with the natural proteins and may therefore be used for diagnosis of Type I allergy. Major advantages of RAs are they are well defined and can be produced in unlimited amounts. In general RAs can be used in the same way as natural allergens to establish *in vitro* diagnostic tests both for IgE and lymphocyte tests (19). However, less is known on *in vivo* diagnosis (15, 17).

The use of RA for the diagnosis of allergic conditions may improve the diagnosis of allergy since some natural allergens are rapidly denatured during or after their extraction (e.g. apple) (20), others exist in very low concentrations in the extracts (e.g. cypress pollen allergens) (21), others are poorly extracted or the amount of allergens extracted varies according to climatic conditions (at least for some pollens) (22). Natural allergen preparations may contain different other allergens and lead to false positive results. (examples: cat or dog allergen preparations may contain mite particles, weed pollen preparations may contain grass pollen). Use of single RA may provide useful tools to characterize the patient's sensitivity to all allergens to which he is allergic and may lead to treatment with extracts tailored for the sensitivity of each individual.

The use of RAs for any diagnostic purpose requires that a number of relevant allergens can be defined. Due to extensive structural similarities and cross-reactivities within the major tree and within grass pollen allergens or in case of the pan-allergen profilin (23), it seems that a realistic number of RAs could be produced for diagnosis and treatment.

Recently, RA have been used in a commercial IgE test. Two tests are now available on CAP System (Pharmacia Diagnostics) including two components of birch pollen (Bet v1 and Bet v2). These tests are not available for diagnostic procedures but to assess the allergy profile of the patients.

1.2.2. Disadvantages. Only a few RA have been synthetized and their IgE-binding capacity may be less than that of the corresponding natural allergens both in vitro (11–14) and in vivo (24). Differences in IgE-binding activity were shown to be variable according to the patient's reactivity.

The use of RAs for the diagnosis of allergic conditions provides an elegant method as was recently demonstrated in case of birch (7, 8) or grass (25) pollen allergy. However, birch pollen and cross reactive Betulaceae pollens (26) may be unusual as compared with other allergen species by having only one dominant and a few minor allergens. Thus, the numbers of RAs to be produced for all allergen species may be very high and will need very important resources.

1.3. Improvement of Allergen Standardisation Using Recombinant Allergens

The introduction of molecular cloning techniques may be considered as a real breakthrough in the field of allergen standardisation. RA perfectly characterized can be obtained in unlimited amounts and consistent high quality. RA may serve as standard molecules. It would therefore be desirable to have available recombinant standard allergens for the production of monoclonal antibodies which then can be used for standardising extracts. Furthermore it would be possible to compare the stability of natural allergens in the extracts with recombinant reference molecules (27).

1.4. Immunotherapy (IT) with RA

IT with purified allergens has been examined in controlled studies using Amb a I for ragweed pollen allergy and a single grass pollen allergen. It has been shown that Amb aI represents an effective alternative to IT with the whole extract (28), these favourable results were not however confirmed in grass pollen allergy (29). Thus, although IT with RA cannot be implemented at present, this may be a future opportunity particularly for selected allergies such as birch pollen because of the availability of Bet v I RA and the small number of allergens of birch pollen. For more complex aeroallergens such as grass pollens, the major allergens Lol p I, Lol p II, Lol p III and Poa p IX have been cloned and these RAs might also be used in IT trials (30, 31). For most other allergen species IT cannot be envisioned soon because of the complexity of the allergen extracts, a perfect characterization of the repertoire of major allergens and the availability of their recombinant counterparts. However, RA represent a therapeutic potential (32).

2. EPITOPES

2.1. Immunotherapy (IT) with T-cell Epitopes

The rationales for IT with T cell epitopes are based on the most recent developments of Immunology and the differentiation between B cell and T cell epitopes (2, 3). T cell epitopes are not conformational but sequential and as such may not be recognized by IgE. They are immunogenic through their interaction with specific T cell receptors without inducing systemic reactions when injected to allergic individuals as they may not bind IgE (33–35). The IgE immune response is linked with the Th2 phenotype of T-cells resulting in an enhanced production of IL-4, IL-5 and IL-10. It is proposed that T-cell epitopes may lead to an anergic response (Th0) inducing the lack of responsiveness of the patient and therefore decreased IgE and IgE-mediated inflammatory responses. Allergen-specific human T-cell clones can be rendered non-responsive to subsequent allergen challenges by incubation of supra-immunogenic doses of antigenic peptides in the absence of antigen presenting cells. Ideally one would like to administer high concentrations of T cell activation inducing allergen-derived peptides. Several T-cell epitopes have been identified for allergens (36, 37).

Although IT with T-cell epitopes may represent a major improvement in the treatment of allergic patients, our knowledge is still limited. The diversity of the IgE immune response is of importance and it might be estimated that a total of at least 10,000 epitopes is needed to cover the entire spectrum of all allergens in all allergic patients [Bousquet, 1994 #1595]. However, due to their relative importance some "dominant" epitopes may exist and only 200 might be useful for allergen specific IT. The design of the peptides may lead to an even smaller number of relevant epitopes since they may be clustered on small portions of the whole molecule and there may be some epitopes regulating the whole sequence. Studies on egg lysozymes have observed "dominant" epitopes possessing a tolerogenic activity (38). Alternatively the modification of some epitopes may lead to the suppression of the whole immune response to a given allergen. However, more studies are needed to support these hypothesis.

The ability of peptidic fragments to modulate the immune response to intact molecules has been studied in the IgE-immune system using bovine serum albumin (39) and shown to downregulate the IgE immune response. Peptides have already been used in the treatment of allergic patients. Urea-denaturation of Amb a I creates two peptide chains which have lost much of their tertiary folding. The denatured peptides induced tolerance in mice but not in humans (40). Litwig et al (41) attempted to downregulate the specific IgE response to bee venom phospholipase A_2 by injecting to allergic patients fragments of this allergen. Although they did not examine the clinical effect of this treatment they showed that skin tests were reduced and specific IgE and IgG declined rapidly.

The safety of any immunologic treatment has to be carefully assessed. Although theoretically T cell epitopes do not bind to IgE, recent data show that some small peptides can bind to IgE (42) and even trigger basophils (43) or platelets (44). Moreover, T cells can produce histamine releasing factors priming basophils and mast cells. Thus, the safety of vaccination with T cell epitopes is critical.

2.2. Immunotherapy (IT) with T-cell Reactive Peptides Derived from Allergens

Small peptides containing several T-cell epitopes have been prepared for IT. The first peptides which have been prepared include Fel d1, Cry J1 and Amb a1 (4). The complete primary structure of Fel d I has been determined and shown to be comprised of two separate polypeptide chains (designated chain 1 and 2) (45, 46). Overlapping peptides covering the entire sequence of both chains of Fel d I have been used to map the major areas of human T cell reactivity. Three non-contiguous T cell reactive regions of under 30 amino-acids in length were assembled in all six possible configurations using PCR and recombinant DNA methods. These six recombinant proteins comprised of defined non-contiguous T cell epitope regions artificially combined into single polypeptide chains have been expressed in E. coli, highly purified, and examined for their ability to bind to human cat-allergic IgE and for human T cell reactivity. Several of these recombined T cell epitope-containing polypeptides exhibit markedly reduced IgE binding as compared to the native Fel d I (47). Importantly, the human T cell reactivity to individual T cell epitope-containing regions is maintained even though each was placed in an unnatural position as compared to the native molecule. In addition, T cell responses to potential junctional epitopes were not detected. It was also demonstrated in mice that s.c. injection of T cell epitope-containing polypeptides inhibits the T cell response to the individual peptides upon subsequent challenge in vitro (48). These recombind T cell epitope-containing polypeptides, which harbour multiple T cell reactive regions but have significantly reduced reactivity with allergic human IgE, constitute a novel potential approach for desensitisation to important allergens. The first phase I and phase II studies have show that these peptides were efficient for a dose of 750 μg per injection but elicited side effects which were unexpected. They were usually mild and their onset was ranging between 60 and 180 min without any immediate reaction. The nature of these side effects is still unknown but they may be related to a T-cell activation inducing a secondary histamine release.

3. HEALTH ECONOMICS

The preparation of high-tech, high-cost recombinant allergens, epitopes or peptides should also be discussed in terms of health economics. When the introduction of biotechnology-derived pharmaceuticals is providing live-saving opportunities for conditions for which there was little alternative or no hope for a cure, the high costs of these products can be cost-effective. However, although allergic diseases bear a significant burden for the affected individuals, they are not usually life-threatening and alternative treatments are often available at a lower cost. It may therefore be important to demonstrate that these high-tech, high-cost preparations are highly effective and safe in the short term and can alter the natural course of the disease in the long term to show their cost-efficiency.

REFERENCES

1. Scheiner O, Kraft D. Basic and practical aspects of recombinant allergens. Allergy 1995;50:384–92.
2. Schou C. T-cell epitopes of allergen molecules. Arb Paul Ehrlich Inst Bundesamt Sera Impfstoffe Frankf A M 1994;87:247–9.
3. Valenta R, Vrtala S, Laffer S, et al. B-cell epitopes of allergens determined by recombinant techniques; use for diagnosis and therapy of type I allergy. Arb Paul Ehrlich Inst Bundesamt Sera Impfstoffe Frankf A M 1994;87:235–46.
4. Wallner B, Gefter M. Immunotherapy with T-cell reactive peptides derived from allergens. Allergy 1994;49:302–8.
5. Bousquet J, Breitenebach M, Dreborg S, Kenimer J, Løwestein H, Norman P. Diagnosis of allergy and specific immunotherapy using recombinant allergens and epitopes. In Kraft D, Sehon A, eds. Molecular biology and immunology of allergensBoca Raton, Fl: CRC Press, 1993:311–20.
6. Bousquet J. Clinical use of recombinant allergens and epitopes. Arb Paul Ehrlich Inst Bundesamt Sera Impfstoffe Frankf A M 1994;87:257–62.
7. Valenta R, Vrtala S, Ebner C, Kraft D, Scheiner O. Diagnosis of grass pollen allergy with recombinant timothy grass (Phleum pratense) pollen allergens. Int Arch Allergy Immunol 1992;97:287–94.
8. Yang M, Olsen E, Dolovich J, Sehon AH, Mohapatra SS. Immunologic characterization of a recombinant Kentucky bluegrass (Poa pratensis) allergenic peptide. J Allergy Clin Immunol 1991;87:1096–104.
9. Valenta R, Vrtala S, Ebner C, Kraft D, Scheiner O. Diagnosis of grass pollen allergy with recombinant timothy grass (Phleum pratense) pollen allergens. Int Arch Allergy Immunol 1992;97:287–94.
10. Valenta R, Sperr WR, Ferreira F, et al. Induction of specific histamine release from basophils with purified natural and recombinant birch pollen allergens. J Allergy Clin Immunol 1993;91:88–97.
11. Breiteneder H, Ferreira F, Hoffmann-Sommergruber K, et al. Four recombinant isoforms of Cor a I, the major allergen of hazel pollen, show different IgE-binding properties. Eur J Biochem 1993;212:355–62.
12. Chua KY, Dilworth RJ, Thomas WR. Expression of Dermatophagoides pteronyssinus allergen, Der p II, in Escherichia coli and the binding studies with human IgE. Int Arch Allergy Appl Immunol 1990;91:124–9.

13. Greene WK, Thomas WR. IgE binding structures of the major house dust mite allergen Der p I. Mol Immunol 1992;29:257–62.

14. Rafnar T, Ghosh B, Metzler WJ, et al. Expression and analysis of recombinant Amb a V and Amb t V allergens. Comparison with native proteins by immunological assays and NMR spectroscopy. J Biol Chem 1992;267:21119–23.

15. Moser M, Crameri R, Menz G, et al. Cloning and expression of recombinant Aspergillus fumigatus allergen I/a (rAsp f I/a) with IgE binding and type I skin test activity. J Immunol 1992;149:454–60.

16. Moser M, Crameri R, Brust E, Suter M, Menz G. Diagnostic value of recombinant Aspergillus fumigatus allergen I/a for skin testing and serology. J Allergy Clin Immunol 1994;93:1–11.

17. Förster E, Müller U, Dudler T, Suter M, Aberer W, Urbanek R. Recombinant bee venom phospholipase A2 releases histamine from basophils and elicits positive skin reactions in allergic individuals. In: Kraft D, Sehon A, ed. Molecular biology and immunology of allergens. Boca Raton: CRC Press, 1993: 307–10.

18. Lynch NR, Thomas WR, Chua Y, Garcia N, Di-Prisco MC, Lopez R. In vivo biological activity of recombinant Der p II allergen of house-dust mite. Int Arch Allergy Immunol 1994;105:70–4.

19. Bond JF, Garman RD, Keating KM, et al. Multiple Amb a I allergens demonstrate specific reactivity with IgE and T cells from ragweed-allergic patients. J Immunol 1991;146:3380–5.

20. Bjorksten F, Halmepuro L, Hannuksela M, Lahti A. Extraction and properties of apple allergens. Allergy 1980;35:671–7.

21. Bousquet J, Knani J, Hejjaoui A, et al. Heterogeneity of atopy. I. Clinical and immunologic characteristics of patients allergic to cypress pollen. Allergy 1993;48:183–8.

22. Barber D, Carpizo J, Garcia-Rumbao MC, Polo F, Juan F. Allergenic variability in olea pollen. Ann Allergy 1990;64:43–6.

23. Valenta R, Duchene M, Ebner C, et al. Profilins constitute a novel family of functional plant pan-allergens. J Exp Med 1992;175:377–85.

24. Lin KL, Hsieh KH, Thomas WR, Chiang BL, Chua KY. Characterization of Der p V allergen, cDNA analysis, and IgE-mediated reactivity to the recombinant protein. J Allergy Clin Immunol 1994;94:989–96.

25. Laffer S, Vrtala S, Duchene M, et al. IgE-binding capacity of recombinant timothy grass (Phleum pratense) pollen allergens. J Allergy Clin Immunol 1994;94:88–94.

26. Larsen JN, Stroman P, Ipsen H. PCR based cloning and sequencing of isogenes encoding the tree pollen major allergen Car b I from Carpinus betulus, hornbeam. Mol Immunol 1992;29:703–11.

27. Bousquet J, Michel F. Standardization of allergens. In: Spector S, ed. Provocation testing in clinical practice. NY: Marcel Dekker, 1994: 15–50. (Kaliner M, ed. Clinical Allergy and Immunology;

28. Norman P, Winkelwerder W, Lichtenstein L. Immunotherapy of hay fever with ragweed antigen E: comparisons with whole extracts and placebo. J Allergy 1968;42:93–108.

29. Østerballe O. Immunotherapy in hay fever with two major allergens 19, 25 and partially purified extract of timothy grass pollen. A controlled double blind study. In vivo variables, season I. Allergy 1980;35:473–89.

30. Zhang L, Kisil FT, Sehon AH, Mohapatra SS. Allergenic and antigenic cross-reactivities of group IX grass pollen allergens. Int Arch Allergy Appl Immunol 1991;96:28–34.

31. Mohapatra S. Structural motifs as a basis of cross-reactivity among pollen allergens. In: Kraft D, Sehon A, ed. Molecular biology and Immunology of Allergens. Boca Raton, Fl: CRC Press, 1993: 69–82.

32. Sehon A, Mohapatra S. Therapeutic potential of recombinant allergens. In: Kraft D, Sehon A, ed. Molecular biology and immunology of allergens. Boca raton: CRC Press, 1993: 113–22.

33. O'Hehir R, Higgins J, Jarman E, Lamb J. T cell epitopes, MHC antigens and their application. In: Kraft D, Sehon A, ed. Molecular biology and immunology of allergens. Boca Raton: CRC Press, 1993: vol 63–8).

34. O'Hehir RE, Hoyne GF, Thomas WR, Lamb JR. House dust mite allergy: from T-cell epitopes to immunotherapy. Eur J Clin Invest 1993;23:763–72.

35. Schad VC, Garman RD, Greenstein JL. The potential use of T cell epitopes to alter the immune response. Semin Immunol 1991;3:217–24.

36. Thomas WR. Mite allergens groups I-VII. A catalogue of enzymes. Clin Exp Allergy 1993;23:350–3.

37. Knox K, Taylor P, P PS, al. e. Pollen allergens: botanical aspects. In: Kraft D, Sehon A, ed. Molecular biology and immunology of allergens. Boca Raton: CRC Press, 1993: 31–8.

38. Gammon G, Sercarz E. How some T cells escape tolerance induction. Nature 1989;342:183–5.

39. Ferguson TA, Peters T Jr., Reed R, Pesce AJ, Michael JG. Immunoregulatory properties of antigenic fragments from bovine serum albumin. Cell Immunol 1983;78:1–12.

40. Norman PS, Ishizaka K, Lichtenstein LM, Adkinson N Jr. Treatment of ragweed hay fever with urea-denatured antigen E. J Allergy Clin Immunol 1980;66:336–41.

41. Litwin A, Pesce AJ, Michael JG. Regulation of the immune response to allergens by immunosuppressive allergenic fragments. 1. Peptic fragments of honey bee venom phospholipase A2. Int Arch Allergy Appl Immunol 1988;87:361–6.

42. van-'t-Hof W, Driedijk PC, van-den-Berg M, Beck-Sickinger AG, Jung G, Aalberse RC. Epitope mapping of the Dermatophagoides pteronyssinus house dust mite major allergen Der p II using overlapping synthetic peptides. Mol Immunol 1991;28:1225–32.

43. Jeannin P, Didierlaurent A, Gras-Masse H, et al. Specific histamine release capacity of peptides selected from the modelized Der p I protein, a major allergen of Dermatophagoides pteronyssinus. Mol Immunol 1992;29:739–49.

44. Cardot E, Pestel J, Callebaut I, et al. Specific activation of platelets from patients allergic to Dermatophagoides pteronyssinus by synthetic peptides derived from the allergen Der p I. Int Arch Allergy Immunol 1992;98:127–34.

45. Morgenstern JP, Griffith IJ, Brauer AW, et al. Amino acid sequence of Fel dI, the major allergen of the domestic cat: protein sequence analysis and cDNA cloning. Proc Natl Acad Sci U S A 1991;88:9690–4.

46. Bond JF, Brauer AW, Segal DB, Nault AK, Rogers BL, Kuo MC. Native and recombinant Fel dI as probes into the relationship of allergen structure to human IgE immunoreactivity. Mol Immunol 1993;30:1529–41.

47. Rogers BL, Morgenstern JP, Garman RD, Bond JF, Kuo MC. Recombinant Fel d.I: Expression, purification, IgE binding and reaction with cat-allergic human T cells. Mol Immunol 1993;30:559–68.

48. Briner TJ, Kuo MC, Keating KM, Rogers BL, Greenstein JL. Peripheral T-cell tolerance induced in naive and primed mice by subcutaneous injection of peptides from the major cat allergen Fel d I. Proc Natl Acad Sci U S A 1993;90:7608–12.

68

DIAGNOSTIC AND THERAPEUTIC USE OF RECOMBINANT ALLERGENS

D. Kraft

Institute of General and Experimental Pathology
University of Vienna Medical School
AKH, Vienna, Austria

Ladies and Gentlemen, Dear Colleagues and Friends:

First of all, I would like to thank you all for your participation and persistence over the last 4 days, which has led to the successful outcome of this symposium. Before taking the opportunity to thank Prof. Sehon and Prof. Herbert and his team for the excellent organization I would like to give you my personal view on the diagnostic and therapeutic use of recombinant allergens in the future.

THE USE OF RECOMBINANT ALLERGENS FOR DIAGNOSTIC PURPOSES

The future use of recombinant allergens for diagnosis of IgE mediated allergies is quite clear and simple to me. We will have to use about 40 allergens, depending on various geographic areas, causes of allergies etc. Most of these allergens have been cloned over the last 6 years (1):

- for tree pollen allergies we need two allergens, Bet v 1 and Bet v 2, in most parts of Europe; in the Mediterranean countries an additional allergen, Ole e 1, maybe necessary. In North America an additional allergen, and in Japan Cry j 1 and Cry j 2 have to be added to the panel of allergens
- regarding grass pollen allergies, 5 recombinant molecules will be enough for testing, for example Phl p 1, Phl p 2, Phl p 4, Phl p 5, and grass profilin
- in the case of weed allergies, 3 allergens for mugwort and 3 molecules for ragweed in North America should be sufficient for diagnosis
- in the case of mite allergies 5 to 6 molecules seem to be enough
- in the case of cockroach allergies 3 allergens seem to be sufficient
- in the case of pets, for each type of pet 2–3 allergens with the use of albumin as a cross-reacting allergen should be used

New Horizons in Allergy Immunotherapy
edited by Sehon et al. Plenum Press, New York, 1996

471

- in the case of bee, wasp, yellowjacket allergies etc., each requires 3 allergens
- in the case of mould allergens the situation is more difficult, apparently 4 to 6 allergens for each fungus, but there are many cross-reacting allergens which should bring down the number of allergens (2). However, we need more results to clarify the necessity of some molecules
- finally, in food allergy 3 pollen-associated allergens and 7 other allergens seem to be of major importance.

In summary, a limited number of recombinant allergens are sufficient for diagnostic tests and these recombinant molecules can be produced in high quality and quantity (3).

New results show that major allergens exist in various isoforms with different IgE-binding capacities and this has led to some confusion. In my opinion, it's absolutely useless to clone an incredible number of isoforms by PCR for diagnostic purposes. It is like in the field of monoclonal antibodies. If you choose the wrong hybridomas you will never end up with the right antibodies. You have to decide on your targets at the right time: which epitope, which isotype, affinity constant etc. you are interested in. In the case of recombinant allergens for diagnostic procedures, we have to pick up molecules with maximal IgE-binding capacities only. Only those molecules will behave exactly the same as the natural ones in the diagnostic tests. This was shown for Bet v 1 and Bet v 2 *in vitro* as well as *in vivo* (3), and also in new studies for the Phleum pratense allergens Phl p 1, Phl p 2, Phl p 5 and Phleum profilin, using sera from Europe, Canada, and Australia (4). Similar results were obtained with vegetable food-associated allergens in pollen-allergic patients(5).

In my opinion, recombinant allergens are excellent tools for standardized diagnostic tests and will bring the same revolution as was observed in Clinical Chemistry and Clinical Immunology with monoclonal antibodies. It is also important to note that a second generation of recombinant molecules produced by site directed mutagenesis and again chosen for their maximal IgE- binding capacity as reported at this Symposium by F. Ferreira et al and Alisa Smith et al will help us enormously.

THE USE OF RECOMBINANT ALLERGENS FOR IMMUNOTHERAPY

Despite the great progress in the diagnosis of IgE-mediated allergies much bigger problems are connected with recombinant allergen-based therapy. There is a nice sentence from Johann Wolfgang von Goethe who said: *"A hypothesis is very similar to scaffolding. When we have obtained enough results, the house is finished and the scaffolding can be taken down"*. In the case of recombinant allergen-based therapy, we are still at the hypothetical stage. I have always been in favour of an allergen-specific way of modulating the immune system. Allergen-unspecific immunotherapy seems to affect our whole defence system too strongly. There are too many receptors, interleukins, antagonists, etc. involved in this network. It is more instinct than science, but I prefer the allergen-specific way. In this context, the results of the work with T cell epitopes containing polypeptides, which harbour multiple T cell reactive regions but have significantly reduced or no-reactivity at all with IgE from allergics, are encouraging (6,7).

In 1992 at our last Symposium in Vienna, I stressed the point that a lot more studies regarding IgE regulation should be carried out on healthy people. You may remember my words. In the meantime, a limited number of studies have been undertaken. We now have discovered identical T cell epitopes of allergens in healthy people as observed in allergics (8), although important questions with regard to IgE as well as IgG epitopes of allergens in allergy free individuals have yet to be answered.

It is astonishing that during this meeting only few results have been reported, which address the same questions in patients undergoing hyposensitization treatment. We should never forget that allergologists have the unique opportunity to repeat continuously a successful experiment on humans without knowing the reason for its success. This gathering here mainly involves researchers interested in fundamental immunology. The effects of classical hyposensitization should be their targets too and not be restricted to clinicians. The knowledge in fundamental immunology gained over the last three years will strongly influence the design and parameters of new studies. I know that collaborations of researchers from theoretical institutes with clinicians are time-consuming and difficult, but still we have to do this to solve the problem.

Now to a more exotic topic. I grew up in the Salzkammergut in Upper Austria, where worm diseases are common. In this region, worm infections have a long history, going back 3000 years. Microbiologists have investigated the faeces of workers of one of the oldest salt mines in the world in Hallstatt near Salzburg in Upper Austria. The faeces of the people of the Hallstatt-Period — 1000 to 300 BC — working in this salt mine were full of eggs of *Trichuris trichiura* and *Ascaris lumbricoides* (9). I was living there after the Second World War from the age of 7 to 10. Hygiene had not really changed since the old times of the salt mine and my friends and I were full of worms. I remember very well a nice conversation with two pretty girls: How many worms did you count today in your faeces? Only one or two? Much less than the 5 you counted yesterday!!! – – Looking at the poster of Faux et al., telling skin test and specific IgE results in *parasitized aborigines*, I have remembered that my friends and I have never suffered from IgE-mediated allergies. Evolution created the IgE system as a defence mechanism against parasitic diseases (10). For years I have had the idea that *"bringing back"* the worms could result in polyclonal IgE-production and in dampening of IgE-mediated allergies as a result of overcrowding the mast cells and basophils with IgE antibodies to worm allergens and thus inhibiting the fixation and/or cross-linking of IgE antibodies to common allergens on these cells. Maybe, we should produce more unconventional ideas. I am looking forward to our next symposium in three years, maybe we will have results at that time.

Finally, I would like to express my sincerest thanks to Prof. Jaques Hebert, Dr. Yvan Boutin, Mrs. LiseHardy, and many others of the local organizing comittee for their excellent work and the warm hospitalité Quebecoise. We all have had a marvellous week with our colleagues from Quebec. Last but not least I would like to thank most cordially my Cochairman Alec Sehon for his persistent efforts to organize a Symposium of this caliber. It was not easy for him to raise the necessary funding, our times are tough and the understanding of some pharmaceutical companies for our field is apparantly very limited. Nevertheless, he managed it. Congratulations, and thank you very much indeed.

REFERENCES

1. Scheiner O. and Kraft D. 1995. Basic and practical aspects of recombinant allergens. Allergy 50: 384–391.
2. Achatz G., Oberkofler H., Lechenauer E., Simon B., Unger A., Kandler D., Ebner C., Prillinger H., Kraft D., and Breitenbach M. 1995. Molecular cloning of major and minor allergens of *Alternaria alternata* and *Cladosporium herbarum*. Mol Immunol 32: 213–227.
3. Valenta R. and Kraft D. 1995. Recombinant allergens for diagnosis and therapy of allergic diseases. Curr Op Immunol, in press.

4. Laffer S. and Valenta R., in preparation.
5. Ebner C., Hirschwehr R., Bauer L., Breiteneder H., Valenta R., Ebner H., Kraft D., Scheiner O. 1995. Identification of allergens in fruits and vegetables: IgE cross-reactivities with the important birch pollen allergens Bet v 1 and Bet v 2 (birch profilin). J Allergy Clin Immunol 95: 962–969.
6. Wallner B.P. and Gefter M.L. 1994. Immunotherapy with T-cell-reactive peptides derived from allergens. Allergy 49: 302–308.
7. Ferreira F., Hirtenlehner K., Jilek A., Godnic-Cvar J., Breiteneder H., Grimm R., Hoffmann-Sommergruber K., Scheiner O., Kraft D., Breitenbach M., Rheinberger H.-J., Ebner C. 1996. Dissection of IgE and T lymphocyte reactivity of isoforms of the major birch pollen allergen Bet v 1: Potential use of hypoallergenic isoforms for immunotherapy. J Exp Med, in press.
8. Ebner C., Schenk S., Najafian N., Siemann U., Steiner R., Fischer G.W., Hoffmann K., Szépfalusi Z., Scheiner O., Kraft D. 1995. Non-allergic individuals recognize the same epitopes of Bet v 1, the major birch pollen allergen, as atopic patients. J Immunol 154: 1932–1940.
9. Asböck H., Flamm H., Picher O. 1973. Intestinal parasites in human excrements from prehistoric salt mines of the Hallstatt period (800–350 B.C.). Zentralbl. Bakteriol. Orig. A. 223: 549–558.
10. Locksley R.M. 1994. Th2 cells: help for helminths. J Exp Med 179: 1405–1407.

INVITED CONTRIBUTORS

Aasmul-Olsen, S.	Horsholm, Denmark
Achatz, G.	Freiburg, Germany
Agerlin Olsen, A.	Bagsvaerd, Denmark
Arosio, P.	Milano, Italy
Arruda, L.K.	Charlottesville, USA
Astwood, J.	St. Louis, USA
Bannon, S.	Little Rock, USA
Barnes, C.	Kansas City, USA
Batard, T.	Fresnes, France
Becker, A.	Winnipeg, Canada
Becker, W.M.	Borstel, Germany
Befus, D.	Edmonton, Canada
Bjerke, Torbjorn	Aarhus, Denmark
Blaser, K.	Davos Platz, Switzerland
Blocki, F.	Chaska, USA
Borga, A.	Uppsala, Sweden
Boulet, L.	Pointe-Claire, Quebec
Boulet, L.-P.	Ste-Foy, Quebec
Bousquet, J.	Montpellier, France
Breitenbach, M.	Salzburg, Austria
Breiteneder, H.	Vienna, Austria
Bufe, A.	Borstel, Germany
Byers, V.	San Francisco, USA
Campbell, D.A.	Leeds, UK
Caraballo, L.	Cartagena, Colombia
Carlsson, M.	Uppsala, Sweden
Chapman, M.	Charlottesville, USA
Chua, K.-Y.	Taipei, PRC
Cookson, W.	Oxford, UK
Côté, J.	Ste-Foy, Quebec
Crameri, R.	Davos Platz, Switzerland
Davies, F.	Houston, USA
Deichmann, K.	Freisburg, Germany
de Vries, J.	Palo Alto, USA
Dreborg, S.	Uppsala, Sweden

Elfman, L.	Uppsala, Sweden
Fernandez-Caldez, E.	Tampa, USA
Ferreira, F.	Salzburg, Austria
Fiebig, H.	Reinbek, Germany
Frick, O.L.	San Francisco, USA
Gelfand, E.	Denver, USA
Ghanem, R.	Totowa, USA
Grönlund, H.	Uppsala, Sweden
Hamid, Q.	Montreal, Canada
HayGlass, K.	Winnipeg, Canada
Hébert, J.	Ste-Foy, Canada
Hellman, L.	Uppsala, Sweden
Helm, R.M.	Little Rock, USA
Heusser, C.H.	Basel, Switzerland
Hill, M.	Oxford, UK
Hong, S.-J.	Seoul, Korea
Horner, W.E.	New Orleans, USA
Inacio, F.	Setubal, Portugal
Ishizaka, K.	La Jolla, USA
Iwasawa, Y.	San Diego, USA
Jardieu, P.	S. San Francisco, USA
Jordana, M.	Hamilton, Canada
Kapsenberg, M.	Amsterdam, The Netherlands
Kettelhut, B.	Cincinatti, USA
Kikutani, H.	Suita, Japan
Kinet, J.-P.	Rockville, USA
Klysner, S.	Horsholm, Denmark
Kraft, D.	Vienna, Austria
Kricek, F.	Vienna, Austria
Lamb, J.R.	London, UK
Lang, G.	Winnipeg, Canada
Larsen, J.N.	Horsholm, Denmark
Laviolette, M.	Ste-Foy, Canada
Lehrer, S.	New Orleans, USA
Lidholm, J.	Uppsala, Sweden
Liebers, V.	Bochum, Germany
Liedstrand, P.	Uppsala, Sweden
Lipscomb, M.F.	Albuquerque, USA
Lombardero, M.	Madrid, Spain
Lowenstein, H.	Horsholm, Denmark
Luehr, C.	Chaska, USA
Magnusson, C.	Stockholm, Sweden
Malkiel, S.	Worcester, USA
Marsh, D.	Baltimore, USA
Martin, J.	Montreal, Canada
Mathison, D.	La Jolla, CA
Mazer, B.	Montreal, Canada
Mello, J.F.	Sao Paulo, Brazil
Mikayama, T.	Maebashi, Japan

Moffatt, M.	Oxford, UK
Moon, H.-B.	Seoul, Korea
Moqbel, R.	London, UK
Morrison, J.	Leeds, UK
Müller, W.-D.	Jena, Germany
Murphy, K.	St. Louis, USA
Nontasut, P.	Bangkok, Thailand
Norman, P.	Baltimore, USA
O'Brien, R.	Kew, Australia
Oh, J.-W.	Seoul, Korea
Okudaira, H.	Tokyo, Japan
Okumura, Y.	Tokyo, Japan
Pauli, G.	Strasbourg, France
Peltre, G.	Paris, France
Petersen, A.	Borstel, Germany
Plunkett, G.	Spokane, USA
Polo, F.	Madrid, Spain
Poulsen, L.K.	Copenhagen, Denmark
Raulf-Heimsoth, M.	Bochum, Germany
Reese, G.	New Orleans, USA
Renz, H.	Berlin, Germany
Rode, H.	Ottawa, Canada
Romagnani, S.	Firenze, Italy
Ruffilli, A.	Napoli, Italy
Saint-Remy, L.-M.	Brussels, Belgium
Schenk, S.	Vienna, Austria
Scheynius, A.	Stockholm, Sweden
Schmidt, M.	Stockholm, Sweden
Schou, C.	Horsholm, Denmark
Sehon, A.	Winnipeg, Canada
Seger, R.	Zürich, Switzerland
Shen, H.-D.	Taipei, Taiwan
Sidoli, A.	Milano, Italy
Singh, M.B.	Parkville, Australia
Singhamany, V.	Bangkok, Thailand
Skamene, E.	Montreal, Canada
Song, C.	Torrance, USA
Spangfort, M.D.	Horsholm, Denmark
Stadler, B.M.	Bern, Switzerland
Suphioglu, C.	Parkville, Australia
Tamborini, E.	Parkville, Australia
Thomas, W.	West Perth, Australia
Tomaz, E.	Lisbon, Portugal
Valenta, R.	Wien, Austria
Van der Ploeg, I.	Stockholm, Sweden
van Hage-Hamsten, M.	Stockholm, Sweden
van Ree, R.	Amsterdam, The Netherlands
Vijay, H.	Ottawa, Canada
Wallner, B.	Waltham, USA

Wills-Karp, M.   Baltimore, USA
Wilson, B.   Albuquerque, USA
Yssel, H.   Palo Alto, USA

INDEX